Queen Square: A History of the National Hospital and its Institute of Neurology

Queen Square: A History of the National Hospital and its Institute of Neurology

Simon Shorvon
UCL Institute of Neurology, London

Alastair Compston
Department of Clinical Neurosciences, University of Cambridge

With contributions by
Andrew Lees
UCL Institute of Neurology, London

Michael Clark
King's College London

Martin Rossor
UCL Institute of Neurology, London

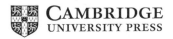

CAMBRIDGE
UNIVERSITY PRESS

University Printing House, Cambridge CB2 8BS, United Kingdom

One Liberty Plaza, 20th Floor, New York, NY 10006, USA

477 Williamstown Road, Port Melbourne, VIC 3207, Australia

314–321, 3rd Floor, Plot 3, Splendor Forum, Jasola District Centre, New Delhi – 110025, India

79 Anson Road, #06–04/06, Singapore 079906

Cambridge University Press is part of the University of Cambridge.

It furthers the University's mission by disseminating knowledge in the pursuit of
education, learning and research at the highest international levels of excellence.

www.cambridge.org
Information on this title: www.cambridge.org/9781107100824
DOI: 10.1017/9781316181430

First published 2019

Printed in the United Kingdom by TJ International Ltd. Padstow Cornwall

A catalogue record for this publication is available from the British Library.

Library of Congress Cataloging-in-Publication Data
Names: Shorvon, S. D. (Simon D.), author. | Compston, Alastair, author. | Rossor, M. (Martin), author. |
Lees, Andrew, author. | Clark, Michael, author.
Title: Queen Square: A History of the National Hospital and its Institute of Neurology / Simon Shorvon, Alastair Compston ;
with contributions by Martin Rossor, Andrew Lees, Michael J. Clark.
Description: Cambridge, United Kingdom ; New York, NY : Cambridge University Press, 2019. |
Includes indexes.
Identifiers: LCCN 2018022381 | ISBN 9781107100824
Subjects: LCSH: National Hospital, Queen Square – History. | National Hospitals for Nervous Diseases
(London, England) – History. | Neurology – England – London – History.
Classification: LCC RA988.L82 S56 2018 | DDC 362.1109421–dc23
LC record available at https://lccn.loc.gov/2018022381

ISBN 978-1-107-10082-4 Hardback

To those who made Queen Square; and especially to the memory of Joe Shorvon and lan McDonald

Contents

Figures

Preface

The National Hospital for the Relief and Cure of the Paralysed and Epileptic, as it was first officially named, was founded in November 1859, and opened its doors for business in 1860 as the first specialist neurological hospital in the world. It quickly gained a reputation as the 'mecca of neurology' and soon became a place of pilgrimage for neurologists from many countries. The book celebrates the fluctuating fortunes and history of the hospital from foundation to eventual amalgamation with University College London Hospital (UCLH) in 1996 and absorption of the Institute of Neurology into University College London (UCL) in 1997.

Our book leans heavily on the remarkable archive of the National Hospital, which provides a rich source of hitherto unpublished material. The illustrations, unless otherwise stated, are from the unique and very large collection of images in the same archive. We have also plundered the unpublished papers, memories and memoirs of individuals for records of contemporaneous events, and have used the annual reports and other written documents covering the work of the hospital, its medical school and the Institute of Neurology. We are also advantaged by the bequest to one of us of the large collection of uncatalogued material relating to Queen Square formed by Ian McDonald. In addition, we have made reference to a variety of other published documents and secondary sources. Although recognising that these are uneven in places, we have annotated the narrative with footnotes in order to add anecdote or detail and to provide context and comment without interrupting the flow of the text.

We have adopted a few conventions to which we draw the reader's attention. Biographical sketches are provided for many of the deceased staff. These do not necessarily appear at first mention of each individual and with some obvious exceptions, their placement either in the main text or footnotes is not a statement on the relative contributions of these individuals. As Gordon Holmes elected to do in his 1954 book on the National Hospital, we have not referred to living persons, except in passing. This is because the snow is too fresh to provide a suitable footprint, and our policy both spares the blushes and avoids the reprimands of our colleagues. We recognise that not referring to living persons lessens the impact of the story for recent decades, and we accept that this decision much underplays the significant achievements of those associated with Queen Square who are still alive. We hope those affected by this decision will accept this with forbearance. Their work is for others to describe in due course.

For the same reason, we do not extend our account beyond 1996/7 as this was a natural point at which to end our account, even though much of interest and importance has happened since.

In the interests of space and readability, we have decided not to provide excessive references to many of the minutes or records in the hospital archives. These are freely available in the Queen Square library to any reader interested in further detail, and many can be easily accessed from the online archive. For the same reasons, we have not provided references to biographical details which lean heavily on conventional sources, such as *Plarr's Lives* and *Munk's Roll* or obituaries in the *British Medical Journal* and *Lancet*, as these are also freely available online. In some instances, we have adapted our own previously published biographical accounts of specific individuals. We have also tried to avoid multiple citation of the same source, leaving some quotes apparently unsupported when their provenance is generally clear from earlier text.

We have added dates of birth and death of individuals mentioned in the text in the index, but have restricted this detail to those who have a direct bearing on the hospital's history or on British neurology.

We have generally used the abbreviated term 'National Hospital' to refer to the hospital (the official name of which changed a number of times), and 'Queen Square' to refer both to the hospital and its medical school and institute. Similarly, we have in general given the first name and surname of individuals at their first appearance in a chapter and just the surname subsequently. However, we have varied these two conventions many times for purposes of style or emphasis. Finally, at times throughout this book, in the absence of a suitable umbrella term, we have used the term 'neurology' as shorthand for other specialties in the clinical neurosciences. We hope that our distinguished colleagues working in these specialist areas will be forgiving and not feel too disenfranchised.

We would like to acknowledge the assistance of many people in the production of this book. The National Brain Appeal[1] provided financial support to the publishers, and we are grateful for their assistance and particularly to the Chief Executive, Ms Theresa Dauncey. Ms Sarah Lawson and her colleagues in the Queen Square medical library and archives provided enormous assistance in our search for information and in the provision of illustrations. Drs Christopher Gardner-Thorpe and Michael O'Brien both kindly read and commented on early drafts, and Dr O'Brien also provided invaluable help in producing the maps in

Chapter 2. Others to whom we are grateful for their comments and information include: Dr Gordon Bird, Dr Anthony Dayan, Dr Stanley Hawkins, Dr Lee Illis, George Kaim, Professor David Miller, Dr Nicholas Murray, Dr Yoko Nagai, Dr John Silver, Nadeem Toodayan, Professor Michael Trimble, Dr John Walshe, and Julian Axe, Nick Ayres, Jennifer Gough-Cooper, Michael and Dr Nicholas Slater and Peter Zimmerman. The work of Simon Shorvon is partly supported by the estate of Mrs Susan Wright, and part of this work was undertaken at University College London Hospitals/University College London, which received a proportion of its funding from the Department of Health's National Institute for Health Research Biomedical Research Centres funding scheme. We also finally thank our long-suffering copy-editor, Leigh Mueller, who much improved the manuscript, and our publishers, Cambridge University Press, and in particular to Mr Nicholas Dunton, Ms Anna Whiting, Ms Charlotte Brisley and Ms Jade Scard for all their expertise, generous assistance and understanding in what has been a project that has endured many delays and shifting timelines.

Despite so much help and guidance, in the end we have necessarily written this book in line with our own perspectives, prejudices and preferences. Others would undoubtedly have written a story different in emphasis, style and content. We have included as much original and archival material, not previously accessed, as seemed appropriate and have aimed for a faithful account of the fame and fortunes of the National Hospital and Institute of Neurology. At the very least, we hope that this provides a factual record of the evolution of an institution that witnessed the beginnings, and contributed much to the development, of a major medical specialty – that of diseases of the central and peripheral nervous systems – in the shifting medical and social contexts of its times.

---

[1] National Brain Appeal raises funds to advance treatment and research at the National Hospital for Neurology and Neurosurgery and the Institute of Neurology. For more about the charity, visit www.nationalbrainappeal.org or telephone 020 3448 4724. The charity can also be found and followed on: Twitter @BrainAppeal, Facebook TheNationalBrainAppeal, and Instagram Brain_Appeal. The National Brain Appeal is the working name of the National Hospital Development Foundation – Registered Charity No. 290173.

Introduction

The period of the history of Queen Square covered in this book is from the foundation of the National Hospital in 1859 until its absorption into the University College London Hospital (UCLH) Trust in 1996, and that of the Institute of Neurology into University College London (UCL) in 1997.

We have two main objectives in writing this account. First is to present a comprehensive narrative history of the hospital using primary and secondary material. We have not spared the reader detail and have amalgamated information from diverse sources, much previously unpublished, into a single work of reference for the convenience of those with an interest in Queen Square and the history of medical institutions. Our second objective is to place this story of the famous hospital within the wider contexts of British social history and the development of British neurology in the modern age. The history of the National Hospital is not by any means straightforward. It is self-evident that the narrative and interpretation of factual events will vary depending on the perspective taken. We are reminded of the analogy of the mountain, which has an unvarying structure but appears entirely different from separate slopes and viewpoints, and whose faces are changed over time by shifting snows and glaciers. The predominant themes that we have explored, and the different vantage points from which the narrative of Queen Square can be considered, are summarised below. In particular, we have deliberately steered away from the temptation of being overly biographical and adopting the Carlylian method of viewing the historical record simply as the sum of the deeds of exceptional people. We have also tried to avoid excessive hagiography in telling the story of Queen Square, which has often been accused of endlessly polishing its own halo. As a result, our account is at times far from complimentary. Nonetheless, by any yardstick, the hospital and some individuals on its staff made exceptional and distinctive contributions to neurology, and provided succour to generations of persons afflicted with neurological diseases.

Chronology

A broadly chronological approach has been adopted in our narrative. The story of the hospital seems naturally to be separated into three distinctive periods, each of about 40–50 years.

1859–1902: The foundation of the National Hospital was followed by a rapid and linear rise to achieve the status of, and reputation as, one of the leading neurological hospitals in the world, perhaps indeed *primus inter pares*. In these years, the hospital was the crucible of notable scientific and clinical achievements, and it is no exaggeration to say that a significant part of modern neurology was created within Queen Square. A series of remarkable figures in the world of medicine and science worked at the hospital and were largely responsible for establishing its high reputation. Neurosurgery was essentially born there and a medical school formed. It was a voluntary hospital, funded by philanthropic donations but, by the end of the nineteenth century, this source of funds was becoming inadequate and the finances increasingly fragile. The period ended with an explosive conflict between the medical staff and administration over issues that were nationally debated, and resolved with victory for the medical staff.

1903–45: The history of the hospital during this period was, in contrast, a bumpier ride. The punishing avalanche of history included the two World Wars, each of which presented the National Hospital with exceptional difficulties and threatened its existence. The inter-war years were punctuated by financial crises and twice the hospital came close to bankruptcy, on one occasion beginning the process of closure before being rescued by a large government grant. In this period, a series of major figures in neurology dominated life at the National Hospital and who, despite the erratic course and financial vicissitudes, provided the hospital with a growing reputation for clinical skills and acumen, and the teaching of neurology. A systematic approach to clinical neurology had been developed – the Queen Square method – which was used throughout the world. The style of clinical practice was patrician, focused on diagnosis, not treatment, and on the esoteric, not the common. Teaching was prominent and both patients and postgraduate doctors arrived from all parts of the country, the Empire and the rest of the world. As its clinical reputation soared, the first priority of the medical staff was their clinical practice, and research activity faltered, unnoticed at first but, by the mid-1930s, becoming an increasing source of concern. This was a complacent period when the hospital became adept at self-aggrandisement, but during which its contribution to academic life atrophied. By the end of this period, the reputation of the hospital was once again at risk.

1946–97: This was a time of great administrative change, dominated initially by incorporation of the National Hospital into the National Health Service (NHS), the forced merger with Maida Vale Hospital, and the transformation of the medical school into an institute within the British Postgraduate Medical Federation. The machinations of NHS policy and state control, with repeated organisational and policy change and almost continuous financial stringency, were chaotic. The hospital administration found itself often snow-blind in a blizzard of bureaucracy, trekking Sisyphus-like up and down rock faces with little onward purpose, and occupied by what, with the benefit of hindsight, was largely useless expenditure of energy. At the same time, neurological units developed widely elsewhere in the country and neurology was modernised. To maintain its position at the top of the pile, the hospital focused on highly specialised clinical services, the provision of tertiary opinion, teaching and – just in time – on academic development. The specialised clinical services retained their traditional high standards and the hospital hung on to its training role. The renewed emphasis on research and investment in academic medicine was a deliberate policy change not welcomed by all, as was clear from the controversy surrounding the proposal for creating a

professorship of neurology. There was an initially slow, but then rapid, academic flowering, with research activity taking an increasingly prominent role. By the 1980s, now nurturing a strong portfolio of research work, Queen Square had again resumed its place among academic leaders worldwide.

Our disaggregation of the fortunes of Queen Square into these three periods is necessarily contrived and at times impossible to maintain as the historical narrative becomes more detailed. The boundary between the second and third periods is especially blurred but, in broad terms, the division holds true. The book is organised generally along these chronological lines, with Chapters 1, 3 and 4 devoted largely to the first period; Chapters 5 and 6 to the second; Chapters 7, 13 and 14 to the third; and with Chapters 2, 8, 9, 10, 11 and 12 straddling two or all three periods. Inevitably, there is material that is distributed across these chapters, and many of the more prominent names appear repeatedly in different contexts. We have chosen not to provide cross-referencing in the text, leaving those who read individual chapters to use the index in searching for comprehensive coverage of people and events.

Themes

Within the overall arrangement of the book – largely, but not entirely, chronological – certain themes (our vantage points) are developed which have on repeated occasions influenced the course of the history of the hospital and its reciprocal engagement with the wider national and international community. These provide different viewpoints, and to help the reader we signpost ten of these prominent themes in the hospital's history:

The Tripartite Role of the National Hospital: The provision of a clinical service, training and research have been the three fundamental roles of the hospital. Their relative importance changed over time and, in fact, over-neglect of, or over-focus on, one or another injured the hospital's prospects at various points in its historical trajectory.

The Struggle to Maintain Independence: The hospital was, until 1948, a 'voluntary' – i.e. a charitable foundation with independent governance. However, it became increasingly reliant financially on the state in the twentieth century as social mores and conditions changed, causing friction and argument. Even after incorporation into the NHS in 1948, it often attempted solo performances, and its ambitions for retaining independence and self-governance within a centralised system caused continued difficulties.

Recurring Financial Problems: As a voluntary hospital, income was initially entirely philanthropic. By the end of the nineteenth century, this source of funding was proving inadequate, and financial crises dogged the hospital throughout the early twentieth century. Despite initial hopes, the crises continued after incorporation into the NHS, when the hospital's finances became intimately bound up with national policy and fortune.

The Context of British Social and Political History: The hospital's role and position have been determined to a large extent by the social and political course of the country. Although often overlooked internally, these forces frequently trumped any attempt at autonomy and proved impossible to resist.

The Importance of Individual Members of the Consultant Staff: The reputation of the hospital to a great extent depended on the quality of the clinical and academic work of individuals on its consultant staff. The consultant body's power and influence on hospital policy have been important ingredients in the success of Queen Square. This influence was predominant in the first 100 years but progressively weakened in the later twentieth century. Strikingly, too, the consultant body was small and highly selected, at least until recent times, and this conferred an elite status.

Academic Contribution to Neurology: An enduring legacy of the hospital has been the written contributions of its staff to the practice and scientific basis of clinical neurology and related disciplines, and the evolution of the hospital's clinical method.

Maintaining Dominance in Neurology and Queen Square's position within the wider context of British neurology: The hospital aspired to prominence and dominance nationally and internationally throughout its history. By monopolising national teaching and professional policy-making bodies, its staff worked to maintain an elite position that did not always make for friendships but, by any objective analysis, was seldom seriously challenged.

Specialism and the Relationship of Neurology to General Medicine and Psychiatry: The National Hospital led in developing specialism and, later, subspecialisation of neurology in Britain, and this became the single most important justification for its existence as an independent hospital. As neurology specialised and became divided along disease lines into subspecialties, its relationship with general (internal) medicine and psychiatry became difficult. Ultimately there were differences in policy which could not be reconciled. Throughout the twentieth century the difficult personal relationships between neurologists, physicians and psychiatrists contributed to a schism between the disciplines.

The Relationship of Neurology to Neurosurgery: The attitude of the hospital physicians to neurosurgery, after the death of Victor Horsley, resulted in loss of leadership in the subject, at least for a while. This threatened the hospital's position when, stimulated by events in the Second World War, neurosurgery led the development of services outside London, and neurology followed. In more recent times, neurosurgery has grown at the expense of neurology – clinically, if not academically – and the relationship between the disciplines remains fragile.

The Estate and Lack of Space: The limitations of space in Queen Square have been an important factor in determining the course of the hospital. Much management time and effort were expended on property and estate development. The Queen Square 'brand' has always been dependent on its location, and repeated proposals to move the hospital or its institute fortunately failed once it was recognised that co-locating the National Hospital and its institute in Queen Square was central to its success.

The Name of the Hospital

The naming of the National Hospital has always caused some difficulty. At its foundation, the hospital was referred to as the National Hospital for the Paralysed and Epileptic or the National Hospital for Paralysis and Epilepsy, but its first set of rules printed in March 1860 refer to it by the official name, which was followed in all subsequent reports for the next 50 years – the National Hospital for the Relief and Cure of the Paralysed and Epileptic. Of course, having 'National' in the name was a clever and somewhat bold decision, and a feature closely guarded in sub-sequent name changes. Some people inaccurately referred to the Royal National Hospital, and certainly this might have been a possible formulation in view of its level of royal patronage and the award of a Royal Charter in 1903 (the re-launch of the hospital then might have been the best opportunity for this parti-cular name change, but this did not happen). Its name was rather a mouthful and even Hughlings Jackson occasionally got it wrong when he reversed the order of 'paralysed' and 'epileptic' in an article in 1864. By the end of the nineteenth century, it was being referred to in day-to-day conversation simply as the National Hospital, the National Hospital Queen Square, or just either the National, or Queen Square.

In 1926, the first formal name change occurred, to the National Hospital, Queen Square, for the Relief and Cure of Diseases of the Nervous System, including Paralysis and Epilepsy, a curiously inept attempt to recognise the longstanding practice at the hospital of treating all neurological diseases and not just epilepsy and paralysis (the name change required a supplementary royal charter). This name was then often abbreviated to the National Hospital for Nervous Diseases, not least as the inclusion of epilepsy and paralysis was deemed a 'deterrent to the public' by some of the medical staff. Then in 1948, at the time of incorporation into the NHS and the merger with Maida Vale Hospital, the official name was again changed, this time to the National Hospitals for Nervous Diseases. The inclusion of 'Nervous Diseases' was widely unpop-ular and the hospital was still often known in casual conversation as the National Hospital, or Queen Square, or the National Hospital Queen Square. The latter was the title Gordon Holmes gave to his book, published in 1954, on the history of the hospital, presumably reflecting his own dissatisfaction with the official name. In the latter part of the twentieth century, almost no one referred to the hospital by its full name, and in 1980 the fund-raisers of a new building cam-paign urged a change in name in view of the fact that, to the public, nervous diseases were the same as neurotic disorders. A similar debate had occurred in the 1950s, but change was then rejected.

In 1988, however, the chairman of the Board sug-gested a new name, the National Hospital for Neurosciences. The Medical Committee considered other potential changes (including a suggestion by Roman Kocen, ahead of his time, that the hospital simply be called Neurocare) but no clear decision was reached, and more than 50 per cent of its members responding to a ballot requested no change. Slowly, a consensus came round to the name the National Hospital for Neurology but this was violently opposed by the professor of neurosurgery, and the Board ulti-mately agreed to compromise and change the name to the National Hospital for Neurology and Neurosurgery, a designation that was formally ratified in Parliament in May 1990. One has to say that the new name is no less clumsy than its predecessors and this decision was another lost opportunity. More recently, further moves by the Medical Committee to name the hospital simply as the National Hospital Queen Square, as Holmes did, have been made, but were seemingly of no interest to UCLH. In practice, it remains almost universally known in conversation as either the National or Queen Square by most people around the world. Part of the difficulty arises because there is no umbrella term which encompasses all the neuro-specialties or neuro-medicine: neuroscience, which is the nearest we have, seems inappropriate, by not reflect-ing the clinical or societal aspects of day-to-day practice.

It is interesting to note in passing that similar diffi-culties were experienced by the other two specialised neuro-hospitals established in London. The London Infirmary for Epilepsy and Paralysis, founded in 1866, changed its name to the Hospital for Diseases of the Nervous System (1873), then to the Hospital for Epilepsy and Paralysis (1876), then to the Hospital for Epilepsy and Paralysis and Other Diseases of the Nervous System, Maida Vale (1900), and then to Maida Vale Hospital for Nervous Diseases including Epilepsy and Paralysis (1937) and was then merged with its cousin at Queen Square. The other hospital was the West End Hospital for Diseases of the Nervous System, Paralysis and Epilepsy which changed its name to the West End Hospital for Nervous Diseases. The confusion between the names of these hospitals was a source of tension, and at one stage threatened litigation. On several occasions, it was not clear to which hospital would-be benefactors were leav-ing bequests when their will referred to the Asylum for Paralytics or the Hospital for Epilepsy and Paralysis.

Previous Histories of the National Hospital

The first published account of the hospital was written by Benjamin Burford Rawlings, *A Hospital in the Making: A History of the National Hospital for the*

Paralysed and Epileptic (Albany Memorial) 1859–1901 (London: Sir Isaac Pitman & Sons Ltd, 1913). This is a highly autobiographical account of the development of the hospital, emphasising his own fundamental role. He writes in the preface: 'I have endeavoured to thwart any attempt to read into the text a meaning injurious to the hospital … the records of a past controversy, which though of much more than personal or passing import, is given no undue prominence in these pages.' This is a reference to the explosive events leading up to the Fry Inquiry and the text is inevitably an attempt to justify his position and importance.

The first comprehensive history of the hospital from the medical point of view was proposed in December 1906 by William Gowers when he wrote to the Board of Management suggesting that such an account be written and asking the Board to meet the cost; but it responded that 'there are no funds at the Board's disposal which can be devoted to this project'. Gowers never wrote the history and there is no further reference to it in the minutes. In February 1921, Heathcote Hamilton wrote to the Medical Committee stating that 'he was on the authority of the Board writing a short account of the history of the Hospital' and inviting the Committee 'to nominate someone to write an account of the medical aspect of the Hospital's work'. The Committee decided to ask Joseph Ormerod whether he would undertake this part of the work but it is not clear whether anything came of it and there does not seem to be any follow up. Certainly, Hamilton's book, *Queen Square: Its Neighbourhood and its Institutions* (London: Leonard Parsons, 1926) is mainly concerned with local history, architecture and antiquity, and contains little about the medical or even administrative aspects of the National Hospital and its work. Hamilton also completed a second manuscript ('Tales of the National', c. 1940), which exists in unpublished form, and provides a series of impressionistic anecdotes of hospital life during his time as hospital secretary between 1902 and 1939.

It was left to Gordon Holmes to write the first authoritative book, *The National Hospital Queen Square 1860–1948* (Edinburgh and London: Livingstone Ltd, 1954), with a foreword by Sir Ernest Gowers. This is a concise and accurate, but dry, account, of only 95 pages, with a relatively narrow scope and focusing mainly on medical personalities.

A History of Maida Vale Hospital for Nervous Diseases (London: Butterworth & Co., 1958) was written by Anthony Feiling, and again contained a foreword by Gowers. This was a scholarly but short account of Maida Vale Hospital from foundation in 1866 to amalgamation with the National Hospital in 1948. The book is notable too for its appendices, among which is otherwise-unpublished information about the 1934 Jubilee commemoration dinner celebrating Rickman Godlee's 1884 brain operation, including the transcript of an address by Wilfred Trotter.

Queen Square and the National Hospital 1860–1960 (London: Edward Arnold Ltd) was published in 1960. It too had a foreword by Gowers, and, although written anonymously on behalf of the Chartered Society of Queen Square, it is widely acknowledged that the author was Macdonald Critchley. It is a short but lively impressionistic work, essentially a medical and social-historical miscellany, written in Critchley's elegant prose and published to mark the centenary of the hospital. It provides brief biographies of the founders, some donors and selected doctors, and some interesting anecdotes about Queen Square itself. As a brief hagiographical and amusing account, it is hard to beat, and generations of students at Queen Square have left the hospital with this little book in their luggage.

The final book, *The National Hospitals for Nervous Diseases 1948–1982*, was written by Geoffrey Robinson, and privately published by the Board of Governors of the Hospitals (1982). It is a rather uncritical and brief, and at times inaccurate, collection of narrative sketches focusing mainly on non-medical topics. Robinson was secretary to the Board of Governors between 1959 and 1980, and (we jealously note) was given six months paid leave on retirement to write the book.

No other synoptical histories have been written, although articles have appeared from time to time in the medical journals on various aspects of the hospital, its work or its staff; and, indeed, these seem to be increasing in number as the microscope of history is being applied to neurology in particular. All of these have converged to produce what is the rather mythologised reputation that the hospital currently enjoys, as a mountain peak rising higher than all others in the turbulent ranges of neurology.

Foundation and Making of the National Hospital

When, in 1859, Johanna Chandler and her family founded a hospital for 'the relief of paralysis, epilepsy and allied diseases', which became designated as the National Hospital, she staked a claim that no one else in the United Kingdom was in a position to contest. For this was the only hospital that confined its activities to diseases thought to result primarily from damage to the brain and spinal cord. From this it should not be understood that neurology did not exist outside the National Hospital, or that its staff restricted their practice to neurology. Each consultant held an appointment practising general medicine, usually at a London teaching hospital, and the staff played crucial roles in shaping the emerging disciplines of neurology and neurosurgery away from the National Hospital. Nevertheless, in the field of diseases of the brain and spinal cord, Queen Square led where others followed.

The National Hospital was the earliest of the Chandlers' charitable schemes for the paralysed and epileptic. Prominent features of the hospital, such as its name and floral emblem symbolising the aspiration to provide care for needy patients from all parts of Great Britain and Ireland, show their influence.[1] The 'Charity', as it soon became known, was made up of more than just the hospital at Queen Square. In 1861, the Ladies' Samaritan Society was founded to provide various kinds of practical assistance for poor patients, and to assist

their recovery and, where possible, re-integration into the working world. In 1862–3, in accordance with the Chandlers' original intentions, a Pensions Fund was also created to support incurable patients who could no longer benefit from hospital treatment. At the Chandlers' insistence, in 1870, the Finchley Convalescent Home, or 'the Country Branch' as it was often known, was purchased to provide convalescence for National Hospital patients – in practice, almost all of them female and epileptic – and this continued to function until 1999.[2] After the Chandlers' time, further

---

[1] Burford Rawlings later wrote that the name of the hospital was 'not well chosen'. He viewed it as too long and not comprehensive, and furthermore the 'title awakened a sense of hopelessness deregatory to an institution devoted in chief part to curative treatment, while in its orthographical intricacies it made demands not always complied with even by the erudite'. It was often even then known as the 'Queen Square Hospital', and he relates how the postal workers had delivered letters addressed to the 'Fits Hospital, London', the 'Hospital for Paralis' and the 'Eliptic Hospital, Holborn': B. Burford Rawlings, *A Hospital in the Making: A History of the National Hospital for the Paralysed and Epileptic (Albany Memorial) 1859–1901* (London: Sir Isaac Pitman & Sons Ltd, 1913).

[2] On 26 July 1870 the hospital opened the Home. It was situated first in The Elms, a pair of semi-detached villas in East End Road, East Finchley. According to Burford Rawlings, 'Few more attractive and cheery homesteads could be found within the suburban limits … a wealth of leafage, with jasmine and clematis about the porches, roses everywere and the hum of bees in the colour-laden and scentful borders.' This was purchased for £1,500 from the appeal, which raised £3,000, and the 20-bedded home was initially intended primarily to accommodate female patients with epilepsy. After 25 years of usage, the home was proving too small and there was also a need to accommodate a wider range of patients. Thus, on June 16 1897, the Duchess of Albany opened a newly constructed purpose-built premises designed by Langton Cole, off the Bishop's Avenue, and, in the words of its dedicatory plaque, it was for 'the benefit of a class of patients inadmissable to any other convalescent home in the kingdom'. It cost £11,000 to build and furnish, and to lay out the gardens. The appeal was launched with a donation of £2,000 from Mrs Margaret Gibbins, whose mother had been treated at Queen Square. It was in the style of a country house, with its spacious wards and entrance hall adorned with watercolours. It had then 40 beds for women and children. The grounds contained large lawns, herbaceous and other plants, shrubberies, fruit and vegetable enclosures and newly planted specimen trees – cypress, poplar, fir, holly and pine. Trees were also planted to screen the Home from the railway. A pond turned out to be a deep spring, one of the sources of the River Brent, and became a feature of the garden, with bamboos, bullrushes, ferns, irises and weeping willows. The convalescent home was enlarged in 1896 and opened in a grand ceremony by the Duchess of Albany in June 1897. In the early 1900s, wards had had to be closed for financial reasons, and by 1910 there were 36 beds and cots.

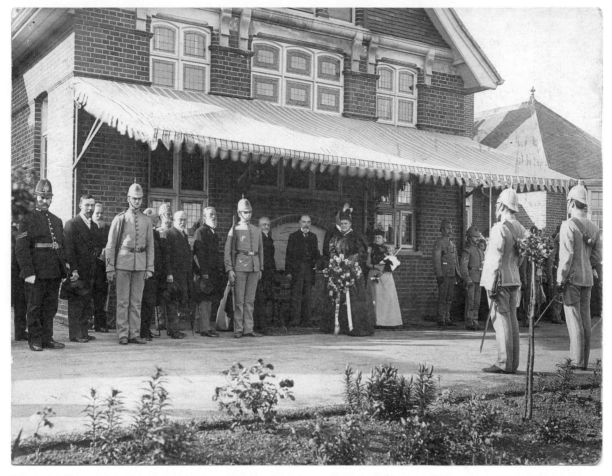

Figure 1.1 The opening of the new and enlarged Finchley Convalescent Home by the Duchess of Albany on June 16 1897.

charitable endeavours linked but external to the National Hospital were launched. In 1894, an Epileptic Colony was established at Chalfont St Peter, Buckinghamshire, for male long-term patients, which, although run by a separate charity, was closely associated with the National Hospital, and that association continues. In 1917–18, the hospital also took over management and care provision at Lonsdale House in Clapham, south London – a centre for paraplegic soldiers and sailors – and of Bray House near Maidenhead in Berkshire – for convalescent neuropsychiatric casualties of war. In parallel to its caring role, the doctors at the hospital contributed much to the development of scientific medicine, and assumed leadership in the emerging

specialties of neurology and neurosurgery. Perhaps inevitably, there were clashes between the ethos of philanthropy, on which the hospital was originally founded, and the doctrines of scientific medicine. As a result, tensions developed between the lay board and the clinicians, which resulted in a damaging and public conflict in the first years of the twentieth century that brought the National Hospital to the brink of closure.

The Age of Equipoise

The historical moment of foundation was to prove decidedly advantageous for the National Hospital. The years 1859–60 were almost the high point of the so-called mid-Victorian 'age of equipoise', the brief period of relative social harmony, peace, security and growing prosperity that separated the severe economic crises and intense social and political upheavals of the 'Hungry 40s', and the international conflicts

In 1948, it was incorporated into the NHS, and by 1961 had 25 beds. In 1967, it became the Rehabilitation Unit of the Hospital. It closed in September 1999.

and imperial wars of the early 1850s, from the growing social and political tensions and renewed economic difficulties of the 1870s and 1880s. Following the apparent failure of the Chartist and Trades Union agitations of 1848–52 and the split in the Conservative party over repeal of the Corn Laws in 1846 by Sir Robert Peel, the political system appeared to have stabilised around a 'natural' Whig–Liberal Parliamentary majority led by Lord John Russell and Viscount Palmerston. Although a new Reform Bill was under discussion in 1859, few members of the political classes expected more than fine-tuning to the political system created by the 1832 Reform Act. The end of the 1850s saw the first major steps towards the national unifications of both Germany and Italy, but neither posed a serious threat to British interests in Europe; and the diplomatic rapprochement between Britain and the French Second Empire in 1859–60 appeared to have removed the only serious external threat to homeland security. The American Civil War seemed far away. British naval supremacy remained unchallenged; and, after defeat of Russia in the Crimean War of 1853–4 and the suppression of the Indian 'Mutiny' in 1856–7, there were no obvious impediments to Britain's imperial dominance.

In the middle decades of the nineteenth century, technological change, population growth and agricultural and industrial innovation, which had driven the Industrial Revolution and made Britain into the 'workshop of the world' during the previous century, continued, and Britain's economic supremacy seemed secure. Far from undermining the dominant position of the land-owning classes, as predicted by Marx and Engels, industrialisation was tightening its grip, and in 1859–60 the English landed aristocracy was enjoying unbridled social influence, political power and economic prosperity.

Not all of this wealth was channelled into the more usual forms of conspicuous consumption and, as a result, medical philanthropy flourished – perhaps surprisingly, since there was little public support for state-funded collective action to tackle social or public health problems and most medical care was privately funded. Any major development was largely dependent on financial backing and patronage by the aristocracy. Low inflation and price stability at a time of rising living standards created an economic climate that encouraged the foundation of new charitable institutions. The reduced cost of food and overall price stability made it easier for institutional administrators to balance the books of fledgling charitable institutions that had little or no endowment. It was generally held that charitable benevolence towards the poor and needy was an important duty for what Benjamin Disraeli called the 'classes' towards the 'masses'. Benefaction was seen as a comparatively small price to pay for continued social and political dominance. The new philanthropy of the respectable middle classes also reflected piety and religious duty as much as enlightened self-interest. Charity became a powerful and passionate impulse for many, giving meaning to a pious life and gratifying the Victorian sense of responsibility and muscular citizenship. It was in this climate of political stability, good works, relative social harmony and auspicious economic and financial conditions that Johanna, Louisa and Edward Chandler founded the National Hospital under circumstances ensuring its survival during gestation and infancy, and allowing the institution to grow rapidly over the next few years.

For all these reasons, the response to charitable appeals in the 1860s and early 1870s consistently exceeded expectations. But the period of abundance in which the National Hospital was founded was not to last. By the 1880s and 1890s, the economic and financial climate had altered for the worse and the age of evangelical philanthropy was passing, as was the paternalistic and evangelical approach to hospital management. A more technological and scientific practice of medicine gained ascendancy and, risky as it turned out to be, the National Hospital was at its forefront.

The Founders of the National Hospital

The foundation of the National Hospital for the Paralysed and Epileptic is conventionally dated to the public meeting called by the Lord Mayor of London, David Wire, held at the Mansion House in the City of London on 2 November 1859 and attended by a number of city businessmen, lay philanthropists and members of the medical profession. A resolution proposed by the Liberal MP and social reformer John Villiers Stuart Townshend, Viscount Raynham MP,[3]

---

[3] See F. M. L. Thompson's biographical account in the *Oxford Dictionary of National Biography* for an excellent appreciation of his life and work, even though the account does not mention Raynham's connection with the National Hospital. The figure of £800 pledged to the hospital at the meeting is given in the article 'Johanna Chandler' from *Good Words* (August 1866).

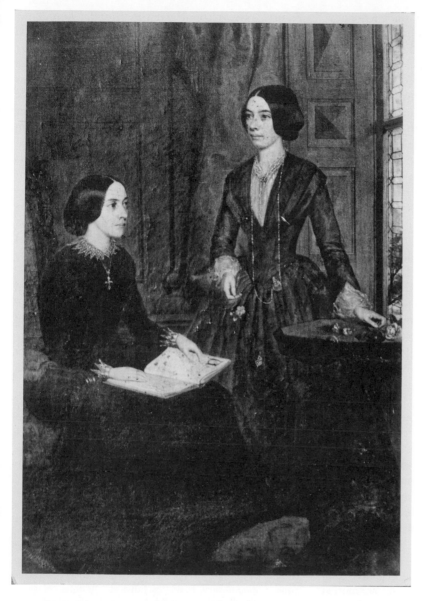

Figure 1.2 The sisters Johanna and Louisa Chandler who inspired the foundation of the National Hospital.

to establish a new hospital 'for the relief of the paralysed and epileptic' was carried by acclamation, and more than £800 pledged in subscriptions and donations. An informal steering committee was soon constituted which, in December 1859, became the first Board of Management of the new hospital.[4] Less than

---

[4] The first two meetings minuted in the first volume of the *Board of Management of the National Hospital*, 25 November and 5 December 1859, are described as 'Committee' meetings. However, the next recorded meeting, held on 29 December 1859, is designated a 'Board' meeting, and thereafter the title 'Board of Management' was used for all subsequent meetings (pp. 1–5ff.).

six months later, more than £4,000 had been raised. A house in Queen Square had been rented to accommodate the new hospital, physicians and surgeons had been appointed, and the first patients admitted for treatment. By April 1861, the number of outpatients treated already exceeded 1,000, and, by the summer of 1866, the expanding hospital was able to accommodate up to 70 inpatients.

The move to establish a new hospital specifically for the 'Relief and Cure of the Paralysed and Epileptic' certainly attracted a good deal of medical and public interest at the time, and was undoubtedly attended by a level of expectation not normally associated with the foundation of new hospitals. Indeed, there was nothing very unusual about the establishment of yet another specialist hospital in London. As well as the National Hospital, more than ten others opened in London during the decade 1850–9, including the nearby Great Ormond Street Hospital for Sick Children. Before the National Hospital was 25 years old, it had been joined by no fewer than three others in Queen Square alone. However, few – if any – of those who attended the Mansion House meeting in November 1859 or took part in the early Board of Management meetings and fund-raising initiatives could have anticipated that the new hospital would prove so successful in terms of its institutional growth and development, or that it would subsequently play such an important role in the emergence and development of a whole new clinical specialty.

The prime movers in the establishment of the National Hospital were the three children of an intensely evangelical London middle-class household, Johanna and Louisa Chandler and their brother Edward. Surprisingly little is known about the Chandlers, at least before the summer of 1859, other than details subsequently incorporated into published narratives of the history of the hospital. Louisa Chandler's posthumously published poems[5] contain some occasional references to her earlier life, but no solid biographical information. Johanna Chandler's near-contemporary account of the foundation of the hospital, 'The Story of the Institution', has not survived, except for a fragment taken out of context and reprinted on the preliminary leaves of the early annual

reports.[6] The account given in *Hospital Jottings*, or *Reminiscences of the Rise and Progress of the National Hospital for the Paralysed and Epileptic*, is described by Chandler as 'a lucid and concise narrative of the events connected with [the foundation of] this Institution', but it is not the work of any of the people primarily involved and it was written some years later for a different purpose.[7] There are inconsistencies in the fragmentary accounts of the hospital's origins that do survive, so that even some of the most basic facts concerning the Chandlers and their role in the foundation of the National Hospital cannot be relied upon. However, to the extent that the facts can be ascertained and a plausible narrative constructed, the following account, compiled from several different sources, would seem to provide a reasonably accurate version of the sequence of events.

At the start of the 1850s, Johanna, Louisa and Edward Chandler were three unmarried middle-class siblings living in the St Pancras district of London with their grandmother, Mrs Pinnock, who had been largely responsible for their upbringing after the children were orphaned while still very young.[8] In

---

[5] Louisa Chandler, *Evaline, Madelon and Other Poems*, ed. Johanna Chandler and Edward Chandler (London: John Bumpus, 1861). Taken as a whole, the poems are morbid in the extreme. The author gives the impression of having been much enamoured of 'The cold, calm loveliness of Death' ('Madelon', Pt III, Stanza 16, on p. 62). Death marks the culmination of almost every poem, long and short, and actually features in several of the titles. Other themes are the seduction and betrayal of innocent young women (usually followed by an illegitimate birth), prostitution, poverty, the heartless exploitation of female and child labour, emigration, 'consumption' (the disease from which Louisa Chandler died), the beauties of southern Italy, the consolations of religion, and the cold hypocrisy lurking just below the surface of much conventional religion and 'Christian charity'. There is a great deal of (mainly unspecified) illness and death, but no discernible references to 'nervous' disease or paralysis as such, nor to hospitals or medical care.

[6] Johanna Chandler, 'The Story of the Institution', in *National Hospital for the Relief and Cure of the Paralysed and Epileptic … 3rd. Annual Report* (London: Harrison & Sons, 1864). The same extract is reprinted on the preliminary leaves of several subsequent annual reports of the hospital published in the 1860s. The title given may simply be an abbreviation or paraphrase of one of the many occasional articles about the hospital that Johanna Chandler wrote for magazines published in Britain and the USA during the 1860s, none ever compiled or fully listed.

[7] 'Johanna Chandler', in Edward Chandler, comp., *Hospital Jottings: or Reminiscences of the Rise and Progress of the National Hospital for the Paralysed and Epileptic, Queen Square, Bloomsbury*, hereafter Edward Chandler, *Hospital Jottings* (London: R. Folkard & Sons, 1872). The article itself is stated in the preface to be by '… a distinguished author … one intimately associated with the most important charities of the metropolis'. Although this sounds rather like Charles Dickens, who at the time lived less than half a mile away from the hospital in Tavistock Square, Dickens is not known to have written for *Good Words*.

[8] For the early life of the Chandler siblings, see the article 'Johanna Chandler' in *Hospital Jottings*, pp. 5–6; Johanna Chandler, 'The Story of the Institution', p. 2; Burford Rawlings, *A Hospital in the Making*, pp. 1–3; G. Holmes, *The National Hospital Queen Square, 1860–1948* (Edinburgh and London: E. & S. Livingstone Ltd, 1954), pp. 8–9; Anon. (Macdonald Critchley), *Queen Square and the National Hospital 1860–1960* (London: Edward Arnold Ltd, 1960), pp. 8–9.

the surviving fragment of 'The Story of the Institution', Johanna describes her mother as 'a woman of strong mind and active habits, [whose] daily prayer was to live only while she retained the use of her limbs'. But since she must have been very young to form such a judgement at the time of her mother's death, and as both she and her brother Edward elsewhere refer to their grandmother as their mother, it is not at all clear to whom this description applies. In any event, in 1852 or 1853, Mrs Pinnock had a stroke, which doubtless left the family in straitened circumstances. Shortly afterwards, Johanna Chandler witnessed first-hand the tragic case of a carpenter unable to work after being struck down by paralysis, whose wife then died of consumption brought on, it was believed, by overwork, anxiety and the prospect of destitution. These circumstances served to concentrate the minds of the Chandlers on the role of paralysis as a potential cause of impoverishment for middle-class families and of destitution for working-class households. However, it was not just the first-hand knowledge of the misery caused by paralysis that spurred the Chandlers to action, but their intense evangelical piety and sense of duty. In a characteristic moment combining religious reflection and a highly practical sense of unmet social need, Johanna Chandler recalled that, on seeing the dead body of the paralysed carpenter's wife laid out by a workhouse nurse

> Mentally I repeated, 'these are they who came out of much tribulation, and have washed their robes and made them white in the blood of the lamb', and the thought arose in my mind, 'there are charities in London for the relief of nearly every class of human affliction, but the sufferings of the paralysed have been most strangely overlooked', and with that thought came the strong resolve that, God helping me, I would devote my life to endeavouring to supply this great want.[9]

Johanna and her sister Louisa's response to these experiences initially took a somewhat unusual but characteristically Victorian form. They began to make artificial flowers, beads and ornaments from Barbados rice shells[10] to sell to their friends, and by this modest means laboriously built up a fund of some £200 over the next three or four years. This was not intended to provide the sole resource for a new charitable 'Institution for Paralytics' but rather, as Johanna subsequently explained, to trigger a certain emotional and practical response on the part of those in more fortunate circumstances, which might in turn lead on to greater things. The sisters conceived the idea of founding a charity for the especial benefit of persons afflicted by paralysis, but they were not rich, and they knew, too, that the worthy and benevolent were besieged with applications, and rightly judged that theirs would be cast aside. 'We know a little art', said the elder sister (Johanna), 'we will practise it until we have gained 200 [pounds]; we will offer that in earnest of our sincerity, and God will incline some kind heart to take up the cause.'

Sometime during the late 1850s, the sisters appear to have made the acquaintance and enlisted the support of Viscount Raynham, who was subsequently to become the National Hospital's first treasurer and an important member of the Board of Management during its early years.[11] A decisive breakthrough came in the summer of 1859, when Johanna Chandler met, and secured the highly influential backing of Alderman David Wire – solicitor, magistrate and benefactor of numerous London charities, with many wealthy and influential contacts in the worlds of business, philanthropy, city politics and medicine. Crucially, Wire was at that time Lord Mayor of London, and it was his ability to call the Mansion House meeting and thus provide a public platform for the hospital appeal that set the wheels of press publicity and business philanthropy in motion, and gave the Chandlers their entrée to London society, civic activism and the medical profession. Wire himself had recently suffered a stroke and was partially paralysed. Although he died a year later after a second episode, his energetic intervention on behalf of the Chandlers proved decisive in establishing the hospital late in 1859.

---

[9] Johanna Chandler, 'The Story of the Institution'; and Edward Chandler, *Hospital Jottings*, p. 6, where it is stated that this expression of Johanna Chandler's thoughts is based on a note that she made at the time.

[10] A number of these ornaments have been preserved in the National Hospital archives.

[11] The importance of Raynham's role in forming the organisational coalition of businessmen, city worthies and philanthropists who helped to establish the hospital in 1859–60 is apparent from a letter of August 1859 to Johanna Chandler, in which he congratulates her on the success of her recent interview with David Wire, and observes that 'We may now look forward to the Institution being shortly established on a much more extensive scale than we could have hoped at our last meeting.' Accompanying these papers is a first draft outline of a constitution for the proposed 'Institution for the relief of poor persons afflicted with paralysis', signed by Raynham and in his own hand.

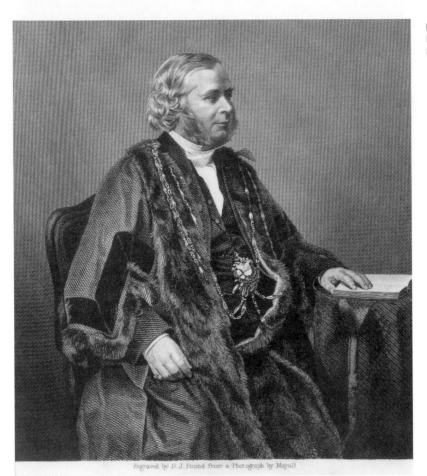

Figure 1.3 David Wire, Lord Mayor of London and chair of the first Board of Management of the National Hospital.

Engraved by D. J. Pound from a Photograph by Mayall

Contingency and chance played a very large part in events that created the National Hospital for the Relief and Cure of the Paralysed and Epileptic. Thus, one might (as did the hospital's founders themselves) emphasise the importance of the Chandlers' experience of paralysis in their own family, and of the misery and hardship that it could bring upon whole households. Yet it is doubtful whether these experiences alone were sufficient to initiate the foundation of a charity for the paralysed and epileptic, had it not been also for the powerful sense of civic duty imparted by their religious faith. Even these forces would probably not have sufficed had it not been for the fortunate accident of Johanna Chandler's meeting with David Wire in August 1859, because it was he who steered the Chandlers towards the foundation of a hospital, rather than an asylum for incurables.[12] The Chandlers were not acquainted with the medical world and, without

Wire's intervention and the influence of his 'medical friends', their wish to do good might never have been expressed in this way. Moreover, if the meeting had been scheduled to take place only a few months later, it would not have happened before Wire's fatal stroke. His active support was crucial in helping to launch the initial fund-raising appeal. This was recognised later by the managers naming one of the principal wards at the National Hospital in his honour.

It is tempting to argue, as did many Victorian commentators, that the conditions of rapid urbanisation and industrialisation which intensified commercial development and accelerated social change also encouraged a great increase in the frequency of particular diseases, including neurosyphilis.[13] Certainly,

---

[12] Burford Rawlings, *A Hospital in the Making* (1913), p. 5.

[13] Mrs Brewer, 'National Hospital for the Paralysed and Epileptic', Hospitals and Hospital Work 10, *Sunday at Home: A Family Magazine for Sabbath Reading* **34** (1887); Michael J. Clark, 'The Data of Alienism: Evolutionary Neurology, Physiological Psychology and the Reconstruction

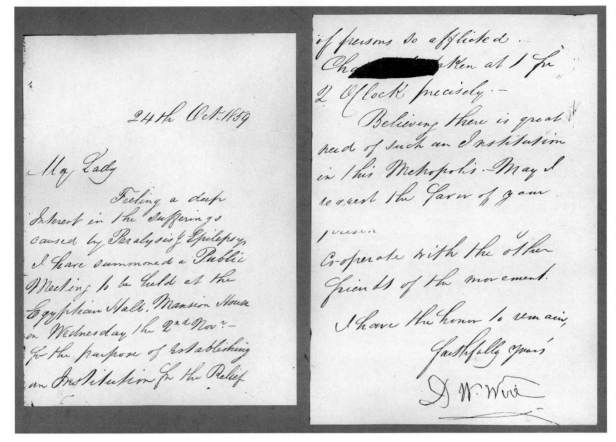

Figure 1.4 A letter from David Wire announcing the Mansion House meeting at which the National Hospital was founded.

the founders of the National Hospital seem to have believed this, to judge from the phraseology employed in some of the early annual reports. As late as 1888, the secretary, Burford Rawlings, writing in the official Report to the Governors and subscribers on the recent rebuilding of the hospital, proclaimed that 'nervous diseases are the concomitants of nineteenth century civilisation, the bitter fruits of a restless and palpitating era'.[14] It could also be argued that these economic and social forces tended merely to increase the awareness of epilepsy and paralysis as disabling conditions in working-class households, and that progressive extension of the New Poor Law and 'workhouse

system' after 1834 focused attention on the importance of medical causes of chronic poverty, which in turn acted as a welcome spur to private charitable action. Johanna and Edward Chandler's own writings appear to lend some credence to this analysis.

Although the original philanthropic impulse that created the National Hospital sprang from a small family circle whose motivations were religious and highly personal, momentum and critical mass were achieved only when benefaction associated with city philanthropy became focused on medicine. This was the association that enabled the initiative to raise funds rapidly and become a going concern. There was also a certain timeliness and resonance in the hospital's avowed dual aims of addressing contemporary socioeconomic conditions and advancing medical interest in the physiology and pathology of the brain and nervous system. These factors each contributed to the initial success of the enterprise and its favourable reception by the press and medical profession. Importantly for the subject, in the 1860s

---

of British Psychiatric Theory, c. 1850 – c. 1900' (unpublished DPhil thesis, Oxford University, 1982).

[14] National Hospital for the Paralysed and Epileptic (Albany Memorial), *Report Upon the Rebuilding* [of the Hospital], *with Statement of Receipts and Expenditure, and List of Contributors* (London: Chiswick Press, 1888), foreword ('Note') (unsigned, but clearly the work of Burford Rawlings), p. 1.

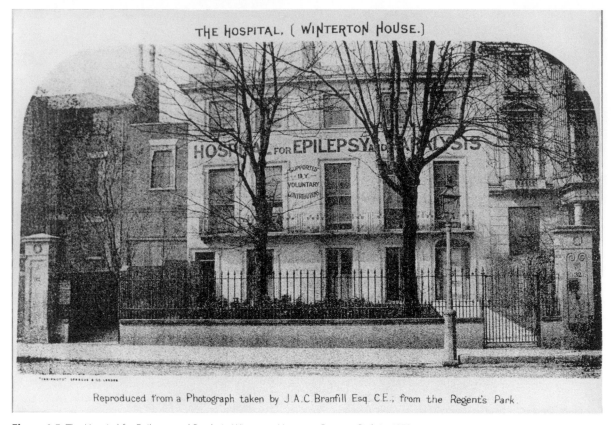

Reproduced from a Photograph taken by J.A.C. Branfill Esq. C.E., from the Regent's Park.

Figure 1.5 The Hospital for Epilepsy and Paralysis, Winterton House, at Regents Park, in 1873.

there was no conflict between philanthropy and medicine; and for some time afterwards, this climate stimulated the development of clinical neurology as a distinct medical specialty, thereby providing an environment that encouraged physicians such as John Hughlings Jackson and William Gowers, each with emerging interests in diseases of the nervous system, to join the hospital staff, use its resources to build up their own practices, and achieve professional eminence as neurologists.[15] More generally, at a time when specialist medicine was still very much in its infancy, physicians with an interest in designated specialties needed all the help and support they could get from lay people and opinion leaders within the profession. As is apparent from the early reports and publicity, the lay managers and benefactors of the National Hospital were fully persuaded that medical progress was key to relieving the plight of paralysed and epileptic individuals. Philanthropy and the practice of medicine were mutually supportive and advancing together – though it was tension and hostility between these same elements that had almost destroyed the hospital at the turn of the century.

[15] Although the term 'neurology' was coined by Thomas Willis, exactly when the designation 'neurologist' was adopted is less clear. The *Oxford English Dictionary* (1971) gives a citation from 1832 from J. Thomson, *An Account of the Life, Lectures and Writings, of William Cullen*, Vol. I, p. 443 (William Cullen was a leading physician of the Enlightenment, and a professor of medicine in Edinburgh). Thomson wrote, in relation to Professor Paul Joseph Barthez and the mind–body debate, that Barthez considered it essential that the phenomena of living beings should not be regarded as having their origins 'either in the powers of the mind, as had been conceived by the Stahlians, or in the properties of the organized body, as had been believed by the mechanical school and still more recently maintained by the Neurologists who he terms the Solidists' but considered it rather a property of 'the Vital Principle'. Whether the word 'neurologist' derives from Thomson, Cullen or Barthez is not clear from this text. The use of the term to define a physician specialising in the treatment of neurological disease, though, seems to have arisen at some point in the late nineteenth century, with obscure provenance.

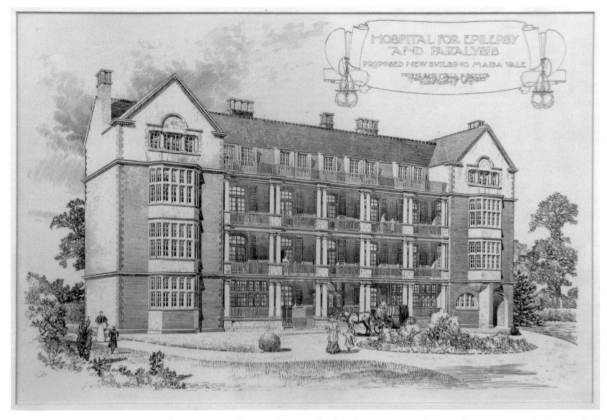

Figure 1.6 Maida Vale Hospital. Undated architect's drawing of the façade of the building, opened in 1902, by Keith Young of Young and Hall Architects.

The Rivals of the National Hospital

Throughout the first 50 years of its existence, the National Hospital had to face competition from several rival hospitals. In 1866, the German medical exile Julius Althaus founded the 'London Infirmary for Epilepsy and Paralysis' in Blandford Place, Marylebone, which, after two moves and several changes of name, eventually merged with Queen Square in 1948 under the auspices of the National Health Service to form the National Hospitals.[16]

During the whole period from the late 1860s to the end of the First World War, the London Infirmary was, in effect, a direct competitor with the National Hospital, claiming to offer specialist treatment and facilities for similar conditions, appealing to the same potential benefactors and patrons, and with each of its successive name changes serving only to underline the extent to which the two hospitals were competing for identical business. In fact, a whole series of instructive comparisons may be drawn between the National Hospital and its best-known London rival. At least initially, both hospitals worked primarily on epilepsy and paralysis. Each offered treatment regimens in which electrotherapeutics and massage, or 'medical rubbing', played important roles. And, almost from the start, lay administrators, nurses and doctors moved readily from one institution to the other as opportunities arose for career advancement. Thus, George Reid, the first secretary of the National Hospital, resigned from his position in January 1865, ostensibly on the grounds of ill health, only to become the first secretary of the new London Infirmary in 1867. Conversely, in February 1880, David Ferrier, who since 1878 had been an assistant physician at what had then become the Hospital for Epilepsy and Paralysis, Portland Terrace, Regent's Park, was appointed physician to outpatients at the National Hospital, but only on condition that he resigned forthwith from his position at the rival institution.

---

[16] Anthony Feiling, *A History of the Maida Vale Hospital for Nervous Diseases* (London: Butterworth & Co. for the Board of Governors of the National Hospitals for Nervous Diseases, 1958).

Also, in 1880, having failed to secure appointment as assistant physician to outpatients at the National Hospital under controversial circumstances, William Allen Sturge[17] was promptly appointed assistant physician at the Regent's Park Hospital for Epilepsy and Paralysis. Throughout the last decades of the nineteenth century, both hospitals suffered from chronic shortages of funds and space, each struggling to attract wealthy supporters and patrons and, where possible, to offer free treatment. But although the National Hospital was the inspiration of lay evangelical philanthropy, Maida Vale Hospital[18] was the product of medical entrepreneurs and almost entirely controlled during the nineteenth century by its medical staff.

There were other would-be rivals. The Charity Organisation Society's 1889 inquiry into the funding of voluntary hospitals in London listed four institutions specialising in nervous diseases: the National Hospital; the Portland Terrace Hospital for Epilepsy and Paralysis; the National Hospital for Diseases of the Heart, Brompton, founded in 1868; and the West End Hospital for Diseases of the Nervous System, Paralysis and Epilepsy, Welbeck Street, founded in 1878.[19] Others followed, including the Empire Hospital for Nervous Diseases, Vincent Square, founded in 1913 (and closing in 1919). Almost from the first, the National Hospital was buffeted by these competitors. In March 1868, the Board of Management was much vexed by the prospectus issued by the fledgling Infirmary for Epilepsy and Paralysis in the name of their former secretary, George Reid, so that the deputy

chairman, Thomas Parker, solicitor, 'promised to see Mr. Reid on the subject'. Four years later, in January 1872, Burford Rawlings, together with Messrs Parker, Lee & Haddock, solicitors to the hospital, took legal advice from Mr Napier Higgins, QC, of Lincoln's Inn, on their chances of successfully applying for an injunction against the recently established National Hospital for Diseases of the Heart '[for] … assum[-ing] a title calculated to confound it with this Hospital'. However, on being advised that they stood little chance of success, the Board decided instead to follow Higgins' advice and insert notices in the press warning the public of the danger of confusing the two hospitals, and writing to the president of the Heart Hospital, the Earl of Dudley, 'calling his Lordship's attention to the successive alterations in the title of the Institution and begging his interference to prevent the further use of the words Paralysis and Epilepsy and the subsequent confusion of the two Hospitals'. Most annoying of all, perhaps, in a move strangely reminiscent of Reid's defection to the 'London Infirmary', Herbert Tibbits, medical superintendent of the National Hospital since 1868 and one of the leading British advocates and practitioners of electrotherapeutics in the treatment of nervous diseases, resigned from his position at the hospital in 1877, ostensibly on grounds of ill health, and was elected 'honorary medical superintendent' by the Board, only to re-emerge as principal co-founder of the new West End Hospital a year later. Presented with a prospectus for the new hospital issued by Tibbits in June 1878, the Board understandably decided 'to consider his connection with the proposed Institution as an act of resignation of the honorary post to which he had previously been elected'. Six years later, when the new buildings in Queen Square had just been completed, overtures were made by the West End Hospital with a view to effecting a merger between the two institutions. But the Board refused to consider the proposal (similar moves were again made in the 1920s and 1930s). By this time, although the National Hospital had already developed as a distinctive institution in a class of its own intellectually and was acclaimed nationally and internationally in medical and scientific circles, for the lay public it remained just another specialist hospital not readily distinguishable from its competitors. On more than one occasion, would-be benefactors left money in their wills to the 'Asylum for Paralytics' or the 'Hospital for Epilepsy and Paralysis', but in such vague terms that the National Hospital was eventually forced to share the

---

[17] Sturge described what has become known as Sturge–Weber disease. Rejection of his application to join the staff of the National Hospital was a lost opportunity. He had served as resident medical officer and registrar from 1874 to 1876.

[18] The Regent's Park Hospiltal for Epilepsy and Paralysis was renamed Maida Vale Hospital when it moved in 1903. The new hospital was designed by Keith Young of Young and Hall Architects, of 17 Southampton St, Bloomsbury (close to Queen Square). They had an interest in hospital building and, in 1900, the partnership had entered the competition to build Glasgow Royal Infirmary, but was unplaced in the competition.

[19] *Memorandum on the Medical Charities of the Metropolis, with special reference to the Proposal for an Inquiry in regard to the Administration and Common Organisation of Voluntary Hospitals and Dispensaries, and Poor Law Infirmaries and Dispensaries, by a Select Committee of the House of Lords* (London: Charity Organisation Society, 1889), pp. 16–17.

benefaction with one or other of its competitors, thereby acknowledging the gulf between medical perceptions of the National Hospital as an elite institution and the public perception that hospitals for nervous diseases were all more or less interchangeable.

As late as 1901, the administrative secretary of the rival Hospital for Epilepsy and Paralysis openly sought to take advantage of the opportunity presented by the apparent turmoil into which the National Hospital had been thrown by the conflict between the Board of Management and its honorary medical staff to entice paying customers and potential benefactors away from Queen Square to the Regent's Park Hospital.[20] The relative ease with which doctors moved between the National Hospital and its competitors by the late nineteenth century also reflects the gradual acceptance of clinical neurology as a unified specialty, with a shared clinical knowledge base and transferable skills

Administrating the National Hospital

Responsibility for running the National Hospital, and the other beneficiaries of the Charity, was vested in various management committees, administrative officers and unofficial networks of lay activists, supporters and patrons. The roles of some of these, such as the Board of Management and the secretary, were specified in the Rules and Bye-laws; but those of others, including the (mainly female) networks of benefactors, fund-raisers and patrons, were not explicitly formalised. All played a part in the formation and development of the National Hospital.

The Board of Management

Although their special status as founders of the institution is universally acknowledged, the Chandler siblings did not act alone. Indeed, the institution owed much of its rapid progress during the 1860s to early recognition of how much help they needed from influential and experienced men and women in the worlds of medicine, business and philanthropy. They succeeded handsomely in enlisting this support. In August or September 1859, Viscount Raynham suggested forming a small steering committee to direct the campaign to raise funds for the new hospital; and, after the Mansion House meeting of November 1859, this group formed the nucleus of the future Board of Management.[21] The radically minded Raynham had initially proposed that the committee should include both men and women, particularly Johanna Chandler and her friend and fellow-worker Miss Elizabeth Bevington, but Johanna preferred to stand back in favour of her brother Edward, leaving the new committee exclusively in the hands of the hospital's male supporters, although she herself took the Ladies' Committee and subsequently the Ladies' Samaritan Society as her preferred spheres of action. This may have benefitted both the hospital and Johanna Chandler, because, for much of the 15 years of active

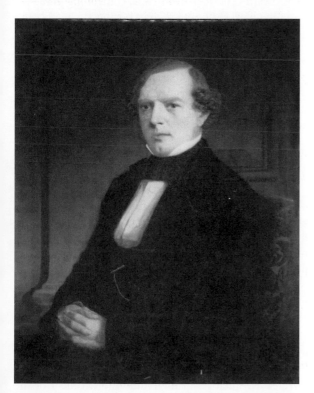

Figure 1.7 Oil painting (artist not recorded) of Edward Chandler, the elder brother of Johanna and Louisa and member of the first Board of Management.

---

20 See H. Howgrave Graham, secretary to the Regent's Park (later Maida Vale) Hospital for Epilepsy and Paralysis, letter to *The Times*, paraphrased in an editorial note of 13 August 1900 (issue 36167).

21 The Board of Management retained ultimate control of the Charity, and over time created other committees which reported to it, including the Ladies' Committee, the House Committee, the Finance Committee, and the Medical Committee (in 1878), and other *ad-hoc* subcommittees.

life that remained to her, the Ladies' Committee was no less busy than the Board of Management, and it seems probable that she enjoyed more freedom of action and was able to accomplish far more as an independent fund-raiser than as a member of the Board.

With the notable exception of Viscount Raynham, the first Board of Management chaired by the then Lord Mayor, Alderman David Wire, was composed largely of evangelically minded city solicitors, accountants, businessmen and philanthropists, such as Thomas Parker, Richard Barton, Alderman (later Lord Mayor) Warren Stormes Hale and Edward Chandler. Mainly low-church or non-conformist in religion, and Liberal in politics, they represented a cross-section of the established commercial middle classes, united as much by piety and philanthropic concerns as by shared business interests or any sense of class identity. Subsequently, the Board became more diversified in its origins and affiliations. Military men, such as Captain (later Colonel) George Porter, Captain Leonard Shuter, Major-General the Hon. Sir Percy Herbert, KCB, MP, and Lieutenant-General Sir Walter Walker, KCB, began to take over from the city solicitors and accountants; and the influence of the aristocracy and men of leisure also became more evident. There was still financial, business and professional presence on the Board, represented by those such as the solicitor John Pearman. These representatives of finance and the professions gained in influence, as in the case of the Hon. Dudley Ryder, for many years the acting treasurer and also titular head of Coutts Bank before briefly succeeding his brother as fourth Earl of Harrowby in 1900. Similarly, Lord Halsbury was a member of the Board of Management for more than 15 years, from 1884 to 1900, despite serving three terms as Lord Chancellor during this period. Low-church and evangelical opinions continued to be strongly represented, notably through the Hon. George William Erskine Russell, Liberal MP for North Bedfordshire, sometime member of the London County Council, and chairman of the Board of Management for much of the 1890s. So too were some high churchmen such as the Revd John Back and the Hon. Dudley Ryder, who were on the Board of Management for many years from the early 1870s. After the deaths of David Wire and Warren Hales, and the *de facto* withdrawal of Viscount Raynham after 1866, the political centre of gravity of the Board moved in a more conservative direction, notably during the 1870s and 1880s when General Sir Percy Herbert, the Hon. Dudley Ryder and Lord Halsbury were all prominent members. This shift in affiliation contributed to the crisis that occurred at the end of the century.

The 1860s and 1870s also revealed tensions between Johanna and Edward Chandler and the newly appointed members of the Board of Management. Edward was increasingly at odds with the Board over the proposed enlargement of the hospital and particularly the accommodation of needy middle-class contributing patients in separate wards. There were clashes on the Board between 'traditionalists' and 'modernisers' over the future role of women in the Charity, although the Ladies' Committee and the Ladies' Samaritan Society both retained some independence. From the mid-1870s onwards, and especially after the virtual withdrawal of Edward Chandler from 1879, controlling influence on the Board shifted to men of business – notably the secretary Benjamin Burford Rawlings (of whom, much later); the Board's longest-serving member and chairman, Captain Porter; the Hon. Dudley Ryder, treasurer; and the Hon. George W. E. Russell, MP. In addition, although an infrequent attender at Board meetings, Lord Halsbury also exercised much influence behind the scenes during the late 1880s and 1890s by virtue of his powerful connections and legal and political eminence. Board meetings became less frequent and were attended by fewer Board members, whereas more and more business was effectively delegated to the secretary-director (as Burford Rawlings' title became in 1885), or decided informally by him together with one or two other experienced Board members. House and Finance Committees were established in the early years; *ad-hoc* subcommittees and working groups proliferated; and the Board delegated its power over appointments and clinical matters to the increasingly independently minded Medical Committee. At the same time, the hospital was becoming more reliant on the external funding provided by the Saturday and Sunday Funds and the Prince of Wales' Hospital Fund for London (antecedent of the present-day King's Fund). For the first time, these changes gave external bodies other than the Charity Commissioners and the Local Government Board leverage over the Board's decisions. From time to time, ordinary members of the Board could still reassert their authority *vis-à-vis* the secretary-director, as, for example, in the arguments over investment policy in the mid-1880s. But, by the mid-1890s, the power-base had shifted and the Board was increasingly forced to refer to other bodies and interest groups both inside and outside the National Hospital.

Of the founders, both Johanna and Edward Chandler were, in their different ways, highly effective fund-raisers and financial planners. Indeed, together with some of her fellow workers on the Ladies' Committee, notably Miss Bevington and Miss Sophia King, Johanna Chandler proved herself to be a fund-raiser and volunteer organiser of genius. After her death, the Ladies' Committee raised so little new money that its continued existence was seriously called into question. In the 1880s and 1890s, the financial strains imposed by the building of the new hospital were to have far-reaching consequences for the fortunes of the National Hospital over the next years. The House and Finance Committees of the Board of Management were perfectly capable of dealing with the day-to-day domestic and financial affairs, but there was neither a specialist fund-raising officer nor an in-house investments adviser, so that, although Burford Rawlings had his own ideas about how to increase the financial returns on the investment portfolio, he was largely unsuccessful in his attempts to persuade the Board to focus on fiscal issues during the 1880s and 1890s. Time and again, the Board deferred any in-depth discussion of the investment portfolio and strategy; and significant opportunities for boosting the hospital's income and capital reserves for future expansion were missed.

In the early years, when the National Hospital was still a small institution, the relationships between benefactors, governors, Board members, physicians and patients were close. Thus, for example, in January 1865, Edward Chandler informed the Board that the late Mrs Elizabeth Morgan of Aldershot, Hants, had left a legacy of £1,000 to the hospital. Mrs Morgan's executor, Mr John Back, was the father of the Revd John Back, governor and future Board member, as well as himself being a patient of Dr Charles Radcliffe. Three years later, by which time Mrs Morgan's executors had agreed to settle a further £10,000 on the National Hospital in the form of a special trust, the Board voted to rename Ward Number 2 as 'Morgan ward' and to elect Mrs Morgan's executors as Honorary Vice-Presidents of the Charity. Six months later, the deputy chairman, Thomas Parker, a keen amateur artist, presented a portrait of the late Mrs Morgan painted by himself

to the hospital. When John Back died, he left a further £5,000, and was in turn commemorated by a memorial window. His son, the Revd Back, was elected to the Board six months later, subsequently serving as deputy chairman as well as acting as chaplain to the hospital until a permanent appointment was made. A ward was named after him. Similarly, when in May 1869 Major-General Herbert and his wife Lady Mary Herbert offered £285 towards the purchase of two villas in East Finchley to serve as the Convalescent Home, to which they later added a further £124 4s 2d, plus 2,000 rupees'-worth of India Stock, the Board of Management readily accepted Herbert's stipulation that he be elected a member of the Board – of which he subsequently became chairman – and appointed him 'Treasurer of the Convalescent Home Fund'. In July 1870, the Board agreed to name one of the three wards in the new Home after Lady Mary Herbert. Even in later years, close relationships of this kind existed for certain Board members, hospital officials, benefactors and patrons, but, increasingly, as the National Hospital grew into a significant player on the London medical scene, such informal ties became constrained by hospital bureaucracy and regulations laid down by the Charity Commissioners. As a result, by the late nineteenth century the National Hospital was transformed from being small and domestic into a large and more conventionally regulated institution.

Benjamin Burford Rawlings

In the first 50 years of the National Hospital, the most important lay administrators turned out to be its secretaries or honorary secretaries and not its treasurers, as was the case with most of the great public hospitals in London. George Reid was appointed secretary in December 1859 at a salary of £50 p.a., subsequently increased incrementally to £150 p.a. He appears to have performed his duties conscientiously over the next five years, but there is nothing to suggest that he ever saw his role as anything more than acting on the instructions of the Board of Management. There was then no clear demarcation of duties between the secretary and the honorary secretary, Edward Chandler, who was also a leading member of the Board of Management and the House Committee, and in these early years Chandler played a critical role in the daily running of the hospital, writing letters to potential donors and sponsors, ordering bed-linen and furnishings for the new wards, and dealing with tradesmen and the water company. Chandler also excelled at fund-raising, an activity to which Reid contributed rather little. In January 1865, Reid resigned, and was succeeded by Cyrus Edmonds. He was described by Burford Rawlings as 'a gentleman of literary attainments', and was paid a salary of £150 p.a. However, there are indications that the performance of the new secretary and the division of labour between Edmonds and the honorary secretary were causing concern, because, in November 1866, Viscount Raynham, now Marquis Townshend, treasurer of the hospital, proposed abolishing the honorary secretaryship. This he considered to be 'bad in principle', urging 'that an efficient paid secretary be engaged forthwith so that in future the services of an honorary secretary [can] be dispensed with'. Burford Rawlings was subsequently informed that, during his brief time in office, '[Edmonds] had been thwarted and rendered miserable in the discharge of his duties by never-ceasing interference and obstruction by the founders', Edward and Johanna Chandler. However, Burford Rawlings clearly had some doubts as to the truth of this report and, other than Marquis Townshend's motion to abolish the post of honorary secretary, which attracted little support from other members of the Board, no independent evidence was found to support this claim.

Whatever the truth of the matter, Edmonds soon became embroiled in a dispute with the Board over the £175 commission that he claimed was owing to him for subscriptions and donations secured during his time in office. He resigned in March 1866, to be replaced temporarily by his assistant Thomas Boughton who, however, had already fallen under suspicion of peculation and, after months of discreet surveillance, was summarily dismissed in October 1866 for the alleged theft of £28 by means of false accounting. In February 1867, the hospital auditor, Frederick Maynard, reported that 'the deficiencies of Mr. Boughton' in fact amounted to £215 6s 7d, and the Board was informed that Boughton had now left the country. Nor was this the only case of fraud and theft in the early history of the National Hospital. In October 1873, it was reported that William Whitmore, who had acted as collector for the hospital from October 1868 to March/April 1873, 'had been given into custody by the authorities of the Hospital for Women for irregularities in his accounts'. Burford Rawlings tried to assure the Board that, thanks to the National Hospital's system of internal accounting,

any 'deficiency' in its accounts could not exceed £40, but this issue does not appear to have been resolved definitively.

Burford Rawlings, an Essex-born Londoner, who had previously tried his hand as both man of letters and tin-mining promoter, was engaged as secretary in November 1866. Most previous accounts of the early history of the National Hospital relegate him to a footnote but, in fact, throughout the tenure of his appointment, Burford Rawlings became the dominant figure in the hospital. He started at a salary of £150 p.a., the same terms as those offered to Cyrus Edmonds in January 1865 – although Burford Rawlings was not at first awarded the 5 per cent commission on any sum exceeding £500 above the average yearly total of subscriptions and donations (exclusive of legacies) to which Edmonds had been entitled. By 1870, Burford Rawlings' salary had increased incrementally to £250 p.a., with £50 payable at Christmas in each year. When, in May 1873, he asked for yet another rise, the request was turned down. Burford Rawlings was reminded in passing that he should be on duty in the hospital by 10.00 a. m. each weekday morning. However, he did not give up so easily, and at the very next Board meeting he presented 'a statement showing the average receipts before and since his appointment & the amount of subscriptions and donations obtained directly by his individual exertions', at which a suitably impressed Captain Porter 'expressed his surprise at the figures submitted & his conviction that the Board generally were uninformed of the financial results accruing from the Secretary's labour'. At the next Board meeting, held in July 1873, Edward Chandler proposed that the secretary's salary be increased to £300 p.a., 'and that an opportunity be given him to gain some additional remuneration … equivalent to 5% upon all sums received in reply to his appeals', much as in Cyrus Edmonds' case. This was duly approved by the Board. However, Burford Rawlings evidently did not care much for this arrangement, which smacked rather too much of trade, and moreover seemed likely to preclude receipt of the annual £50 gratuity to which he aspired. Shrewdly, he neglected to claim any of the commission on donations and subscriptions to which he was entitled during the next 18 months; and, in January 1875, persuaded the Board to appoint a subcommittee to report on the amount of commission deemed owing to him since July 1873, and his future remuneration. The subcommittee recommended keeping the existing commission on donations and subscriptions received, with a payment of £25 (eventually increased to £41 16s) in settlement of any monies owed since July 1873. But Burford Rawlings somehow managed in effect to reinstate his annual £50 bonus, in the guise of a lump sum paid in lieu of outstanding commissions. The yearly £50 Christmas bonuses were frequently supplemented by additional payments in recognition of his efforts in organising festival dinners and other fund-raising events. In August 1878, his salary was increased to £400 p.a., provided that he resigned his part-time secretaryship of the Iron & Metal Pension Society (worth £100 p.a.) and devoted himself full-time to the affairs of the National Hospital. With further pay increases, by March 1893, to £600 p.a., but without the Christmas bonuses, he was earning four times as much as the assistant secretary and three-and-a-half times that of the hospital dispenser. Burford Rawlings also enjoyed a generous, and apparently flexible, annual leave allowance; and, in 1899, he persuaded the Board to pay his salary and that of certain other hospital officers without deduction of income tax. Even after his enforced retirement in January 1902 (see below), Burford Rawlings continued to live very comfortably on the National Hospital's bounty. The Fry Commission of Inquiry of May–June 1901 recommended that he be pensioned off with an allowance of £350 p.a., increased to £450 p.a. at a special general meeting of the governors held on 12 December 1901. Even so, his supporters among the governors and outgoing Board of Management were not satisfied and succeeded in voting him an honorarium equivalent to one year's salary in addition to his annual pension, 'in recognition of his past special services to the Charity'.

It would be wrong, however, to conclude from this that Burford Rawlings was simply a money-grabbing administrator who used the hospital to feather his nest. Whatever his faults, as even his most inveterate enemies conceded, he was an energetic and usually efficient manager and a tireless fund-raiser, completely devoted to the National Hospital, furthering what he conceived to be its best interests, and more than willing to assume a leading role in its development.

Possessed of a great deal of energy, a considerable measure of strategic vision, and a steadily growing sense of his own importance in the scheme of things, Burford Rawlings was the prime mover, and, in effect, project manager, for the massive expansion and wholesale rebuilding of the hospital during the early 1880s. In subsequent decades, he implemented extensive reforms of the medical and nursing organisation, the management of its finances and investment portfolio, and its administrative and policy-making procedures, as well as securing royal patronage for the Charity and undertaking several major revisions of the Rules and Bye-laws. From modest beginnings as a hard working, loyal servant of the Board who readily identified with the hospital's philanthropic traditions, Burford Rawlings gradually built up his position to become the driving force behind the Board of Management and the dominant influence in the National Hospital. The Board granted him the title of 'Secretary and General Director' in January 1885 shortly before the opening of the new hospital – one imagines, at his instigation – and he considered this just reward, given the scope of his post. By then, he saw himself not merely as chief clerk to the Board of Management, but also chief executive officer of the National Hospital.

Burford Rawlings was responsible for a multitude of routine administrative tasks within the hospital, including the admission and discharge of patients; dealing with the medical, nursing and domestic staff; corresponding with patients' families, subscribers and patrons; and calling meetings, preparing agendas and papers, and taking minutes of the Board of Management, the House Committee and general meetings of governors and subscribers. In addition, he solicited legacies and donations; liaised with the Saturday and Sunday Funds; negotiated with local authorities, utility companies and tradesmen for rate, tariff and price reductions; organised the purchase, rental or sale of properties; and represented the hospital at Parliamentary and other official enquiries or legal proceedings. He loved organising evening concerts and other entertainments for the patients, and socialising with royal and aristocratic patrons at fund-raising dinners and other events, such as the opening ceremonies for new extensions to the National Hospital, but does not seem to have felt any comparable need to socialise with doctors.

Gregarious, sociable, optimistic and naturally curious about people in all walks of life, Burford Rawlings had an instinctive sympathy with many of the patients and nursing staff, but not with the younger generation of consultants, such as Victor Horsley. All these duties he undertook with enthusiasm and a large measure of success, although his natural conservatism, sentimental attachment to the founding traditions of the National Hospital, and instinctive concern to safeguard his own position and power stopped him from pursuing fundamental reforms of the Charity's decision-making structures. Shrewd, resourceful and well versed in all the bureaucratic arts of delay, diversion, compromise, committee management and concealment of errors and misjudgements, and not one to be discouraged or deflected by initial resistance or other temporary setbacks, Burford Rawlings was a master of the long-game in hospital politics. Had he not succumbed to the fatal error of clinging on to power for too long, he might well have retired with his reputation intact as the principal architect of a prototypical nineteenth-century hospital, instead of becoming a symbol of everything that the medical staff of the National Hospital, as well as other public and media figures, found most outmoded and objectionable in hospital administration and governance.

While still in post, Burford Rawlings was described as 'the doyen of English hospital secretaries', and even those who accused him of serious mismanagement of the affairs of the National Hospital, and of presiding over a grave decline in standards of patient care, were ultimately unable to prove him guilty of any serious misdemeanour that would have warranted dismissal. The factors that ultimately led to his downfall were not so much matters of performance or dereliction of duty, but, rather, certain character traits and a mind-set that seemed increasingly at odds with the changed hospital environment of the 1890s. Although he could be a formidable adversary, Burford Rawlings was not a devious plotter and schemer. He was, however, officious, self-important and jealous of his own authority, and frequently tactless and abrasive to the point of downright rudeness towards those who did not share his Victorian values and vision.

Burford Rawlings had little real understanding of developments in science and medicine over the last three decades of the nineteenth century or of the place that, by the 1890s, medical and surgical research had come to occupy in the work of the National Hospital. As was the case with his predecessor Cyrus Edmonds, Burford Rawlings was a man of literary tastes and, though he shared the prevailing Victorian belief in science and progress, he did not understand it and could not relate to the kind of experimental animal work with which Horsley, Ferrier, Charles Beevor and others were engaged in the 1880s and 1890s. His concept of medicine was essentially rooted in expectant treatments and what would now be termed 'supportive care'. For him, medicine corresponded essentially to the early Victorian psychiatric idea of 'moral treatment', in which rest, nourishing food, good nursing care, kindness, gentle mental stimulation and recreation were the chief instruments of recovery. Burford Rawlings was clearly sceptical about the benefits of drug treatments and, particularly, of neurosurgical procedures. Feeling increasingly ill at ease in the hospital during the 1890s, Burford Rawlings concentrated on rebuilding at Queen Square and refurbishment of the Convalescent Home at Finchley; the semi-rural surroundings of the latter, together with the virtual absence of any active medical presence and the dominant emphasis on nursing care, allowed him to escape for a while into the nostalgia of how the National Hospital once had been.

With such an inadequate appreciation of medical science, it is hardly surprising that Burford Rawlings should have appeared out-of-touch and an obstacle to progress for many younger members of the medical and surgical staff. Nor did he have much understanding of late nineteenth-century medical politics. He failed to grasp the implications of the profession's rise in status and growing self-confidence towards the end of the century, and could not understand why former medical friends and supporters such as Sir James Crichton-Browne, Robert Brudenell Carter and John Hughlings Jackson had by 1900 turned against him. When his competence to hold office and the Board's right to direct the hospital's affairs were challenged, Burford Rawlings' lack of interest in medical science and failure to appreciate the medical profession's need for recognition of its importance in the life and work of the National Hospital left him isolated and vulnerable to attack by the medical staff and their supporters in the medical press and profession at large.

Burford Rawlings' unofficial memoir *A Hospital in the Making* (1913) is not in any way impartial – or even, in places, factually accurate – but it does not make for dull reading. Garrulous, opinionated and self-important, Burford Rawlings' account of the first 40 years of the National Hospital is rich in colourful anecdote, description of strong and eccentric personalities, and has touches of dry humour. Although saying very little about himself or his opinions, Burford Rawlings' personality comes across as overbearing. Like him or loathe him, he was the dominant personality in the hospital for much of the first four decades of its existence. His influence shaped much of its development and continued to be felt long after Burford Rawlings had been forced out of office.

Royal and Aristocratic Patronage

Although the National Hospital depended for its routine management on the work of its paid administrators, and on the dedication of the Board of Management, it also relied heavily in its first 50 years on the active support of royal and aristocratic patrons and subscribers. In a society where the social standing and respect due to the medical profession were far from universally acknowledged, patronage was one of the principal means whereby a new institution such as the National Hospital sought to establish its respectability and credentials. This was particularly important among those sections of the middle classes who were accustomed to following the leaders of Victorian society, and whose own self-image was greatly enhanced by association with so many of the great and the good. Subscriptions and donations, professional knowledge and connections, and the organisational and administrative abilities of the middle class were necessary for prudent and efficient running of the Charity. However, over and above any direct financial support, upper-class and royal patronage endowed the National Hospital with a prestigious public image and high standing among the other specialist hospitals, and it attracted less illustrious donors and supporters.

Even during the lean years, the Chandler sisters' rice shell ornaments and the cause they supported attracted the attention of the Duchess of Cambridge and Princess Mary Adelaide of Teck – both of whom later became patronesses of the hospital – and well-known aristocratic philanthropists and social reformers including Viscount Raynham and the Earl of Shaftesbury. The Mansion House meeting of November 1859 was attended by members of the aristocracy and gentry; and the landed classes were well represented among the National Hospital's initial tranche of governors and subscribers. From 1861, royal and aristocratic patronage also extended to the Ladies' Samaritan Society. The annual report for 1872 listed no fewer than 31 additional 'Lady Patronesses', including 4 duchesses, 6 marchionesses, countesses and baronesses, and a further 13 titled ladies, together with 14 male vice-presidents, of whom 3 were dukes and a further 7 were earls, marquesses or viscounts. In 1874–5, the Ladies' Samaritan Society was similarly described as being 'Under the Especial Patronage'.

The same pattern of patronage was reproduced in the many fund-raising events and activities organised by the Ladies' Samaritan Society during this period, including the 'Grand Amateur Musical Soirées' held in London organised by Miss Bevington, and the various 'Fancy Goods' sales, 'Garden Fêtes' and bazaars organised by Johanna Chandler and her Lady Samaritans at various places in London and the home counties in the 1860s and 1870s.

Festival dinners, a key element in the National Hospital's fund-raising strategy, were usually presided over by some well-known aristocratic figure, such as Viscount Enfield, MP, Lord Taunton and the Marquis of Lorne, KT, MP. Honorary stewards at these events were largely recruited from the hospital's aristocratic subscribers. Thus, the 45 honorary stewards listed on the programme for dinner held at The Albion, Aldersgate, on 10 April 1872 included two dukes, two marquesses, two earls, one viscount, a baron and two baronets, as well as three MPs and a German baron. On these occasions, even the more Liberal members of the Board of Management did not hesitate to show the most blatant sycophancy towards the nobility, apparently in the interests of the Charity. Thus, at the first festival dinner held at the London Tavern in March 1862, Alderman Warren Hale, future chairman of the Board of Management, lauded the honorary president, Lord Taunton, a Tory

> Like himself [the company at dinner] could not fail to be delighted that one connected with so distinguished a body as the House of Lords had stepped [down] from his exalted position to attend the first anniversary of this infant Institution ... They ought, indeed, to be highly honoured that a peer of the realm had come among them ... in order to augment the funds of this excellent and highly deserving charity ... Lord Taunton ... did not shut himself up in frigid exclusiveness, saying that he would do nothing beyond the circuit of his daily life, but was at all times anxious to aid in the promotion of all good works ... and much more in a similar vein.[22]

As with other public and ceremonial occasions connected with the National Hospital, festival dinners were among the rituals whereby Victorians publicly celebrated the hierarchical order of society and reaffirmed their belief in the nature and moral justification of the class system, but they were also reminders to the aristocracy and gentry of their charitable responsibilities.

---

[22] Contemporary press cutting (source not identified) in Queen Square Archive (NHNN/EF/1/2).

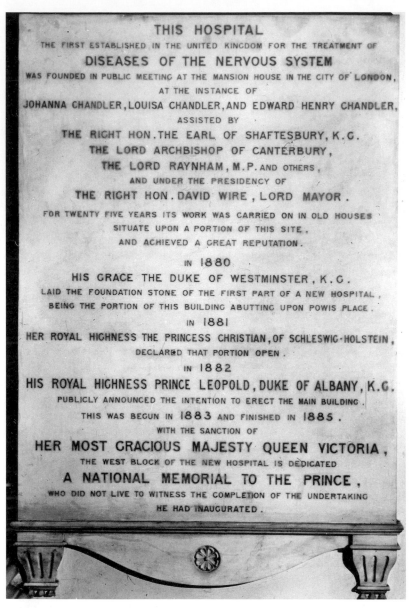

THIS HOSPITAL
THE FIRST ESTABLISHED IN THE UNITED KINGDOM FOR THE TREATMENT OF
DISEASES OF THE NERVOUS SYSTEM
WAS FOUNDED IN PUBLIC MEETING AT THE MANSION HOUSE IN THE CITY OF LONDON,
AT THE INSTANCE OF
JOHANNA CHANDLER, LOUISA CHANDLER, AND EDWARD HENRY CHANDLER,
ASSISTED BY
THE RIGHT HON. THE EARL OF SHAFTESBURY, K.G.
THE LORD ARCHBISHOP OF CANTERBURY,
THE LORD RAYNHAM, M.P. AND OTHERS,
AND UNDER THE PRESIDENCY OF
THE RIGHT HON. DAVID WIRE, LORD MAYOR.
FOR TWENTY FIVE YEARS ITS WORK WAS CARRIED ON IN OLD HOUSES
SITUATE UPON A PORTION OF THIS SITE,
AND ACHIEVED A GREAT REPUTATION.
IN 1880
HIS GRACE THE DUKE OF WESTMINSTER, K.G.
LAID THE FOUNDATION STONE OF THE FIRST PART OF A NEW HOSPITAL,
BEING THE PORTION OF THIS BUILDING ABUTTING UPON POWIS PLACE.
IN 1881
HER ROYAL HIGHNESS THE PRINCESS CHRISTIAN, OF SCHLESWIG-HOLSTEIN,
DECLARED THAT PORTION OPEN.
IN 1882
HIS ROYAL HIGHNESS PRINCE LEOPOLD, DUKE OF ALBANY, K.G.
PUBLICLY ANNOUNCED THE INTENTION TO ERECT THE MAIN BUILDING.
THIS WAS BEGUN IN 1883 AND FINISHED IN 1885.
WITH THE SANCTION OF
HER MOST GRACIOUS MAJESTY QUEEN VICTORIA,
THE WEST BLOCK OF THE NEW HOSPITAL IS DEDICATED
A NATIONAL MEMORIAL TO THE PRINCE,
WHO DID NOT LIVE TO WITNESS THE COMPLETION OF THE UNDERTAKING
HE HAD INAUGURATED.

Figure 1.8 Plaque of 1885, in the entrance hall of the hospital, commemorating the opening of the new hospital building and the dedication of the west wing as a national memorial to HRH Prince Leopold, the Duke of Albany, who did not live long enough to witness the opening of the new building in 1885.

In 1880, the Duke of Westminster, shortly to become honorary president of the Charity, presided over the opening of the Powis Place building that housed the outpatients' department. And in March 1882, Queen Victoria's youngest son Prince Leopold, Duke of Albany, who suffered from mild epilepsy as well as haemophilia, gave a keynote speech in support of the Rebuilding Fund appeal at the Freemasons' Hall, London.[23] This was widely reported in the press, and thereafter both the Prince and his young wife, Princess Helena of Waldeck, Duchess of Albany,

in form and usually followed a serious episode of bleeding. Queen Victoria went to great lengths to keep her son's epilepsy secret, in view of its social stigma. It had been claimed that some of Leopold's speeches and appeals for funds were written by Dean Stanley, the dean of Westminster, but he died in 1881, and it is now thought that Leopold's extensive charitable work was all of his own making (details taken from C. Zeepvat, *Prince Leopold: The Untold Story of Queen Victoria's Youngest Son* (Stroud: Sutton Publishing, 1998)).

---

[23] Leopold's epilepsy was said to have started in childhood. Jenner was his physician and he recorded that the fits were infrequent, usually no more than 1–2 a year, and were mild

became closely involved in fund-raising for the hospital. Prince Leopold was making a name for himself as a serious and committed advocate of social and educational reform and, had he lived longer and been able to extend further his brief association with the National Hospital and its work, might well have brought many more tangible benefits to the Charity. After the Duke's untimely death[24] in the south of France in March 1884, Queen Victoria agreed to the Board's request 'to constitute the Western Pavilion [of the new hospital] as a Memorial to H.R.H. the late Duke of Albany' – hence the frequently used term 'Albany Memorial' for the main hospital building, the familiar façade of which faces Queen Square. A terracotta memorial plaque was installed for the official opening ceremony in July 1885, which remains *in situ* to this day as a reminder of the Duke's energetic, if short-lived, contribution to the growth of the National Hospital.

In February 1887, the Queen herself agreed to become patron of the hospital, sending a donation of £50, and the official *Report Upon the Rebuilding* (of the National Hospital), published in 1888, listed the Queen and five other members of the royal family – the Duke of Edinburgh, the Duchess of Albany, the Duchess of Cambridge, Princess Mary Adelaide and Princess Christian of Schleswig-Holstein – as co-patrons. This impressive tally was echoed in the names given to three of the four pavilions constituting the new hospital: in addition to the Albany Memorial wing facing onto Queen Square was now the Princess Christian pavilion, housing the outpatients department on Powis Place, and the adjacent Princess Alexandra or Princess of Wales pavilion situated between the Albany Memorial and Princess Christian wings. Inpatient wards were named in honour of Princess Christian and Princess Helena, Duchess of Albany, who continued her late husband's involvement and, over the next three decades, became one of the hospital's most ardent supporters. The Duchess took a special interest in the rebuilding and enlargement of the Finchley Convalescent Home in the 1890s and, as chairman of the Hospital Diamond Jubilee Committee established in August 1907, played

a major role in the committee's fund-raising campaign during the next 18 months. Princess Alice, later Countess of Athlone, daughter of Leopold and Helena also took an active role in supporting the hospital, and in 1904 she became both patroness and president of the Ladies' Samaritan Society. Princess Alice presided over the official opening of the Queen Mary wing in 1938 and continued her family's benevolent association with the hospital and the Ladies' Samaritan Society until the mid twentieth century.

In early 1900, Burford Rawlings and the Board of Management sought further to enhance the hospital's prestige by petitioning the Crown to incorporate the Charity by Royal Charter. In April 1900, the solicitors Messrs Bower, Cotton & Bower were instructed to prepare the necessary documentation, but the project had to be left in temporary abeyance when the conflict between the Board and the honorary medical and surgical staff escalated. A draft memorandum and articles of association for the re-founded Charity drawn up by Messrs Paine and Paine, the new hospital solicitors, were submitted to the Board in November 1902, and in March 1903 the National Hospital finally obtained its cherished Royal Charter together with the patronage of the new monarch, King Edward VII, who (as the then Prince of Wales) had officially opened the new hospital in July 1885. In January 1907, the King agreed to subscribe 10 guineas per annum to the hospital funds. Together, these official marks of royal favour set the seal on the re-branding of the National Hospital after the long and damaging internal conflicts of 1900–1, and helped reaffirm its standing in Edwardian London.

Aristocratic patrons and patronesses could, however, be very demanding. During the last two decades of the nineteenth century, Burford Rawlings and the Board of Management repeatedly bemoaned the number of wealthy and influential supporters of the hospital who wrote requesting the admission of their relatives, clients or dependants as inpatients, without feeling obliged to make any contribution towards the financial costs of treating them. This was a problem which many voluntary hospitals faced from their subscribers, but, at Queen Square, the high rank of the subscribers made this worse.

Nor were patients the only people with powerful backers among the hospital's patrons and patronesses. In November 1895, the Board persuaded the lady superintendent of nurses, Miss Louisa East, to resign on grounds of ill health after an extended leave of

---

[24] He died in a convulsion and it is assumed that he had a cerebral haemorrhage due to the haemophilia. It was recognised that the fit was not of his usual type and Dr John Russell Reynolds was called after his death to give an opinion. His view was that nothing further could have been done to save the prince.

absence, and voted her a retirement pension of £30 p. a. However, Miss East had influential friends, who evidently felt that she had been shabbily treated, because, at the next Board meeting, on the motion of Ryder and Russell, Burford Rawlings was instructed '[to] convey to H.R.H. the Princess Christian and the Duke of Westminster an explanation of the circumstances attending the resignation of Miss East, who has their sincere sympathy, and inform H.R.H. and his Grace that the question of pension has been considered with a desire to assist Miss East to the utmost extent [that] the circumstances allowed'. Burford Rawlings was further instructed to draft a 'suitable Testimonial' for Miss East, which was duly approved and signed by Colonel George Porter as chairman of the Board in February 1896. However, this was only the start of Burford Rawlings' problems with the superintendent of nurses. In January–February 1896, he and the Board of Management moved swiftly to advertise Miss East's vacant position, short-list and interview candidates, and offer the post to Miss Rosalind Fynes-Clinton before discovering that this had already been promised to the acting lady superintendent, Miss Rachel Tweed, who also had influential friends on the Board. Faced with the strong possibility that either Miss Fynes-Clinton or Miss Tweed might bring legal action against the hospital, and that the Board would turn on him for mismanaging the whole affair, Burford Rawlings was forced once again to go cap-in-hand to the Duke of Westminster, this time to seek his help and that of Lord Halsbury in persuading Miss Fynes-Clinton to withdraw in favour of Miss Tweed, with the promise of a personal letter of recommendation for other applications signed by the Duke as president of the National Hospital.

Finance and Fund-raising

As a voluntary hospital and charity without endowment of its own, entirely dependent on generating funds from subscribers and well-wishers, the need for a revenue stream dominated the agenda of the Finance Committee during the early years. As Burford Rawlings stated in 1882, 'active and persistent begging must enter largely into any scheme for maintaining hospitals under the voluntary system'. In the early 1860s, responsibility for raising funds rested on Johanna and Edward Chandler, the secretary Reid and members of the Board of Management (notably Aldermen David Wire and Hale), and the solicitors Richard Barton and Thomas Parker, with the bulk of the work being undertaken by the Chandlers. It was not until March 1863 that a regular Finance Committee was constituted, as part of a series of measures taken by the Board to improve internal financial control and auditing. Edward Chandler exemplified the attitude of the institution's founders towards finance and fund-raising when, in a speech to hospital governors and subscribers at the tenth election of pensioners in July 1875, he declared his belief 'that God will always send you funds as they are needed, for God rules over everything in this world for the best, … such is the feeling of sympathy for the incurable in this country that the means for their relief will always be provided'.

For the first 25 years of its existence, the National Hospital grew slowly but steadily and without falling into debt or having to close wards or lay off staff to reduce costs. Fund-raising campaigns regularly exceeded their targets. Indeed, the annual reports of the Board of Management documented year-on-year increases in the hospital's reserve funds and a healthy balance on the current account. Between 1865 and her death in 1876, Johanna Chandler promised the Board of Management to deliver at least £2,000 a year in funds raised through personal appeals and by the Ladies' Committee, and every year she succeeded in fulfilling her undertaking. Only after completion of the rebuilding, which cost a great deal more than anticipated and, for the first time, incurred debt, did financial constraints hamper continued growth of the institution.

During the first four decades, income came principally from four main sources: annual subscriptions, special appeals, fund-raising events and festival dinners, and legacies and donations. The initial expectation seems to have been that income from annual subscriptions, which entitled subscribers and governors of the hospital to vote at general meetings and made them eligible for appointment to the Board of Management, would cover the bulk of ordinary expenditure. However, this source never provided more than a fraction of the income necessary to cover ongoing expenditure – much less to finance growth of the hospital. For this purpose, special appeals were necessary. From the 1860s, a festival dinner, usually presided over by a well-known aristocratic politician or philanthropist, was held biennially in London and, as well as raising funds, helped to maintain the National Hospital's public profile.

These events frequently raised more than £2,500 in a single night, but were costly and time-consuming to organise and, after the first few years, reached a level of expenditure that proved almost impossible to sustain.

Burford Rawlings devoted much effort in securing a few substantial donations in order to stimulate wider fund-raising appeals for hospital expansion. Not only was the coaxing of donations time-consuming and frequently unrewarding, but donors often made their intentions unclear, making it necessary to seek legal assistance in realising funds left to the Charity. Thus, in August 1870, Burford Rawlings reported the receipt of a legacy of £173 19s 0d, 'being the amount ... bequeathed by Mr. Wood to the "Paralytic Society"', but only after Messrs Parker, Lee & Haddock, solicitors to the Charity, had successfully appealed to the Courts on the hospital's behalf to have the legacy paid to the National Hospital. Again, for example, in November 1871, a Mrs Frances Shaw left £50 in her will to 'the Asylum for Paralytic Persons', so vague a description that it might have referred either to the National Hospital or to the Portland Terrace (Regent's Park) Infirmary for Epilepsy and Paralysis. Although a 50/50 split between the two hospitals was first proposed in November 1871, agreement was not finally reached until July 1888, by which time the value of the legacy had increased to nearly £80 with accumulated interest.[25]

Faced with the uncertainty, unforeseen legal problems and disproportionate effort associated with soliciting subscriptions, legacies and donations from a reluctant public, Burford Rawlings and the hospital managers increasingly turned to alternative means of fund-raising. Chief among these were four schemes to boost capital funds: an arrangement whereby particular regions or towns could endow beds or cots in the National Hospital and Convalescent Home for the use of their own residents; reinvestment of the Charity's funds in higher-yielding investments; creation of a fund for donations carrying life annuities; and institution of a system of partial payment for medicinal treatment by outpatients. These expedients all proved difficult and costly to administer and, in the case of the institution of payment for medicines by

outpatients, ultimately contributed to the downfall of the old regime in the hospital.

The idea of a special fund for donations carrying life annuities (the 'D. A. Fund', as it became known) was first mooted in 1889, and officially launched at the Annual General Meeting of May 1890. In its original form, the idea was that, in exchange for gifts of at least £50, invested in gilt-edged securities, the Board of Management would undertake to pay donors or their adult nominees an annuity equivalent to an interest rate of between 4 and 5.5 per cent maximum, depending on the age of the annuitant and when the donation was made. As Burford Rawlings explained in his prospectus for the fund, 'By this means, Donors, while materially helping the Charity, may still derive an income from the money during their lives, or the lives of their Nominees.' The 'Annuities Fund' had separate trustees from the general hospital funds, and was maintained by the new Board of Management, constituted in January 1902. This contributed between £1,300 and £1,400 p.a. to hospital income in the first years of the twentieth century, complementing, in 1902, the annual subscription income of about £1,540 and a combined total of £1,232 from the Saturday and Sunday Funds. The Donations Carrying Life Annuities Fund thus made a significant contribution to the hospital at an exceptionally difficult time for the Charity and its new Board of Management, and continued to do so up until the outbreak of the First World War, but it failed to attain the levels hoped for by Burford Rawlings; and, as with other fund-raising schemes from this period, the results were modest in relation to the overall need for funds and the cost and effort expended in securing them.

Attempts to introduce much greater flexibility and 'market-responsiveness' in the management of investments met with very modest success. As early as 1880, Burford Rawlings had become convinced that, in an era of price deflation and slowdown in the growth of the British economy, more income could be squeezed out of the National Hospital's investment portfolio by reinvesting in higher-yielding stocks and shares and by more market-sensitive fund management. At a special general meeting held in June 1881, amid general agreement 'that in dealing with the funds of the Charity greater scope and liberty should be given to the Board of Management than had been the case hitherto', he persuaded the governors and subscribers to agree to a modification of Section 8 of the Charity's Rules

---

[25] See minutes of Board of Management for 7 November 1871, on p. 192, and minutes of Board of Management for 10 July 1888, on p. 108.

whereby 'the funds of the Charity may be invested in any Security sanctioned by the Court of Chancery'. This would enable the Board to invest hospital funds in higher-yielding colonial government stocks and railway bonds, in addition to the British government stocks and central London real estate, which had hitherto accounted for the bulk of the investment portfolio. However, this new investment strategy clearly caused alarm among the more cautious governors and Board members. At a meeting in January 1882, John Pearman argued successfully that the motions passed in June 1881 be rescinded and 'That the funds of the Charity may under the direction of the Board of Management, be invested in any Security usually allowed for the investment of Trust Funds', a much more restricted list consisting largely of landed property and mortgages, Treasury stock, English municipal government bonds, East India Company stock, British and Irish bank stocks and colonial government stocks guaranteed by the Imperial government. In May 1882, these motions were duly passed and incorporated into the rules of the Charity at the next general meeting. Pearman's motions were clearly designed permanently to reduce the overall level of risk associated with the hospital's investment portfolio, and to curb Burford Rawlings' growing tendency to make important decisions without the prior consent of the Board. But they almost certainly had the effect of restricting the potential income stream.

Last, but by no means least, the Board made a number of attempts to charge certain patients for part of the costs of inpatient treatment, or, in the case of outpatients, their medicines. The medical staff were strongly opposed to any attempt by the Board to recover the costs of treatment in this way. Thus, at a Board meeting in April 1871, Jabez Ramskill drew attention to 'the payment of 5/- for the renewal of an expired patient's card, in lieu of bringing a [subscriber's] letter of recommendation', a practice that he described as 'unworthy of the Charity, and injurious to its interests'. At the next meeting, he moved that these payments should be abolished. However, Ramskill's motion was opposed by Edward Chandler, the *de facto* hospital treasurer at this point, on the grounds 'that the sums so received were paid over to the [Ladies'] Samaritan Society, and do not go to the [general] maintenance of the Hospital'. Although there was support for Ramskill's position, on Chandler's motion the charges were merely suspended, but not

abolished. Ever since the mid-1860s, Johanna and Edward Chandler had both felt that the hospital was making insufficient provision for a group of the 'genteel poor', as Edward Chandler described them – middle and lower-middle class patients and their families who felt humiliated by the thought of having to enter the hospital as 'charity' patients but lacked the means to pay for more than a fraction of the costs of their treatment. In 1874, after much discussion at Board level, Edward Chandler secured agreement to create two 'In Memoriam' wards for 'contributing patients'. These were originally dedicated to the memory of Louisa Chandler and, following her death in January 1875, also to Johanna. These wards proved a source of almost constant friction and vexation not only between members of the Board and the administrators, but also with the medical and nursing staff.

By the turn of the century, the National Hospital's financial reserves were held in a number of separate funds, the relative size and importance of which varied considerably over time. The trusteeship and administration of these funds had become a complex and often difficult affair. They included:

The 'Hospital Endowment Fund', intended to provide a permanent source of income for general purposes, the origins of which went back to the early fund-raising efforts of Johanna and Edward Chandler, and the nominal value of which in stocks, shares and ground rents amounted to just over £32,400 by 1902.

The 'Country Branch Endowment Fund', created to support the Home for Convalescent Patients at East Finchley, amounting to £3,412 in 1902.

The 'In Memoriam Pension Fund for the Incurable', described in 1902 as 'really a separate charity', amounting to £32,000 in stocks, shares and ground rents, the income from which was paid out to around 90 'incurable sufferers from Paralysis, Epilepsy, or kindred nervous disease' in pensions worth between £10 and £22 10s p.a.

The 'Commemoration Fund' established to mark the Diamond Jubilee of Queen Victoria in April 1897 which, by 1902, had raised more than £8,100 towards the costs of enlarging the outpatients' department, providing more and better accommodation and amenities for the nursing staff, and to support an airing court for the male inpatients.

There were also separate funds for the chapel and the hospital chaplaincy, amounting to more than

£3,400 in 1902, and for the Ladies' Samaritan Society, which then held investments worth almost £6,000 administered quite independently of the general hospital funds. In 1881, when Edward Chandler had rather pointedly left a bequest of £1,000 to the Ladies' Samaritan Fund, rather than to the Rebuilding Fund, Burford Rawlings had taken legal advice as to whether this legacy might be diverted into the hospital's general purposes fund, but the advice was that the terms must be respected, and thereafter the Samaritan Fund remained inviolate.

The Ladies' Committee

The long-drawn-out conflict between the honorary medical staff and the lay Board members and secretary of the 1890s was not the only struggle for power within the hospital during this period. A serious dispute also arose among the lay Board members and administrators over the role and value of the Ladies' Committee. Representing the wealthiest and socially most influential female supporters of the Charity, together with the Finance and House Committees this had been recognised in the constitution of the hospital as one of three standing committees. During the years in which Johanna Chandler remained influential, the Ladies' Committee performed a vital function in raising money for the National Hospital by organising and promoting bazaars, fancy goods sales, and charity soirées and concerts, as well as regular collections and special appeals. Its offshoot, the Ladies' Samaritan Society, provided after-care and social aid for ex-patients and holders of hospital pensions. The Ladies' Committee was often decisive in the appointment of matrons and nursing sisters. In December 1864, the Board of Management delegated final say in the design of the nurses' uniform to the Ladies' Committee. Fund-raising and almonry work of the Ladies' Committee and the Ladies' Samaritan Society featured prominently in the annual reports. Their aristocratic membership and the active support of society hostesses such as the Marchioness of Thomond and the Countess of Abergavenny conferred great social prestige on the Charity and its work. In May 1886, Burford Rawlings calculated that, between November 1859 and the death of Johanna Chandler in January 1875, the Ladies' Committee had raised £20,450 for hospital funds. This was almost certainly a significant underestimate since it did not take into account the purchase price of

freeholds for the hospital premises at 23 and 24 Queen Square and Powis Place.

However, the position of the Ladies' Committee in the governance of the hospital, especially its powers in connection with the matron and the House Committee, had never been clearly defined. Already, in May 1862, there had been an abortive attempt to bring the Ladies' Committee and its funds firmly under the control of the Board of Management and the secretary; and, after the death of Johanna Chandler, the very existence of the Ladies' Committee became a flashpoint for arguments between factions on the Board of Management. Traditionalists such as Edward Chandler and Pearman were strongly attached to the Ladies' Committee and the values of voluntarism and paternalism that it represented. Modernisers such as George Porter, and reforming hospital managers including Burford Rawlings, saw the committee's independence as undermining the authority of the Board; and they believed that the influence of the committee deterred capable and experienced candidates from applying for senior nursing positions.

A bone of contention was meaningful representation of the Ladies' Committee on the House Committee. In March 1876, after considerable discussion, proposals and counter-proposals, the Board had resolved 'That ... [in] future the House Committee [shall] consist of seven members, four of whom shall be gentlemen and members of the Board of Management, and that the Ladies' Committee be invited to nominate three of their number to fill the remaining vacancies'. This represented a qualified victory for those who, like Edward Chandler, wished to strengthen the position and influence of middle- and upper-class gentlewomen in the domestic life of the hospital, and thereby preserve the lay-philanthropic tradition of the founders of the Charity. It was, however, a setback for those who saw the domestic concerns and sometimes fierce feminine rivalries of the Ladies' Committee as obstacles to the rationalisation and modernisation of the National Hospital. They resented its independence from Board of Management control and, against the evidence, doubted its ongoing capacity to raise funds. In May–June 1879, different members of the Board brought forward proposals to change the composition of the House Committee, either enlarging or curtailing the role of the Ladies' Committee in governance of the hospital. After prolonged and sometimes heated debate, the Board was split down the middle. In a partial victory for the supporters of greater control by the all-male Board of Management, a compromise resolution sponsored by Pearman and Chandler was passed, which provided that, in future, the Ladies' Committee be invited to nominate six of its members to serve on the House Committee, all of whom had to be approved in advance by the Board of Management, but, conversely, that all members of the Board should *ex officio* be entitled to sit on the House Committee.

This compromise lasted until shortly after the completion and opening of the new hospital, during which time the Ladies' Committee continued to raise funds, albeit on a more modest scale than in the days of Johanna Chandler. However, in July 1885, when asked by Colonel Porter why there had been so few suitable candidates for the recently advertised post of lady superintendent of nurses, Burford Rawlings 'stated that he ... had been told by two or three persons intimately acquainted with hospital work that the existence of a Ladies' Committee operated to prevent the application of the most eligible class of candidates'. In the following year, arguments resurfaced between those who wished to reconstitute the House Committee with all-male membership drawn from the Board, and others who promoted feminine influence in the domestic life and governance of the hospital. This ongoing dispute came to a head at a bad-tempered special meeting of the Board held on 4 May 1886 'to consider the origins, status and duties of the Ladies' Committee'. Burford Rawlings argued that there was no clear basis in either the early resolutions of the Board or the rules of the Charity for the position of the Ladies' Committee, and inferred that its work, which he claimed was by now almost entirely restricted to that of the Samaritan Society, was implicitly carried on at the Board's 'pleasure'. In contrast, Radcliffe argued that the Ladies' Committee was not under the authority of the Board of Management, but answerable only to the governors at a general meeting. Colonel Porter, since 1879 chairman of the Board, and Captain Leonard Shuter gave notice of a motion to be put to the governors and subscribers restricting activities of the Ladies' Committee to the work of the Samaritan Society. In answer, calling for a return to the *status quo ante* as of May 1879, Pearman (supported by several governors) gave notice of a counter-motion censuring the Board's proposal 'to exclude the members of the Ladies' Committee from a share in the management of the internal arrangements of the Institution' as 'subversive of the Constitution of the

Charity and injurious to its best interests'. Colonel Porter and his supporters wanted to replace the Ladies' Committee with hand-picked hospital visitors appointed by the Board, and Burford Rawlings had already approached several suitable ladies asking them to fill this role. However, Pearman and his supporters among the governors and subscribers were determined to prevent the demise of the Ladies' Committee, and took exception to Burford Rawlings' minutes of the acrimonious special Board meeting of 4 May 1886 and its associated resolutions, which the ordinary Board struck out a week later. Faced with the prospect of the Board presenting a dis-united front to the governors and subscribers at the rapidly approaching general meeting, tempers cooled somewhat during the next few days, and both Pearman and Porter agreed to withdraw notice of their motions. All that happened at the general meeting held on 20 May 1886 was an innocuous vote of thanks to the Ladies' Samaritan Society, proposed jointly by Colonel Porter, Captain Shuter and Pearman. Although it became more or less indistinguishable from the Ladies' Samaritan Society over the next few years, no further attempt was made either to reform or to abolish the Ladies' Committee during the remaining years of the old regime in the hospital. Perhaps the Marchioness of Abergavenny, president of the Society in the 1880s, hit the right note when she accused it of 'interminable twaddle'.

Nursing at the National Hospital

Before 1859 no institutional experience could be used on which to model the organisation and practice of nursing care in a specialist hospital for paralysis and epilepsy.[26] It is not surprising therefore that the hospital founders and early Board of Management had no preconceived plan for the organisation and delivery of nursing but, rather, had to improvise and learn from experience as they went along. At first, the size and limited resources of the National Hospital, together with the particular demands made by patients with paralysis and seizures, suggested a more informal,

---

26 With the notable exception of Thomas Aird's article on the origins of neuroscience nursing in the UK (Thomas Aird, *British Journal of Neuroscience Nursing* 1 (2005): 28–31), very little has been published since the centenary celebrations in 1960 on the nursing history of the National Hospital. The relevant archival sources remain largely unexplored and a full investigation of the nursing history of the hospital, although desirable, lies beyond the scope of this book.

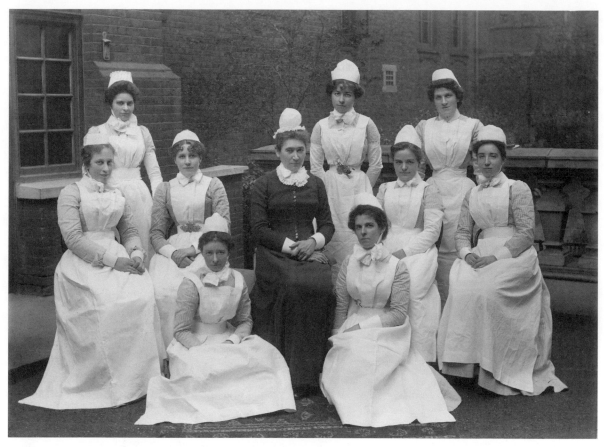

Figure 1.9 Lady superintendent and senior nurses and ward sisters in 1886.

and less hierarchical and orthodox approach to care than that favoured by contemporary nursing reformers in large general hospitals. The chronic nature of the patients' illnesses and the legacy of the original 'asylum' concept also favoured a more domestic style of care. As a result, no clear distinction was made by hospital administrators between nursing responsibilities and housekeeping aspects of hospital life when making appointments to senior nursing positions.

Nursing at the National Hospital quickly developed other distinctive features. As early as June 1860, the Board of Management asked the physicians to 'be good enough to provide a man to act as Night Nurse in the Male Ward' and, according to Burford Rawlings, by the late 1860s, 'the nursing of the male patients was largely in the hands of men'. From the 1880s, the National Hospital was the only civilian voluntary and specialist hospital to be accredited for the training of male nurses in the State Certificate in Nursing. Furthermore, by the late nineteenth and early twentieth centuries, the National Hospital was

also unique in that female ward sisters were routinely in charge of all-male nursing staff on the male wards. Taken together, the purpose of the hospital, its type of patients and the nursing and domestic organisation made for a highly distinctive nursing experience.

In March 1860, the new Board appointed a 'Superintendent Nurse', Miss Agnes Gower, at a salary of £20 p.a. The first ward nurse, Ann Marsh, was engaged the following month, at a salary of £14 p.a. plus 1s per week 'for Tea & Sugar and one pint of beer per diem', in time for the first female patients to be admitted. However, only a week later, at a meeting of the 'Furnishing' (later House) Committee, it was 'resolved, that another nurse be forthwith procured, as the present one is quite incapable for the post'; and although it was acknowledged subsequently that the committee had exceeded its authority, Nurse Marsh's dismissal was confirmed by the full Board in May 1860. The Board of Management had little more success with the appointment of a matron. In May–June 1862, and again in November–December of that year, personality

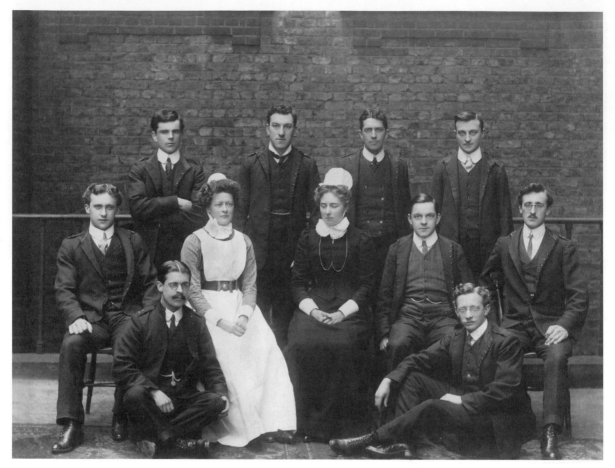

Figure 1.10 Lady superintendent, matron and male nurses, 1905.

clashes, allegations of financial irregularities and conflicts of authority between the then matron, Mrs Kitsell, and other senior members of the domestic and nursing staff brought the work of the hospital almost to a standstill; and the Board seemed unable either to reconcile the warring parties or to dispense with their services. Between early 1860 and the spring of 1864, the National Hospital saw four matrons come and go before, in March 1864, Edward Chandler and Richard Barton secured the appointment of a subcommittee to visit elsewhere 'for the purpose of taking further steps to get a Matron'. In the event, the subcommittee seems only to have visited King's College Hospital, then located in Norfolk Street near the Strand. However, the visit turned into a fairly wide-ranging inquiry into many aspects of contemporary nursing organisation in London hospitals.[27]

The subcommittee found the domestic and nursing organisation of King's College Hospital, as explained to them by the lady superintendent, Miss Jones, to be highly centralised, authoritarian and infused throughout with the evangelical-Protestant ethos then characteristic of that institution. The entire domestic and nursing organisation of the hospital was under the absolute control of the lady superintendent. She supervised five sisters, all unpaid 'Gentlewomen', each of whom was in charge of a ward and its qualified and trainee nursing staff. All nurses were paid on the same salary scale, varying from £10 10s to £20 p.a., according to length of service. They were expected to live a highly regulated, quasi-monastic life in the adjoining St John's

---

[27] The report is found in the minutes of the Board of Governors, March 1864. The subcommittee was formed by

three members of the Board (Mears, Sangster and Barton) and, although two physicians were also said to have been invited, it is not clear who these were and no physicians were signatories of the report.

House, receiving free board, lodging, washing and medical attendance, as well as uniform and attendance allowances. Each nurse was responsible for 15 beds, and was expected to work a 10½-hour shift, either by day or by night, with one meal allowed and a little tea, bread and butter, and beer for the night nurses. Only nurses trained at King's College Hospital were taken on as salaried staff, after a year's probation. Trainee nurses had to be spinsters or widows aged between 25 and 40 years, literate and members of the Church of England – no Dissenters or Roman Catholics being acceptable. All the nursing and domestic staff came under direct authority of the lady superintendent and might be summarily dismissed without notice. Finally, members of the subcommittee were informed that there was no Ladies' Committee at King's, 'one having been tried at first but it entirely failed'.

The subcommittee concluded that the 'Communal system' of nursing in operation at King's College Hospital was not at all suited to the requirements of the National Hospital. This was not so much on account of its narrow evangelical–Anglican religious ethos, which the representatives of the National Hospital largely shared, or even the salary levels that Superintendent Jones deemed necessary to secure and retain reliable and competent nursing and domestic staff, but most crucially, to what Thomas Parker and his colleagues described as 'the total want of control on the part of the Board [of Management] over the Matron, nurses and servants, and the domestic affairs of the Institution'. Although the autonomy and independent authority enjoyed by the lady superintendent at King's College Hospital were anathema to the National Hospital Board members, subsequent experience was to show that, even when the heads of the nursing and the domestic staff were both under the control of the House Committee and the Board of Management, there was still plenty of scope for conflicts of authority. As Burford Rawlings was later to remark, disputes between successive matrons and superintendents of nurses became a familiar feature of the domestic life at the National Hospital across the first 40 years of its existence.

In the short term, the Board decided to advertise for a matron who would be 'a well-educated and competent Protestant Lady of Evangelical principles, aged from 30 to 45'. They appointed Mrs Tysser, formerly of the Middlesex Hospital, at a salary of £40 p.a., rather than the £50 p.a. minimum recommended by Superintendent Jones. In August 1868, Mrs Tysser resigned, to be replaced by Miss Jane Keddell, nominated to the post by the Ladies' Committee in September 1868. But, when she also resigned in November 1869, the Board decided to abolish the post of matron, and appointed Mrs Ryan as 'Superintendent Nurse', at a reduced salary of £40 p.a. The new appointee was expected to maintain 'active superintendence of the Wards of the Hospital and … the nursing of the patients', and carry out domestic duties previously performed by the matron. Indeed, it is noticeable that, even as late as the 1890s, hospital administrators continued to use the terms 'Superintendent Nurse' and 'Matron' indiscriminately in referring to the position and its responsibilities, reflecting a sense of philanthropic sentimentality. Thus, according to Burford Rawlings, 'the office of matron is … all important to the inner life of a hospital. The holder exercises an influence which reaches to every corner … no possible authority could govern well without her capable co-operation … her office embodies in peculiar degree the philanthropy of the institution'.

The first version of the rules and bye-laws in 1860 have very little to say about either the nursing staff or the matron but, from 1867 onwards, the revisions became much more explicit about the duties and discipline of the former. The 1867 bye-laws contain 21 paragraphs referring specifically to the nurses and 24 to the matron, as opposed to only 13 dealing with physicians and assistant physicians, and 16 with the medical superintendent. Together with female servants, nurses were under the authority of the matron, who controlled the reception of inpatients and was expected 'as much as possible, to promote among the inmates habits of piety, kindness and self-respect', as well as to 'assist personally in … carrying out any portion of the medical treatment, galvanism, etc.'. Nurses must be able 'to read [and, from 1871 onwards, to write] handwriting well', and were not to be taken on, even as probationers, 'without a proper character for honesty, sobriety and kindness'. In general, the bye-laws were highly prescriptive on duties, responsibilities, hours of attendance and conduct, as indeed they were for all hospital staff below the level of physician and secretary. The nurses' hours of waking and 'retiring to rest' were regulated; they could not leave the hospital without permission; they were expected to attend morning and evening prayers daily; and they were not allowed to receive money or gifts from patients or their families, on pain of dismissal.

We learn something of the experience of being a nurse at the National Hospital from a letter by Mrs Lucy Holt from Jersey.[28] She was employed, aged 24 years, from September 1897 at a salary of £25 p.a. Lucy was woken by a bell at 6 a.m. and worked, with a break of two hours, until the evening, with one day off work each month. New recruits were interviewed on arrival by Dr Arthur (this is presumably Howard Henry) Tooth for details of recent illnesses and dates of vaccination. The 'unpleasantness' of the wards followed the nurses to the dining room where the plates were all embossed with 'National Hospital' in the centre and 'For the Paralysed and Epileptic' round the edge. The Irish sister on David Wire ward was a bully. She asked Lucy's opinion on a letter seeking volunteer nurses to manage the plague in India. Mrs Holt saw an opportunity to rid the hospital of a tyrant and encouraged her to apply, which the sister did: but 'she caught the plague and died. Poor girl. I felt that I was partly responsible for her death.' The two junior doctors, James Purves-Stewart and James Collier accompanied William Gowers, 'a gruff old grizzly bear', on his rounds. Collier jumped up when Gowers ordered the blind to be drawn – '"not you Collier, let the nurse do it" … none of us looked forward to his visits'. On night duty, the nurses looked after the young doctors: Collier ate tea with bread and butter; Purves-Stewart had Bovril and toast. But night sister kept a watchful eye on these intimacies, much to the younger nurses' amusement. Work in the children's ward was happier but Lucy felt 'heartbreak for those poor darling babes who should never have been born'.

In the February 1871 revision of the bye-laws, the matron's title was changed to that of 'Superintendent of Nurses and Housekeeper', assisted by a deputy superintendent or 'Sister', and reference made for the first time to 'Male Attendants or Nurses'. Significantly, the nurse superintendent and sister were now answerable to the House Committee and the secretary, and no longer to the Ladies' Committee.

Nursing organisation and supervision, especially at ward level, remained a recurrent problem, mainly through lack of proper training and failure to appoint sufficient nursing staff to keep pace with growth of the hospital. In July 1878, a lay member of the Board visiting the wards in the company of the secretary

'found the Male Epileptic Wards … without an attendant, whilst a patient was struggling in a fit, surrounded by other patients and strangers, it being visiting day'. However, when Burford Rawlings 'remonstrated with the Superintendent Nurse [Mrs Ryan]', she 'denied all knowledge of the Attendant's absence and added that it was impossible for her to see that all the Wards were not neglected'. Later that month, Rawlings persuaded the Board of Management to appoint a subcommittee consisting of Edward Chandler, Major Porter and J. Netten Radcliffe, later joined by James Sangster, Charles Radcliffe and Thomas Buzzard, to enquire into 'arrangements for supervising the nursing staff and for the control of the Nurses and Attendants, and other matters concerning the regulation of the Wards'. The subcommittee found 'that the Superintendent Nurse did not – so far as [the resident medical officer] was aware – take any part in nursing care either in the Male or Female Wards', and this was confirmed by Radcliffe and Buzzard, and by the deputy superintendent or 'Senior Sister', Alice Jones. The two physicians further stated 'that the Nursing in the Male Wards was unsatisfactory where acute cases of illness were concerned', whereas Burford Rawlings reminded the subcommittee that the Medical Committee had already recommended that patients in the new Powis Place 'pavilion' should be nursed by women alone.

In order to resolve the problem of overlap between nursing and domestic roles highlighted by Sister Jones, Burford Rawlings proposed combination of the posts of superintendent nurse and senior nurse, and that a housekeeper be appointed 'who should perform all duties in respect of the House, Kitchen, Stores, Furniture, Linen, Diets, [and] the charges of the servants … so that the attention of the Head of the Nursing Staff should be exclusively directed to the Nursing of Patients, the condition of the Wards & the control of the Nurses and Attendants'. However, this was resisted by Edward Chandler, who counterproposed the appointment of a temporary superintendent of nurses, pending wide-ranging review of the rules relating to the nursing staff and supervision, and a storekeeper (subsequently changed to housekeeper) 'who shall be subordinate to the Superintendent of Nurses, but with charge of the House, Household effects, Furniture, Linen, Diets, Stores and Kitchen, and [be] in control of servants other than Nurses', at a salary of £25 (later increased to £30) p.a. This alternative fell far short of what Burford Rawlings had

---

[28] McDonald archive: transcript dated 29 February 1960

proposed, and of 'alterations in the arrangements of the hospital' suggested by Sister Jones, but the proposal to appoint a storekeeper 'to relieve the Superintendent of Nursing of Housekeeping duties' was adopted by the Board of Management in April 1879. Burford Rawlings and the subcommittee were charged with re-drafting the rules for the post of superintendent of nurses and, after consultation with the Ladies' Committee, Mrs Wadham was appointed housekeeper later in the same month. Shortly afterwards, Mrs Ryan, who had previously been thought of as a possible temporary superintendent of nurses at Queen Square, was appointed superintendent of nurses and housekeeper at the Convalescent Home in Finchley, at a salary of £40 p.a. Sister Alice Jones, who had tendered her resignation in February 1879, was appointed superintendent of nurses at the National Hospital at a salary of £60 p. a. The Board also decided formally to recognise the long and faithful service of nurses Wells and Morris, who had worked in the hospital for 10 and 11 years, respectively, by conferring on each the title of senior nurse and increasing their salaries by £3 p.a.

Although this appeared to deal with some of the problems highlighted by the nursing subcommittee's investigations, Burford Rawlings was not entirely satisfied with the outcome. As he himself later admitted, by the time that the major rebuilding and enlargement of the hospital were undertaken in 1883–5, the arrangements for nurses' meals, recreation and accommodation were 'mere makeshifts' which compared unfavourably with the facilities provided by other London hospitals, and the organisation and supervision of the ward nursing also left much to be desired. When the new hospital opened in May 1885, Burford Rawlings took the opportunity to remodel the nursing arrangements, so that 'a head sister, fully trained, was placed in control of the nursing, with charge and staff nurses in each ward [while] probationer nurses were [also] appointed, some of them … men'. What he failed to mention was that one of the primary objectives of these new arrangements was to reduce the overall cost of nursing care to the National Hospital. In August 1887, Burford Rawlings presented 'a statement concerning the nursing establishment of the hospital – past, present and future' to the Board, 'showing a scheme for nursing at a cost in wages reduced from £5 to £3.15s. per head, and with probable reductions of the latter figures by the employment of paying probationers and the granting of

instruction in massage, etc.'. Although approved by the Board, it is not clear precisely how far Burford Rawlings' scheme was actually implemented, and it seems highly unlikely that any of the anticipated savings were realised.

With opening of the new hospital, the managers must have anticipated the dawn of a more expansive era in its medical and nursing work. But the hospital filled up almost immediately, and many of the improved facilities soon proved inadequate to meet outpatient activity and the intensive medical and surgical interventions for inpatients. The increased number and activity of physicians and surgeons made extra demands on the nursing staff and, for the first time, hospital managers had to delegate or relinquish much of their authority over nursing practice to the honorary and resident medical staff. During the 1890s, a number of interrelated factors combined to make nursing one of the most challenging aspects of hospital administration and a potential flashpoint in the escalating conflicts between lay administrators and medical staff. First, the last years of the century saw a considerable increase in the number of paralytic and acute patients confined wholly or almost entirely to bed, each requiring heavy lifting and intensive nursing. Thus, according to the Board of Management's own subcommittee of inquiry into allegations of mismanagement and neglect of patient care, brought by the medical staff in the spring of 1900, 'It is nothing unusual for a Ward of 16 beds to contain 12 Patients in an entirely helpless condition … requiring everything to be done for them in bed.' Second, the amount of treatment, especially massage and electrotherapy, ordered by the physicians increased, so that, as the subcommittee of inquiry observed, 'formerly, massage was usually prescribed for alternate days … in recent times daily massage is frequently ordered while in some cases massage twice daily is ordered'. Admittedly, the Board of Management's subcommittee of inquiry was not shy about finding excuses for any apparent shortcomings in care of patients; but the Fry Commission of Inquiry Report of May 1901, which had no such agenda, confirmed that 'in recent times the amount of massage and electrical treatment ordered both for in- and outpatients has increased; and … the staff of nurses now in the hospital, … is insufficient for the present demands [made] upon it'.

Furthermore, expansion of the nursing staff resulting from the increase in the number of patients, together with the intensity of care, made it necessary to institute more rigorous performance monitoring and training programmes for hospital nurses. Raising professional standards in turn implied acceptance, and even encouragement, of a higher level of independent professionalism among the nursing staff. Burford Rawlings was desperate to enlist the support of nurses in his struggle with the medical staff, and to promote loyalty to the National Hospital and its lay philanthropic and volunteer traditions. This made him sympathetic towards nurses and, during the 1880s and 1890s, he became involved in a number of initiatives to improve recruitment and training both of male and female nurses and to raise standards of care on the wards. However, he was strongly opposed to the attempts currently being made by the Royal British Nurses' Association 'to elevate nursing into a profession'. This he described as 'disastrous ... from a business point of view'. According to Burford Rawlings

> The nurse who is too completely surrendered to the professional idea ... no longer identifies herself with the hospital where she is employed, she no longer regards the hospital as her home, nor is she content to perform the good work which comes ... her way. Her attitude is that of the medical student, whom she is apt to imitate ... She is concerned chiefly with her own advancement; she looks upon the time spent in this or that hospital as employed educationally; and she regards the patients ... less as sufferers to be ministered to, than as 'cases' from which something is to be learned.

Such attitudes, he believed, inevitably resulted in unnecessarily high levels of staff turnover and declining standards of care. Alarmed by what he perceived as the growing tendency for nurse trainees to 'look for their rules of general conduct to the house-doctors rather than to the matron', Burford Rawlings sought to strengthen the authority of the matron, 'who more than any other ... embodies in her own person and actions the philanthropic principle to which all else in hospital life should be subsidiary', in order to serve as a counterweight to what he saw as the growing medicalisation of the institution. 'Sisters and nurses who endeavour to exalt their own position by becoming mere ... satellites of the doctor', he believed, 'only sacrifice a large part of their usefulness and not a little of their womanhood and humanity', thereby losing 'the all-powerful sentiment of sympathy, without which the most skilful nursing lacks something essential'. Burford Rawlings

certainly wanted to improve nurse training and standards and to attract a better class of nursing recruit, but he did so in the hope of strengthening the nurse's sense of vocation and loyalty to her (or his) hospital rather than to promote the profession and, still less, to support the progress of medical science. By the end of the 1890s, his partisan engagement in the unfolding political struggle with the medical staff, having what he regarded as the 'soul' of the hospital at stake, completely dominated his views on nurse training and professionalism. For this reason, it was impossible for him either to accept many of the changes taking place in nursing within the hospital or to play a constructive role in the ongoing development of nursing at the National Hospital during the first years of the new century.

With all these considerations in mind, it is difficult to reach any firm conclusions as to the overall condition of nursing at the National Hospital during the last years of the nineteenth and the early years of the twentieth century. The 1890s saw the introduction of formal systems of staff reporting, along with some basic accreditation and certification of the conduct and competence of both probationers and staff nurses, which at the very least suggests a growing awareness of the increasing complexity of nursing work, staff development and the need to foster higher professional standards. When, in August 1900, Sir Henry Burdett, a governor and authority on hospital planning, organisation and management, made a thorough inspection of the hospital in the company of his fellow-governor the Honourable Sydney Holland, he found 'good evidence of the loyalty and efficiency of the nursing staff', whereas 'the good order and cleanliness throughout the [whole] establishment were as remarkable as they were satisfactory'. The report of the subcommittee of inquiry appointed by the Board of Management in July 1900, to investigate the allegations of maladministration and neglect of patient care made by the hospital medical staff, acknowledged that nursing resources were under huge and growing strain. Evidence presented to the Fry Commission in the following year suggests that the nursing establishment was seriously under-strength and standards low. In April 1901, Wilfrid Harris, the outgoing senior house physician, made serious criticisms of the nursing care available in the hospital during the nine months since his appointment in July 1900. According to Harris

The number of Nurses both male and female ... is barely sufficient to discharge the ordinary working duties of the Wards and if as ... frequently occurs a Nurse is off duty ... or special Nurses are required for any particular purpose the work which they should in the ordinary way be discharging falls upon others who are already more than fully occupied.

By comparison with other hospitals where he had worked, Harris was 'impressed by the low class of Nursing at the Queen's Square [sic] National Hospital ... the class of Nurses provided', he alleged, 'is of distinctly a lower standard than in any other Hospital with which I am acquainted and it is ... difficult to educate them to a proper sense of their duties so as to enable them to ... take an intelligent interest in their work'.

The educational level of the nurses, he believed, was inferior, and they were often 'totally ignorant of the bare facts concerning ... patients which a Nurse is expected to know', especially the night nurses and those assigned to temporary ward duties in the absence of the regular ward sister. Consequently, wards were frequently left unattended at night for long periods. Treatments that had been ordered by the physicians were often deferred, performed very perfunctorily or not carried out at all, due to the chronic shortage of properly trained and competent staff, while at the same time patients, especially children, who ought to be up during the day were kept in bed, to the detriment of their health and well-being, again due to the lack of trained staff to look after and supervise them. Finally, the accommodation, dining and recreational facilities for both nurses and domestic staff were inadequate and depressing, and afforded little or no privacy, which, in his view, further deterred well-educated and well-brought-up young ladies from applying to work as nursing probationers in the hospital. Harris' evidence is difficult to assess objectively, as he had been in service in the hospital for only nine months, does not give any specific examples of his charges against the hospital management, and was about to leave the country to serve in the Boer War at the time his evidence was submitted. However, it is difficult to believe that he would have gone to the trouble of making a statutory declaration to the Fry Commission on the eve of his departure without genuine concerns. Whatever the case, Harris' criticisms certainly resonate with those expressed by other contemporary observers, lay and medical, and make it difficult to believe that

standards of nursing work and the quality of nursing experience at the National Hospital at the end of the nineteenth century did not leave much to be desired.

Harris' criticisms may have been somewhat ill judged and exaggerated, but the final report of the Fry Commission of Inquiry published in June 1901 bore out much of his evidence, and further confirmed the earlier findings of the Board of Management's own subcommittee of inquiry in the spring of 1900. Overall, the Fry Commission concluded that 'the nursing [of the hospital] is carried on with efficiency, so far as the staff is able ... the sisters are ... both competent and zealous, and the nurses fairly efficient'. But this general conclusion was highly qualified in two important respects. First, even though Burford Rawlings and the subcommittee had claimed that the nursing staff had been increased from 42 to 52 for the same number of beds between 1893 and 1900, the Fry Commission found that the complement was 'distinctly below the requirements of the Hospital'. This resulted in shortfalls in treatment, notably in respect of massage, and 'some few occasions occurred when the aid to paralytic patients by catheterisation was not properly given, and bed-ridden patients were washed less frequently than they should have been', findings that appeared very largely to bear out Dr Harris' strictures of April 1901. Second, the duties that the hard-pressed nurses were called upon to perform were, in the Commission's view, simply too onerous, especially when the male and female nurses, who had been on night duty until 8.45 a.m., were required, 'after half-an-hour's pause for their morning meal, to assist in the massage of the out-patients ... and are frequently occupied in this duty from 9.15 to 10.30 or even 12'. Worse still, 'on Tuesdays, and sometimes on Fridays, when operations are performed, three or four nurses who have been on night duty are required to attend in the theatre and to assist ... the operations, as there is no male dresser and only one male nurse provided to assist the surgeon'. These operating theatre duties sometimes continued until 1 p.m. The committee also found the nurses' dining room and sleeping accommodation to be barely adequate, although they did not believe that it was detrimental to their health or that the nutritional quality of their food was 'seriously defective', as had been alleged. The Fry Commission concluded that the hospital must choose 'between the reception of a large number of patients with inadequate accommodation, and the provision of adequate accommodation for a smaller number of sufferers', and that, if provision for the current number of patients was to be maintained, 'the nursing staff both male and female ought forthwith to be considerably increased'. Substantial increase in the number of nurses employed in the hospital, more effective and less demanding organisation of nursing work, and improved accommodation and recreational facilities thus became part of the substantial agenda for change that the Fry Commission bequeathed to the new incoming Board of Management and hospital administrators in January 1902.

Patients and Their Care

During the whole period up to the early 1900s, the National Hospital remained essentially a private charitable institution and, as such, care of patients was its main purpose. Patients were at once the *raison d'être* and, by evoking the compassion and generosity of supporters and patrons, a source of income. Viewed from a slightly different perspective, they were also a persistent problem for the hospital management and a source of tension between the medical and nursing staff and the lay hospital administrators.

Even though, as the medical superintendents, resident medical officers and house physicians often noted in their reports, the turnover of patients at the National Hospital was much less rapid than in an ordinary acute general hospital, as a group the patients were numerous and diverse – medically and in their geographical origins and socioeconomic profiles.[29] Based on the minutes of the Board of Management meeting for 14 March 1861, which recorded her reported cure, Margaret Warwick, of 7 Hayes Court, Soho, was, in April 1860, the first patient to be admitted to the National Hospital. It is said that she burst into tears on finding herself alone in a large ward.[30] However, as the minutes of the

Board meeting of 19 April 1860 show, Warwick was in fact one of five women who, on the recommendation of the physicians, 'were ordered to be admitted on Monday next as In Patients'. At the same time, the application to admit a young man from Hastings as an inpatient had to be deferred for a month because the ward for male patients was not yet ready. In the event, the first male patient, John Powell, was not admitted until Tuesday 3 July 1860. In January 1861, case numbers 397, Mary Gilfillan, and 451, Ann Kelly, were both refused admission as inpatients 'for want of room', although Mary Gilfillan was 'reported cured' two months later. Less fortunately, case 394, William Trench, who had been refused admission at the December 1860 Board meeting for the same reason, 'was reported by Mr. Chandler to have "gone mad"'. In fact, the minutes of the Board of Management meeting for 1861 contain several references to patients being refused admission 'for want of room'; and, in October 1861, the Board resolved 'that the attention of the Physicians be called to those patients who have been more than 6 months in the Hospital with a view of determining whether it might not be advisable to discharge them in order to make room for New Cases'. At the same time, the Board became concerned that Ramskill and Charles-Édouard Brown-Séquard were admitting patients on their own authority between Board meetings. It followed that the purpose of the newly formed House Committee was no longer primarily to supervise domestic arrangements of the hospital but, rather, to keep a check on the admission of new inpatients between Board meetings.

In the first year of activity, when all new admissions were supposed to be approved directly by the Board of Management, the minutes contain many references to individual patients, but these became relatively infrequent after 1862, and reference is then made usually in the context of complaints, or misconduct resulting in summary discharge, rather than the circumstances of admission or outcome of treatment. The physicians and hospital managers soon found that many inpatients failed to get well after a decent interval, and that the hospital was rapidly filling up with long-stay patients who showed no signs of recovery. In May 1872, Edward Chandler drew the Board's attention to 'the condition of several patients in the Hospital', more especially in the ward 'for Paralytic Male Patients', urging the physicians 'to select for admission none but cases which, in their judgment,

---

[29] Richard Hunter and Louis Hurwitz highlight the medical-historical interest and importance of clinical case notes, and studies have been published based on the case histories of patients diagnosed with particular neurological conditions such as migraine and shell-shock, or on the case notes of particular physicians: R. Hunter and L. Hurwitz, 'The Case Notes of the National Hospital for the Paralysed and Epileptic, Queen Square, London, before 1900', *Journal of Neurology, Neurosurgery, and Psychiatry* **24** (1961): 187–94.

[30] Manuscript notes by Sister Magnusson (undated), McDonald archive.

are amenable to medical treatment'. Only gradually did the hospital managers and physicians come to realise that this comparatively slow turnover of patients would become a more or less permanent feature of life at the National Hospital, and seek to adapt their expectations and ways of working accordingly. As well as those who outstayed their welcome, some patients, especially females on the 'In Memoriam' wards, appeared singularly ungrateful for their treatment and the standard of comfort provided. Others, in the opinion of the hospital administrators, should never have been admitted, because they were either deemed 'ineligible' under the rules, too well-off to be appropriate objects of the Charity's benevolence, or believed to have procured their admission by corrupt means. Thus, in November 1864, Edward Chandler 'called the attention of the Board to the admission of patients whom he considered ineligible on account of their good social position'; and, in February 1887, the Medical Committee alleged that, during the previous year, some patients had in effect bribed subscribers and governors to provide them with letters of recommendation for inpatient treatment. At the same time, it was by no means uncommon for contributing patients to default on their weekly payments.

Throughout the first four decades of the hospital's existence, one of the most problematic categories of patients with which it had to deal was that of children. Sometimes unaccompanied, they were treated both as out- and inpatients. Thus, in December 1860, George Parker, aged 3 years, was discharged 'as … too young for the Ward of a Public Hospital'; whereas, in May 1862, the minutes of the Board of Management refer to a 'boy from Carlisle' and a 'boy from Scarborough' admitted on the recommendation of Dr Brown-Séquard. The rules and bye-laws of the 1860s and 1870s do not mention child patients, but it is apparent from the minutes of the Board of Management that the special problems associated with admitting younger patients did not diminish with time. In the mid-1870s, there were a number of beds or 'cots' especially reserved for children dispersed among the wards of the hospital. But, by this time, there was a good deal of support among both the physicians and some lay Board members for the establishment of a children's ward; and, in June 1878, a subcommittee of the Board, consisting of Colonel Porter, C. Radcliffe, his brother J. N. Radcliffe and Edward Chandler, was appointed 'to consider and report how

accommodation could be provided for the reception of young children as In patients'. However, the issue of providing special accommodation for children, preferably at 25 Queen Square, became embroiled in the increasingly bitter hospital politics surrounding the 'In Memoriam' wards for contributing middle-class patients, established two years earlier. At a time when there was intense competition for the very limited space available in the hospital, Edward Chandler saw the proposed children's ward as a potentially dangerous competitor for his beloved 'In Memoriam' wards (dedicated as they were to the memory of his sisters) and steadfastly opposed the proposal. But, despite Chandler's opposition, in July 1878 the subcommittee recommended 'that it is desirable that accommodation be provided without delay for the reception of children between 4 and 8 years of age and that a special ward should be assigned for the purpose'. In deference to Chandler, initially they recommended only that two cots be placed in each of the female wards for the next six months, rather than immediately commandeering space on the upper floor of 25 Queen Square as originally envisaged. This was implemented in January 1879. Chandler threatened to take the 'In Memoriam' wards out of the hospital altogether, but his influence and health were fast declining and, in January 1880, on the motion of C. Radcliffe, the Board unanimously agreed (Edward Chandler being absent) 'that the Cots for Children be collected into one ward apart by themselves'. Thus began what was eventually to become, in the new hospital, the Duchess of Albany children's ward.

However, the inpatient accommodation and treatment of child patients remained a highly sensitive issue during the 1880s and 1890s. Perhaps in response to growing press coverage and philanthropic attention addressing child welfare in the late nineteenth century, Burford Rawlings seems to have become increasingly aware of the potential for adverse legal consequences if the hospital allowed the medical staff to retain children indefinitely without meaningful consent from a parent or guardian, especially those whose mental development was significantly impaired. In January–February 1890, at the same time that lack of representation of the honorary medical staff on the Board of Management was first becoming a serious issue, a heated dispute arose over a child named Olive Griffin. Although rule changes were made, further disputes also arose, especially in relation to the case of Grace Bridges, described by Burford Rawlings as 'a half idiotic child', admitted at the instance of Horsley and Hughlings Jackson late in 1893 as a 'surgical' case, and subsequently kept alone in a separate room for several months without any active treatment or continuous nursing supervision. The Medical Committee apparently did not see this as a problem, but Burford Rawlings argued that, if anything happened to the child, 'grave charges' might be made against the hospital; and, moreover, that keeping her indefinitely while awaiting a second operation might allow the perception 'that the child was only retained for scientific purposes ... with a very uncertain prospect of a beneficial result'. In the end the view of the Medical Committee prevailed over the Board of Management, a sign of the increasing power of the physicians.

These disputes over the admission of children with significant mental impairments continued until the showdown in 1901, but the children's ward itself did not long survive the final victory of the medical and surgical staff. In 1902, the Duchess of Albany children's ward contained 21 beds, with a further single child's cot in the surgical wards. But, in April 1903, the ward was finally closed, following two outbreaks of diphtheria and scarlet fever in 1900–1 which necessitated temporary ward closures and disinfections. At the suggestion of the senior house physician, Stanley Barnes, the cots were again redistributed among the female wards and the space formerly occupied by the children's ward converted into a new ward for adult female patients, thereby reverting to the arrangement that had existed prior to 1879. Several more decades were to pass before the hospital was to make any further special provision for child patients.

Some adult patients were also regarded as unsuitable on account of their supposedly bad character and morals. In March 1879, the Board received a formal request from the secretary of the Royal Albert Hospital, Devonport, to admit a young woman named Kate Dingle, who was stated to have been 'at one time of immoral character but since September [1878] the inmate of a Home and recently attacked with Epilepsy'. At first, the Board resolved 'that subject to the Rules as to eligibility and medical fitness, the patient be admitted', affirming 'that antecedent circumstances should not be allowed to militate against a person needing medical

relief as long as his or her conduct in the hospital was satisfactory'. However, this resolution was vehemently opposed by Edward Chandler, who threatened to publicise details of Miss Dingle's past if she were admitted; and, only four weeks later, the Board was forced to reverse its decision in the face of determined opposition from Radcliffe and Ramskill who 'advised the Board that ... from a medical point of view, the patient was unfitted for admission'. The minutes of the Board meetings indicate that the case provoked 'considerable discussion', and the form of words used makes it plain that most of the lay members of the Board, led by the chairman and deputy, and supported by the secretary, were unhappy with the attitude of Radcliffe and Ramskill but seemed unable to go against the physicians in matters of this kind. Other patients were deemed unsuitable on account of their violent behaviour, a problem often encountered with male epileptic patients. In May 1894, the Board reluctantly agreed to a request from Hughlings Jackson to admit an epileptic patient named Boddy 'who had been in a lunatic asylum'. The day after admission, 'he became extremely violent and attempted to stab the attendant with a dinner knife', whereupon he was immediately discharged by Burford Rawlings with the approval of the Board, who 'considered the case well illustrates the value of the rule [not to admit recent psychiatric patients] which had been relaxed in this instance'.

Suicide is a reminder of the violent despair into which patients with nervous diseases could easily fall and, although uncommon, this was by no means unknown.[31] There were also occasional instances of death in the hospital that suggested the possibility of poor care or medical neglect.[32] Although the Board investigated serious incidents and complaints, their enquiries usually failed to shed light on the circumstances.

---

[31] For instance, in November 1870, Burford Rawlings informed the Board that 'a patient named Skelton ... left the Hospital a few days since without notice, taking with him a pistol, which he had discharged in the street ... [and] was now in the hands of the police on a charge of attempted suicide', although 'There had been no signs of mental aberration during his residence in the Hospital.' Suicides amongst inpatients were reported also on April 1889 and in June 1908.

[32] An example in June 1880 was of a patient named Hart, who died under Dr Radcliffe's care. Questions were raised about possible medical neglect, and whether or not an attendant had been present in the ward at the time of death.

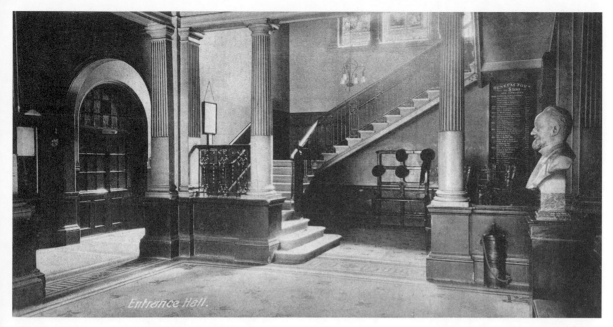

Figure 1.11 Entrance hall of the National Hospital (undated, around 1900).

The investigation of complaints was a persistent problem throughout the first 50 years of the hospital's existence, one that successive Boards of Management and secretaries found difficult to handle satisfactorily. In July 1900, the House Committee heard a report from Burford Rawlings of a complaint made by an (unnamed) patient in David Wire ward 'who had been discharged for rudeness to the acting Sister'. However, Burford Rawlings stated that 'the patient was wholly to blame', and no further discussion took place. Less than a month later, the House Committee heard another complaint made by a male patient named Greer, 'concerning the quantity of the chicken diet supplied him, and also the quality of the mutton'. Burford Rawlings and the House Committee clearly thought that the patient might have had a fair point as regards the chicken, but dismissed the further complaint, observing that none of the other patients who had eaten mutton from the same joint had complained, and that 'The Sister and Nurses gave Mr. Greer the character of a constant grumbler.' In his April 1901 article 'Doctors in Hospitals',[33] Burford Rawlings argued that it was necessary to maintain the supremacy of lay authority for the sake of the patients, because medical men could not be trusted impartially to investigate or decide on complaints made by patients against other doctors or surgeons

> If [a] patient has, or supposes he has, a cause of complaint against his medical attendant, it would be useless for him to make it known to the resident house-physician or to a clinical assistant [while] in the reverse case it would be almost equally useless for the patient to complain to the visiting [physician or surgeon] … concerning the house-physician. Complaints by patients are certain of consideration only when communicated to the lay authorities … whose authority and independence of medical constraints should be well understood and constantly made manifest.

However, the scant evidence of investigation of complaints during the last two decades of the nineteenth century offers little support for this claim. Unless made by someone of high social standing or influence in the hospital, or without an ulterior motive – as in the case of Burford Rawlings' investigation of the complaints made against Horsley in 1895 and 1899–1900 for neglecting patients' urgent treatment – the hospital managers seem not to have taken complaints seriously. The need to safeguard the good name of the National Hospital seemed uppermost in their minds.

[33] Benjamin Burford Rawlings, 'Doctors in Hospitals', *London Nineteenth Century and After – A Monthly Review* **49** (1901): 290.

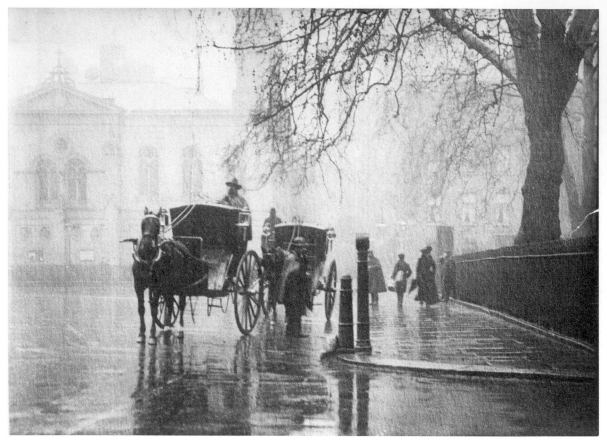

Figure 1.12 The south-west end of Queen Square c. 1900.

Tensions between Administrators and Medical Staff

By the late nineteenth century, the institution had become progressively more 'medicalised'. Although it was increasing felt, by the lay members of the Board particularly, that the welfare of patients had yielded too far to the medical and scientific interest in rare and unusual cases, and that the doctors saw the hospital less as a charitable institution for the relief of patients than, rather, as a court of appeal in clinical neurology, all were agreed that the scientific perspective was important, and in the 1895 annual report of the Board of Management, for instance, it was stated with some pride that:

> A large and increasing proportion of Patients [are] sent here on the recommendation of medical practitioners and from other hospitals for an authoritative diagnosis of obscure and difficult

cases ... distinguished members of the profession ... have from time to time borne testimony to the value of the Hospital as an Institution where the Patient will obtain 'an opinion beyond which there is no appeal ... he will be candidly told whether his ailment be curable or incurable, and, if curable, he will have the best means which science at the present day can afford towards his restoration to health'.

At one level, the medical achievements were a badge of pride for the Board, and, in August 1884, the four serving physicians for inpatients (Ramskill, Radcliffe, Buzzard and Hughlings Jackson), together with three former physicians (Brown-Séquard, John Russell Reynolds and Edward Sieveking), were all made honorary life governors. In June 1890, this privilege was further extended to the senior physicians for outpatients (Charlton Bastian, William Gowers and Ferrier) and to one outgoing surgeon (William Adams). When Adams resigned as surgeon to the National Hospital in December 1890, it was even

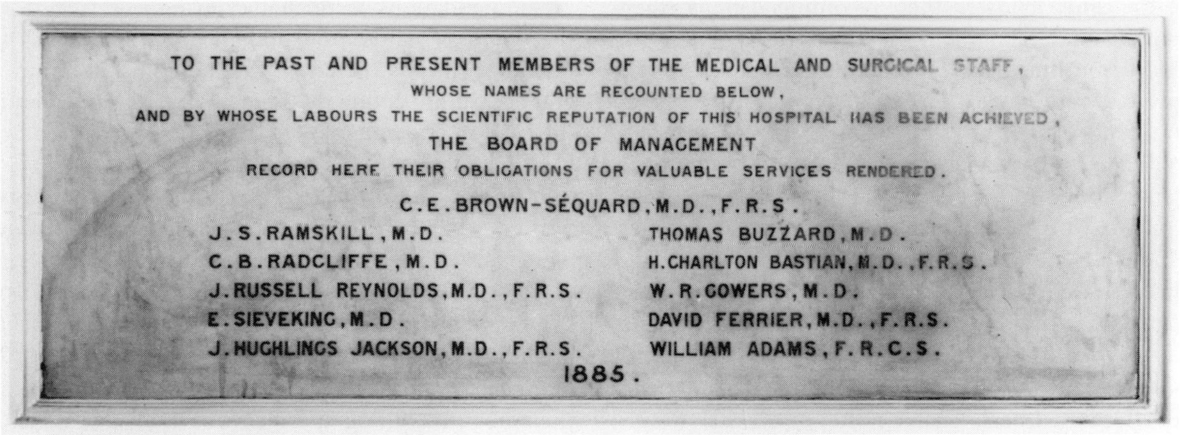

TO THE PAST AND PRESENT MEMBERS OF THE MEDICAL AND SURGICAL STAFF,
WHOSE NAMES ARE RECOUNTED BELOW,
AND BY WHOSE LABOURS THE SCIENTIFIC REPUTATION OF THIS HOSPITAL HAS BEEN ACHIEVED,
THE BOARD OF MANAGEMENT
RECORD HERE THEIR OBLIGATIONS FOR VALUABLE SERVICES RENDERED.

C.E.BROWN-SÉQUARD,M.D.,F.R.S.

J.S.RAMSKILL,M.D.   THOMAS BUZZARD,M.D.
C.B.RADCLIFFE,M.D.   H.CHARLTON BASTIAN,M.D.,F.R.S.
J.RUSSELL REYNOLDS,M.D.,F.R.S.   W.R.GOWERS,M.D.
E.SIEVEKING,M.D.   DAVID FERRIER,M.D.,F.R.S.
J.HUGHLINGS JACKSON,M.D.,F.R.S.   WILLIAM ADAMS,F.R.C.S.

1885.

Figure 1.13 Plaque listing the 11 members of the medical and surgical staff in 1885, in the entrance hall of the hospital.

proposed to elect him to the Board of Management, but the solicitors advised that this would violate the rules of the Charity.

However, the fundamental tension that existed between the medicalisation of the Charity and the founders' philanthropic tradition of care and welfare was a rent which could not be papered over. It resulted in tensions and clashes between the Board and the medical staff in relation to their terms of contract and, particularly, to the control of the admission and discharge of patients. In the latter two areas, dissent was stirred up by Burford Rawlings who, strongly supported by the traditionalist members of the Board, began to take an increasingly hostile stance towards the medical staff, and in response the doctors began to become more organised in opposition.

In relation to medical appointments, though, the doctors and the administration were at one. The Board of Management was aware of the importance of appointing physicians and surgeons highly regarded for their knowledge and expertise in the field of nervous disorders. In a speech to the festival dinner of May 1866, Edward Chandler said that, in appointing Russell Reynolds to the honorary medical staff in the previous year, the Board 'had sought the best men they could find'. In a speech to another festival dinner held in 1873, he claimed further that 'from the very commencement of the institution the object had been to associate with it all who were distinguished in the treatment of paralysis and epilepsy', in which respect 'he did not think they had been disappointed'.

Appointments were made on the basis of personal knowledge and recommendation, and drawn largely from the circle of medical men known personally to members of the Board. At first, the process was very informal. Ramskill, the first physician appointed to the National Hospital, who lived and practised in Bishopsgate in the heart of the city, almost certainly owed his preferment to the fact that he had been the personal medical attendant of both Johanna Chandler and David Wire. Ramskill in turn knew Brown-Séquard and Russell Reynolds, to whose five-volume *System of Medicine* (1866–79) Ramskill contributed a number of chapters. He supported Hughlings Jackson when his fellow Yorkshireman arrived in London in 1861, helping him to secure positions at the London Hospital and then Queen Square. Ramskill also knew C. Radcliffe, another northerner with strong Yorkshire connections. Shortly after Radcliffe's appointment as physician in succession to Brown-Séquard in 1863, his brother J. N. Radcliffe, a surgeon and public health reformer, was appointed first medical superintendent to the hospital. When Netten Radcliffe resigned from this post in April 1869, he was promptly elected to the Board of Management, where he joined Ramskill and his brother Charles. Collectively, these three served as physicians and superintendent to the National Hospital for more than 65 years, and as Board members for more than 75 years, between 1860 and 1897.

In the early 1870s, the process for making appointments became more formalised as the hospital grew in size and complexity, with advertisements being placed in the medical press, and formal applications and testimonials sought from candidates. However, lay members of the Board still took advice from the physicians and, unusually for London voluntary hospitals at the time, followed their recommendations when making medical appointments. Even by 1901, the Board continued to seek and almost invariably followed the advice of the Medical Committee in selecting staff. One interesting controversy arose when William Allen Sturge (1850–1919) – a graduate of Bristol Medical School and University College London, who had studied in Paris for two years after graduating and was the nephew of the Quaker philanthropist George Sturge, one of the hospital's most loyal and generous lay benefactors – applied for one of two vacant positions as assistant physician to outpatients. He came with strong recommendations from his French teachers, Charcot and Fournier. However, Sturge was also known to be a strong supporter of women's entry into the medical profession, and was married to Emily Bovell, one of the first women to be admitted to the Edinburgh Medical School and subsequently to qualify as a doctor in Britain. Although his application was accompanied by a letter 'in which he disavowed any intention to take action in the question of admitting lady doctors to the hospital', the Board was 'irremediably divided in regard to the desirability of electing Dr. Sturge', as was the Medical Committee, and, in the end, after much manoeuvring, the far less well-qualified candidate, Dr Peter Horrocks, was appointed.

The contractual terms of the medical staff appointments, and in particular the policing of attendance at the hospital, became a source of serious grievance. It should not be forgotten that the medical staff were honoraries (i.e. unpaid), and perhaps this lay at the back of what appeared to the administration an insouciant attitude to their duties. But the heavy-handed approach to this issue taken by Burford Rawlings created tension. The first serious attempt to ensure adequate medical attendance both for in- and outpatients was made in December 1870, when the Board approved a subcommittee memorandum that the senior physicians should attend at least once a week and confine their attention to the inpatients under their care; that the two senior assistant physicians should also attend weekly and be entirely responsible for the outpatients on their days of attendance; and that the two junior assistant physicians should be present twice weekly. No more than lip service may have been paid to this demand, and there were further complaints, leading, in 1875, to the formation of another subcommittee 'to enquire into the attendance of the Medical Staff'. Detailed

recommendations were made, laying out rules for the doctors. Matters did not improve, and Burford Rawlings was instructed to write to Ramskill on several occasions, stating that the 'Board are grieved and disappointed to find that the rules are not observed by him', and demanding an undertaking that these lapses 'shall not recur in future'. Similar letters were also written to Charlton Bastian and Charles Elam, which, in the latter's case, provoked an indignant reply and his subsequent resignation. In the 1870s, the Board then adopted the practice of getting new medical appointees to give a formal undertaking to obey all the hospital rules and bye-laws relating to their post, including specified hours of attendance, but problems relating to medical discipline recurred frequently. In January 1880, the Board appointed yet another subcommittee to 'take into consideration the whole subject of the Medical administration of the Hospital and advise the Board generally as to … [how] an adequate attendance upon In- and Out-Patients may be secured'. From the chair, Major Porter 'reminded the Board that a large portion of the Out Patients were seen and prescribed for by the Resident Medical Officer in contravention of the Bye-Laws', and, he feared, 'to the injury of the Institution, by reason of the dissatisfaction aroused amongst patients and subscribers'. According to Burford Rawlings, 'the feeling that the Board must insist upon an observance of the Rules was general'. However, these strictures were largely ignored by the medical staff, and their main effect was to sour relations between Burford Rawlings and the doctors. As relationships between the medical staff, secretary-director and lay Board members deteriorated during the 1890s, the issue of non-attendance by physicians and surgeons took on a personal and political aspect. Indeed, it is not difficult to conclude that Burford Rawlings increasingly saw the problem as a challenge to his own authority.

The matter which perhaps most soured relations between the doctors and the Board (in the person of Burford Rawlings) was the question of who had responsibility for the admission and discharge of patients. Burford Rawlings clashed particularly with Victor Horsley, and their arguments became increasingly personal and acrimonious. As introduced above, in February–March 1890, the two became embroiled in a long correspondence over Olive Green, aged 5 years, admitted with epilepsy at Horsley's insistence. He had already failed to have the child admitted in

November 1889, and had protested about Burford Rawlings' reluctance to comply at a meeting of the Medical Committee. When Olive was finally admitted on 3 February 1890, Burford Rawlings promptly had her discharged because she appeared to him to be 'an idiot' and thus ineligible for inpatient treatment under the rules. Horsley – who considered this to be an infringement of the bye-laws, inconsiderate treatment of a patient (and her mother) and a calculated snub to himself – then operated on her successfully 'in a private home'.[34] He absented himself from the National Hospital without leave for nearly six weeks, supposedly suffering from 'recurrent influenza', and did not resume his surgical duties until the end of March. From this time onwards, it is clear that the secretary was on the lookout for another opportunity to discipline and humiliate Horsley. A number of minor incidents saw them squaring-off against each other over such matters as delayed or cancelled operations. In early 1900, a complaint was made by Miss Dunn, who alleged that it had taken Horsley three weeks to see and treat her after admission in December 1899. Horsley's explanation was 'that there was nothing wrong [with Miss Dunn] either medically or surgically … and that there might be some gynaecological trouble present'. He referred to her as 'quasi-hysterical'. The Board took a more serious view and instructed Burford Rawlings to inform Horsley that 'the House Committee does not entertain the complaint against him without inquiry'. Burford Rawlings did his best to make Horsley feel as uncomfortable as possible, but by the time this incident occurred he no longer commanded the full respect of the medical staff and his influence was waning.

From the early 1880s onwards, the medical staff were, at least in theory, organised and represented as a distinct body within the hospital through the Medical Committee. Ironically, in the light of subsequent events, this had been established by the Board itself, in order to 'confer with the Board upon all matters … refer[ring] to the medical arrangements of the hospital'. When first constituted, in January 1880, the Medical Committee had as members all the serving medical and surgical staff, and two representatives of the Board of Management. By May 1880, with tension rising between the Board and the new committee, Burford Rawlings and the two Board of Management representatives asked to be allowed to

withdraw from their dual roles. After a series of apparently petty disputes with Burford Rawlings in the early 1890s over the right to use the Board room for meetings, the Medical Committee began to meet in the houses of its senior members, and increasingly to follow its own agenda in dealing with the hospital management. By 1900, it had more or less abandoned any pretence of seeking consensus or compromise solutions to the hospital's growing internal problems, and instead had become the principal focus for orchestrating medical opposition to the authority of the Board of Management and the secretary.

The Schism and the Fry Report

The history of the National Hospital in the nineteenth century ends with an episode that nearly closed it down. During its first two decades, relationships amongst the administrative and medical staff were reasonable and, as a result, the hospital ran well but, as we have seen above, in the 1880s matters began progressively to deteriorate. Discord was catalysed by the personality and behaviour of Burford Rawlings, but at its core the problems represented a power struggle between two different ideologies. The eventual resolution of this storm amounted to a virtual re-foundation of the hospital. These events reflected a wider change in social attitude that had been wrought in British society between 1860 and 1900. It was a crisis that was slow to catch fire, but that, when finally ignited, proved powerful and highly inflammable.

This was a period in which science was beginning its long ascendency in a society previously dominated by religious thought. The Board of Management retained the philanthropic and Christian ethic of the National Hospital and, as such, was becoming increasingly outmoded. The public rows over evolution were a sign of the swing in societal opinion towards science and technology and, by 1900, the essence of mid-Victorian philanthropy, patrician and rooted in religiosity, was in retreat. The figure of Burford Rawlings was an incarnation of this increasingly old-fashioned point of view; and his domineering style, which was bound to rub against the rising power of the physicians – also arrogant and seeking to place neurology on a new and scientific footing – did not help. Burford Rawlings had a complex and contradictory attitude to medicine and to doctors – alternatively very supportive and, at other times, entirely hostile. He defended his opposition by pointing out that scientific work was identified with vivisection,

---

[34] Horsley, like other surgeons of the time, often operated in the patient's home.

and this offended charitable giving. Whilst no doubt partly justified, this stance seemed a manifestation of his desire to keep science in its place, and of personal enmity towards doctors in general and Horsley in particular. The row was symptomatic also of the rising power, influence and prosperity of the middle classes, including doctors, and the challenge this represented to existing authority.

In his new position as secretary-director, and with the backing of the Board, Burford Rawlings began to take increasingly uncompromising positions that, to the medical staff, exceeded his authority. With growing tension over the admissions policy and attendance, a flash-point was the Board's decision to introduce charges for outpatients, flagrantly ignoring the strongly expressed disapproval of this policy by the Medical Committee. In the mid-1890s, the doctors began to unite, as never before, in their opposition to Burford Rawlings' behaviour and, having previously lacked much interest, now demanded more influence in the daily management of the hospital. The Medical Committee requested that the doctors should be represented on the Board of Management. The idea was brought up informally in different settings, and voiced, for instance, by Sir James Crichton Browne in his toast at a 'festive dinner'. Finally, the request was made officially to the Board in 1899; and, on 24 October of that year, it convened a special meeting which unanimously rejected this request, writing a five-page minute clearly reflecting recognition that this was potentially a crucial decision – as indeed it turned out to be.

Burford Rawlings' account shows the gulf that seems to have developed. The Board

> had to learn by painful experience that the medical mind when in disputation with the laity has no arrestments and no misgivings. Therefore it reserves no place for conciliation, and turns with aversion and impatience from thought of compromise. In things purely professional, the medical bent is right. Between the practiser of an occult art and the world of ignorance beyond, no mental commerce is possible. But the disposition of not a few professors of medicine, especially as represented in hospitals, is to maintain this unyielding attitude when rights and interests other than their own are present, and the conditions call for reciprocity. Hence a chief difficulty in hospital administration, where lay labours and lay responsibilities are inherent and irremovable.[35]

Rawlings was right about one thing – that the medical staff would not let this decision go unchallenged. The rejection of their seemingly innocuous request was followed by a blistering attack on the Board by Buzzard, and a 16-page printed document sent in May 1900 by the Medical Committee (17 doctors in all) directly to the Board of Governors and members of the Charity, which, in its preamble, stated that the medical staff had experienced 'difficulties from the Board of Management in the real appreciation, or permanent redress, of the evils prejudicing the institution'; and that they were therefore 'compelled to cease communication with the Board' and to communicate directly with the governors. The signatures were Jackson, Buzzard, Bastian, Gowers, Ferrier, Ormerod, Beevor, Tooth, Taylor, Risien Russell, Turner, Batten, Semon, Horsley, Ballance, Gunn and Cumberbatch. The document then laid out a series of concerns about the diet offered to patients, their care and treatment, the nursing standards and the maladministration of the hospital. In regard to the latter, the document pointed to the lack of lines of communication with the Board of Management, and the additional friction caused by appointing an intermediate office of secretary-director (or general director, as he was also sometimes known), arguing that 'no such office exists in any other London hospital and its existence proves prejudicial to the National Hospital'. In an appendix, the document also complained about the system of payments by outpatients, set up in defiance of medical opinion.[36]

On behalf of the Board of Management, Burford Rawlings then wrote to the Board of Governors reporting that subcommittees had been set up to look into the complaints, and also that the 'extraordinary character of the announcement is enhanced by the fact that the Board had already considered and complied with many of the recommendations of the staff, but that they cannot consent to the actions of the staff in anyway abrogating their function'. The chairman of the Board of Management (Colonel Porter) also wrote, in support of its refusal to have medical staff on the committee, stating that they would 'be resisting encroachments calculated to destroy the religious and philanthropic nature of the hospital and to subordinate to purely professional objects institutions

---

[35] Burford Rawlings, *A Hospital in the Making* (1913).

[36] The *British Medical Journal* then published a letter from 18 of the hospital medical staff, which enclosed the report: *British Medical Journal* **2** (1900): 333.

maintained by the benevolent for benevolent purposes'.

The row reached the pages of the medical and national press, especially in the months between July and October 1900, and acrimonious letters on the topics in *The Times* and the medical journals continued into the next year.[37] Burford Rawlings was repeatedly called to defend the Board of Management from a range of attacks by the senior medical staff and others. He was unyielding in his criticism, saying, for instance, that the 'medical staff were engaged in one great effort to injure the hospital financially'.[38] One of the most brilliant polemics was the powerful three-column letter by Brudenell Carter, who had recently retired from the staff, containing a very strongly worded personal attack on Burford Rawlings and the Board. It ended

> The case lies in a nutshell. The proper reform of the constitution of the hospital would leave it in the very van of curative work in the growing science of neurology; whilst a victory of the Board would reduce it to a receptacle of incurable paralytics and hysterical imposters living in an establishment controlled by a Secretary-Director and nominally under the medical care of weak and incompetent medical practitioners.[39]

At this stage, further problems arose. The Sunday Fund and Prince of Wales' Fund each wrote to the hospital suspending their annual grants because of the disputes. The Board then announced that it would set up an 'Independent Inquiry' into the complaints about the running of the National Hospital, with Sir Ford North, an ex-Lord Justice, in the chair. However, according to Burford Rawlings' account, 'the complainants again refused to take part in the proceedings, upon the plea that Sir Ford North's services had been given at the invitation of the Lord Chancellor who was a member of the Board'. The medical staff were certainly not

prepared to accept this form of inquiry and when, in October 1900, Sir Ford North attended the hospital to open the inquiry, with Mr Alfred Lyttelton, Mr Boydell Houghton and Mr George Bower and the secretary-director attending from the Board, no representative of the medical staff appeared. The proceedings had to be adjourned *sine die*.

There was further publicity, and the Board of Governors and members of the Charity then met. A new proposal was made and accepted – that a committee of inquiry be set up, truly independent and under the chairmanship of Sir Edward Fry FRS. Burford Rawlings describes the meeting in colourful and bitter terms:

> The proposal before the meeting was to appoint a committee of seven, whose sole function should be to provide a tribunal for the investigation of the charges, and afterwards to receive and pass on to the governors in general meeting the report of the investigating body. This proposal, though it encountered no opposition, was productive of much speaking, and as time went on, one and another speaker raised controversial issues until feeling rose high. On the doctors' side the stupendous assertion was made that 'the Board had been trying to get rid of this magnificent staff.' Upon the other hand, Mr. George Russell, either misunderstanding the nature of the agreement arrived at, or refusing to be fettered, delivered a powerful and not unprovoked attack. It was magnificent and it was war, but the meeting was to have been one of peace, and in the end the full power of the exiguous majority of governors present, was exercised. The Lord Chancellor [Lord Hailsbury, chairman of the Board of Governors] had appreciated the position, but the course of procedure agreed upon not having been followed, he refused to intervene. A Committee was appointed then and there; not representative of both parties, but composed of persons mostly strangers to the hospital, every one of whom was an avowed opponent of the Board, who accepted in silence the decision of a meeting comprising less than five per cent, of the whole body of governors, and acquiesced without a protest in the committal of their case to the adjudication of their opponents. In deference to the wishes of the Lord Chancellor and the Board generally, backed by the solicitor, I had remained silent during the meeting. What the Chancellor thought of the upshot he kept to himself; what the staff thought of it was made plain by their jubilation. My view found expression in a letter I addressed to the solicitor directly after the meeting separated, in which I placed upon record the fact that of the seven governors chosen only one had

---

[37] See, for instance, the 21 letters and papers in the Lancet: 156 (1900): 34, 412–3, 463, 351–2, 551–8, 630–1, 751, 769, 1222, 1380–1; 157 (1901): 798–800, 950–1, 981–7, 1837–8, 1855; 158 (1902): 91–92, 110–14, 1755–57; 159 (1902): 181, 184–185, 1614. Also, the other letters and editorials which appeared in other newspapers and journals, including the *Guardian*, *Westminster Gazette*, *Westminster Budget*, *Hospital*, *Echo*, *Christian World*, *Queen*, *St James Gazette*, *British Medical Journal* and *Nursing Record*.

[38] See *The Times*, 9 August 1900.

[39] See *The Times*, 20 August 1900.

contributed substantially to the hospital funds, and that long ago; while four had contributed nothing at all, being 'honorary governors.' Not one of the seven had given, during the forty years before the disagreement, a sign of interest in the hospital's work or progress.

Burford Rawlings continued, accusing the committee of being as 'autocratic as any Court of Assize' and to have been profoundly ignorant of the running of a hospital, and with some members inherently biased.

Sir Edward Fry was a distinguished retired Court of Appeal judge, and member of the Council of University College London. He had a track record in chairing a Royal Commission on the Irish Land Acts; as arbitrator in the Welsh coal strikes of 1898 and, later, other industrial disputes; and also as arbitrator at The Hague in international disputes between the USA and Mexico, and between France and Germany.[40] Thus, he was no stranger to major spats and a good choice for this affair, which he probably considered a minor local difficulty.

The Fry Commission met on 12 occasions from 1 May 1901, and heard evidence from 43 witnesses, ranging from Lord Lister to the hospital cook.[41] The function of the committee was to inquire into 'the allegations made by the medical staff in their statement of May 1900; the facility of inter-communication between the medical staff and the Board,

including the demand of the former for direct representation on the Board; the position, function, and acts of the secretary-director; and the constitution, rules, and management of the hospital generally'.

The Commission investigated complaints on issues ranging from the diet of patients and the quality of the food, to the supply of linen and cleanliness. It noted that payment had not changed the character of the outpatients department or resulted in any manifest ill effects despite the doctors' protests. It concluded that the nursing was substandard, largely because the establishment was too small and the duties required of nurses excessive.

On the question of representation by the medical staff, the Board of Management informed the Fry Commission that this would give 'undue emphasis to the scientific element in the hospital, and tend to subordinate the immediate benefit of the patients to the pursuit of medical knowledge'. In support of this view, the Board cited grounds for suspicion that, in one case of which they were aware, the sufferings of the patient (Olive Griffin) had been prolonged in the interest of medical science. The Commission dismissed this assertion and reinforced the view that Olive's admission was justified, and that Burford Rawlings had shown a 'gross error of judgment' in challenging care deemed suitable by a physician and surgeon. The Board then argued that any increase in medical representation 'would leave less room for the religious care of the patients' but this position was also rejected, with the Commission pointing out that medical staff were represented on the Boards of most of the other London hospitals, presumably without any increase in ungodliness. Overall, in upholding the request that doctors should be represented on the Board, the Commission argued that, had this been in place, it 'would be to the great and permanent benefit of the hospital ... [and] the present schisms in the body would never have arisen, or would speedily have been healed'.

Finally, the Commission turned its attention to the 'secretary-director', Burford Rawlings. It concluded that his powers were too wide, and that he hindered appropriate communication between the medical staff and Board. They recognised that Burford Rawlings had 'devoted much energy and ability, and [had] been a valuable and faithful servant of the institution', but that he did 'not possess all the exceptional combination of qualities essential to the performance of the wider duties he had assumed, and that he

---

[40] The *Dictionary of National Biography* notes that 'he was renowned for his painstaking scrupulosity, for his passion for justice, and for his unusual versatility, [but that he] was seen by some other judges as pedantic and overly scrupulous'.

[41] Witnesses were Lord Lister, Sir William Broadbent, Sir Sydney Waterlow and Mr C. S. Loch; three members of the Board of Management; two medical officers of the hospital; seven present and past house physicians; eight present and past lady superintendents and assistant matrons; the head of the Convalescent Home, Finchley; eight present and past sisters; five present and past nurses, male and female; the chaplain, the sanitary officer, the secretary and general director, the assistant secretary, the auditor, the steward, the cook, the late clerk to the Samaritan Society and the dispenser. The committee also made a surprise visit to the hospital. Dr Ormerod represented the hospital, assisted by Sir Felix Semon and Sir Victor Horsley, and Boydell Houghton was appointed as counsel for the Board of Management.

Documents, papers and newspaper reports regarding the Fry Commission are to be found in the Queen Square archives: NHNN/A/35.

had on many occasions shown a tendency to amplify his jurisdiction beyond its legitimate bounds'. The committee recommended that the office of general director be abolished and replaced by a secretary performing a more traditional role. Before endorsing this recommendation, they sounded out Burford Rawlings, who stated simply that he would resign immediately if this was the conclusion of the report.

Sir Edward noted disapprovingly that Burford Rawlings had recently published an article entitled 'Doctors in Hospitals'.[42] This was an excoriating and extraordinary attack in which he pointed out that all voluntary hospitals risk the possibility of friction between 'two essentially conflicting influences' – the philanthropic and the professional – due mainly to the arrogant attitudes of doctors. He thought that many physicians consider the hospital 'in pawn' to them but, in fact, the 'obligation the profession owes to the hospital is immeasurably greater'. Doctors consider administrators at most to be 'hewers of wood and drawers of water', whereas doctors 'do all the real work'. Burford Rawlings noted that doctors, 'many of whom amass great wealth', rarely provide financial assistance to hospitals, and that neither duties nor ethics stand in the way of private practice. In his opinion, doctors consider all men who are not medical as distinctly inferior, an attitude reinforced by medical journals which engage in 'undiluted laudation' of the profession. He considered that doctors work in hospital because they 'supply wide fields for study and experiment, and are most important as a means of advertisement'; and that the ideal hospital patient, in their view, is commonly 'one for whom … little or nothing can be done, but whose condition affords opportunity for clinical instruction, the elucidation of theory or for carrying out a brilliant operation'. The metropolitan consultant 'exalts himself high above his professional brethren of the provinces and the suburbs', and 'as a judge not a barrister, or a bishop (or higher) amongst priests'.

This was an extremely badly timed attack and showed the depth of Burford Rawlings' feelings. Although he subsequently claimed that his polemic was a general description and nothing to do with the National Hospital, Burford Rawlings had no managerial experience other than at Queen Square and it is not possible to see his comments as anything other than aimed at its staff, and Horsley in particular. An anonymous author (possibly Brudenell Carter) rubbed salt

in the wound by publishing a stinging attack on Rawlings[43] which ended 'but fortunately hospitals can exist without secretary-directors, and the medical profession can afford to despise the petty spite of vaulting ambition which has o'er leaped itself'. His difficulties were compounded when the chairman of the Board of Management, Colonel Porter, died just before the inquiry started. He was an aged and deeply conservative man, whose view of the medical professional was much in accord with that of Burford Rawlings, and he might have been able to strengthen the case.

As reported by the *British Medical Journal*, the inquiry 'in summary found the most serious allegations to be true, whist others were exaggerated or unsupported. The commission also found that the Medical Committee's action in complaining directly to the governors and Members of the hospital, without first doing so to the Board was also justified.'[44] The Commission's condemnation of the Board of Management and of Burford Rawlings was overwhelming and unanimous.

The effects of the report, which the governors accepted, were devastating, and a chain of actions followed. New rules were drawn up for the hospital and a general meeting held on 9 January 1902 to vote in a new Board of Management. Two members of the old Board agreed to be nominated,[45] but their candidature was voted down by the governors present. They then demanded a ballot of all governors, the *Lancet* reporting in a review of events at the general meeting that the demand for a ballot was characteristic of the methods employed all through the controversy by the Board of Management, 'who were not content with defeat of their candidature at the meeting but sacrificed the time and the money of the Charity by demanding a ballot'. The editor expressed the hope that the vote would not be reversed and the new Board would 'carry out the many reforms which are so urgently needed and which have been so bitterly opposed'. The *Lancet* did, however, express approval of the appointment of the Earl of Dudley who, it was felt, could be 'relied

---

[42] Burford Rawlings, 'Doctors in Hospitals', *The nineteenth century and after: a monthly review* (1901), 611.

[43] Anon., 'The Wrath of Burford Rawlings', *British Medical Journal* (6 April 1901): 847.
[44] *British Medical Journal* 2 (1901): 85 (and, further, 2: 1821).
[45] Frank C. Capel and John Pearman. Burford Rawlings also mentions that he himself was nominated but that this 'little understood the feeling actuating the victors'.

upon to play a most important part in rescuing this deserving hospital from the brink of ruin'.[46]

Burford Rawlings duly resigned and his post was abolished. He wrote

> Having enclosed my keys in a packet addressed to the newly-elected President, the Earl of Dudley, I went forth. I encountered nobody, I was the solitary occupant of the footway, and glad of the solitude, even though it meant no kindly anaesthetism of solace to dull the pain of severance from a prized task and of the putting off of harness, which, if it gripped often, never had galled.

The narrative of the next few years had several different interpretations. Burford Rawlings felt vindicated, two years after 'the revolution', that the 'exchequer was empty' and the finances of the National Hospital in disarray. The new Board was, as he put it, 'made up of strangers. Many of them to this time had not passed the hospital doors. Not one had lived through the bracing days when the institution was in the making, and of the cost in toil and treasure of the heritage to which they were succeeding, the newcomers could have no adequate conception.' He claimed that, had the 'revolution' not taken place, the hospital would have increased its association with Finchley, 100 new beds would have been offered on that site in the Jubilee year, and great sums of philanthropy would have been made available. As he ended his book:

> No greater misfortune could be suffered by the sick poor than the severance of hospital work from its religious and benevolent bases and its subjection to purely economic and scientific ends. Many cherished institutions are threatened, and if hospitals remain unscathed, it will be, not because they are spared as outposts of science, but because they have maintained their claim to sanctity as homes of beneficent tradition born of philanthropic service.

Gordon Holmes took a more optimistic line.[47] He noted that many changes were made to modernise the National Hospital. There was a revised diet for patients; a larger and better-trained nursing staff was put in place; new drainage and heating arrangements were made; and electric lights and an internal telephone system were installed. Better accommodation for nurses and resident servants was provided and the kitchens and household departments were enlarged – improvements that were all in line with the recommendations of the Fry Commission. Contradicting the assessment of Burford Rawlings, Holmes noted that the new Board inherited considerable debt and declining revenue, but it was possible to carry out the improvements through a loan from the hospital bankers. In fact, the Board managed to purchase new property in Powis Place and Queen Square; and in 1904, a new operating theatre was built. The outpatients area was enlarged, and a gymnasium built. An appeal during the 50-year anniversary celebrations in 1909 assisted.[48]

Whichever version is accepted, what is clear is that the events surrounding the 'revolution' were symptomatic of the times, and that the management at the National Hospital had become increasingly old-fashioned in its outlook and out-of-touch. The rise of science and of the professions, the decline of patronage, the de-linking of philanthropy from a philosophy of 'benevolent care', and the retreat of religion had passed them by. Societal mores had changed over the 40 years since the hospital's foundation, and what emerged into the twentieth century after the traumas of the previous year was now more modern in outlook, and forward-looking in attitude. The subsequent decades were to prove even more adventurous, but, as Burford Rawlings had put it, by 1901 the National Hospital was at least 'made' and it proved durable enough to survive.

---

[46] *Lancet* **159** (1902): 181.

[47] Holmes, *The National Hospital Queen Square* (1954).
[48] Financial problems did continue to plague the administration, and these are described in the next chapter.

Chapter 2

Queen Square, the Salmon Pink and Other Hospital Buildings

The Origins of Queen Square

In 1926, Godfrey Heathcote Hamilton began his history of Queen Square by describing Bloomsbury up to the time of Henry II as 'wooded and swampy and frequented by wild animals',[1] and it is with this thought in mind that we start this survey of the building history of the square in general and the National Hospital in particular. Ownership of the land has in fact been recorded since the thirteenth century and, by 1700, it was in the possession of Sir Nathaniel Curzon, fourth Baronet of Kedleston. It then consisted of arable pastures and a stream known as the 'Devil's conduit' which took its origin in or near the north-west corner of what was to become Queen Square and ran into the River Fleet, providing a supply of sweet pure water for the celebrated pump which still stands on the south-west end of the square.[2]

London was expanding westward, and Curzon decided to develop the area – possibly, it is said, through the agency of Nicholas Barbon[3] – in the form of a square named originally Devonshire Square but quickly changed to Queen Square in honour of Anne, the reigning monarch (between 1702 and 1714). The name has lasted.[4] The Curzon family sold off the square in 1779, to pay debts, allowing the freeholds to be taken up by residents. As it turned out, this diversification of ownership made it easier to change usage of the buildings, a process that facilitated the nineteenth-century development in contrast, for instance, to nearby estates of the Duke of Bedford, where licensing for residential or commercial purposes was more heavily restricted. Detailed records remain, and the history of the square is well documented in various sources.[5]

The earliest building, dating from around 1706, was the Church of St George the Martyr. The first houses were built on the south and east sides between 1713 and 1725, and on the west side slightly later, mainly by the surveyor Thomas Barlow. The land was set out as a square in 1716. The north end was left open, and late eighteenth-century prints show the

---

[1] Godfrey Heathcote Hamilton, *Queen Square: Its Neighbourhood and its Institutions* (London: Leonard Parsons, 1926), p. 4. His description has echos of academic neurology today.

[2] For the 'Devil's conduit', see Hamilton, *Queen Square* (1926), pp. 4–7, 27; and Anon. (Macdonald Critchley), *Queen Square and the National Hospital 1860–1960* (London: Edward Arnold Ltd, 1960), pp. 38–9, with photos of the walls. The conduit was accessible through a trap door in the garden of no. 20 Queen Square until its demolition in 1911–13, but the stone walls are apparently preserved by the Metropolitan Water Board. For the Queen Square pump, see Hamilton, *Queen Square* (1926), pp. 33–4, and Anon. (Macdonald Critchley), *Queen Square* (1960), pp. 42–3.

[3] Nicholas Barbon was a physician and notorious developer, who made his fortune by the aggressive redevelopment of London in the aftermath of the Great Fire. He died before the Queen Square development started and so it is not clear whether he was in fact responsible for the plans. It is rather appropriate that Queen Square may owe its origins to a Fellow of the Royal College of Physicians.

[4] Although it is often, and erroneously, misspelt Queen's Square. This mistake seems to have been made repeatedly from the eighteenth century onwards (see, for instance, the example of J. Noorthouck, *A New History of London: Including Westminster and Southwark* (London: R. Baldwin, 1773)), and continues to be made. At one stage, the square may also have been named 'Queen Anne Square'.

[5] These include: the Land Registry; the Camden Historical Society; Hamilton, *Queen Square*; E. Walford, *Old and New London: A Narrative of its History, its People and its Places* (London and New York: Cassell, 1878), Vol. IV; Anon. (Macdonald Critchley), *Queen Square and the National Hospital 1860–1960* (London: Chartered Society of Queen Square, 1960); R. Ashton, *Victorian Bloomsbury* (Newhaven, CT: Yale University Press, 2012); the Leaverhulme-funded 'Bloomsbury project' of UCL; N. Black, *Walking London's Medical History* (London: Royal Society of Medicine Press, 2006); R. Thames, *Bloomsbury Past* (London: Historical Publications, 1993); G. Holmes, *The National Hospital Queen Square, 1860–1948* (Edinburgh and London: E. & S. Livingstone Ltd, 1954). This account is based on these sources.

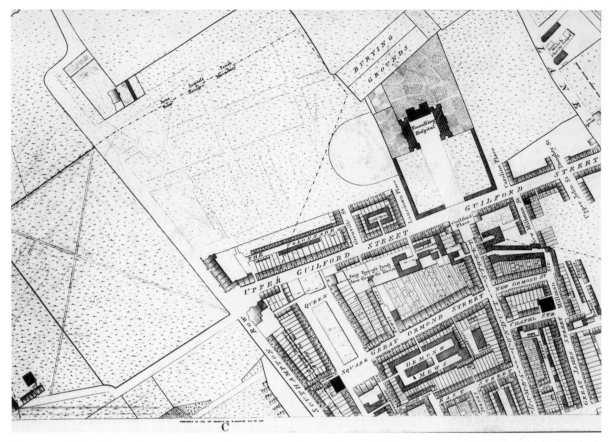

Figure 2.1 A plan of Queen Square and surrounding area in 1799, showing the early buildings in Upper Guilford Street and the fields to the north and west.

result – a wide and spacious area, surrounded on three sides by elegant Georgian terraces and demarcated to the north only by iron railings. The square rapidly became fashionable and popular due to its reputation for promoting good health because its open north side allowed uninterrupted draught of the north wind across what was then open countryside up to the rising land of the hamlets of Hampstead and Highgate.

Many of the early residents were wealthy aristocrats, lawyers, clergymen and doctors, and also men of letters, architects, artists, writers and intellectuals.[6] French refugees also frequented the area, giving this part of Bloomsbury an increasingly cosmopolitan feel, and towards the end of the eighteenth century a number of bookshops, publishers and print-sellers set up business there.

portrait painter; Dr Charles Burney, Fanny Burney's father; Hannah More, poet and religious writer and philanthropist; Martin Folkes, President of the Royal Society; Mr Hoare, the banker; Sir Rickman Godlee, the neurosurgeon; Jerome K. Jerome; Baron Sir (Jonathan) Frederick Pollock, judge and Governor of the Foundling Hospital; and Elihu Yale, after whom that university was named. Hamilton (*Queen Square*, p. 57) mentions that Hughlings Jackson lived at no. 5 Queen Square in the 1860s, where Rickman Godlee had been born, but there seems to be no corroboration of this. The Catholic bishop, Dr Richard Challoner, had his home in the square ransacked during the Gordon Riots. Another important early resident was the physician Anthony Askew, a bibliophile and protégé of Mead, who lived on the site of Powis Place. It was recorded that 'Our house in Queen Square was crammed full of books. We could dispense with no more. Our passages were full; even our garrets overflowed.'

[6] Hamilton and Critchley list, among the residents in the eighteenth and nineteenth centuries: the Bishops of Carlisle, Chester and Chichester; Lord Windsor and Lord Kingston; Lord Scarsdale; Lord Thomas Denman, the Lord Chief Justice; Sir Robert Fowler, Lord Mayor of London and MP; Mr Justice Bathurst, the Lord Chancellor; Lady Gainsborough; Lady Farnaby; Jonathan Richardson, the

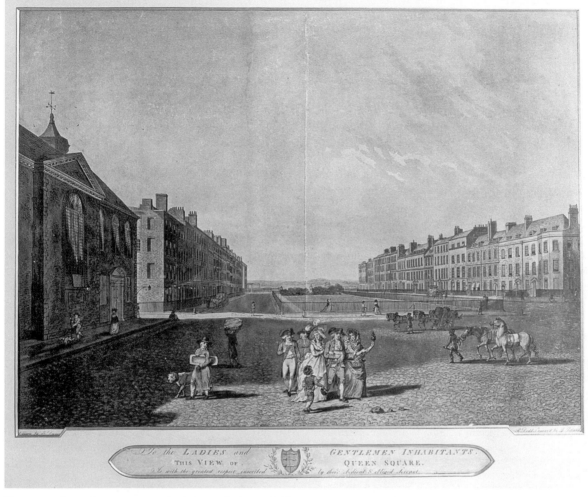

Figure 2.2 Queen Square engraving by Robert Pollard, 1790 (Wellcome Images, L0012093).

Written in 1773, the *New History of London* by John Noorthouck contains the following description of St George the Martyr and the square:

St. George the martyr. Queen's square: On the west side of Queen's-square near Great Ormond-street, stands the church of St. George Queen's-square, which was erected in 1706, by private subscription, as a chapel of ease to St. Andrew's Holborn … it was consecrated in the year 1723 and dedicated to St. George, in compliment to Sir Streynsham Master, one of the founders of it, who had been governor of Fort St. George in the East-Indies.

Queen's square. The square this church stands in has been observed to be an area of a peculiar kind, being left open on the north side for the sake of the beautiful landscape before it, terminated by the hills of Hampstead and Highgate: this open exposure renders the square remarkably airy and agreeable to the inhabitants of the other three sides; and though the distant beauties have occasioned the decoration of the area to be overlooked, a walk round it is as pleasant as any of the public gardens, none of which can boast so fine a prospect.[7]

---

[7] Noorthouck, *A New History of London*. Queen Square has interesting East India Company and Derbyshire connections. Hamilton mentions that 'There is some evidence that this area of Bloomsbury was a favourite residential quarter for retired Nabobs.' Sir Streynsham Master was the first East India Company Agent in Madras from 1675 to 1681, where he made his fortune and was involved in the foundation of St Mary's, the oldest church in Madras. The church in Queen Square may have been so named by Master in memory of Fort St George in Madras. Elihu Yale was the second Company Agent in Madras and had lived in the

In a similar vein, Fanny Burney wrote in her novel *Evelina* (1776) of the 'beautiful prospect of the hills, ever verdant and smiling' seen from her house in Queen Square. In Hawkins' *Life of Johnson* (1787) we read that Dr John Campbell's residence was 'a new built house in the North West Corner of Queen Square [number 20] whither, particularly on a Sunday evening, great numbers of persons of the first eminence for science and literature were accustomed to resort for the enjoyment of conversation'. Dr Samuel Johnson told Boswell that on one evening Campbell had drunk 13 bottles of port (although Boswell doubted the veracity of this) and that he was 'the richest author that ever grazed the common of literature'.

When houses were built on the north side of Guilford Street at the end of the eighteenth century,[8] obstructing the view, trees began to be added to the square, which up until this time was simply a lawn. Then a lead statue of Queen Charlotte[9] was erected

in April 1775 at the north end. By 1812, Ackerman's coloured aquatint shows how much vegetation had grown up, and, by 1926, Hamilton mentions planes, poplars, mountain ash, lime and a fig tree in the north-west corner, which, to this day, produces fruit. Several of the larger trees fell in the storm that swept through London on 15 and 16 October 1987.

That the square itself still retains its gardens is due in part to the Act of Parliament passed in 1832 to protect the 'squares and gardens within the united parishes of St Andrew, Holborn above Bars, and St George the Martyr'. Under this Act, the commissioners nominated and appointed resident householders as trustees to maintain, ornament and improve the gardens. These trustees claimed expenses from the commissioners, who in turn charged the surrounding houses a levy. Although repealed by the Local Government Act of 1899, this method of land management continued and the gardens and amenities of Queen Square are still managed by trustees, among whose members are included a nominee of the National Hospital. A testing time for Queen Square was when a bomb was dropped by a Zeppelin on 8 September 1915,[10] landing on the grass about 30 yards from the main entrance of the National Hospital, a spot marked now by a circular plaque embedded in the ground (one of the few such commemorative plaques in London). At the south end of the gardens is a concrete flower bowl, erected in 1978 to celebrate the Queen's Silver Jubilee,[11] and on the paving stones surrounding this is inscribed a quatrain by Philip Larkin: '1952–1977 / In times when nothing stood / But worsened or grew strange / There was one constant good / She did not change'.

Square, as had Laurence Sulivan, chairman of the East India Company, who was nicknamed 'the old man of Queen Square'. On returning from India, Master acquired Codnor Castle and lived in London and Derbyshire. Other aristocratic Derbyshire connections include Sir Nathanial Curzon of Kedleston Hall who, as noted above, owned the land on which Queen Square was built, and whose grandson George was the first Viceroy of India; and Thomas Denman, first Baron of Dovedale, whose seat was Middleton Hall and who became Lord Chief Justice of England in 1832.

[8] By the Foundling Hospital estate. This redevelopment of Guilford Street and surrounding areas, decided upon by the governors of the hospital because of its financial difficulties, was very unpopular and caused great commotion at the time. The houses were largely the work of the speculative builder James Burton, who is said to have built over 600 houses between 1792 and 1802 (see Oxford Dictionary of National Biography: James Burton). The poor quality of the building work of the houses in Guilford Street was to present recurring problems for the National Hospital when they leased or later acquired them.

[9] The Queen originally held a sceptre, as shown in early twentieth-century drawings, but this has disappeared – taken, it is said, by medical students during a riotous party. Critchley points out the irony that Queen Charlotte's grandson, Sir Augustus Frederick d'Este, developed multiple sclerosis, and states that this case was 'indeed the first instance of the disease'. Queen Charlotte's counsel at one time was Thomas Denham (see above), another inhabitant of Queen Square, who made, during his impassioned pleas on her behalf in the House of Lords, an unfortunate *faux pas* implying she was a sinner. This was the inspiration for the famous doggerel 'Most Gracious Queen, we thee implore / To go away and sin no more / Or if that effort be too great / To go away at any rate'.

[10] Interestingly, this was the most devastating of all the Zeppelin raids. The damage was caused mainly by L13 which meandered across central and east London and, on this one occasion, caused more than half the material damage resulting from all the Zeppelin raids against Britain in 1915. The hospital's annual report for 1919 mentions permission to report on this attack, prohibited at the time because this might have lowered morale. The blast was said to have broken window glass and glazing bars, and damaged the brickwork, but there were no injuries. Had the bombs landed a few yards farther east, the hospital would probably have been destroyed.

[11] It had been intended to build a fountain, and an appeal for this was launched but failed to reach the target sum. The flower bowl was all that could be afforded. It was dedicated for the use and enjoyment of the public by Audrey Callaghan, the wife of the then Prime Minister, in July 1978.

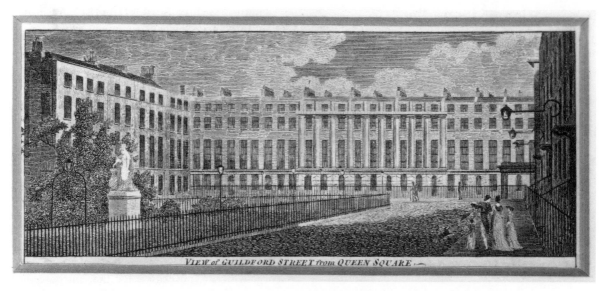

Figure 2.3 Engraving of the north end of Queen Square and Guilford Street (undated, *c.* 1800).

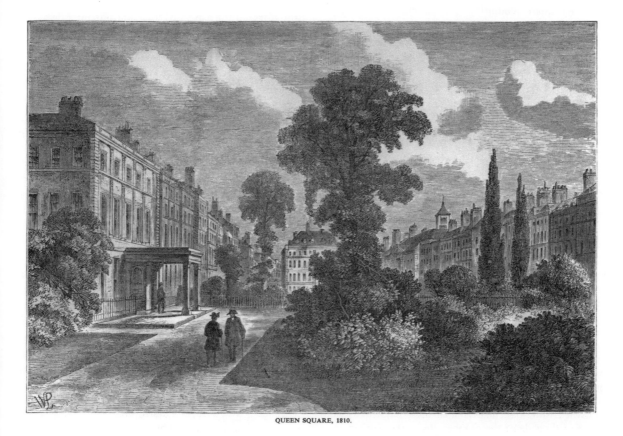

Figure 2.4 An etching of Queen Square in 1810 from the north end, showing the Queen Square House portico, Queen Square Gardens and the extent of planting in the previous 2 decades.

The Invasion of Institutions

In 1850, the square still consisted almost entirely of its original four- or five-storey residential Georgian houses, in terraced lines on the east, south and west sides,[12] but, in the next three decades, a remarkable transformation took place. With great rapidity, a procession of institutions devoted to health, education and other social purposes arrived. Massive reconstruction occurred rendering the scene of Georgian domesticity unrecognisable. Indeed, in the whole square, only St George the Martyr and numbers 1, 2, 6, 7, 13–15 and 42–43 now retain any trace of the original buildings, even as a shell, and only the name, Queen Square, reminds us of the eighteenth-century origins.

Nevertheless, the square retained its peaceful quality, now laced with philanthropic grace. Robert Louis Stevenson is said to have written, in 1874:[13]

> Queen Square, Bloomsbury is a little enclosure of tall trees and comely old brick houses ... It seems to have been set apart for the humanities of life and the alleviation of all hard destinies. As you go round it, you read, upon every second door-plate, some offer of help to the afflicted. There are hospitals for sick children [the Alexandra Hospital], where you may see a little white-faced convalescent on the balcony talking to his brothers and sisters and the baby, who are below there, on a visit to him and obstruct our passage not unpleasantly ... There is something grave and kindly about the aspect of the square that does not belie the grave and kindly character of what goes on there day by day.

Another version of this text is published in Stevenson's novel *The Dynamiter*, where Queen Square is described as a:

> fine and grave old quarter of Bloomsbury, roared about on every side by the high tides of London, but itself rejoicing in romantic silences and city peace ... Queen Square, sacred to humane and liberal arts, whence homes were made beautiful, where the sparrows were plentiful and loud and where groups of patient little ones would hover all day long before the hospital, if by chance they might kiss their hand or speak a word to their sick brother at the window.

The four hospitals in the square (the National Hospital, the Italian Hospital, the Homoeopathic Hospital and the Alexandra Hospital) all developed in a similar fashion. Each began its work in a single Georgian house, purchased for that purpose. Each then expanded and acquired neighbouring properties. And each was then pulled down and replaced with custom-built hospital buildings. These institutions transformed the aspect of the square from a domestic setting, with terraces of uniform commodious Georgian houses and gardens and stables, into its current state of buildings of different styles and sizes, all extending backwards away from the central square with the loss of garden and green spaces behind them. These developments carried the risk of oppressive over-urbanisation, and the fact that the square retains its magical tranquility and 'secret' quality is due to the ownership of the gardens by the trustees, and to its difficult vehicular access limited by narrow roads from the south and east, and pedestrian-only access by narrow passageways (Cosmo Place – once Little Ormond Street – and Queen Anne's Place).

The speed of development was remarkable and, by 1900, most buildings in the square had become home to various institutions. Although the mid-Victorian period was marked by the establishment of many educational and social charities intended to benefit the deserving poor, the almost complete institutionalisation of Queen Square was still a notable phenomenon. Part of the reason was financial. By 1860, Queen Square had lost its earlier social cachet, and Bloomsbury had for some decades been in transition from an aristocratic and upper-class quarter to one that was more bohemian and artistic in character, with some poor neighbourhoods and neglected housing subdivided into low-rent accommodation for artisans. The relatively low rents appealed to newly established medical

---

[12] As shown in the 1789 aquatint by R. Dodd based on the drawing by Edward Dayesand, engraved by R. Pollard.

[13] This piece is cited by Hamilton who noted it to be in a draft of an article for the *Academy* magazine in October 1874, which Stevenson wrote on behalf of the Working Women's College (based at 29 Queen Square). The passage, however, does not appear in the published piece. It also forms the dedication in Anon. (Critchley), *Queen Square and the National*. Robert Louis Stevenson often visited the square, as he wrote passionate letters to Frances Sitwell (addressed as Madamina or Madonna), a resident of Brunswick Row – a small lane in those days off Queen Square at the side of the number 20s – who worked as a secretary at the College. In one letter, he wrote 'I was several times very near Queen's Square but went away again. I once went down Southampton Row, and felt in a fine flutter in case you should come out of Cosmo Place. But you didn't'.

and private charitable institutions, which were also perhaps attracted by the adjacent presence of University College, itself a flag bearer of radicalism and social reform.

The institutions in Queen Square were in general of three types. First were the voluntary hospitals, the earliest to be established being the 'Private Spinal Institution', in existence around 1850 (the exact date of its foundation is not known). Second were the charitable educational institutions, many of which focused on education for women, stimulated by University College which had in 1878 become the first English university to offer degrees for women. The third were residential institutions for the poor or disadvantaged, or those who had fallen on hard times, most of which focused on providing employment or training, in the high Victorian manner of philanthropic self-help, as well as shelter.

By the 1880s, institutions occupied 60 per cent of buildings in the square, and, by 1950, the whole of the north, east and south, and most of the west sides. The evolution of Queen Square in the middle of the nineteenth century was an extreme example of developments seen elsewhere in Holborn; and, so named by Nick Black,[14] Bloomsbury became 'the cradle of reform', with the foundation of hospitals and other charitable foundations in the Euston Road, Great Ormond Street, Gray's Inn Road, Hunter Street and Tavistock Square.

The Buildings in Queen Square and Their Links to the National Hospital

The National Hospital had a powerful influence on life in Queen Square and slowly many of the buildings in the square were either incorporated into or involved in some way with the hospital. No doubt it would have suited the hospital eventually to have owned everything, but this was prevented in part by lack of vision and limited finances, together with a short-term approach to planning. Had more of the buildings been acquired when they became available, many crises of the last 50 years might have been avoided.

The West Side

The west side of Queen Square originally consisted of houses numbered 1–22, constructed sometime after 1725 as a typical Georgian terrace, each house usually of five storeys with basements, attic rooms, large chimneys and iron work, and with gardens behind and a mews (Brunswick Row) between numbers 19 and 20. The houses remained largely intact into the nineteenth century and thus witnessed the birth and spawning of the rising salmon of the National Hospital on the other side of the square.

At the south-west end is the church of St George the Martyr, built in 1706, and beautifully embellished by Nicholas Hawksmoor in 1718–20 with money from the Fifty New Churches Act of 1711 to become a parish church. Unfortunately, it was massacred architecturally in 1867 by Samuel Sanders Teulon, who removed the Grecian porches (of 1813), plastered and stuccoed the walls, added Gothic windows and a spire, and made numerous internal changes (Teulon was also responsible for the neighbouring Gothic-style St George's Schools at the Queen Square end of Old Gloucester Street). Number 1, now the Queen's Larder public house, is one of the original buildings, founded around 1710, so named because it was said to be where Queen Charlotte stored food for King George III, although this seems improbable. In 1861, it was a beer shop, and possibly a welcome relief from all the charitable and good works that were springing up around it. Two other alehouses and Burr's Hotel existed around the square.

Numbers 2, 3 and 5 were demolished in 1926, rebuilt as offices and became the home of Faber & Faber with only the facade of number 2 retained. This publishing house moved out on 19 January 2009 to Great Russell Street, and some of the building was reconverted into residential use (extraordinarily expensive luxury flats[15]). No doubt it was proximity to their publishers, and the poetry editor T. S. Eliot, that led Ted Hughes and Sylvia Plath to be married at St George the Martyr's church in 1956. Publishing and bookselling had previously also been a feature of the square and, in the eighteenth century, the famous 'Golden Head' bookseller was based there. At number 4 had been the Gordon College, founded in 1868 to teach women German, and which seems to have lasted only a few years.

Number 5 had a series of interesting residents. The glamorous and famous 'gaiety girl' Nelly Farren had lived there. 'Principal boy' roles allowed Nelly to show her legs in tights, encouraging a popular following among young men of the time, but sadly – and

---

[14] N. Black, *Walking London's Medical History* (2006).

[15] In 2014, a two-bedroom penthouse flat leasehold was on sale for £5m.

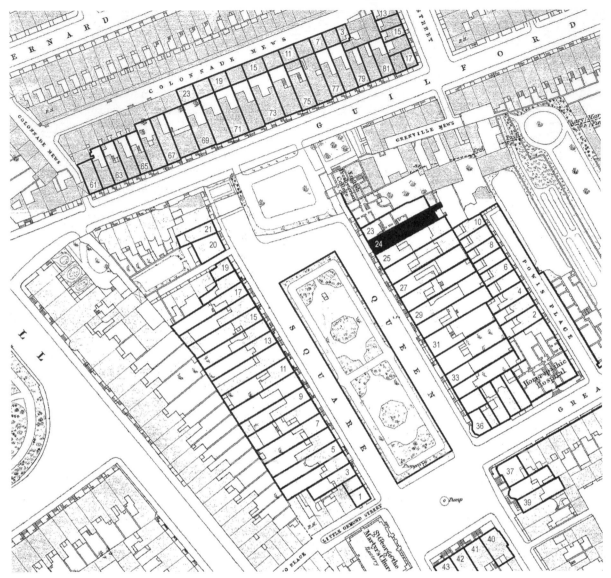

Figure 2.5 Five maps of Queen Square area showing the footprint of the National Hospital (shaded) in 1860 (above), 1868 (page 59), 1888 (page 60), 1979 (page 61) and 1997 (page 62).

perhaps predictably – she later developed locomotor ataxy, thus ironically securing a connection to the National Hospital. Sir Rickman Godlee was born in the house, and Hughlings Jackson may have lived there briefly in the 1860s. Arthur Conan Doyle found solace in the meeting rooms of the London Spiritualist Alliance at number 5, hoping to make contact with his family on the other side. Conan Doyle mentions the Light Publishing Company at number 6 Queen Square in his book *The Vital Message*, and it also seems possible that he consulted

Gowers' *Manual of the Diseases of the Nervous System* as source material for the Sherlock Holmes adventure *The Resident Patient*.[16] The St Margaret's Home and Industrial School for Girls, a Catholic charity, was established in 1861 at number 6, but two years later moved to number 31, and then relocated in 1866 to Finchley. It was replaced in 1869 by the Alexandra Institute for the Blind, providing aid to 21 inmates

[16] A. J. Lees, 'The Strange Case of Dr. William Gowers and Mr. Sherlock Holmes', *Brain* **138** (2015): 2103–8.

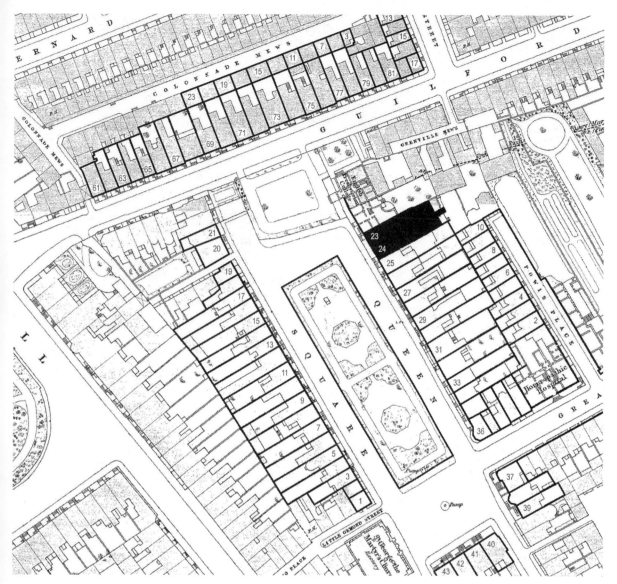

Figure 2.5 (cont.) Map, 1868.

and 10 outworkers. It is not clear when this establishment closed down. In 1884, the Art Workers Guild was founded and this has occupied number 6 ever since. The building still retains its panelling and many original features, including an eighteenth-century staircase with twister balusters and carved tread ends. It has a charming panelled meeting hall, top-lit, built in 1914 by F. W. Troup, to the rear over what was once the garden area. This is now the most charming room in the square with sensitive arts and crafts decoration, many paintings, and sculptures of members. Presiding over the room is a splendid bronze bust of

William Morris, made by Conrad Dressler in 1892, in a niche above the master's chair. Around the hall are a remarkable collection of paintings, dominated by a large group portrait above the fireplace, with the architect Gerald Callcott Horsley RA, Sir Victor's brother and a founder member of the Guild, in the centre.

Number 7 was leased by the National Hospital from the Royal College of Physicians, and housed the personnel and treasurer's departments from 1977, at which point they moved out of number 23. In 2001, University College London (UCL) bought the freehold from the hospital, and the Education Unit of

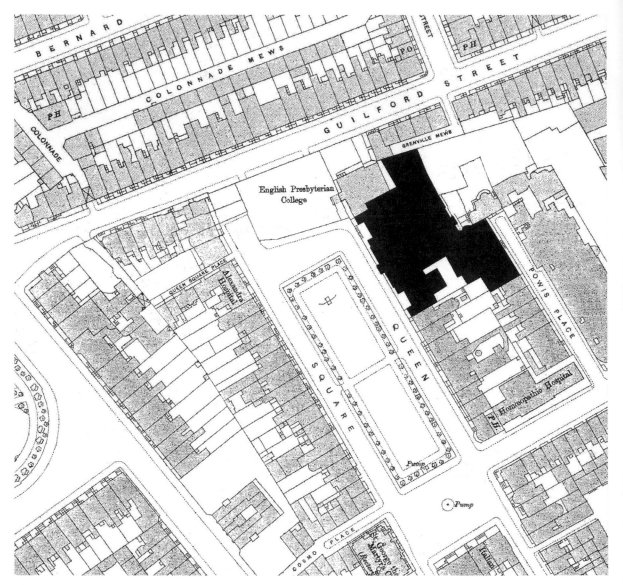

Figure 2.5 (cont.) Map, 1888.

the Institute of Neurology is currently based there. Although it is one of the few remaining Georgian buildings in the square, with original doors and cornices, extensive changes have been made to the interior and an extension built onto the back. These are insensitive and clownish modifications and give the whole an appearance of depressing muddle.

Numbers 8–11 were pulled down and rebuilt as the examination halls of the Royal Colleges of Physicians and Surgeons in 1909 and served this purpose for over 70 years. Many doctors living today will

recall the sense of agitation on entering the forbidding building. It is a large but rather routine seven-storey neo-Wren pile, and its size and dominance marked the death knell of the Georgian style on the western side of the square. A competition for the design was held among ten architects, of whom Mr Andrew Prentice[17] was chosen, with a tender from Messrs

[17] Andrew Noble Prentice was a Scottish architect who won the Soane Medallion in 1888 and published a famous folio of *Renaissance Architecture and Ornament in Spain* (1893). He was elected FRIBA in 1902, proposed by Collcutt, Spiers and

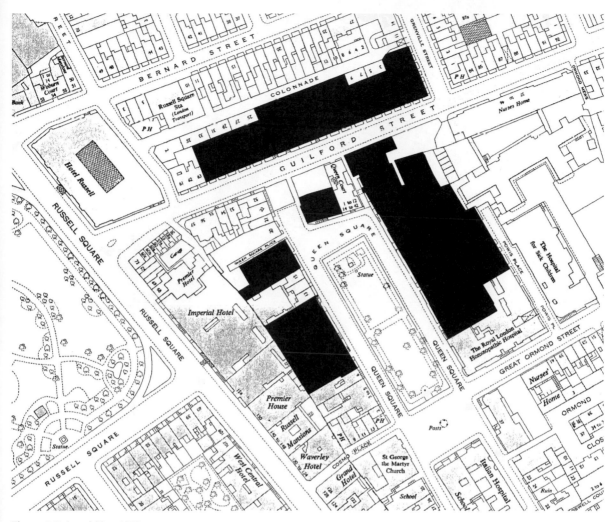

Figure 2.5 (cont.) Map, 1979.

Holland and Hannen of £27,644 for the building work. Not all was plain sailing, and the works severely damaged the neighbouring buildings on both sides, with repair costs of £1,100, so that expenditure overran by £4,000. In 1938, the Imperial Cancer Research Fund occupied the top two floors. The Royal College

---

Aston Webb. With his friend Voysey, he was a founder of the Imperial Arts League, now the Artists' League of Great Britain, in 1909. He had a large and very successful portfolio, mainly of grand houses, and worked in his earlier years in an early- to mid-seventeenth century style, but then later adopted a more classical early Georgian approach with tall roofs and big stacks (the examination halls is a good example) with arts-and-crafts influence. With this pedigree, it is easy to see how Prentice was chosen for the Queen Square commission.

of Physicians obtained the freehold a few years before selling it to the National Hospital for £1,375,000 in 1982. It was then renamed Sir Charles Symonds House, and initially housed the outpatients department on the ground floor and offices above, but it has since been extensively remodelled and currently has an MRI suite in the basement, modernised offices and seminar rooms and the neuromuscular centre and dementia research group offices on the ground and first floors, and offices of the hospital departments above. Of the 1909 building, the façade and the staircase remain, and the crest of the Royal Colleges is still displayed in the interior. The rest was largely destroyed. The building had the first Portland stone and red-brick façade to intrude into the square

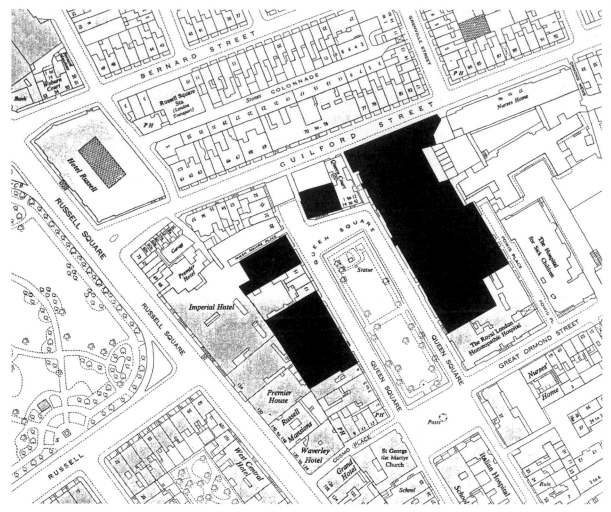

Figure 2.5 (cont.) Map, 1997.

(although a common feature of large institutions elsewhere in Bloomsbury), and numbers 17–19 and 23 followed suit.

The Georgian remnants of number 12 were altered in a major way by the South African architect Eustace Frere in 1907 when the building became the new headquarters of the St John's House Sisterhood, the Catholic nursing organisation attached to St Thomas' Hospital from which Florence Nightingale recruited nurses to accompany her to the Crimea.[18] The conversion is a sympathetic arts-and-crafts design with two storeys of plain stone and yellow brick above,

retaining Georgian proportions and sensibility, and with a charming wrought iron railing and central niche containing a statue of St John hollowed out of stone by Frederic Lassore.[19] After 1948, it was owned by the Department of Social Services and still used as a hostel for nurses from St Thomas', before being acquired by the National Hospital in 1967. The building was then bought by the Wellcome Trust, on behalf of the Institute of Neurology, and altered extensively in 1994–5 to house the Functional Imaging Laboratory. Its quiet and restrained neo-Georgian exterior gives no hint of the glitzy imaging machines inside, which included a Positron Emission Tomography scanner in commission until 2004,

---

[18] Geoffrey Robinson mentions that it was a copy of a building in Norfolk built in 1859, which was dismantled brick by brick and used for the current building.

[19] Hamilton, *Queen Square* (1926).

magnetic resonance imaging scanners and, most recently, a magnetoencephalography suite.

Numbers 13–15 retain some of their original features, although these have been extensively remodelled with new fronts. The doorway of number 14 has disappeared, so that numbers 13 and 15 seem to be neighbours. This remnant of a terrace now houses 16 separate flats. There is a photograph of number 19 with a bay frontage (misidentified in the photograph in the hospital archive as number 26) but the building is long gone.

Numbers 17–19 now comprise a rather routine neo-Georgian red-brick building with Portland stone dressing, dating from 1899. Previously it had been the House of Relief for Children with Chronic Diseases of the Joints, then in 1881 the Alexandra Hospital for Children with Hip Disease. The houses were demolished in 1899 and replaced by the current structure which was originally a purpose-built hospital. It was vacated in 1920 and the building converted into offices. Its lease fell vacant in 1960 and the National Hospital was offered the freehold, but considered this too expensive (£140,000) and took it on a 21-year lease at £9,000 per annum jointly with the Institute of Neurology. It housed the histology and chemical pathology departments, the medical library and residential accommodation. The hospital had to vacate the property when the lease expired in 1981 and it reverted to the Imperial Hotel, which faces onto Russell Square and still owns the freehold. Later the building was leased to UCL and accommodates the Institute of Cognitive Neuroscience and Gatsby Computational Neuroscience Unit. Again, extensive renovation has taken place and none of the original interiors remain.

There was originally a mews, Brunswick Row, between numbers 19 and 20, but this too has disappeared. Number 20 Queen Square was said to be the finest house on the west side. It occupied the northwest corner, with windows out onto Guilford Street as well as Queen Square, and with Bloomsbury gardens in front. It had been the house of Dr Campbell (of bottles of port fame) in the eighteenth century, and then of the Swiss 'count' Mr Heidigger who, among other things, managed the Royal Opera House. Other nineteenth-century inhabitants included Mr Rowlandson and Mr Plumptre, and from 1866 to 1882, the remarkable and indefatigable Miss Louisa Twining, philanthropist and poor-law reformer. She converted the building to St Luke's House in April 1866 for use as a home for epileptics and the elderly, where Radcliffe and Russell Reynolds were the medical attendants. In her time, the house was described as a charming and spacious mansion, with a noble old oak staircase and a large garden at the back with fine trees.[20] She also mentions in her autobiography that Sir Walter Crofton had opened a home for discharged female prisoners in Queen Square, but it is not clear where this was situated. After 1882, the house became the home of Thomas Henry Wyatt,[21] president of the Royal Institute of British Architects, who died just before Manning's new building rose up opposite. The house was demolished around 1960 to make way for the truly ghastly back elevation of the building of the President Hotel. Of number 21, nothing now remains.

The North Side

The north side of Queen Square comprised open space and gardens, known as Bloomsbury Gardens, and fronting onto Guilford Street. In 1929, it was reported with regret that the efforts of the hospital to persuade the London County Council and Holborn Council to prevent Queen Square House gardens, the open space 'with its fine trees' at the north end of Queen Square, being built upon were in vain, and in 1931 what is now known (confusingly) as number 23 Queen Square was constructed to house the Institute of Public Health and Hygiene. On either side of its entrance are still a pair of lamps on top of handsome painted iron standards. These depict the *caduceus*, a staff with two entwined snakes, the symbol of Hermes. This is no doubt a mistake, as the intention was almost certainly to portray the rod of Aesclepius, which should be encircled by a single snake only.[22] Ironically, given the hospital's initial trenchant opposition to the building, when the second floor became vacant in 1962 it was leased to the Institute of

---

[20] L. Twining, *Recollections of Life and Work, Being the Autobiography of Louisa Twining* (London: Edward Arnold, 1893).

[21] Wyatt's own buildings include Knightsbridge Barracks of 1878, the Brompton Hospital of 1879 and the Adelphi theatre of 1858.

[22] In *Walking London's Medical History*, Black points out that a similar mistake was made by the US Army Medical Corps, which adopted the wrong symbol in 1902, and the same error is repeated in the current lamp standards in front of the Royal Society of Medicine.

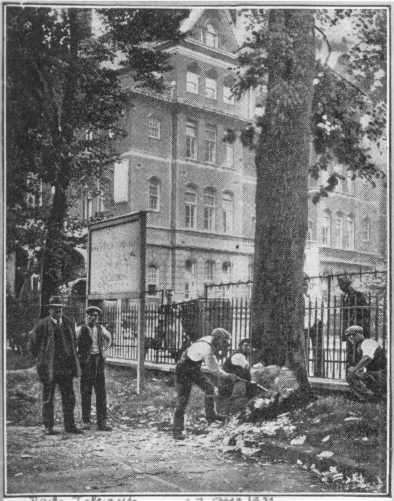

VANISHING BLOOMSBURY GARDEN.—The axe is being laid to the fine plane trees in Queen's-square. The site is being cleared for the new offices of the Royal Institute of Public Health.

Figure 2.6 Photo from the *Daily Telegraph*, 27 August 1931, showing the destruction of the 'fine plane trees' and site clearance of Queen Square gardens to make way for the building of 23 Queen Square.

Neurology and occupied by the professorial department of clinical neurology, treasurer's office and the supplies department, before this moved again to numbers 8–11. In 1980, the Royal Institute of Public Health put the building up for sale, and with the financial support of the University Grants Committee (UGC) and the Secretary of State, it was purchased for the Institute of Neurology. From August 1981, it has been occupied entirely by the National Hospital and Institute of Neurology. The Rockefeller library, offices and some residential accommodation were moved from Alexandra House when the lease expired, and currently the building also houses the private outpatients department on the ground floor, and the medical library on the first floor (and its stacks in the attic).

Originally at the north-east corner of the square was the imposing mansion Queen Square House. It had spacious grounds and a large stone porch, which opened up onto gardens that formed the north end of the square. When it was built in 1779, the square had open countryside to the north, known as Conduit Fields, but soon afterwards the Georgian houses in Guilford Street began to be constructed. Its inhabitants included the doctor said to be treating King George III and, from 1844 to 1864, Charles Edward Pollock, Baron of the Court of the Exchequer and Serjeant-at-Law. Its owners had a famous row with

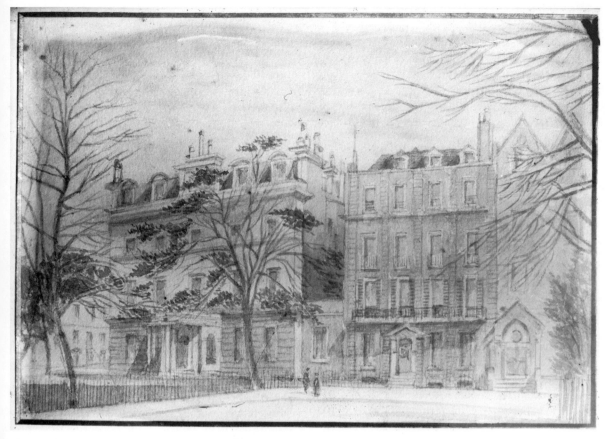

Figure 2.7 Queen Square House. Drawing by Dennis Flanders RA, who lived in Great Ormond Street and was a frequent visitor to the Art Workers Guild in Queen Square.

the National Hospital in which legal action was threatened to stop patients sitting on chairs outside the railings of his house, after they had been barred from using the gardens. The house was leased to the Presbyterian College in 1864 (which moved there from number 29), and from 1900 it housed Jews' College until the lease expired. Then, in 1932, the lease was held by the Foundling Estate, which used the house as flats for ladies, until it was acquired by the National Hospital in 1948. The mansion was pulled down in 1970 after a mammoth struggle with the planning authorities, and the current brutalist building, also named Queen Square House, was constructed. The disastrous saga of construction works in the 1960s and 1970s is described below. Queens Court was built in the 1930s, architecturally wholly undistinguished, and this reduced the grand entrance space of the old Queen Square House to the narrow Queen Anne's passage, thereby closing up once and for all the north end of the square.

The East Side

Many houses on the east side of Queen Square were acquired by the National Hospital during its rebuilding programmes. Most had been small charitable or voluntary educational establishments. Some were finding it hard to maintain their finances and this made them ripe for picking-off by the National Hospital. Many were in poor states of repair, but they retained fine architectural features and their wholesale destruction by the hospital would nowadays be met with dismay by conservationists, far more it seems than was the then contemporary mood. At number 22, the Ladies' Charity School (also known as the Ladies' Charity Home for Girls, or Ladies' Charity School for Training Girls as Servants) was established around 1859. In 1861, there were 28 girls between the ages of 7 and 11 living there, and in 1871, 50 girls between the ages of 8 and 14. In 1881, the charity had only six residents and it moved out to

Notting Hill Gate, and the building was taken over by the National Hospital. It was said to have had a noble staircase (sold), painted ceiling (broken up) and mahogany doors and marble chimney pieces (lost), before its acquisition by the hospital. Number 23 had been owned by celebrated lawyers and judges working in the nearby Inner Temple, had a large garden with mulberry trees, and was occupied by John Eustace Grubb, barrister and Parliamentary agent, and his family, before its purchase in 1864 by the National Hospital. It accommodated the offices of the Ladies' Samaritan Society, originally set up by Johanna Chandler to support families of the patients at the National Hospital. The charity still exists, now based in the hospital offices. In the census returns of 1841 and 1851, at number 24 there was a school registered, with 17 girls between the ages of 12 and 17 resident in 1851, but this had closed by the time the National Hospital bought the lease in 1860. A solicitor and his family had occupied number 25 in 1841, and then in 1851 the Industrial Home for Gentlewomen[23] was established at numbers 25 and 26, providing a refuge, employment and support for the 'widows and daughters of private gentlemen, officers in the Army or Navy, professional men, bankers and merchants, suffering under the reverses of fortune'. In 1861, there were 13 'gentlewomen' listed amongst the 22 occupants. By 1872, the home had disappeared, and the building was leased to the National Hospital by 1875. Number 26 was then occupied from 1861 by William Morris' firm and bought by the National Hospital in 1881 at a cost of £3,000.[24] Morris himself lived there from 1865 to 1872 and Esther Maynell describes the arrangements:

> A large ballroom had once been built at the end of the yard and it made an admirable workshop. In the long corridor that led to the ballroom, the glass painters worked, and there was a kiln. Above dwelt the family, in rooms made as bright and gay as possible with white-wash and white paint, lovely embroidered hangings and cushions, and painted furniture.

Queen Square had undoubted attractions. There was a fine garden with immense plane trees, where the two little Morris girls [Jane Alice and Mary] spent much of their time. Needless to say, they also haunted the workshops to watch what was going on there whenever there was a chance.[25]

Of numbers 27 and 28 not much is recorded, and these were demolished in 1881. The Presbyterian College occupied number 29 from 1858 to 1864, followed by the Working Women's College founded by Elizabeth Malleson in 1864, and supported by John Ruskin and Charles Kingsley to offer education for shop assistants, dressmakers, milliners, domestic servants, secretaries, bootmakers, laundresses and others. In 1874, it became coeducational and changed its name to the College for Men and Women but ceased to exist in 1901. Numbers 29 and 30 were owned by the National Hospital at the time of the rebuilding but not incorporated into the Albany wing (see below). They retained their Georgian structure and were known as 'the Annexe'. Photographs of its elegant interior show marble columns, painted friezes and a fireplace in the Adams style. Hamilton mentions an eighteenth-century ceiling painting, which had been taken down, restored and installed in the Board room (from where it has since disappeared). In 1936, however, the houses were demolished to make way for the Queen Mary wing.

The first hospital established in the square opened its doors at number 31. This was the Private Spinal Institution, founded by Joseph Amesbury. The building became the headquarters of the Aged Poor Society, a Catholic charity associated with the Society of St Vincent de Paul, in the 1860s, and the charity remained there until 1881, later occupying number 41. The Anglican order of the Sisters of St Margaret of East Grinstead ran a hospital in their convent (also known as St Katherine's), initially at number 32. The convent then bought number 33, where it also ran a school of ecclesiastical embroidery; and a little chapel was built in the grounds at the back of the house but, tragically, pulled down in 2008 to make way for a lecture theatre. In 1850, before its sale

---

[23] Also known as the 'Industrial Home for Gentlewomen suffering under the Reverse of Fortune', and the 'Industrial Home of Indigent Gentlewomen'. It had the royal patronage of Queen Victoria and capacity for 57 women. By 1861, the rent was 10s a week for each resident.

[24] The hospital is in possession of the 1868 deeds of number 26, leasing the building to Messrs Morris and Marshall, and the counterpart is signed by Ford Madox Brown, Charles Joseph Faulkner, Edward Burne-Jones, Peter Paul Marshall, William Morris, Dante Gabriel Rossetti and Philip Webb.

[25] E. Maynell, *Portrait of William Morris* (London: Chapman, 1947). Interestingly, Jane Alice ('Jenny') Morris, William's daughter, suffered from epilepsy, and William himself had a nervous disposition and has variously been described as suffering from Tourette's syndrome and epilepsy, although definitive evidence on these points is lacking.

to the convent, number 33 was occupied by Abraham Bensusan and his children and grandchildren.[26] It was rebuilt after a fire in 1896 and remained in the ownership of the convent. It was then vacated and became the site of a book publishing business owned by Mr B. Herder. In 1960 it was purchased by the Department of Health for the joint use of the Royal Homeopathic Hospital and the National Hospital, which adapted it for their telephone exchange and linen room. On the door posts of the convent were charming carvings of a Catherine wheel, created in 1896, but which disappeared during the rebuild of 2008. The Homeopathic Hospital moved from Golden Square in 1859 into a building in Great Ormond Street and, in 1909, it purchased and demolished the neighbouring numbers 34–36 Queen Square, as well as the Queen's Head public house in Great Ormond Street, to make way for its new Sir Henry Tyler wing. This building, by E. T. Hall,[27] still stands, an imposing edifice in English Renaissance style, seven storeys high, and including amongst its innovations an electric lift and a roof garden. It was partly incorporated into the National Hospital in 2005.

At number 38, the London Society for Teaching the Blind to Read, a residential school for blind pupils, existed between 1842 and 1848 (it then moved and became the Royal London Society for Blind People). At number 39 was the Bessbrook Homes for Sandwich Men, founded in 1893 as a 'home for broken-down men' who were then found work carrying sandwich boards.[28] Numbers 37–39 (and neighbouring houses up to number 61 Great Ormond Street) were demolished in building the nurses' home of the Royal London Homoeopathic Hospital in 1911, also designed by E. T. Hall. This was notable for its

badminton court, but this was destroyed in the Blitz. At the time of writing, these buildings have been reincarnated as Barclay House and York House, offices of the Great Ormond Street Hospital.

The South Side

On the south side of Queen Square, at number 41 was the Home for Youths, run by the Society of St Vincent de Paul for about 30 boys, who were employed as clerks and servants, and in various trades. It existed from 1881 and seems to have moved out when the building was bought by the Italian Hospital in 1883. At number 42, the College of Preceptors was established in 1846 and remained there until 1882. Number 43 was occupied by the Female School of Art in 1861. Somewhere in the square was the office of the Society for Promoting the Employment of Women, which rented rooms around 1860, and was founded to teach book-keeping and law copying.

The Italian Hospital (Ospedale Italiano) was founded in 1884 by Commendatore Giovanni Ortelli. He had owned several houses in Queen Square, and then bought numbers 40 and 41, a pair of very handsome large Georgian buildings, and converted these into the hospital. We are fortunate to have a watercolour by J. P. Emslie from 1882 showing these five-storey houses with elegant doorcase and powerful elevation. As was the typical pattern, that hospital outgrew its buildings, and these were duly demolished in 1899 to be replaced by the current 'renaissance' pile designed by the architect Thomas William Cutler. He in fact lived at number 5 Queen Square for many years, and thus had the pleasure of daily sight of his masterpiece. The Ospedale has a four-storey façade of stone and red bricks, with giant pilasters and one or two nice touches, including the large cartouche over its door with a coat of arms, and a smaller one on the corner of its elevation in honour of the founder, an inscription ('Charity knows no restriction of country'), and nice bold lettering announcing the hospital name around its upper storey. It was extended in 1911 into Boswell Street[29] by the architect J. Dench Slater,[30] and, in the process, three more Georgian houses were demolished. Hamilton mentions the striking and familiar sight of nurses of St Vincent de Paul, who tended the sick in the Ospedale Italiano until 1923, parading in the square in

---

[26] By extraordinary coincidence, while researching this book, one of the authors (SDS) discovered that Abraham Bensusan (born 1799) was his great-great-great-grandfather, who lived in number 33 with his daughter Emily, the author's great-great-grandmother, and her daughter Miriam, the author's great-grandmother.

[27] Edwin Thomas Hall, afterwards vice-president of the Royal Institute of British Architects, is remembered most as the architect of Liberty & Co., the department store in Regent Street, the extensions to the Dulwich College Old Library, and various hospital buildings, including the Manchester Royal Infirmary (with John Brooks).

[28] The home housed 50 men when it was visited for the Booth poverty survey update in May 1894, and a veritable battalion of sandwich boards must have enlivened the square in those days.

[29] As now named, although until 1927 the street was Devonshire Street.

[30] Father of the J. Slater who was architect for the National Hospital's Queen Mary wing extension.

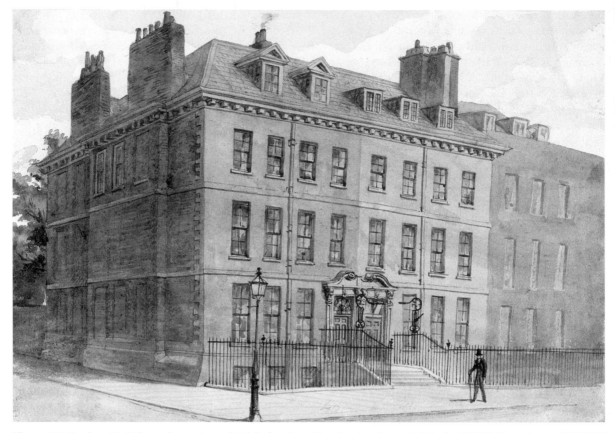

Figure 2.8 Numbers 40–41 Queen Square, immediately before demolition. A watercolour by J. P. Emslie, 1882 (Wellcome Images V0013477).

their stiffly starched head-dresses and dark stuffed gowns. The hospital had a temporary connection with the National Hospital, housing its private patients in ground floor wards until the 1980s, but it closed in 1990 and was taken over by the Hospital for Sick Children as a residence for parents of children admitted to the hospital. The interior has been extensively altered but the façade remains.

The leases of numbers 42–43 Queen Square were granted on 19 June 1703 to William Hawkins, and these were the first houses to be built in the square, around 1713. These were considerably remodelled towards the end of the eighteenth century, when the front elevation took its present form, along with various interior features. The two houses have a fascinating history, devoted to female education. Although originally residences, in 1846 the College of Preceptors (the first professional body for teachers) established itself at number 42. The Female School of Art, initially based at number 43, took over both houses in 1887. The school was founded in 1842 with the aim

of enabling 'young women of the middle class to obtain an honourable and profitable employment'. It then became part of the Central School of Arts and Crafts in Southampton Row around 1908. The passing of the school was lamented by *The Studio*, which commented that 'the threads of its traditions have been severed by the loss of the stately old eighteenth-century houses in Bloomsbury, in which for nearly half a century the artistic education of London girls was carried on'.[31] In 1910, the houses became the London County Council Day Trade School for Girls, one of several set up for girls leaving elementary schools between the ages of 14 and 16 who wished to enter two-year courses in trades such as lingerie, dressmaking, ladies' tailoring, millinery and photography. At some point in the 1930s, it was turned into a technical college for women and, in the late 1950s, into a secondary school, before becoming part of the Stanhope Institute, affiliated to the Inner

---

[31] Cited by the Bloomsbury Project (from which many details are taken - see www.ucl.ac.uk/bloomsbury-project).

London Education Authority. This closed in 1981 and the property was acquired as the home of the Mary Ward Centre in 1982 for female education. The two houses are still owned by the Royal Female School of Art, a charitable trust that hands out interest on the rent it receives from the Mary Ward Centre as grants to organisations supporting female art students.

The First Buildings of the National Hospital: 1860–1888

We have outlined the architectural and social history of the buildings of the square in some detail to provide a context for appreciating why the National Hospital came to be built there and how it fitted into and integrated with its neighbours.

Before the take-over by the institutions, as we have seen, even as late as 1850 the square was contained on three sides by Georgian domestic terraces. These were very similar to those in other squares and roads in London and in Bloomsbury itself, and examples of similar squares in other parts of Holborn, which have remained largely untouched, can still can be viewed today. On the East side, which is where the National Hospital was to encroach, some of these buildings were grand and others more modest, and several were in a poor state of repair. Most were still domestic residences although several had already become institutions and offices. The new institutions were almost all charitable endeavours and examples of the kind of muscular philanthropy that typified the age. So indeed was the National Hospital, which therefore would have not been out of place in this rapidly-changing and complex mélange (and nor indeed was it the first hospital in the square – that honour belonged to the Private Spinal Institution). However, it was the National Hospital which turned out to be the occupant that was to change the square more than any other.

The records of the committee set up in 1859 to establish the National Hospital, and subsequently those of the Board of Management, provide a rich account of the architectural history. Throughout its first 50 years, the buildings that housed the National Hospital conditioned and constrained the nature and extent of its work, while at the same time reflecting and advertising to the wider world the basic values and self-image of its founders, benefactors and managers.

One of the first acts of the new Board of Management in December 1859 was to place advertisements in *The Times* and *Morning Advertiser* for 'a large

house suitable for a public institution'; and, in January 1860, the Board decided to lease 3 Vernon Place, Bloomsbury, at a rent of £100 p.a. However, for reasons that remain unclear, almost immediately the Board resolved instead to take 24 Queen Square at a rental of £110 p.a. After the lease was signed in February 1860, this four-storey Georgian terraced house near the north-east corner of the square became the nucleus of the hospital for more than 20 years. This building, on the site of the north wing of the current red-brick building, was the first hospital premises, with eight beds for female patients, a consulting room, a waiting room and dispensary and, later in 1860, a ward for ten male patients.

The Original Hospital at Number 24 Queen Square

The first Board meeting to be held in the new hospital took place on 19 March 1860, followed later the same day by the 'First General Court' of the governors and

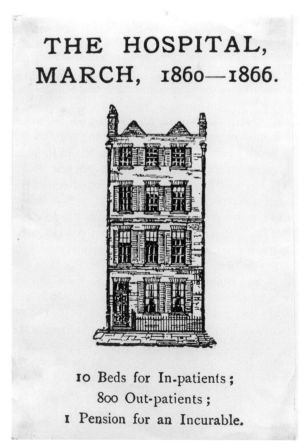

THE HOSPITAL, MARCH, 1860—1866.

10 Beds for In-patients;
800 Out-patients;
1 Pension for an Incurable.

Figure 2.9 The façade of the first building housing the National Hospital 1860–6.

69

subscribers. The first inpatients were admitted just over a month later. By mid-December 1860, there were already 17 patients and, from January 1861, the hospital was regularly having to turn otherwise eligible cases away 'for want of room'.

An appeal launched in November 1859 for £5,000 to open the new hospital was unexpectedly successful. As a result, the Board almost immediately began to explore the possibility of buying or leasing additional space in adjoining properties and also acquiring the freehold of 24 Queen Square. In May 1861, the owners offered to sell the remaining lease for £500 plus two annuities of £50 or £60 p.a. each. In July 1861, Edward Chandler put forward a proposal to purchase the 17-year unexpired term of the lease of Queen Square House for £1,900 plus a ground rent of £25 p.a. Chandler and a fellow Board member, Richard Barton, each offered to lend £300 interest-free for two years towards the price, while Johanna Chandler undertook to lend a further £100 on the same terms. The Board voted by a majority of nine to three in favour of this proposal, but considerable legal delays ensued and eventually the purchase failed.

The first major enlargement of the hospital's estate came only in November/December 1864, when, in response to an urgent plea by Ramskill and Radcliffe for more accommodation for both in- and outpatients, the Board reached agreement with Alfred Shadwell of Lambeth to purchase the freehold of the adjoining house, 23 Queen Square, for £1,500 and also, after prolonged negotiations and debate, in August 1864 the Board finally resolved to purchase the freehold of 24 Queen Square for no more than £1,600 p.a.

In the spring of 1864, Johanna Chandler and the Ladies' Committee were able to hand over or invest sums totalling more than £2,000 towards the purchase price of the freehold and ground rent on 24 Queen Square, which finally came into the hospital's absolute ownership free of all charges in 1868. By this time, the Board had entered into a further agreement to purchase two houses in Powis Place, one of which had already been paid for, again by the efforts of the Ladies' Committee and, by the following year, purchase of the second house was completed. Shortly afterwards, in August 1869, the Board undertook to purchase two houses in Finchley 'for the purposes of the Country Branch [which] the Physicians desire should be established'.[32] Once again, Johanna Chandler and the Ladies' Committee raised £900 of the £1,000 needed

for the purchase of the Finchley properties, and the freehold of the 'Country Branch' was duly acquired in the year before it opened.

As a result of these initiatives and acquisitions, by the end of 1868 the capacity of the hospital, to which 15 beds had been added in February 1863 with the establishment of the Marchioness of Thomond ward on the second floor of 24 Queen Square, had increased from 35 to 64 beds.[33] The opening of the Country Branch at Finchley in July 1870 added a further 25 beds for female epileptic and convalescent patients.

Expansion of the Hospital in Numbers 23 and 24 Queen Square

Nevertheless, the demand for the hospital's services continued to outstrip the available space, a recurring problem in subsequent years. In 1865, it was decided to renovate extensively numbers 23 and 24 Queen Square and rebuild them as a hospital. The conversion began in September 1865 under the direction of the architect Michael Prendergast Manning,[34] and was completed nine months later at a cost of around £6,000, the official opening taking place in July 1866. According to the report presented by the Board of Management to the annual meeting of governors and subscribers held in April 1867, 'The new building offers accommodation for 70 [actually, 60] Inpatients, and is provided with every appliance

---

[32] Minutes of Board of Management for 3 August 1869, on pp. 138–9.

[33] For the growth of the hospital's capacity in the early 1860s, see 4th annual report of the Board of Management [for 1864–5], pp. 13–14. For the increased capacity provided by the conversion of numbers 23 and 24 Queen Square to form the 'New Hospital', see 5th annual report of the Board of Management [for 1865–6], p. 19. For the later increase in bed numbers made possible by the legacy and donations of Mrs Elizabeth Morgan, one of the hospital's principal benefactors in its early years, see 7th annual report of the Board of Management [for 1867–8], pp. 13–14.

[34] Michael Prendergast Manning, a dissenting United Reform Church architect and future member of ARIBA, whose offices were located nearby at Mitre Court Chambers off Fleet Street, was principally responsible for the design of St Mary's Congregational Church, Primrose Hill, Twickenham, and Northwood Cemetery, Cowes, Isle of Wight, but he is now largely forgotten. According to Ruth Waller, unpublished material relating to Manning's architectural practice lies in the British Architectural Library drawings collection (Ruth Waller, *Historic Landscape Assessment of Northwood Cemetery, Cowes, Isle of Wight* (Hampshire and Isle of Wight Wildlife Trust, October 2014), p. 16).

which modern scientific ingenuity has devised for the treatment of disease.' No photographs or drawings showing the interior of the original hospital survive, but a small, finely drawn plan by Manning in the hospital archives, showing the ground and first floors of 23 and 24 Queen Square after their joint conversion for hospital use in 1865–6, gives a good impression of the internal layout of the hospital. The plan shows: the two main wards for female patients, the Sisters' ward on the first floor of number 23, towards the rear, and the Thomond ward on the first floor of number 24 overlooking the square; the David Wire ward for male patients on the ground floor of number 23, towards the rear, with its dormitory and day room; the electrical room and gymnasium adjoining each other on the first floor of number 24, overlooking the airing court for female patients; the waiting room and physicians' consulting room for outpatients, with the dispensary, on the ground floor of number 23; and the Board room and secretary's office on the ground floor of number 24, overlooking the square. It also shows the baths and lavatories at the rear, adjoining the airing court for male patients at the very back of the site, and a padded room, presumably for the restraint of male epileptic patients, at the back on the first floor of number 23 adjoining the day room to the Sisters' ward. The overall impression is one of ingenious adaptation and a tight-fitting, small-scale, domestic establishment, more like a private asylum or nursing home than a hospital. As the annual report for 1865 indicated: 'The internal arrangements are intended to combine all the advantages of a Special Hospital with the comfort of a Private Home.'

In January 1867, the *Lancet* was impressed not only by the excellent medical arrangements of the new hospital, but also by the rich and tasteful character of its furnishings and décor,[35] while the 1867 annual report of the National Hospital claimed that: 'Ignoring the traditions of hospital[s] … generally, the aim has been to impart a home-like character to a public institution, and to afford the poor inmates in … time of sickness, not only the best of medicinal care, but … a happy dwelling and cheerful associations.'

The *British Medical Journal* also approved:

On Thursday, the 7th inst [January 1868], two additional wards were opened at this hospital, each containing twelve beds, two of which are isolated in a separate room, for troublesome or other special cases. To each ward is attached the usual day-room – an improvement introduced in England by this hospital, and which is found to exercise a most beneficial effect on the health and comfort of the inmates. In each day-room there is a library; and everything is furnished in the homely and tasteful manner which characterises the whole hospital. Altogether, the Hospital now numbers sixty beds. In addition to these new wards, bath-rooms have been constructed out of the basement offices of the old houses constituting the hospital, with an ingenuity quite surprising, and reflects the highest praise on the architect, Mr. Michael P. Manning, of Mitre Court. The baths are after the model of the Maison de Santé Municipale in Paris. They consist of hot and cold plunge-baths, shower-douche, sitz [a hip bath], needle, Russian, and sulphur baths, and are arranged in a comfortable and thoughtful manner. The hospital, with its electrical room, gymnasium, and baths, is now furnished with every means for successfully treating nervous diseases, besides the many comforts of a home which it supplies.[36]

In similar vein, Dr Pelman, a German visitor who wrote about a number of English hospitals, visited the National Hospital in 1869 and noted:

The little hospital for poor epileptics and paralytics (Queen Square, Bloomsbury) [is] a pure jewel-case. The hospital contained beautiful baths of every kind including, naturally, a Turkish bath; a spacious room very richly equipped with electrical fittings, and an impressive Gymnasium … The patients' rooms were furnished like the lounges of a first-class hotel, carpets, flowers and pictures everywhere; everything was clean and elegant.[37]

The future hospital secretary, Hamilton, writing in 1926, was less complimentary about the appearance of the renovated 1866 hospital.

Since 1860 the National Hospital had been in possession of … 24 Queen Square and … [in 1865] the Hospital took also [23 Queen Square] and joined the two houses together to make them look something like an institution. The effect, judging from a photograph … was deplorable, and the [two] joined houses were crowned by a row of ignoble gables which must have entirely spoiled the general roof line of the east side [of the square].

---

[35] 'The Hospital for the Paralysed and Epileptic', and 'Description of the New Hospital', *Lancet* **89** (1867): 53–4 and 28–30, respectively.

[36] The National Hospital for the Paralysed and Epileptic. *British Medical Journal* (18 January 1868) i: 57.
[37] Cited in Anon. (Critchley), *Queen Square and the National* (1960).

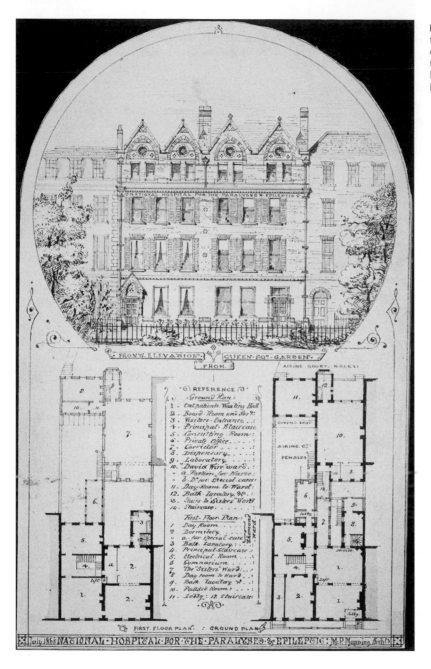

Figure 2.10 The drawing of July 1866, by the architect M. P. Manning, of the plan and elevation of the second building housing the National Hospital. This is the only known illustration of the interior plan of the building.

Furthermore, some of the domestic and sanitary arrangements in the 'New Hospital' were primitive. In February 1866, when the architect (Manning) and the building contractor opened up the drains for cleansing and repair, and attempted to trace their courses and connections, they 'Ascertained that part of the drainage passes through the adjoining premises, and part into a large cess-pool under the post-mortem room; there being no direct communication with any sewer or main drain.'

The architect's elevation drawing and plans of the hospital dated July 1866 give an impression of the façade, as well as a clear picture of the layout of the ground and first floor. Leaving aside the question of aesthetics, the main problem with the buildings was not their appearance but inadequate provision for the growing demands being made on the Charity for both in- and outpatient care. The Board of Governors, with its eye on development, then embarked on a further programme of property acquisition. The first buildings bought were several houses in Powis Place behind the hospital. Then, between 1865 and 1881, the freeholds of the remaining houses between numbers 22 and 32 Queen Square were purchased. Prince Leopold the Duke of Albany helped to acquire several of the houses and, after his death, the governors decided to name the wing in his memory.

The size of the hospital remained roughly constant for some years until in 1875, at the instance of Edward Chandler, an adjoining property, 25 Queen Square, was leased in order to establish an 'In Memoriam' wing for contributing patients, to commemorate Chandler's recently deceased sister Johanna, and formed an extension to David Wire ward. The 'In Memoriam' wing, opened in January 1876, contained another 15 beds, bringing the total number on the Queen Square site to 75,[38] and a vivid picture of the wing and its patients is drawn by Burford Rawlings:

> Painted in delicate and harmonious colours; the floor was covered with linoleum of handsome pattern; each patient was provided with a curtained cubicle; the bedsteads were of brass, lockers were of artistic design, a comfortable Axminster mat lay at every bedside, and the central table of the dormitory was a receptacle of groups of palms, and choice flowers. To the two day-rooms Mr Chandler presented valuable cabinets, the windows were corniced and curtained, the margins of the floors were polished, and there were carpets. The tenants of the wards were mostly educated ladies, the wives and daughters of clergymen, or men of the professional classes, governesses etc. They had the virtues and the defects of their quality; some were among the most amiable and considerate of patients,

gratefully appreciative of the care they received, and frank in acknowledgment. Others, while not wholly wanting in these recommendations, were exacting and prone to complain. They would set an undue value upon their contribution, and not only regard the nurses as their handmaidens, placed there to do their bidding, but were disposed to demand even of the physicians, a regularity and amplitude of service which, under existing conditions, no hospital rules could ensure, and no member of the staff would concede.[39]

The Building of the Salmon Pink (the Albany Memorial) and the Other Two Pavilions (the Powis Place and Princess Alexandra Pavilions)

The eastern side of Queen Square today is dominated by the façade of the National Hospital's Albany Memorial wing (the west wing), built of ornamented salmon pink terracotta and red brick in the then fashionable Queen Anne revival style – a rather undistinguished façade architecturally but which has, with the passage of time, become a familiar and well-loved part of the urban scene. The salmon pink building, with its large central massing and two wings, was something of a Trojan horse for the subsequent heterogeneous jumble of styles and materials that has since replaced other buildings in the square. It was one of three pavilions built around this time in the highly ambitious redevelopment of the National Hospital estate conceived in 1877 and completed between 1880 and 1885. The second pavilion (the east wing), the Powis Place block, also had a central entrance and two wings, in a vaguely French Renaissance architectural style. Between the two pavilions was a third block, the Princess Alexandra pavilion, built behind Queen Square House as a simplified and more vernacular version of the main hospital, with space left for airing courts and a garden. These new buildings occupied land on which previously were numbers 22–28 Queen Square and 6–9 Powis Place.

The idea of a much bigger hospital was clearly taking shape, at least in the minds of some Board members, by the late 1860s; and by mid-1877, the long-running problem of insufficient accommodation for the outpatients' clinic was perceived to have

---

[38] For the 'In Memoriam' wing, see the 14th annual report of the Board of Management (1874–5), pp. 23–4; the 15th annual report (1875–6), p. 9; and the prospectus for the 'In Memoriam' wing printed in the 15th annual report, at p. 30. From the outset, the 'In Memoriam' wing met with stiff opposition from the hospital medical staff, and, instead of generating a net income for the hospital, became a persistent drain on its financial resources and a source of conflict between Edward Chandler and the other members of Board.

[39] Burford Rawlings, *A Hospital in the Making* (London: Sir Isaac Pitman and Sons Ltd, 1913).

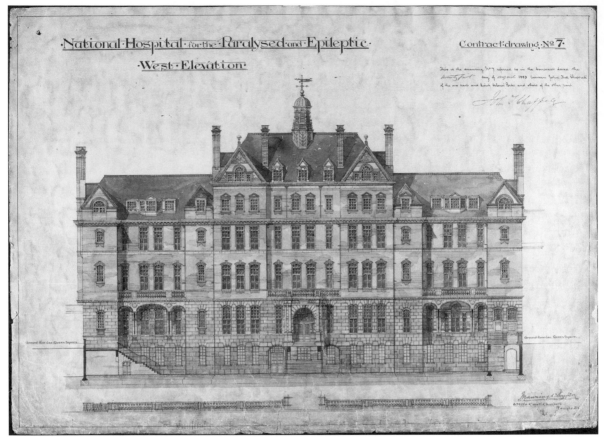

Figure 2.11 The contract drawing no. 7, by the architects Manning & Co., of the west elevation of the Albany wing, 1883.

reached a crisis. In their 16th annual report (1876–7), the Board of Management advised subscribers that 'The insufficient accommodation of the present Out-Patients' Department has become so manifest, and led to so great inconvenience, that the Board have under consideration the practicality of remedying [the] disadvantages which the growth of the Out-Patients' practice renders it more and more necessary to remove.' In June 1877, the Board asked Michael Manning 'to prepare plans for the adaptation of the houses in Powis Place to the requirements of the Out-Patients' department'. A subcommittee formed to examine the merits and demerits of the move met the architect and medical staff in May 1877.

However, in July 1877, Burford Rawlings reported back to the Board that, after careful consideration: 'the Architect had ... deemed the scheme impracticable', whereupon Burford Rawlings was instructed by the Board to carry out a much more

wide-ranging inquiry with local estate agents 'concerning [alternative] sites fit for the erection of a Hospital'. No records of the subcommittee's deliberations or the architect's advice have survived, and, in view of subsequent developments, it seems that Burford Rawlings took advantage of the situation in order to push the Board towards his own preferred solution – rebuilding the hospital on an ambitious scale with himself as project manager. Whatever the truth, in August 1877, Burford Rawlings presented his 'Report concerning a site for the future rebuilding of the Hospital' to a new four-man subcommittee appointed 'to consider and advise the Board as to the selection of a site for the rebuilding of the Hospital when such rebuilding shall be determined upon'. This plan was accepted by a majority vote of the full Board.

Burford Rawlings' report proved to be a key document in the Board's strategic decision to rebuild the entire hospital by enlarging the existing site in Queen

Square and Powis Place, which in turn was to have far-reaching effects on its subsequent development almost to the present day. The report contained five main conclusions and recommendations:

1. That no suitable alternative sites were available, or likely to become vacant in the near future, in the Bloomsbury area.

2. That 'an extension of the Queen Square site is practicable ... at a cost reasonable as a whole and less than I am told is the normal value of land in Central London'.

3. That the best way forward would therefore be: 'to purchase the several adjoining houses [25–27 Queen Square and 6–10 Powis Place] & to authorise the preparation of complete plans for ... rebuilding, such rebuilding to be in part immediate, and in a greater part deferred'.

4. That an immediate start should be made with numbers 7–10 Powis Place, 'which is sufficient to afford accommodation for the Out-patients' practice with ample room for its future expansion', as well as for an estimated 20 to 30 additional beds for acute cases on the upper floors.

5. That the space freed up in the existing hospital be reallocated: 'notably for the sleeping accommodation of nurses and attendants, whose health and comfort are now sacrificed to existing exigencies'.[40]

According to Burford Rawlings, the combined effect of these measures would be to enable a new hospital to be built with a total area of 22,500 square feet, sufficient to accommodate more than 180 beds; and the development in Powis Place would create a much expanded outpatients department of 4,250 square feet, increased from 1,400 square feet in the existing hospital. The total net cost of all the acquisitions proposed was estimated at £11,350 which, according to Burford Rawlings, was well within the total funds available to the hospital (about £14,000). However, a 'special appeal' would be needed to cover additional expenditure on the buildings themselves, and furnishing and equipment. What these unfunded costs might amount to, he declined to say.

These estimates proved optimistic, but it was largely on the basis of Burford Rawlings' report, as

recommended to the Board by three of the four members of the subcommittee (Edward Chandler dissenting), that the crucial decision was taken by the Board on 14 August 1877: 'The site for the future rebuilding of the Hospital shall be that now occupied with such additions as may be required' (Chandler once again opposing). Thereupon, the Board instructed the secretary to begin negotiations with the lease- and freeholders for the purchase of 6–8 Powis Place and 25–27 Queen Square for a sum not exceeding £9,800, with a further £2,700 to purchase the ground rents of 6–10 Powis Place.

In the event, although the broad outlines of the subsequent development did follow closely his recommendations of August 1877, the whole process took longer and cost much more than Burford Rawlings, who assumed the role of manager for the whole rebuilding project, had anticipated. One house, not specified, took a 'full nine years' to acquire, and others five to six years. The price was too high for some, and the condition of others very poor. But a fire in number 26, the business premises of Morris & Co. which encroached on the adjacent old hospital, concentrated the minds of the Board on the urgency of building new premises that would provide for the safety of patients.

Despite the fact that the purchase of the freehold of all the properties had not been fully secured, in November 1877 the Board further resolved, on the motion of John Netten Radcliffe,[41] to invite three

---

[40] 'Report Concerning a Site for the Future Rebuilding of the Hospital', in minutes of 14 August 1877, at pp. 49–53. The five recommendations are to be found at pp. 49–51.

[41] John Netten Radcliffe was the younger brother of Charles Bland Radcliffe. Surgeon and public health expert, he served in the Crimea and was medical superintendent of the National Hospital from 1867 to 1869, but was never appointed to the honorary consulting staff; he was subsequently public health inspector and assistant medical officer in the medical department of the Local Government Board. He was a universally respected doctor known particularly for his reports for the government on public health aspects of cholera and other infectious diseases, written at the behest of Sir John Simon who wrote a fulsome appreciation of Radcliffe on his death. Radcliffe was an important medical influence on the Board of Governors, and a key figure in the building project. For details of his life and work, see obituary notices in the *Lancet* **124** (1884): 524–525, 562–564, *British Medical Journal* (20 September 1884): 588 and *Dictionary of National Biography* (1896), Vol. **XLVII**, pp. 132–3. As well as Buzzard, Netten Radcliffe and his brother Charles Radcliffe, the building committee also included three lay Board members; its subcommittee consisted only of Buzzard and Netten Radcliffe, assisted periodically by Burford Rawlings. The fact that most of the

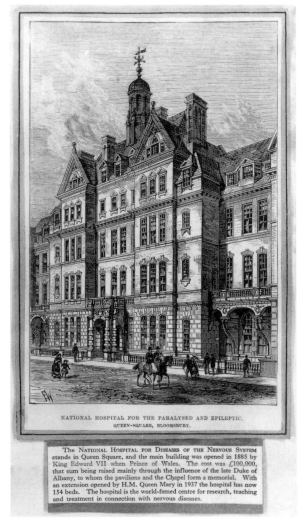

NATIONAL HOSPITAL FOR THE PARALYSED AND EPILEPTIC,
QUEEN-SQUARE, BLOOMSBURY.

The NATIONAL HOSPITAL FOR DISEASES OF THE NERVOUS SYSTEM stands in Queen Square, and the main building was opened in 1885 by King Edward VII when Prince of Wales. The cost was £100,000, that sum being raised mainly through the influence of the late Duke of Albany, to whom the pavilions and the Chapel form a memorial. With an extension opened by H.M. Queen Mary in 1937 the hospital has now 154 beds. The hospital is the world-famed centre for research, teaching and treatment in connection with nervous diseases.

Figure 2.12 Drawing of the Albany wing façade in 1885.

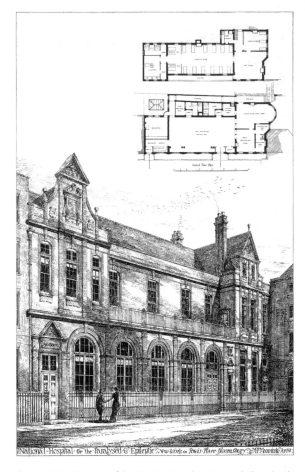

Figure 2.13 Drawing of the Powis wing elevation and plans, by the architects Manning & Co., 1879.

architects, one of whom was Manning, 'to prepare and submit plans for the entire rebuilding of the Hospital with accommodation for 150 In-patients', with an extra 25 beds in separate accommodation to be provided on the Powis Place site; and to invite the medical staff 'to meet … to [consider] … the proposed reconstruction of the Hospital, and to agree upon certain general instructions to the Architects for recommendation to the Board of Management'. The medical staff in turn appointed Gowers and

Buzzard 'to prepare a draft of instructions having reference to the medical portion of the proposed building', which they duly submitted in January 1878. Although most of their recommendations concerned the allocation of beds to different groups of patients and the nursing organisation in the new hospital, rather than any strictly architectural or planning matters, this consultation led to the formation of a building committee on which lay Board members and senior medical staff were represented.

Under the general direction of Netten Radcliffe, who also sought advice on architectural and sanitary matters from his colleagues at the Local Government Board, the building committee played an important role over the next four years in both the eventual choice of architect and the subsequent discussion and modification of the plans and designs for the

meetings of the building subcommittee were held in Netten Radcliffe's office at the Local Government Board in Whitehall, rather than in or near the hospital, is a strong indication of how much influence he had on development of the plans.

new hospital. The Board's 'Instructions to Architects' (undated, but probably finalised in May/June 1878), which incorporated various suggestions made by the medical staff, stipulated that, with respect to inpatients' accommodation, each ward was to consist of a dormitory and a day room, as in the existing hospital; the wards should contain 12 beds each; the minimum space was 1,200 cubic feet per patient in the dormitories, and 1,000 cubic feet in the day rooms; and the wards for male and female inpatients were entirely separated – if possible, in distinct buildings. With regard to the outpatient facilities, the waiting room should be large enough to accommodate at least 200 people in comfort; the physicians' consulting room must allow two physicians to see patients at the same time; and there should be three smaller rooms easily accessible from the physicians' consulting room for special examinations, including one for ophthalmoscopy examinations, another for microscopy, and the third for electrical and gymnastic treatment. Special consideration was also given to the position of the mortuary, 'which should be well lighted from above, and detached from the Hospital, and possess a room for pathological purposes in communication'. More generally, although the Board hoped for 'a simple and harmonious elegance of design', the architects were warned that 'all elaborate and useless ornamentation ... will receive emphatic condemnation'; and that 'as they are resolved to incur no expenditure beyond that which is needful ... their ultimate decisions respecting the plans submitted will be largely influenced by considerations of economy'. No stipulations were made as to either the architectural style of the buildings, or their size, grouping or internal layout. Although it was clearly understood that the new hospital would be built on the pavilion principle, this concept was not defined and no reference made to any existing hospital buildings by way of models for guidance or emulation.

In July 1878, the three invited architects duly submitted plans and drawings for the new hospital, which were then studied by the building committee and the medical staff for more than three months. Although there was relatively little to choose between the three plans in terms of cost or layout, it was hardly surprising that, in November 1878, following the joint recommendations of the medical staff and the building committee, the Board decided provisionally to accept Manning's designs, subject to detailed modification after further consultation. As well as enjoying the great advantage of having already known the hospital, its work and management for more than ten years, Manning's proposals were clearer, more attractively and professionally presented, and evinced a greater unity of design than did those of his competitors.[42] Moreover, although they did not wholly conform to the Board's strictures on unnecessary ornamentation, the 'Queen Anne' style of his drawings for the elevations struck a balance between simplicity and the sense of presence befitting an institution of the National Hospital's standing – one that was likely to appeal strongly to Burford Rawlings and the Board's collective sense of their self-importance and achievement.

Manning's original designs provided for 13 wards (6 male, 6 female, and one for special patients or children), each with 12 beds, making a total of 156 in the main hospital. As explained in his accompanying 'Report on the Design Submitted ... in planning the building I have, so far as the nature of the site and other circumstances permit, arranged wards on the "Pavilion" principle in order to secure on all sides light and air and ... ventilation'. The male wards were placed in the east wing and in the now demolished central (Princess Alexandra) pavilion of the hospital, and over the outpatients department in Powis Place. Female wards were all located in the west wing (the Albany Memorial wing) which also contained rooms for the Ladies' Samaritan Society, the matron and, in the attic, the female nurses and servants. As well as a dormitory and day room, each ward had a self-contained bathroom and water closets with hot and cold water, open fires and additional heating by hot water pipes. The east wing (the Powis Place wing) and central pavilion also housed the electrical and microscopy rooms, and gymnasium. A suite of special baths comprising 'Douche, Shower, Sitz, Needle, Turkish and other Baths' was provided in the basement. The outpatients' waiting hall on the ground floor of the Powis Place pavilion was 'large and lofty ... well ventilated and lighted by ample windows both back and front', although the building committee was soon to complain that it was not big enough and the ceiling too low.[43] The ground floor of

---

42 All have been retained in the hospital archives.

43 For Manning's own description of the outpatients' waiting hall, see his Report, p. 2, para. 6. For the building committee's criticisms, see minutes of Building Sub-Committee for 24 January 1879, n.p.

the Powis Place pavilion also housed the physicians' consulting rooms, each flanked by 'examination chambers' in which every 'needful accessory' was provided; a laboratory and the dispensary; and 'retiring rooms' and lavatories for male and female patients. The outpatient hall had room for 250 patients comfortably seated (in fact, 400 visitors were packed into it at the opening ceremony). The mortuary and post-mortem rooms were in the basement with their own separate entrance and staircase 'entirely detached and removed from the Hospital'. However, this arrangement was severely criticised by the building committee.

In the original plans, a lecture hall occupied much of the ground and first floors of the southern half of the west wing, behind the Board room; but, as eventually approved by the Board, this was replaced by a large and sumptuously decorated chapel. One feature typical of asylums for people with epilepsy, a small retiring room off the chapel for use in case a seizure occurred during a service, was absent. Curiously, for all Burford Rawlings' self-importance and exalted view of his role as the prime mover of the entire hospital, the secretary's office was a small ill-lit room in an awkward corner of the ground floor adjoining the Board room. It was less than half the size of the adjoining clerks' office and no bigger, and worse lit, than the former secretary's office had been in 24 Queen Square. Clearly mindful of the Board's strictures on ornamentation, Manning claimed that 'In the drawings of the Elevations of the Facades … the details are simple and effective, and serve to impart a suitable and distinctive appearance to the building without the use of any elaborate or expensive ornamental details.' Understandably, perhaps, he did not refer to the highly decorative (but now, alas, absent) cupola jauntily surmounting the central pavilion roof of the west wing. Manning's report estimated the total cost of the new buildings at approximately £30,000 (£24,100 for the main hospital, and a further £6,500 for the Powis Place pavilion), significantly less than the £37,000 that Burford Rawlings had been given to expect, but not even half the eventual cost of the completed project.[44]

Meanwhile, Burford Rawlings was at last succeeding in persuading the various residents and owners of the adjoining properties to sign over their rights to the National Hospital. All now seemed set fair for a successful inception of the rebuilding project. However, at this point the project became mired in a series of complex disputes among client, architect and contractors.

The building plans themselves were realised in several stages.[45] First, in July 1880, the Duke of Westminster laid the foundation stone of the new Powis Place wing. This was completed within a year at a total cost of £10,127, including furnishings and fittings. It was opened by, and named after, HRH Princess Christian of Schleswig-Holstein. After something of a hiatus, and despite the Duke of Albany's public announcement in March 1882 that the hospital intended to proceed with reconstruction and enlargement of the main building as soon as possible, not until June–July 1883 were Manning's plans and designs put out to tender, and contracts signed with Messrs Chappell & Phipson. In the second stage, work began on the Princess Alexandra pavilion in August 1883, with completion in December 1884. The third and final stage in the building of the west wing, housing 160 beds, was begun early in 1884 and completed in May 1885. In these building works, 22–28 Queen Square and 6–9 Powis Place were demolished, and a large tablet in the entrance hall of the new hospital recalls that 'For 25 years its work was carried on in old houses situated on a portion of this site.'[46] All three stages were complicated by a series of increasingly bitter disputes involving Manning, Burford Rawlings and John T. Chappell, the principal building contractor, who at one point threatened to abandon the project. Eventually these were resolved and the works were completed more or less on time, thanks in large measure to 'the unusually favourable [weather] conditions which prevailed during the two years the building operations were in progress'.

In the Board of Management's annual report for 1883–4, Burford Rawlings described the rebuilding

---

[44] Between 1881 and 1884, Manning was in partnership with (Sir) John William Simpson (1858–1933), a distinguished architect who became president of the Royal Institute of British Architects. Simpson is often credited with the final plans, in collaboration with Manning, although the nature of their collaboration in regard to the hospital buildings is not known.

[45] The whole complex sequence of the hospital rebuilding works is set out at some length in *Report Upon the Rebuilding with Statement of Receipts and Expenditure, and List of Contributors* (London: Chiswick Press, 1888), pp. 7–9.

[46] The plaque is still *in situ*.

works, a high point in the first 50 years of the hospital's history, as 'the great undertaking to which all that has gone before has in a sense been but a prelude and a preparation', and declared that 'the erection of the New Hospital will mark a fresh era in the study and treatment of ... [nervous] disease'. The hospital was praised for being the first to be built along 'artistic lines', and the façade of the Albany Memorial wing, together with remnants of its fine Victorian interiors,[47] survive as a monument to Victorian lay and medical philanthropy. When first completed, the new building proclaimed the hospital to be among the foremost medical charities of the metropolis. In spite of delayed starts, some major cost over-runs, and fierce arguments and threats of litigation among client, architect and contractors, the whole project had been completed more or less on time and without reducing the Charity to penury, as Edward Chandler (and possibly other Board members and governors) had feared. Indeed, in their official report on the rebuilding of the hospital, published in July 1888, the Board announced that, uniquely in hospital annals, the cost of the building and equipment had already been collected through philanthropic contributions, and declared that

> Among all the noble philanthropic gifts which the Victorian age transmits to posterity, few will transcend the first hospital devoted to the treatment and investigation of those obscure maladies which, while they have been amongst the mysteries of all ages, have gained great and terrible intensity in the present, and it may be safely predicted that the National Hospital will remain a prominent example of utility and practical benevolence.[48]

Interestingly Burford Rawlings informs us that nearly half of the total sum needed was raised from only 23 individuals, and the total number of contributors barely exceeded 1,000.

Notwithstanding his lack of any previous experience of large-scale construction project management, Burford Rawlings had not only originated the whole project but also steered it from start to finish, and the bizarre and contentious new title 'Secretary and General Director' conferred on him by the Board in January 1885, shortly before the official opening of the new hospital, must at the time have seemed no more than just recognition of his apparent all-conquering presence and competence. In the year in which *The Mikado* was first performed, even Gilbert and Sullivan could hardly have imagined a more multi-talented and omnipotent officer.

Completion of the new hospital was celebrated by a grand and prestigious opening ceremony on 4 July 1885.[49] The building was opened by the Prince of Wales (later King Edward VII) and the future Queen Alexandra, in the company of other members of the royal family, the Archbishop of Canterbury, the Prince and Princess Christian of Schleswig-Holstein, Lord Halsbury (Lord Chancellor and future Board member), the presidents of the Royal Colleges of Physicians and Surgeons, and 1,000 guests, 'many eminent in the ranks of philanthropy and science'.[50] The final *Report Upon the Rebuilding, with Statement of Receipts and Expenditures, and List of Contributors*, published by the hospital three years later, described the event in glowing terms, and painted a rosy picture of the financial position and future prospects once all debts had been settled.

However, very Surprisingly, Burford Rawlings' own evaluation of the outcome was distinctly ambivalent and even tinged with regret for missed opportunities. Although he claimed that 'the new buildings have now [as of 1888] been occupied long enough to allow of a definite judgment as to their suitability, and the verdict is wholly favourable', he conceded that 'The rapid progress of science in regard to the treatment of nervous maladies ... has within the past two or three years made so great and unforeseen additions

---

[47] Notably those of the entrance hall and main staircase, with its Victorian stained-glass windows in memory of the Chandler sisters, the chapel, and the former Board room with its rich wood panelling.

[48] *Report Upon the Rebuilding*, p. 11. The report, which speaks with the collective voice of the Board of Management, is unsigned but, as is apparent from the foreword, Burford Rawlings was almost certainly the author, and the 'Report of the Board of Management to the Contributors to the Building Fund' on pp. 6–11 is signed by him.

[49] There is a plaque still in place in the entrance hall of the hospital commemorating the opening of the hospital and the dedication of the Albany wing to the late Prince Leopold the Duke of Albany.

[50] The official opening ceremony by the Prince and Princess of Wales, with the names of the other principal guests of honour, is described in detail in the '*Report upon the Rebuilding*' as are further details of the then patrons of the National Hospital, who now included Queen Victoria herself, as well as the Prince of Wales and five other leading members of the royal family.

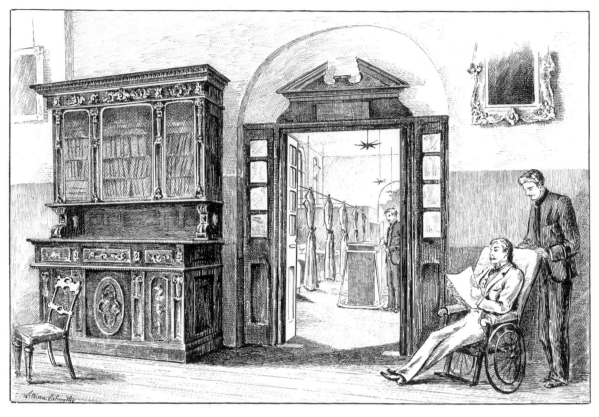

Figure 2.14 Drawing, by Lillian C. Smythe, of the day room of Princess Christian Ward, a paying ward for men, *c.* 1900.

to the surgical work, that it may be regretted [that] the new building does not contain certain accommodation which undoubtedly would be provided were the designs now being prepared.'

It was not merely the lack of adequate facilities for neurosurgical operations that worried Burford Rawlings. As his *Report upon the Rebuilding* acknowledged, the acquisition of the land and property necessary to implement the decision to rebuild the hospital on the Queen Square site had proved very costly. At some stage, Burford Rawlings seems to have concluded that rebuilding on the old site had been a mistake. In November 1881, he informed the Board of Management that the Great Northern Railway Company had been given permission to build a railway extension southwards from King's Cross through the west side of the square – a development which, had it come to pass, would have completely destroyed the relative tranquility and seclusion of the hospital's physical setting and made any further expansion on the Queen Square site almost impossible. Even though

this potential catastrophe failed to materialise, Burford Rawlings himself came to have doubts about the suitability of Queen Square for future expansion and, had he not been forced out of office in 1901, might well have tried to steer the Board of Management towards his preferred policy of long-term expansion at the convalescent home in Finchley.

In the end, the total cost for acquisition and rebuilding was around £90,000, and the project had severely depleted the hospital's finances. The Board was not able to open all the new wards until 1888 and, by the time all the new accommodation was commissioned, the hospital was once again full. A small new operating theatre/lecture theatre and associated facilities were provided in 1891, in what was known as the Westminster wing, but this proved unsatisfactory for the purpose. The room was changed into the pathology department and, in 1904, a new but equally inadequate operating theatre was constructed. The Board spent a good deal of time fruitlessly trying to persuade the Foundling Hospital estate to make over some of its

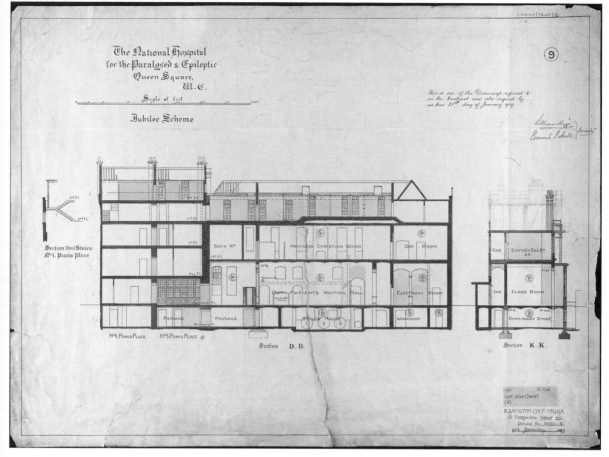

Figure 2.15 Contract drawing no. 9, by the architect R. Langton Cole, of the Powis Place Jubilee scheme renovation, showing the arrangement of rooms in two sections of the building, 1909.

property in order to expand the outpatient facilities and provide more accommodation and better social amenities for the nurses; but, with the exception of rebuilding and enlarging the convalescent branch at Finchley between 1894 and 1895, no further major expansion of the National Hospital estate took place until well into the twentieth century.

Further Development of the Hospital Estate between 1909 and 1950, and the Building of the Queen Mary Wing

Over time, slowly and progressively numerous relatively small-scale modifications and redevelopments replaced the interior layout and structure. As a result, the atmosphere of the original hospital has now been almost completely lost. Only the hallway, the rather grand staircase with stained glass windows, the chapel and the old Board room in the Albany Memorial

wing are undisturbed. Here briefly the most important of these occurring between 1909 and 1950 are listed.

In 1909, during the Jubilee celebrations of the hospital, money was donated to enlarge the outpatient hall, to provide additional consulting rooms, and provide the dispensary with a small manufacturing pharmacy.[51] A lift was installed, and a home created with separate bedrooms for each nurse. In addition, the electrical department and space for ophthalmic and aural examinations were greatly enlarged.[52] These

---

[51] The architect of the Jubilee wing, the operating theatre that opened in 1904, the buildings at Finchley and other small projects throughout the hospital in the first decades of the twentieth century was Robert Langton Cole. He was listed as 'the hospital architect' in the annual reports between 1901 and 1926.

[52] Details from *The National Illustrated* (see Chapter 5, note 29); and Hamilton, *Queen Square* (1926).

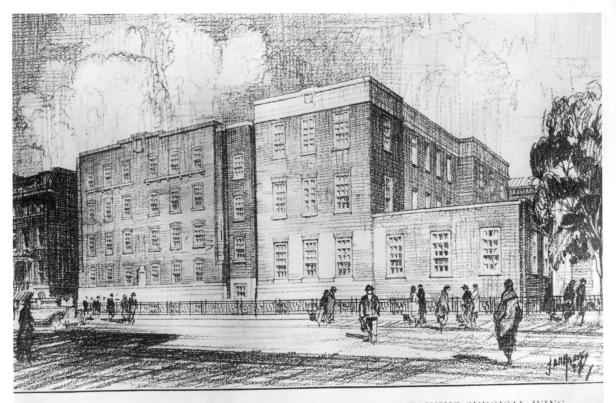

PROPOSED EXTENSION OF THE NATIONAL HOSPITAL, CONTAINING SURGICAL WING,
PATHOLOGICAL AND RESEARCH LABORATORY, ETC.

Figure 2.16 Drawing of the Guilford Street frontage of the proposed extension of the National Hospital, which was to house the surgical wing and the pathology and research laboratories, and the nurses' home, designed by A. H. Moberly but never built.

new facilities were opened by King Edward VII in October 1909. A department for medical gymnastics, 'which is one of the best in London', was the start of a long and distinguished tradition of physiotherapy at the hospital.

Improvements made to the hospital structure over these years included the provision of a sunken pool in the garden, which was then at the centre of the hospital. Designation of the wards changed frequently, and the provision of a day room for the patients, much praised at the time of construction and considered a model for other hospitals, was sacrificed. In the period immediately after the Second World War, the main development was the creation of the Lysholm radiology department in the attic storey in the Albany Memorial wing.

In 1926, the possibility arose of purchasing Queen Square House and numbers 47–50 Guilford Street, as their owners, the Foundling Estate, were relocating out of London. On several occasions between 1860 and 1888, the Board had expressed the wish to own Queen Square House and the opportunity was welcomed. The price was £32,000 and plans were drawn up to build a new surgical wing, pathology laboratories and a nurses' home on the site. A. H. Moberly[53] was commissioned, and his drawing of the proposed building exists showing a fine and solid construction. Sadly, the purchase was never completed and the proposed new wing not built; it was only in 1953 that the opportunity to acquire the property again presented itself, and on that occasion the hospital made sure of the purchase.

The next major rebuilding project was the Queen Mary wing, completed in June 1938 and opened by the Queen. The architectural firm Slater, Moberly and

---

[53] The architect who later designed the Queen Mary wing.

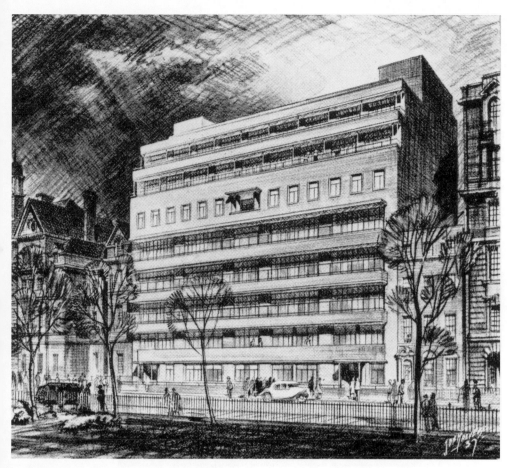

Figure 2.17 Drawing of the Queen Mary wing in 1937.

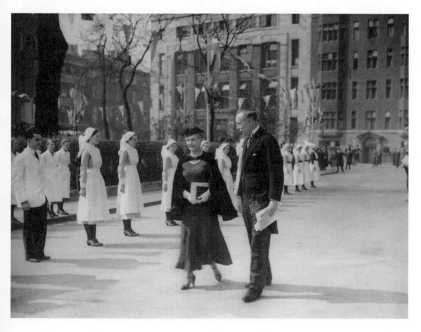

Figure 2.18 The laying of the foundation stone of the Queen Mary wing, on 30 April 1937, by Princess Alice, Countess of Athlone.

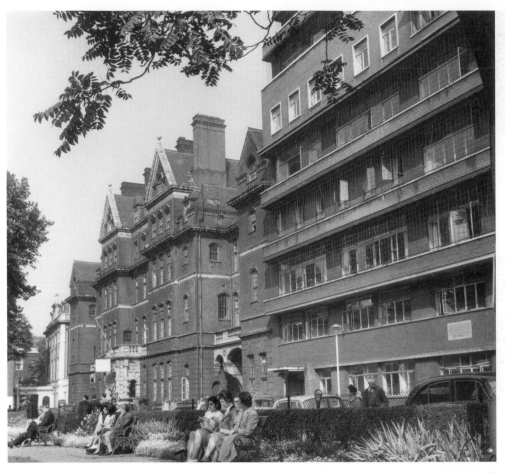

Figure 2.19 The east side of Queen Square in the late 1950s, showing the Queen Mary wing, the main hospital façade and Queen Square House and its portico (soon to be demolished).

Uren[54] designed the building with its sleek horizontal brick bands, which are quiet and rather distinguished compared with its noisy pink neighbour. On the façade, above the doors, are two splendid stone sculptured panels by A. J. Ayres,[55] representing

research and healing.[56] The staircase and many original features remain and have endured well – and, indeed, rather better than some of the later works. The addition of the wing resulted in a change of orientation within the main building, and connecting corridors were built on several levels. The *Architectural Review*[57] remarked that, given the extremely varied usage of each floor, the building required

---

[54] Slater and Moberly were Scottish architects, while Reginald Uren was a New Zealander. Prior to this, Uren had won professional and critical acclaim as the architect of Hornsey town hall in Crouch End, north London, and, subsequently, the successor firm of Slater, Uren and Pike were to become well known as the designers of the John Lewis store in Oxford Street, the former Peter Jones store in Sloane Square, and the former Arthur Sanderson building in Berners Street, W1.

[55] A. J. Ayres worked frequently with the same architectural firm, adding similar sculptural panels, for instance, to Hornsey and Hammersmith town halls. He was a remarkable architectural sculptor, with work in Westminster Abbey and many churches, and the teacher of Anthony Caro.

[56] Healing has Aesclepius' staff, with the correct single serpent, being handed to mankind by the hand of God. Research has an open book displaying the words 'Every addition to true knowledge is an addition to human power' – a quote from Horace Mann, the American educational reformer and abolitionist. Why this particular quote was chosen is unclear.

[57] Anon., 'Extension to the National Hospital to Accommodate New Surgical and Research Departments; Architects: Slater, Moberly & Uren', *Architectural Review* (1938): 99–102.

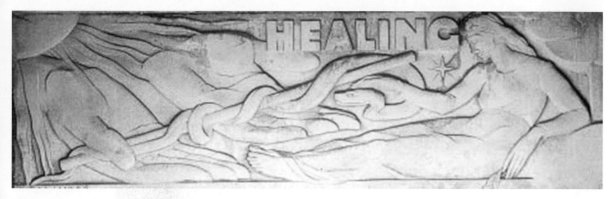

Figure 2.20a Healing. The sculptural panel by A. J. Ayres over the doorway of Queen Mary wing.

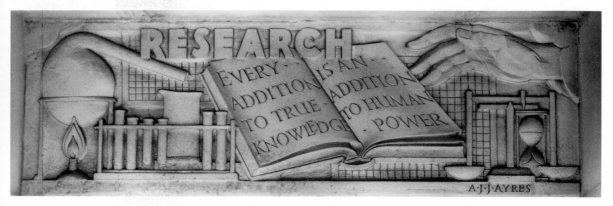

Figure 2.20b Research. The sculptural panel by A. J. Ayres over the doorway of Queen Mary wing.

a complex system of electrical, plumbing and other services concealed in each vertical stanchion. It also noted that the building was faced with 'very hard brick of less obtrusive colour than that of some of its neighbours' (certainly the colour is much more harmonious than Manning's salmon pink). The research department was renamed the 'Institute for the Teaching and Study of Neurology'. It included, on the ground and first floors and in the basement of the new building, consultation rooms, a library, a reading room, space for students, classrooms and laboratories. The clinical area provided four-bedded bays for wards on the second, third and fourth floors, single- and three-bedded bays on the sixth and seventh floors, and two air-conditioned operating theatres on the fifth floor (not at the top as would have been preferred, because of the loss of space from the set-back of the façade). The wards had large folding–sliding windows, opening onto the square, and light metal grilles for security, which are still in place. The basement contained Christian and Jewish chapels, the post-mortem room and various services. The lecture theatre – amphitheatre-style and

later designated the Wolfson lecture theatre – was constructed on the ground and first floors behind the main block.

The building was made possible by a large donation from the Rockefeller Foundation (£120,000 – of which £60,000 was an endowment for research and £60,000 was for buildings and equipment), made on the understanding that the hospital would match this sum.[58] A highly successful fund-raising campaign for this £120,000 was launched and the sum easily reached.[59]

---

[58] The operating theatres and surgical wards were provided with the hospital's share of the funding, as the Rockefeller Foundation pointed out that they did not provide funds for clinical care, but for research, and would only allow this use if the hospital took responsibility for upkeep and these building costs.

[59] The Rockefeller grant was of the greatest importance to Queen Square. It marked a watershed in the hospital's fortunes, and a significant change in its attitude to research and its strategy in relation to neurosurgery. These points are discussed in more detail later in this book.

The laboratories were fully equipped and staffed just before war broke out in September 1939. This put an end to all neurological research; and during the war the laboratories were used by the War Office and the Admiralty for studies of medical problems associated with war.

1950–1976: Rebuilding Queen Square House and the Failed Postwar Development of Queen Square

In the immediate postwar period, another set of extravagant plans to increase the hospital footprint was advanced, but these plans were frustrated in a tortuous serious of negotiations over several decades and never fully realised. As it turned out, with the rapidly rising cost of land and redevelopment, and the recurrent financial crises of the National Health Service, the pace of development seen in the nineteenth century could not be repeated. Plans for rebuilding during the middle years of the twentieth century were also thwarted by bureaucracy, prevarication, planning blight and disastrous labour relations – together forming rather a depressing reflection on Britain in the postwar period.

What was also lacking was the vision and spirit of the original founders and, throughout the 1960s and 1970s, much of the management time was taken up with tortuous discussions around the redevelopment. Despite receiving high priority, these plans were relentlessly pared down. The confusion and delay of this building project are in stark contrast to the rapid completion of construction of the hospital in the 1880s.

A redevelopment plan was first tabled in 1959, in an outline memorandum submitted to the Department of Health, in which it was proposed that the building should take place in two phases at an estimated cost of £1.35 million. This was a time of significant rebuilding projects throughout the National Health Service and each of the three major political parties had made reference in their 1959 election manifestos to renewed hospital construction. The new Minister of Health, Enoch Powell, had announced in 1960 that he would launch a ten-year building plan; and it was in this climate of optimism that the National Hospital made its bid, confident that this would be accepted. In 1962, Enoch Powell's plan for hospital building in England and Wales was presented to Parliament[60] and plans for the

redevelopment of Queen Square gathered pace. This was initially proposed as due to take place in two stages: phase 1 was the construction of a new building for the Institute of Neurology, in collaboration with the University of London, on the site of Queen Square House. This was planned together with the establishment of the first professorship of clinical neurology and is notable as the first time that plans for redevelopment were predicated on academic not clinical grounds – a pattern that became firmly established later in the century. Phase 2 was to be a complex rearrangement which involved taking over the Homoeopathic Hospital, the closing down of Maida Vale Hospital (or at least converting it to a convalescent home) and the merging of the infrastructure and beds of Maida Vale with those of the National Hospital in a completely new building on an enlarged site at Queen Square (known as the island site).

The reasons for redevelopment were summarised in the surprisingly vague 16-page memorandum prepared in 1959 and sent to the Ministry of Health and the University of London, by the Board of Governors.[61] It is worth quoting at length for it is a vision that underpins much of what happened subsequently in a convoluted series of forward and backward steps. The memorandum started with a familiar 'justification' of the hospital (much as had been periodically rolled out in previous times):

> The National Hospitals [now a plural, as the hospitals at Queen Square and Maida Vale were merged in 1948] are the great neurological school of the English speaking world, and … at the time of the outbreak of the war there was hardly a neurologist in the English speaking countries who had not spent some time in the hospital. As these neurologists have returned, either to their own hospitals in this country or to centres abroad, they have carried with them the Queen Square tradition.

The threefold purpose of the hospital was then laid out:

> First to serve as a clinical centre with the greatest concentration of material and facilities and be a training centre for clinical neurologists; secondly to

---

[60]   *A Hospital Plan for England and Wales* (London: HMSO, 1962). Also: Hansard, *The Hospital Plan*, HL Deb 14 February 1962, vol. 237, cols. 472–581. The plan was predicated on a

marked shift from inpatient to outpatient care, and a predicted fall in the number of beds nationally from 150,000 in 1961 to 80,000 16 years later. Powell was particularly keen to see the closure of mental institutions – as he put it, 'There they stand, isolated, majestic, imperious, brooded over by the giant water tower and chimney combined, rising unmistakable and daunting out of the countryside.'

[61]   Minutes of meeting of the Board of Governors for 3 December 1959.

provide a centre for research in new techniques and in the prevention and treatment of neurological disease; and thirdly, to serve as a consultative centre for peripheral units in neurology and general medicine and surgery to whom a range of clinical and research facilities are not available.

The inclusion of research was a sign of how much had changed with respect to the attitude of the hospital to academic work, compared with earlier development plans. The memorandum explained that, in order to achieve these objects, the National Hospitals, along with the Institute of Neurology, must be furnished with academic departments in the major branches of neurology with accommodation for new techniques such as histochemistry, which could be applied to the diagnosis and study of neurological disease. It also emphasised the importance of

> Concentration of clinical material and facilities [which] will make for maintenance of the standard of diagnostic precision required in neurological disease by providing consultants with wide clinical experience and with the invaluable stimulus of the interplay of the critical opinions of several colleagues. … the extensive clinical material will provide unrivalled training for future neurologists, a training they could not obtain in the special department of a general hospital with one or at the most two neurologists.

The memorandum emphasised that, without new space, extension of the current services was impossible and new initiatives would be limited. An outstanding example was the treatment of epilepsy, which had been the subject of a recent government report.[62] It was pointed out that the lack of beds had frustrated attempts to raise the standard of medical care as recommended in the report, and that 'surgery [for epilepsy] is almost non-existent in this country and our attempts to develop it have been hampered by lack of beds and lack of operating time. Of the 1073 new patients with epilepsy who attended as outpatients in 1958, only 212 secured admission (and only 50% of those with epilepsy resulting from tumours).' Similar problems were reported in the stereotactic treatment of Parkinson's disease and acute head injury. The emphasis was on expansion to meet the demands of teaching, as recommended in the Goodenough report.

Ironically, emphasis placed on the inefficiencies of dividing services at Maida Vale from Queen Square ('separated by four miles of busy London streets') contrast with views expressed ten years earlier when the National Hospital objected strongly to merger with Maida Vale.

Together, the new plan provided 68,150 square feet, of which 35,450 was for the care of patients and teaching, and approximately 32,700 for laboratories. The plan was for a total of 280 beds for the National Hospitals (Queen Square had then 207 and Maida Vale 85), and 80 for the academic units, including 20 for a unit of neuropsychiatry; and outpatient accommodation for 60,000 attendances per year. It was noted that running costs would benefit from uniting the two hospitals on one site (although details were very sparse). An additional 7,500 square feet was to be provided by additions to the existing buildings and staff accommodation in Queen Court and on the north side of Guilford Street; and for good measure 300 convalescent beds were to be placed at Finchley. In 1953, the Board of Governors obtained the freehold of Queen Square House using endowments, and this was then sold to the Ministry of Health as part of the development plan.

The new Queen Square House was planned to include academic clinical units in neurology, neurosurgery and neuropsychiatry (including wards, laboratories and offices), and the ancillary departments of neuroradiology and electroencephalography, with extra space for the academic departments of neuropathology and chemical pathology, moved from their present cramped quarters, thus providing both diagnostic services and research facilities with sub-departments of neuroanatomy and neuropharmacology. The architects Richard Llewelyn Davies[63] and John Weeks were commissioned to oversee the work.

By May 1961, it was reported to the Board of Governors that the estimated costs were now: phase 1 – Queen Square House, £600,000 building and £84,000 furnishing and equipment; phase 2 – Homoeopathic site, £500,000 and £45,000 furnishing and equipment, and £1,000,000 for renovation of the

---

62 Central Health Services Council, *Ministry of Health Medical Care of Epileptics: Report of the Sub-Committee of the Central Health Services Council* (London: HMSO, 1956) (Chairman: Lord Henry Cohen).

63 Richard Llewelyn Davies (created a life peer in 1964) was professor of architecture at the Bartlett Institute of UCL, and an expert in urban planning and hospital building (among his buildings were the Nuffield Institute in Regents Park, and Northwick Park Hospital – both with a striking resemblance to Queen Square House). He was the chief architect of Milton Keynes.

original site and £90,000 for furnishing and equipment. Staff accommodation, rebuilding and acquisition of freeholds of adjacent property would be an additional £428,000. The total sum therefore now exceeded £2.5 million.

This was indeed an ambitious plan and initially the Ministry of Health only accepted it on a provisional basis. The hospital hoped that building would start in 1961, but the project became entangled by a series of complications. The root cause seems to have been reluctance of the Ministry to part with funds, but other hurdles were being created and the situation was also complicated by alternative options. External discussions were underway about the role of the London postgraduate hospitals more generally, and especially as to whether these should continue as stand-alone institutions, be grouped together, or be attached to and absorbed into larger teaching hospitals. The advantages of stand-alone hospitals were their ability to focus on one type of medicine, their *esprit de corps* and the concentration of expertise. Their disadvantage was intellectual isolation, faced with the fact that, as medicine was becoming more interconnected, expensive resources were best shared. Sir George Pickering, Regius professor of medicine in Oxford, was asked for advice, and he came down strongly on the side of grouping the postgraduate hospitals. This was also the view of Keith Murray, chairman of the UGC. Internally, too, voices were heard in support of this proposal. Sir Charles Symonds, in his introduction to the 1954–5 annual report of the Institute, defending the role of the special hospitals, wrote:

> I envisage in the remote future instead of Queen Square, Maida Vale, Moorfields, Great Ormond Street, Queen Charlotte's and so on, a single large post-graduate institution for teaching and research that will include them all, and in addition its own departments of Anatomy, Physiology, Biochemistry and Pathology, with appropriate Chairs. This, however, is a dream of Utopia.

In 1960, Wyllie McKissock wrote to the Board of Governors that there may be an opportunity to rebuild the hospitals on the site of the Western Fever Hospital at Seagrave Road, Fulham. This was followed by a letter from Sir Francis Fraser (the then director of the British Postgraduate Medical Federation (BPMF)) proposing that three of the special hospitals and their institutes might move to that site, creating an unparalleled medical enclave.[64]

Promotional material was produced to support the proposal, including a film of the site taken from a helicopter. The cost would be covered, it was proposed, by sale of the current hospital land. This diversion had the potential to postpone rebuilding on the Queen Square site for years and was not likely to be welcomed, but the chairman of the Board wrote to the Minister acknowledging that 'it is an imaginative idea and has very great possibilities ... [but] should not delay work already underway on QSH ... I want to keep a foot in both camps.' The plan came to nothing, not least because the proposed site in Fulham was not for sale. Another plan to group four to six of the special hospitals together also faltered. On 2 May 1961, the Ministry wrote to the hospital accepting that the idea of bringing all the postgraduate hospitals together was impractical.

In the meantime, a working party had been set up at Queen Square in 1961 by the Committee of Management of the Institute of Neurology, comprising Kremer (Chair), Blackwood, Cumings, Gilliatt, Henson and McMenemey, to assess the space requirements of each department. By that time, academic ambitions had increased and the initial rebuilding plans were deemed inadequate. Academic departments of neurology, neuropathology and chemical pathology had been developed. The next urgent priority was to establish further academic departments of neurosurgery and psychiatry; and departments for neurophysiology, neuroanatomy and functional anatomy, experimental pathology and immunology, genetics and epidemiology, and virology were also envisaged. Those developments apart, adequate provision would also be needed for administration, animal housing, central workshops and electron microscopy.[65]

---

[64] This proposal is also mentioned in Francis Walshe's letter to Denny-Brown dated August 1960.

[65] The space to be allocated in the phase 1 plans amounted to a total of 48,800 square feet, leaving 21,200 square feet for circulation space (within the 70,000 square feet of the new Queen Square House). This included: 4,000 square feet each for the proposed departments of clinical neurology, neurosurgery, and psychiatry and psychology; 9,500 square feet for the department of neuropathology (including a museum); 7,500 square feet for the department of neuroanatomy and functional anatomy; 5,000 square feet for the department of neurophysiology; 5,000 square feet for the departments of experimental pathology and immunology; 3,000 square feet for the department of virology; and 1,000

It was now estimated that, in phase 2, the National Hospital would need around 300 beds,[66] and that the outpatient department should provide for 60,000 visits a year (including 9,000 new patients).[67] Adequate space would also be needed for radiography, electro-encephalography, physical medicine, a dispensary, almoners, psychiatric social workers, a library for patients, a chapel, medical records, catering, a works department, linen room and stores, plus space for the nursing school, medical typing office, supplies department, accounts, central sterilising, and hostel and resident staff accommodation. Since there was insufficient space on the current Queen Square site, buildings in the vicinity would have to be purchased. The plan crucially depended on acquisition of the Homeopathic Hospital site, and so the Board was dismayed in July 1961 to hear that the Homeopathic Hospital had been allocated a grant of £200,000 for 'improvements'.

Genuine progress on redevelopment was made when the Ministry of Health agreed to purchase 14 properties in Guilford Street at a cost of £123,000. These were needed to allow the decanting of staff from their existing Queen Square accommodation as a prelude to phase 2 redevelopment, and the hospital had its eye on other adjacent properties in Guilford Street, Glanville Street and the Colonnade. Most had been in private hands since 1947 and in poor states of repair but, slowly, over the next ten years or so, they had been purchased by the National Hospital, the Ministry of Health or the Chartered Society of Queen Square, and held for the benefit of the hospital; or by the University of London with a loan guaranteed by the hospital. These arrangements involved a complex set of financial manoeuvres fraught with frustrating hurdles and delays but, by 1976, the National Hospital owned, leased or had the use of 64–82

Guilford St, 13–17 Grenville Street and 11–23 Colonnade. Attempts were also made to persuade the owners of Queen Court to sell to the hospital. Their refusal had a long-term and detrimental effect. Despite this activity, plans for extensive renovation of the houses in Guilford Street never materialised and, as these properties continued to deteriorate, large sums were spent on minor repairs.

In 1963, despite the fact that it had approved net expenditure of £996,000, the Ministry then informed the hospital that it was not now prepared to start phase 1 until an outline of phase 2 had also been agreed. They suggested therefore a revised starting date for phase 1 in 1966. Thus began a series of prevarications which resulted ultimately in the total failure to enact any of the phase 2 proposals.

In February 1963, the architects (Llewelyn Davies & Weeks and John Musgrove Associates) produced a paper, in response to their discussions with the London County Council in which they were informed that the policy for hospitals in the central London region was that the 'plot ratio' (the gross floor area of the buildings divided by the area of the land) should be around 2:1, with a ratio of 3:1 as the absolute maximum. The plot ratio of plans for phase 2 (even assuming that these included the Homoeopathic Hospital, Queen Court, 25 Queen Square, Alexandra House and 12 Queen Square) exceeded 3:1; and even if 8–11 and 13–15 Queen Square were included in the calculation, the ratio still exceeded 2.5:1. The architects therefore suggested that it would be necessary to extend the hospital's boundaries, and that would require major road alterations.[68] One solution proposed was that Queen Square itself could be turned around at right angles, so that its long axis stretched west of Powis Place (with no loss of area), the hospital being rebuilt on the north side with the extra space reducing the plot ratio below 2.5. Not surprisingly, such a radical plan came to nothing.

On 30 September 1963, Enoch Powell met with the chairmen of the postgraduate hospitals – the Eastman Dental, Royal National Orthopaedic, Moorfields, Royal National ENT, Great Ormond Street and the National Hospitals. He outlined a new plan to group the special postgraduate hospitals into two clusters, one based in Holborn near UCL and the other in the Fulham road near Imperial College (the so-called Holborn and Chelsea clusters). The University of

---

square feet each for the departments of isotopes, genetics and epidemiology; 600 square feet for animal houses; and 800 square feet for lecture theatres. The Institute offices, student accommodation and library were proposed to be housed in Alexandra House.

[66] Initially five neurology firms of 30 beds each, 30 beds for the university department of clinical neurology, 20 beds for the academic department of psychiatry and psychology, 60 beds for neurosurgery, 5 beds for neuro-otology, and 10 private beds.

[67] Outpatient space would be needed for one large teaching room (with side room), three smaller teaching rooms (with side rooms), six other consulting rooms and two special consulting rooms for ENT and ophthalmology.

---

[68] The architects pointed out that there was already a precedent for this in the case of St Thomas' Hospital.

London had agreed in principle to this two-site solution in 1961, but the practical problems of finding a location for development, decanting and relocation of existing accommodation were too great and the costs rapidly seen as prohibitive. Powell was then replaced as Minister of Health in October 1963 by Anthony Barber. He visited Queen Square to discuss redevelopment and suggested selling the Finchley site to pay for developments, but this was opposed due to independent plans to provide facilities there for young chronic sick and some epilepsy patients as recommended by the Cohen Committee.[69] Planning consent was another source of frustration on a number of occasions. For instance, the hospital sought to buy 2 Queen Square as an educational therapy centre for dyslexic children, but the London County Council refused planning permission for this development. There was also a tree preservation order brought by the Borough of Camden for the sycamore at the rear of 13 Grenville Street and an ash tree behind 80 Guilford Street.

In 1964, a further option for reconfiguration was proposed – the possibility of redeveloping Great Ormond Street and the National Hospital together on the Queen Square site. Although this was a departure from the original phase 2 plan, the Institute of Neurology and the National Hospital started to consult with Great Ormond Street and drew up a plan which initially included shared research facilities with the MRC Clinical Genetics Research Unit.

These machinations occurred at a time when the country's financial position was seriously deteriorating and it had become clear that the government's original hospital plans were now unaffordable. The new Labour government of Harold Wilson, in place from October 1964, was faced with an economic crisis, and revised plans were then received by the Board of Governors, in which reference was made only to phase 1, to take place between 1964–5 and 1968–9, but with no mention of phase 2. The new Minister of Health, Kenneth Robinson, wrote to the Board on 14 May 1965, with reference to the central London services: 'There would have to be a much greater degree of coordination of planning in this area than exists at present and this would inevitably involve, in due course, some reduction in the autonomy of the Board of Governors.' A visit by the Minister on 26

June 1965 confirmed that it was not possible to approve the hospital development at that time.

By 1966, the Board of Governors had been informed that the planned start of rebuilding would be delayed until 1968 due to a national review of spending by the government, but finally, in 1967, agreement to proceed with phase 1 at least was given, and, at a meeting on 14 April, the Department of Health agreed to purchase Queen Square House, owned by the endowment fund of the Board of Governors, for £35,000. The estimated cost of phase 1 was now £1,890,700, with space increased to 98,513 square feet – larger than the original January 1963 proposal and the May 1967 revision – and there was even discussion of a proposed epilepsy day hospital. It was intended that decanting should begin in February 1968, with building to start in January 1970. The go-ahead was given to proceed with phase 1, at a total cost of £1,959,236, applying the 'Pater formula', by which 60 per cent of costs were met by the UGC. Later in the year, the Ministry also agreed to proceed with detailed planning for phase 2 of the development, estimating that the island site (which, in the event, never materialised) would now require £11 million.

In 1968, it was announced that demolition was set to start in April 1969, and construction work on phase 1 was scheduled to last two years from January 1970. But everything then stalled again as planning permission was refused on the basis of the historical and architectural importance of the site. The Board of Governors managed to dismiss this objection[70] and consent to proceed seemed imminent, but further planning problems then arose with respect to Grenville Mews.[71] Eventually work did begin on 1

[69] Central Health Services Council, *Ministry of Health Medical Care of Epileptics*. (London: HMSO, 1956)

[70] The historical importance included the fact that George III was said to have stayed there, but Richard Hunter, who had published an account of the life of George III, with his mother, Ida McAlpine, refuted this. This was pointed out by the Board in a letter to the Minister sent on 17 March 1970. The portico was of particular architectural interest, but the hospital claimed that this was not original and had been added in the 1830s. Although this claim seems to have been accepted by the planning authorities, an etching of 1810 does show the portico. It was a fine edifice and its demolition was a travesty.

[71] The buildings of the mews, which was previously used as staff residences, had been demolished but it turned out that the short access road was categorised, unbeknown to the hospital or Ministry, as a public highway. Resolving this required further negotiation.

April 1970 (an appropriate date, as it turned out) with the demolition of Queen Square House.

In his opening address for the academic year 1970–1, Reginald Kelly, the dean, noted the Institute's indebtedness to John Cumings and to Geoffrey Robinson and their committee, without whom the phase 1 demolition and preparation for building would not have been pushed through its 'teething troubles with the Ministry'. Cumings' involvement was again noted in a tribute from the chairman of the Academic Board:

> The first phase of the building to house the Institute of Neurology has been successfully planned, with innumerable and seemingly insurmountable difficulties over fifteen years, and as he [Cumings] leaves, he can see the concrete shape of the ground plan of the new building already laid in Guilford Street ... There cannot have been any step in the development over all those years with which he has not been actively involved. He has been the staff representative on the architects' committees, and every item of space and fitting of the eleven floors has been his direct concern.[72]

In June 1970, the new Conservative government under Edward Heath was elected, and Keith Joseph appointed Minister of Health. More changes were to follow, but initially at least the economic fortunes of the country seemed to have improved and the phase 1 building was allowed to start. The foundation stone was laid on 11 November 1971 by HRH Queen Elizabeth the Queen Mother, who received a silver rose bowl from the National Hospital and Institute of Neurology. The occasion was photographed and prints made available for purchase by staff and patients. But the troubles that the building project faced were not yet done. In May 1972, workers all over the country went on strike demanding a minimum wage, and with a campaign to abolish the 'Lump labour scheme'. By the end of the year, building work was 12 months behind schedule, causing real difficulties for the running of the hospital departments; and the Board of Governors had to ask the Department of Health if they could take parts of the Homeopathic Hospital as temporary accommodation. Nationally, the strike by the Union of Construction, Allied Trades and Technicians (UCATT) caused a 12-week stoppage, and Queen Square was at the centre of publicity when a striker named Kavanagh climbed a 100-foot crane and stayed up there for 11 days, fed by food winched up on a bucket attached to a rope and pulley system. Attempts to restart work on 25 July 1972 led to violence on the picket line. The general building strike lasted into September. The dispute was referred to a standing conciliation panel set up by the Confederation of British Industry (CBI) and the Trades Union Congress (TUC) which met on 31 January 1973, recommending re-employment of the two builders who had lost their jobs, to which the contractors agreed. After lengthy arbitration, work restarted temporarily on 26 February 1973. Later that year, the threatened gas industry strike meant that closure of Finchley had to be seriously considered; and, on the Queen Square site, further disputes also involved the subcontractors. In 1974, there was a national economic crisis, and further industrial action occurred following an objection by the unions to the deployment of a plastering subcontractor, and intermittent stoppages continued until 17 April. A full strike was then referred to the national conciliation panel which found in favour of the contractors.

Work did recommence, but only from 30 May, with a 'go slow' policy. There was discussion around terminating the contract with Lovell's, who were losing large amounts of money on the project, and dispute over costs continued for years after the end of building work. The architects reported at this stage that the site was a shambles of 'rusted steel, broken shutters, general chaos, risk of accidents, disarray of stacked materials, and general disorganisation emphasizing a state of depression'. A confidential letter was leaked to the *Morning Star*, and at one stage there was a break-in at the architects' office. The hospital secretary wrote to Dr David Owen (a former trainee in neurology and now Minister of State for Health in the new Labour government of Harold Wilson), reporting that the project was three years behind schedule and the 'standard of excellence' at Queen Square falling as a consequence of the delay, but no further money was forthcoming.

Further unofficial strike action and stoppages occurred on the site over redundancy notices in 1975. The dean's opening address for 1976–7 reflects the disappointment of not having received a firm date for completion of the construction works, calling phase 1 'the promised land'. Numerous further problems arose and the building was eventually opened on 19 July 1978, by the Queen Mother.[73] The saga was one of

---

[72] Institute of Neurology annual report 1970–1, p. 6.

[73] By 1980, the building housed: basement – electron microscope and post-mortem room; ground floor – lecture theatre

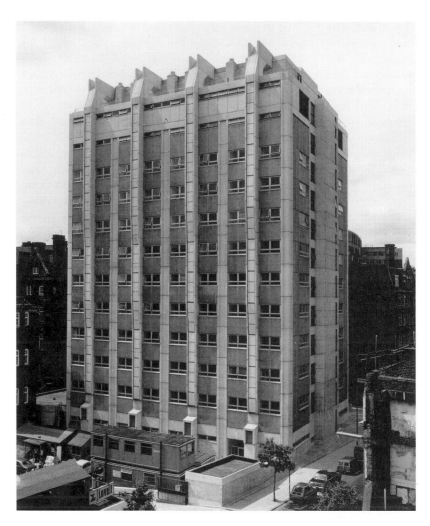

Figure 2.21 Queen Square House by the architect Professor Lord Richard Llewelyn Davies.

the worst examples of labour disruption of its time; and the structure has remained unloved ever since, suffering continual problems due to its unimaginative architectural design and poor quality of the fabric.

Agreement on phase 2 had been repeatedly delayed during the protracted phase 1 building negotiations, but a letter from the Ministry on 25 July 1973 gave the Board approval to proceed to a more detailed

planning stage for the development of the island site jointly with Great Ormond Street. The University Grants Committee also took the view that, although postgraduate hospitals in general should be associated with undergraduate hospitals, 'in view of the money already spent at child health and neurology, the widespread opposition to a move, and the high-cost of rebuilding elsewhere, the only realistic plan is to let the joint development proceed at Queen Square'.

The island site proposals had depended on the incorporation of land and buildings occupied by the Homeopathic Hospital, but a letter from the Department of Health and Social Security (DHSS) indicated that the provision of homoeopathy would continue for as long as it was requested. An impasse had been reached, and then another proposal was made, in 1976, by David Owen suggesting that the National Hospital, Great Ormond Street Hospital and

and reception; 1st floor – clinical pathology; 2nd floor – histopathology; 3rd floor – histopathology, cytogenetics and paediatric neuropathology; 4th floor – neuropathology; 5th floor – clinical neurophysiology and Sobell department of physiology; 6th floor – department of clinical neurology and neuropsychiatry; 7th floor – department of neurosurgery and clinical psychology; 8th floor – pharmacology, drug monitoring unit, Professor John Cavanagh's unit and neurocytology; 9th floor – neurochemistry and specialist clinical pathology; 10th floor – animal house.

the Royal London Homoeopathic Hospital might combine to form a Special Health Authority, contingent on Maida Vale activities also moving to Queen Square. This was a compromise but in the spirit of realpolitik, Peter Gautier-Smith, the dean, supported the proposal and, for the next few years, there was closer cooperation between Queen Square and Great Ormond Street. However, the Homeopathic Hospital resisted closure and stalemate ensued, not least as it seemed that the Department of Health had made a commitment that it could remain where it was. Furthermore, Camden Council would not agree to a three-partner development on the island site.

In the end, the various phase 2 plans never really advanced beyond the drawing board, and huge amounts of bureaucratic time and effort came to nothing. For the next decade, no further plans were made, and there was, perhaps unsurprisingly, no further appetite for embarking on any large-scale building projects for the next ten years.

Post 1998: The Redevelopment of the Powis Place Wing and Closure of Maida Vale, and Later Building Projects

The last major project was the rebuilding of the east wing in Powis Place. In some ways, it can be seen as the phoenix arising from the ashes of the failed phase 2 plans – although, as it turned out, a somewhat flightless bird with wings severely clipped. Both plans shared the idea of closing Maida Vale Hospital and transferring its services to the Queen Square site. Nevertheless, the original phase 2 proposals were more grandiose and sought greatly to expand the bed complement at Queen Square and the National Hospital's footprint. In the finally realised project, Maida Vale did close and its services were transferred, but squeezed onto the Queen Square site without any major expansion of space or footprint, and with no increase in bed numbers. Nevertheless, the redevelopment did result in replacement of an aged Victorian wing with a modern facility and, in so doing, as it turned out protected the National Hospital from more sweeping proposals to move it altogether off-site.

The new plan to refurbish the Powis Place wing was first mooted in 1988. Like its predecessor, the project was to proceed in stages. Phase 1A was the decanting of activity from the existing building into the Examination Halls, the ground floor of the Queen Mary wing, and the

third and fourth floors of the west wing. This process went smoothly and was nearly complete by 1991, although because of poor performance in the latter stages of the contract and conflict over prices, there was a 13-week over-run. Phase 1B comprised the demolition of existing buildings (the 1885 Powis Place pavilion) and construction of the new Powis wing. The contract was put out to tender and by far the most competitive price was £14,107,018 offered by Laing Construction. The contract was duly signed with work due to be completed by May 1993 (actually 12 months earlier than predicted in 1988). Again, everything started well but, in 1992, delays began. The price rose to £14,376,942, with arguments over the contract continuing for several years. Phase 2 comprised the rebuild of the Powis Place wing, improvements to the Queen Mary and Albany wings, the maintenance of the number of medical beds at the same level throughout, and the surrender of the lease and total closure of Maida Vale Hospital, which occurred in July 1993.

The major reorganisation under way in the National Health Service was the backdrop to the plans, and, in particular, the chaos surrounding the provision of care in London (described further in Chapter 14). This constantly blighted successful conclusion of projects for rebuilding, and conflicting options for reconfiguration floated in the air like confetti, including the suggestion that the medical services from Queen Square should be moved entirely off-site to either the Royal Free or University College Hospital sites, and that management should be taken over by one of its larger neighbours. These would inevitably have marked the end of a separate identity for the National Hospital and each was bitterly opposed. As it turned out, one important influence in the ultimate decision not to move the hospital was the fact that a major modern redevelopment programme had already been started.

The contract for rebuilding the Powis Place wing was completed three days before the loss of Crown Immunity in 1991, thus, with Machiavellian haste, avoiding the obstacle of demolishing a listed building in a conservation area. Throughout its course, the project was spearheaded by Rear-Admiral Anthony Wheatley,[74] general manager of the National Hospital. It was a triumph of competence in marked

---

[74] Anthony Wheatley CB was a universally admired general manager of the hospital. His cool determination and focus, under fire, were instrumental in the success of this project. He was appointed as general manager of the hospital in 1988, on the basis that he would guide through the

contrast to the chaos surrounding the earlier postwar building plans, and this was due in large part to the military efficiency and meticulous planning of Wheatley and the strong support he received from John Young and the Board, which retained its focus on the task, despite the turmoil caused by NHS reforms nationally.[75]

The Powis Place redevelopment involved the construction of a new six-storey building, housing 146 beds on the top three floors, with operating theatre suites and a surgical intensive therapy unit (ITU) on the first floor, and medical ITU and outpatients on the ground floor.[76] In addition, space was provided for the neuro-otology unit and various other services. Patients were accommodated in wards of 26 beds, mainly in 6-bedded bays, with additional single and double rooms. Two of the wards were earmarked for neurosurgical use and the rest for neurology. Bed spaces were more generous than usual (2.7 metres wide compared with the 2.4-metre standard). On the top floor was the Nuffield ward for private patients, with 16 single rooms and two high-security suites.

The architects chosen for the work were the Devereux Partnership, and the main contract price was £17,195,000 for a floor area of 10,570 square metres. The total cost ended up closer to £30 million, the Department of Health committing funds on the condition that Maida Vale Hospital was closed and one-third raised by the National Hospital Development Foundation.[77] In 1992, 68 and 69 Guilford Street were sold as part of the overall strategy of realising the value of all the Guilford Street properties. Building work on the site started in May 1991 and HRH Princess of Wales laid the foundation stone on 25 February 1992. Unfortunately, in the summer of 1991, it became clear that there had been fraudulent misappropriation of £1.7 million of hospital development funds by the self-styled 'Lady Aberdour', but this money was subsequently recovered, and the enabling works completed by mid-1991. The building was eventually opened by John Horma MP on behalf of Stephen Dorrell, Secretary of State for Health, on 22 March 1996. In architectural terms, reviews in the specialist press were mixed. The finishes were rather bland and uninspiring, but it was certainly an improvement on the old by then dilapidated Powis Place wing.

A series of other refurbishments and alterations were made to the hospital estate in this period. These included: the siting of a new neuro-rehabilitation unit at Queen Square in the Albany Memorial wing; the transfer of neurosurgical facilities from the Middlesex Hospital by early 1989; the move of private consulting rooms to 23 Queen Square despite concerns of the Institute about limiting their access to the building; the siting of a new ophthalmological unit and EEG telemetry unit in the Queen Mary wing; and the construction of a new outpatients department and a dementia research unit, and then later a neuromuscular centre, in 8–11 Queen Square. Extensive changes were also subsequently made to the new Powis Place wing, including the siting of neurosurgical theatres and intensive care, a brain cancer unit and a unit for respiratory support for patients with muscle disease. These *ad-hoc* rearrangements in the Powis wing have resulted over the years in an over-filled and incoherent space which would have dismayed Wheatley and the original architects.

In 1993, the Functional Brain Imaging Laboratory was established, funded by a grant from the Wellcome

---

redevelopment of the hospital. Five months later, however, the government published its White Paper on the reorganisation of the NHS and, as was later written, 'Rear-Admiral Anthony Wheatley was to need all of his navigational diplomacy to steer the hospital through the minefield of hospital reorganisation' (hospital newsletter: *The National* 10 (summer 1996)). When the studies of London Healthcare began, a freeze was slapped on further development of hospital sites, but the National Hospitals got in just under the wire due to slick and rapid action. As he commented later, the danger was that UCH and the Middlesex would be moved onto the Queen Square site, and the new building would be handed over to Great Ormond Street. His skill in maintaining the existence of the National Hospital, even if two Trust applications failed, cannot be over-estimated. He retired from his post in 1996. Later in his retirement, he had a severe stroke which totally incapacitated him.

[75] John Young, chairman of Young's Brewery and a long-standing supporter, became chairman of the Board, and worked tirelessly for the hospital. His enthusiasm and contacts (which included Princess Diana) were instrumental in the success of the appeal. One of the wards in the new block was named after him. Other philanthropists and supporters included Basil Samuels (the outpatient department was named after him) and the Wolfson family.

[76] It involved the demolition of existing buildings (in the position of the original numbers 4–10 Powis Place). The building abuts on to numbers 2 and 3 which are the only Georgian remains in Powis Place.

[77] By 1989, £7 million of the £10 million was already raised: Institute of Neurology annual report 1988–9, p. 103. The Harris Trust provided £1 million for the intensive therapy unit.

Trust which purchased 12 Queen Square for this purpose, with building work completed and the unit opened in November 1995.

To complete the story of Queen Square development, although outside our designated period, we here briefly mention the projects which have taken place since 1995. In 2004, the lecture theatre in the Queen Mary wing, which had been left untouched in its original 1938 dressings, was refurbished in a disastrous fashion. Although retaining its historic blackboards and tiered seating, the bench seats were daubed an unpleasant red colour and with space far too small for comfort.

The last large-scale infrastructure project, completed at the time of writing, was in 2008, when number 33, the only building on the east side with any original features, was gutted and rebuilt, as the Clinical Neuroscience Centre. This was a narrow infill, with outpatient rooms on the ground floor, and offices, clinical research units and hospital departments on the remaining seven floors, each linked to corresponding levels of the Queen Mary wing and with a new lecture theatre (a third for Queen Square), seating 190 people, squeezed into the basement and linked to the Royal Homoeopathic Hospital. This was a compact design, also by Devereux Architects in collaboration with Allies and Morrison, but unfortunately the major casualties were the destruction of what remained of the chapel of St Katherine's convent and the doorposts of the building with their charming Catherine wheels.[78] Fortunately, one condition of planning consent was that the most important features from the chapel should be retained for display and these are exhibited, in an archeological style, in the 33 Queen Square lecture theatre foyer. The new building was described in *Architecture Today*:

> The facade – an elegant composition of stone and glass – is intended to form a visual link between its two larger neighbours and read as a natural complement to the square and the sensitive context of the Bloomsbury conservation area. The design seeks to extend the adjacent Victorian hospital building by continuing the principal building plane in Portland stone and recalling the articulation of its balconies in the projecting stone and metal details of the new elevation. This encourages a natural transition to the horizontal brick balconies of the 1930s Queen Mary wing. The vertical fins continue the composition of the square as a whole, characterised by a rhythm and proportion borrowed from the original Georgian fenestration. The connection with the red brick Queen Mary wing is underlined by a bronze surface, held by the metal fins, and visible only from the west. [79]

As we write, in 2018, further development is in the planning stage, this time for the repurposing of the unloved brutalist Queen Square House. This follows a failed £300 million bid to replace the building entirely with one having a larger footprint incorporating the goods yard behind the National Hospital – the only piece of land which has never been developed within the whole estate. This repurposing will mean the move of a large part of the Institute of Neurology to the Eastman Hospital site in Grays Inn Road, thus separating the hospital from its institute for the first time in 150 years. Doing so is likely, in the opinion of some, to presage the end of the independent existence of the National Hospital, which, delinked from its research institute, loses much of its reason for existence. Only the passage of time will reveal the consequence of this decision.

Other Property Held by the National Hospital and Institute of Neurology after 1945

After the Second World War, there was a severe problem in providing staff accommodation, not least because of the failure of the pre-war plans for the construction of a large nurses' home, and much attention of the National Hospital estate planning was focused on acquiring and converting houses in Guilford Street, where the terrace comprising numbers 64–82 (between Herbrand St and Grenville St) formed a row of houses that was deemed appropriate and convenient. In 1947, most of these were in a run-down state and used as small hotels, and number 73 was bomb-damaged and vacant. Numbers 74–76, known as Turners Hotel, were owned by the War Office and, in 1946, the hospital acquired and

---

[78] The building won the 2008 Judges Special Award in the Best Hospital Design category at the Building Better Healthcare Awards. The project was noted for its 'importance in the urban context' and was especially praised for the design of the stone and glass façade. The project team was: façade design, Allies & Morrison; lead architect, Devereux Architects; executive architect, Tangram Architects; quantity surveyor, Nisbets; project manager, Inventures; contractor, Eugena.

[79] *Architecture Today* **91** (September 2008): 83.

refurbished this property to house about 50 members of staff and provide a dining room, known as the Wedgewood Suite, for use as the consultants' dining room, a committee room and venue for ceremonial occasions. Numbers 70–72 functioned as a Salvation Army hostel (the Whitehall Hotel) and when they vacated the site in July 1947 the hospital acquired the lease of this building.[80] The houses in Grenville Mews had been demolished before the Second World War and the site formed the goods yard and service structures of the hospital and the new Queen Square House. Other houses in Guilford Street, numbers 13–17 Grenville Street and 11–23 in the Colonnade were also attractive to the hospital.

The manoeuvres whereby the National Hospital gradually acquired much of Guilford Street and nearby properties reflects the role of the Ministry of Health in purchasing buildings for hospital use, but under somewhat restrictive rules and regulations, and the preparedness of the Institute of Neurology and the Chartered Society of Queen Square to secure these *pro tem* as and when opportunities arose. This accumulation of property in the postwar years was a shrewd long-term plan, needed to house support services and residences for the hospital staff, but a slow and tortuous process.

In 1957, the Ministry acquired the freehold of numbers 70–77 Guilford Street, as well as 19–23 in the Colonnade, which seems to have been used mainly for storage, for £80,000. Later that year, the owner of the remaining Guilford Street properties put these on the market and the Ministry of Health bought for the hospital numbers 66, 67, 70, 77 and 82 Guilford Street, and 15 Grenville Street, for £116,750. Queen Court had the same ownership but attempts to buy this, a longstanding aim of the hospital, failed. One flat was leased (Ewart Mitchell lived there in 1958), but later the Chartered Society of the National Hospital did buy the freehold and leased out several flats to senior staff. Unfortunately, in 1981, the Society disposed of the property and the new owner would not lease to the hospital. The remaining properties, 64, 65, 68, 69, 78, 79, 80 and 81, were bought by the Chartered Society and held for the benefit of the National Hospital. In 1962 some were purchased by the Ministry, and 64, 65, 80 and 81 bought by the Institute as a temporary measure. In 1964, numbers 80 and 81 were sold to the Ministry by the Institute, initially on behalf of Moorfields Hospital as a temporary measure, and then these reverted to the benefit of the National Hospital in 1970. In 1973, the Board of Governors purchased numbers 64 and 65 from the Institute using the National Hospital endowment funds, and then asked the Department of Health to purchase them for use in decanting as other projects materialised. The houses were poorly built, and the condition of the whole terrace deteriorated in these postwar years, due to the overcrowding, continual change of use, and also damage caused by vehicles in Guilford Street, which was converted to one-way traffic in the 1970s.

In the 1980s and 1990s, and despite the Herculean efforts expended earlier, it was decided to divest the hospital of all these properties for short-term financial reasons. In retrospect, this seems a gross strategic error and is now a source of much regret, for the obvious potential of future redevelopment of the whole terrace by the hospital, recognised soon after the Second World War, was abruptly lost.

Other property leased by the hospital included 84a Heath Street in Hampstead, which was the site of the Oldrey–Fleming School of Speech Therapy, from 1974, and 59 Portland Place, which housed the West End School of Speech Therapy. Both were in hospital occupation in 1982 but the leaseholds have since been lost. Also, several flats were leased in Bristol House in Southampton Row, where Ewart Mitchell and his wife were accommodated, as well as, for a time, in 5 Handel Street. Number 33 John's Mews was also owned by the hospital and used for relocation of various activities during the redevelopment of Queen Square House. The leasehold of Maida Vale was surrendered when that hospital closed in 1993. Maida Vale also owned or leased 1–17 Cunningham Place, 41 Hamilton Terrace, 5–11 St John's Wood Road, and flats 8, 11 and 14 in Rodney Court, 6–8 Maida Vale.

Property at the Chalfont Centre for Epilepsy was held on leasehold, as were 5–11 St Johns Mews and 1 Wakefield Street. The convalescent home in Finchley had been purchased by the National Hospital in 1870, and this was sold in the 1990s (unwisely, since this has become amongst the most expensive real estate locations in London).

---

[80] The secretary, Ewart Mitchell, learned of the opportunity from a resident asking for work at the National Hospital as a stoker because his job at the Salvation Army hostel was terminating.

Property Held in 1996/1997 by the National Hospital and Institute of Neurology

The saga of purchase and sale of properties makes for dizzy reading as houses came and went. For convenience, the properties owned or leased by the National Hospital and Institute of Neurology in 1996/7, and their current status at the time of writing, are as follows.[81]

- National Hospital (Powis Place wing, west wing, Queen Mary wing): in 1996, the freehold was owned by the National Hospital, and is now by the UCLH Trust.

- Queen Square House: in 1996, the freehold was owned by the National Hospital and part-leased to the Institute of Neurology and the Hospital for Sick Children. It was then transferred to the UCLH Trust, and in 2012 to UCL.

- 23 Queen Square: in 1996, the freehold was owned by the National Hospital. It is now held by joint freehold by UCLH (approximately 46 per cent) and UCL/Institute of Neurology (approximately 54 per cent).

- 33 Queen Square: in 1996, the freehold was owned by the National Hospital (and the building housed staff changing rooms, the linen room and changing rooms in 1997). It was then transferred to UCLH, and on refurbishment 50 per cent is leased by UCL/Institute of Neurology.

- 7 Queen Square: in 1996, it was leased by the National Hospital with the lease extending to 2001. The lease was transferred to UCLH Trust in 1996, and then purchased by UCL/Institute of Neurology in 2001. The UCLH Trust currently lease three floors of the building.

- 8–11 Queen Square: Charles Symonds House. In 1996, the freehold was owned by the National Hospital, and now by the UCLH Trust.

- 12 Queen Square: purchased by the Wellcome Trust from the National Hospital in 1993/4 to establish the Functional Imaging Laboratory and the Wellcome Centre for Neuroimaging. The freehold remains held by the Wellcome Trust with UCL/Institute of Neurology as tenants. The original 20-year lease expired in 2014 and was renewed by the Wellcome Trust.

- 17 Queen Square: Alexandra House. The freehold is held by the Imperial London Hotels. UCL/Institute of Neurology leased the building for the UCL Institute of Cognitive Neuroscience.

- 1 Wakefield Street: in 1996, the freehold was owned by the National Hospital, and it was then transferred to the UCLH Trust. The freehold was then transferred to UCL/Institute of Neurology.

- 66–82 Guilford Street: this was owned by the National Hospital in 1996 but these have since been sold.

- 11–23 The Colonnade: these were owned by the National Hospital in 1996 but have since been sold.

- 115–17 Great North Road, Finchley: leased by the National Hospital in 1997 but have since been sold.

In addition to the above, at the time of writing, parts of the following properties are occupied by the Institute of Neurology on various leasehold and rental bases, which were not part of the estate in 1996/7: Russell Square House, Ormond House, Monomark House, Cruciform building, Francis Crick building, Royal Free Campus and the Chalfont Centre.

---

[81] Details provided by the then Institute secretaries, Mr R. Walker and Ms Helen Crutzen, and from the hospital and Institute's boards of management minutes and reports.

Chapter 3

Queen Square and Neurology 1860–1902

The Medical and Scientific Climate of Victorian London and the Rise of the Voluntary Hospitals

The foundation of the National Hospital in 1859 can, with some justification, be considered to mark the birth of modern neurology in the United Kingdom. Scientific and social revolutions made for a turbulent period in Britain during the last four decades of the nineteenth century. The Industrial Revolution altered the nature of urban life, and science and technology effected permanent changes on society. Patterns of medical practice, including referral between doctors and the bureaucracy of medicine, evolved. The Medical Act of 1858 created an official council (the General Medical Council) to maintain a new register of doctors and to take over certain functions of the Royal Colleges. In turn, these were themselves reformed, their rules for membership were made more equitable and their powers constrained. The standards of education improved, presenting opportunities for specialist institutions such as the National Hospital to offer clinical instruction to the growing number of doctors wanting postgraduate qualifications. Medical training was modernised and examination for Membership of the Royal College of Physicians (MRCP) was introduced in 1859. Florence Nightingale founded a school of nursing at St Thomas' Hospital in 1860, and nursing as a career was revolutionised. Medicine became more internationalised, culminating in the show-piece of the 1881 International Medical Congress in London. In short, Victorian medicine adopted arrangements that remain recognisable today.

In 1852, Marshall Hall called for the establishment of a hospital committed to the treatment of nervous diseases.[1] His own work from the 1830s, and that of

Brown-Séquard in the late 1850s, had stimulated a great deal of medical and public interest in the physiology and pathology of the central nervous system. Books on epilepsy and diseases of the nervous system were published, including those by future physicians to the National Hospital, Charles Bland Radcliffe, John Russell Reynolds and Edward Sieveking. That said, for Gordon Holmes, the parlous state of clinical neurology at the time the National Hospital opened was epitomised by the contents of Russell Reynolds' *Diagnosis of Diseases of the Brain, Spinal Cord, Nerves and their Appendages* (1855).[2]

Although there is no evidence that any of the Chandler family were aware in 1859 of these scientific and medical developments, at least some of their influential advisers were better informed – notably the family doctor Jabez Spence Ramskill,[3] whose clinical skills had impressed Johanna Chandler during a

---

[1] This desire expressed in his Croonian Lectures (1852), republished shortly before his death (1857), was specifically

linked to the foundation of the National Hospital in articles published by the *Lancet* **74** (1859): 624–625 and *Observer* (23 February 1863).

[2] Holmes notes that, although Reynolds was an acute observer, and made a serious effort to define the features of the different afflictions of the nervous system, knowledge was not sufficiently available for the task: 'little was known of either the functions of the nervous system or of the diseases to which it is subject'. He did recognise though that 'the segregation in special institutions of patients suffering with diseases of any organ of the body undoubtedly facilitates investigations into their nature and efficient treatment' and it was this thought, dawning on the medical and scientific community in the mid-Victorian period, that led to the appearance of special hospitals. But, as set out later, we consider Holmes to have been a harsh judge of Reynolds and his writings on neurology in the 1860s.

[3] Jabez Spence Ramskill was a Yorkshireman, trained in medicine at Guy's from 1842 and qualified MRCS in 1846, MB in 1847 and MD in 1849. He was never elected a Fellow of the Royal College of Physicians. He was senior physician at the Metropolitan Free Hospital, where Sir Jonathan Hutchinson was senior surgeon, and in 1859 was assistant physician at the London Hospital, lecturer in pathology at the Metropolitan Free Hospital and, from December 1859,

medical consultation, and David Wire. Ramskill was the first physician appointed at Queen Square (in 1859 just before the first surgeon to be appointed Sir William Fergusson, FRS[4]). He was also senior physician at the Metropolitan Free Hospital, and assistant physician and lecturer at the London Hospital.[5] He worked at Queen Square for the next 38 years but, although he had a successful practice, Ramskill left no intellectual mark on British neurology. However, it was almost certainly Ramskill who persuaded the Chandlers and Wire that the new hospital should include in its remit patients with epilepsy as well as paralysis. Perhaps his greatest contribution to Queen Square was to influence the appointments of Brown-

Séquard and Jackson to the staff. Moreover, it was possibly Ramskill who stimulated Jackson's growing interests in epilepsy and aphasia and, overwhelmed by his clinical workload and contrary to Board of Management rules, Ramskill transferred the care of some patients to his younger colleague. The result of Ramskill's presence in the hospital was that the importance of medical and scientific advances filtered through to the lay founders and helped ensure that they nurtured a medical institution for the diagnosis and treatment of patients with nervous disorders, and not merely a nursing home or asylum for incurables, as might otherwise have been the case.

Another tension had also to be played out. Charles Darwin had published *On the Origin of Species* in 1859, three weeks after the Mansion House meeting, and Francis Galton at the neighbouring University College was developing his theories of inheritance. Thereafter, an interest in heredity became an increasingly important theme of medicine in Victorian Britain, and of neurology at Queen Square. However, the founders of the National Hospital held evangelical Christian beliefs that were challenged by the emerging findings of science, and, whilst the growing interest in physiology and pathology of the nervous system undoubtedly shaped early development of the hospital, the Board of Management was more preoccupied with the perceived dangers of ritualism and Roman Catholicism than scientific doctrine or religious doubt.[6] Although in time the National Hospital was seen in certain quarters as a cradle of scientific materialism and unbelief, its day-to-day management remained almost entirely in the hands of men of sincere and conventional religious belief, ranging from the moderate non-conformist to the high Anglican. Eventually irreconcilable fault lines did develop between the scientific perspective of the medical staff and the religious views of the management, and these lay at the heart of the conflict at the end of the century.

It is not by chance that the first neurological hospital in the world was founded in London. This was then the richest city in the world, but it also had a

---

the first staff member of the National Hospital for the Cure and Relief of Paralysis and Epilepsy. He was described in the *Lancet* as a 'rising city doctor' and was said to be the first of three doctors to start the neurological tradition at the London Hospital (the others being John Langdon Down and John Hughlings Jackson). Ramskill published his lectures on epilepsy, given at the National Hospital in 1863/4, and also on other neurological topics, including vertigo and hydrocephalus, but his published output was small and his written contribution has not endured. He had a private practice in Bishopsgate and was said to be a very genial and kind-hearted man, with many friends inside and outside the medical profession (Anon., 'Jabez Spence Ramskill MD MRCP Lond … MRCS Eng.', *Lancet* **150** (1897): 229; M. Lorch, 'The Unknown Source of Hughling Jackson's Early Interest in Aphasia and Epilepsy', *Cognitive and Behavioral Neurology* **17** (2004): 124–32).

[4] Sir William Fergusson was the first surgeon appointed to the National Hospital (in 1860). In that year, he was consulted by Napoleon III and undertook a secret mission to Paris. As a young anatomist in Edinburgh, Fergusson had given evidence at the trial of the body snatchers Burke and Hare. He was said to operate rapidly and in total silence but with great skill, and to have had 'the eye of an eagle, the heart of a lion and the hand of a lady'. Fergusson was professor of surgery at King's College (1840), and president of the Pathological Society of London (1859), the Royal College of Surgeons (1870) and the British Medical Association (1873). He was elected Fellow of the Royal Society (FRS), made a baronet (1866) and served as sergeant-surgeon to Queen Victoria (1867). It is doubtful that he ever attended Queen Square but his appointment added lustre and respectability to the young hospital.

[5] Ramskill is included on the memorial stone in the main hall of the hospital that commemorates the early physicians; and he is in the middle of the front in the 1886 medical staff photograph. Smartly if conservatively dressed, the only eccentricity being a fine pair of bushy white mutton-chop sideburns, his receding dark hair and serious countenance convey a somewhat unassuming figure compared with Radcliffe, Gowers and Jackson.

---

[6] In the minutes for 17 December 1862, the Board of Management 'expressed a very decided protest against anything of a proselytising or Puseyite practice ever being introduced into the hospital'. A newspaper advertisement for the post of matron at the National Hospital from the early 1860s specified that the successful candidate should be 'a well-educated and competent Protestant lady of evangelical principles'.

rapidly rising population with a growing number of poor, destitute and illiterate people whose health had become a cause for public concern, and yet there was no central or coordinated organisation of health care. The most important medical institutions were the endowed teaching hospitals[7] with their medical schools. These coexisted with various other types of hospital, some run by the London County Council, some in workhouses, some dedicated to maternity care, and some as isolation (fever) hospitals and nursing homes. In this milieu, a number of new voluntary hospitals were established, often small and specialised in scope. These filled a niche not supplied by the large endowed teaching institutions which concentrated on treating acute cases, avoided chronic illness, and specifically excluded certain diseases from admission to their wards. Patients with epilepsy, for instance, were not taken into these hospitals through fear, as it was claimed that seizures might frighten or even infect other patients, and because of the stigma of the condition and its perceived association with possession by evil spirits. Furthermore, although bed numbers were increasing rapidly, the large hospitals found it more and more difficult to cope with the demand for care, and they were ever-fearful of becoming nursing homes for the chronic sick. As a result, patients with stroke and other debilitating neurological conditions were largely ignored. The senior doctors in these hospitals were also keen to preserve their practices and patient flows, and were opposed to specialisation and unwilling to set up individual organ-based departments. The situation was widely recognised as deficient and, as the century wore on, there were strident calls for change.

The establishment of smaller specialised hospitals, all within the voluntary sector, was one response to this crisis. Between 1840 and 1890, 44 specialist hospitals were established in London. For the first time, doctors began to concentrate their practices in specific fields. The National Hospital was one of 16 such hospitals founded in the 1860s. Two other

institutions focusing on diseases of the nervous system appeared soon after: the London Infirmary for Epilepsy and Paralysis[8] in Charles Street, Marylebone (in 1867), and the West End Hospital for Diseases of the Nervous System, Paralysis and Epilepsy[9] in Welbeck Street (in 1878). By 1900, there were 128 special hospitals in England and Wales, most still in London. Their medical staff were usually unpaid, the doctors acting as honoraries, as was the case at the National Hospital, where this arrangement persisted until 1948 with the move to salaried employment by the National Health Service (NHS). Despite the absence of remuneration, appointment to the best hospitals was considered a prestigious prize and an important credential in building up the private practice on which professional income depended.

The voluntary (special) hospitals were invariably established as charitable organisations with funds raised from the general public. The standard of medical care varied but, in the best, scientific inquiry and teaching flourished in a way that would not have been possible in the large general teaching institutions. As Rivett pointed out:

> The usual procedure to found a special hospital was to form a committee, obtain an eminent patron, take a house, appoint medical staff and launch an appeal. Advertisements for funds would appear in the press pointing out how appallingly deficient was the care

---

[7] There were seven teaching hospitals in London by 1800: St Bartholomew's (founded 1123), St Thomas' (1207), Guy's (1721), St George's (1733), the Westminster (1719), the Middlesex (1745) and the London (1740). These were followed in the first half of the nineteenth century by Charing Cross (1818), University College Hospital (1823), the Royal Free (1828), King's College Hospital (1840) and St Mary's (1845). All had medical schools and so, by 1858, there were 12 teaching hospitals in London. These provided 80 per cent of London's general hospital beds.

[8] This hospital, like the National Hospital (and indeed many others) changed its name on several occasions (see p4). It also moved twice – from Charles Street to Portland Terrace and then to Maida Vale (and confusingly for all those who have tried to find the building, Charles Street in which it was originally situated also was renamed Kings Place in 1886 and then Blandford Place in 1937). The first London single specialty hospital was Moorfields Eye Hospital, and for all their faults, the special hospitals had one enormous advantage over all others and that was the concentration of clinical cases. Sir William Lawrence said of Moorfields in 1825 'you may see more of diseases of the eye in this institution in three months than in the largest hospital in fifty years' (cited in R. Kershaw. 'Special Hospitals', Pulman, London 1909). This was even more true of the three special hospitals for neurology, epilepsy and paralysis.
[9] Founded by Dr Herbert Tibbitts and specialising in electrical therapy, and subsequently in psychiatry. It changed its name (in 1915) to the West End Hospital for Nervous Diseases. It established a clinic for stammering (in 1919) and the first school of speech therapy (in 1929). It was closed in 1972 after various amalgamations with other London hospitals.

for certain diseases, but that now as a result of the benevolence of disinterested and far-seeing men the lack might be remedied.[10]

This pattern was followed exactly in the case of the National Hospital. It was founded by lay people on a genuinely philanthropic basis, and although the establishment of other specialist voluntary hospitals was perceived to have resulted from the self-interest of doctors, and heavily criticised on this basis, no such allegation was ever made about Queen Square.

The patients seen within the voluntary hospital system were largely the 'deserving poor', who were indeed the focus of much Victorian philanthropy. The 'undeserving' poor, if treated at all, were admitted to the workhouse, and managed by medical officers under Poor Law legislation: 50,000 such cases were recorded in 1861. Conditions in the workhouse sick-wards were appalling, and it was here that those with chronic neurological conditions unable to support themselves often languished. At the other end of the spectrum, affluent patients were treated at home by a visiting doctor, or as an outpatient in private rooms. They would not have contemplated admission to a hospital, which was perceived as a place of impending death. Even surgical operations were carried out at home.[11] In the United Kingdom census of 1861, only 157 of the 10,414 inmates in voluntary hospitals were classified as professional people (most were government officers, teachers or clergymen), and only 14 as 'persons of rank or property not returned under any office or occupation'.

The growth in voluntary hospitals was on the whole not welcomed by the medical profession at large. Sir Benjamin Brodie cited three reasons against their foundation (curiously, making an exception of hospitals for the eye): diseases were interlinked; special hospitals drained cases from the teaching hospitals; and they were excessively costly. There was also the suspicion that many of these institutions were set up by specialist doctors to increase their referral base, and for reasons of self-interest masquerading as philanthropy or scientific advance. For the *Lancet*:

These excrescencies are being reproduced with all the prolific exuberance characteristic of malignancy and

soon the metropolis threatens to swarm with nuisances of this kind ... next may come a Quinine Hospital, a hospital for Treatment by Cod-Liver Oil, by the Hyophosphites or by the Excrement of Boa-Constrictors.[12]

This particular outburst was prompted by the foundation of the Galvanic Hospital[13] and the Dispensary for Ulcerated Legs, and the Dispensary for Disease of the Throat and Loss of Voice. Other journals were equally vituperative, partly because they also saw the trend as damaging the status and remuneration of doctors, particularly general practitioners.

Although the trend of opening specialist hospitals was in general criticised on the grounds of professional and public interest, this was not the case with respect to founding of the National Hospital. Given the widely condemned lack of care for people with epilepsy and paralysis, its establishment was welcomed by the public, the profession, the national media and the medical journals. The scientific emphasis of the hospital seems also to have been considered a model, and the publicity around its foundation 'as the first hospital in the world established specifically for inpatients with neurological disorders' was wholly favourable. The *Daily Telegraph* expressed public opinion when it stated:

Few persons can have been long familiar with the streets of any great European city without having observed, more or less frequently, a desolate wretch writhing on the ground foaming at the mouth, hissing between the teeth, lacerating the tongue by frenzied clampings, drawing up all the limbs convulsively and then, perhaps smitten into rigidity, as if suddenly petrified. They have been told it was an epileptic patient, and have passed on ... is it credible that none [i.e. no institution] exists for the cure or alleviation of the epileptic and paralytic?[14]

Similarly, the editorials of the *Lancet*, although expressing fierce opposition to most specialist hospitals, were of the view that a special case could be made for epilepsy, and it was also noted that the

---

[10] G. Rivett, *The Development of the London Hospital System 1823–1982* (London: King Edward's Hospital Funds for London, 1986).

[11] See Chapter 5 for a description of the domestic neurosurgery by Victor Horsley, who, for example, regularly operated on the Gasserian ganglion in patients' homes.

[12] Anon., *Lancet* **76** (1860): 89; and Anon., *Lancet* **81** (1863): 183.

[13] Rivett suggests that the London Galvanic Hospital (opened in 1861) was 'little more than a brothel', and it certainly did not survive long.

[14] Leading article, *Daily Telegraph*, 2 November 1859. This was the first example of the knack – repeated over the years – the National Hospital has had for generating good publicity.

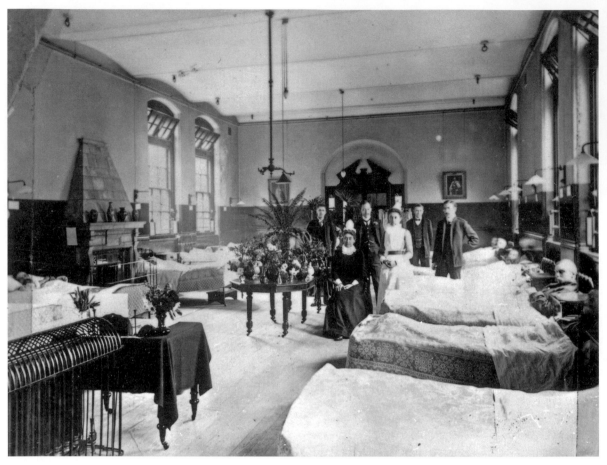

Figure 3.1 John Back ward, *c.* 1900.

appointment of Brown-Séquard, a 'world famous physiologist and clinical scientist', 'would attract to the hospital the earnest attention of the scientific and philanthropic throughout the world'.[15]

Despite the earlier disparagement, later in the nineteenth century both physicians and the public began to see the attractions and advantages of the specialist voluntary hospitals, and specialism grew inexorably in this period. By 1885, of the 195 physicians and surgeons attached to general hospitals in London, only 31 did not also hold a specialist position elsewhere. It seems that the scientific advantages and improved clinical care that resulted from the foundation of specialist hospitals were by then being widely appreciated.

15 Anon., 'The Argument for Founding a Hospital for Epileptics', *Lancet* **74** (1859): 624–5.

The Medical Staff and the Practice of Medicine at the National Hospital

The reputation of hospitals has always been (and still remains) dependent to a very large extent on the quality of their clinicians, and their standing within the medical profession. The National Hospital, at its inception, was especially fortunate in this respect. During its first 50 years, the medical staff consisted of no more than ten physicians (senior and junior) at any one time. Each consultant held a part-time appointment only, all were attached to other London teaching hospitals and each had an extensive private practice. They were (or became) a very distinguished group. Of the first 20 physicians at the National Hospital (appointed between 1859 and 1886), seven were elected FRS, five were knighted, three were appointed as physician to the royal household, and three served as president or vice-president of the

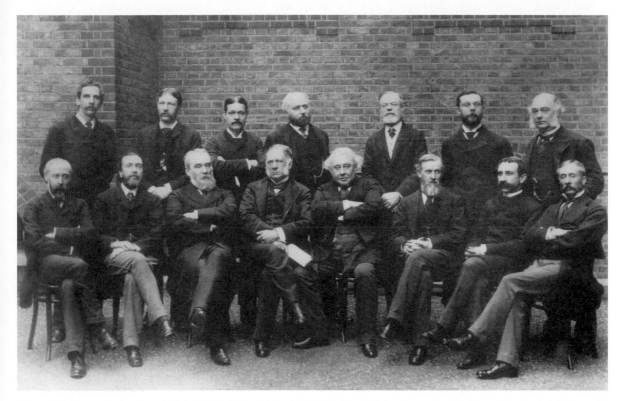

Figure 3.2 The medical and surgical staff at the National Hospital, 1886 (left to right: back row – Horsley, Beevor, Cumberbatch, Buzzard, Brudenall Carter, Ormerod, Adams; front row – Gunn, Bastian, Jackson, Ramskill, Radcliffe, Gowers, Semon, Ferrier).

Royal College of Physicians. Although several practised at the hospital for only a short time – Reynolds (five years), Brown-Séquard (four years), Sieveking (three years) and Laurence (one year) – others held appointments for many years, including Jackson (44 years), Bastian (40 years), Buzzard (39 years), Gowers (38 years), Horsley (30 years) and Ferrier (27 years). Their enormous contribution to both academic knowledge and clinical practice was unquestionably facilitated by working in a specialist hospital, with its concentration of instructive patients and the contact with like-minded colleagues. These pioneers shaped the emerging specialty and ensured the independence and status of neurology across that period.

In total, 33 physicians or surgeons were appointed to the National Hospital between 1859 and 1900. Their lives and contributions are described throughout this chapter and five are covered in more depth in Chapter 5.[16]

appears that he rarely, if ever, attended the hospital. He wrote a monograph *On Cerebria and Other Diseases of the Brain* (1872). D. M. Maclure was appointed assistant physician (1870–9); he is said to have contributed nothing to research or teaching. William Adams was surgeon to the National Hospital from 1872, before the development of neurosurgery, but little is known of his activities at the hospital or when he left the staff. Peter Horrocks was obstetric physician to the National Hospital (1880–3). James Anderson was appointed as assistant physician to the National Hospital (1886) and full physician in succession to Gowers (1893). He was considered to have a promising future career, but died suddenly aged 40, a few weeks after his appointment. Sir John Rose Bradford was born in London, educated at University College Hospital (1889), and appointed assistant physician there (in 1889) and at the National Hospital (from 1896 to 1899). He had a distinguished career, but not in neurology, being elected FRS for his work on the kidney. In 1895, he was appointed professor-superintendent of the Brown Institution and later became professor of medicine at UCH and president of the Royal College of Physicians from 1926 to 1930. He was created a baronet in 1931. His appointment to Queen Square no doubt was more to do with prestige than neurological practice.

---

[16] Six are not mentioned in detail elsewhere. Charles Elam was appointed physician to outpatients (1870–7). It

Charles-Edouard Brown-Séquard

Of its first appointees, one in particular epitomises the combination of experimental work and clinical practice that shaped the style and stature of the National Hospital. Charles-Edouard Brown-Séquard was born in Port Louis in Mauritius to an American father and French mother. He attended the Royal College in Mauritius and graduated in medicine in Paris. He had already been elected FRS for his work on the physiology and pathology of the nervous system when he was appointed to the National Hospital, three weeks after Ramskill. In the years after graduation, Brown-Séquard's scrupulous observations of patients with spinal cord trauma injured by machetes in the sugar fields of Mauritius, and his animal lesion experiments in Paris, working in the clinical services of Trousseau and Rayer, led him to question existing dogma on the transmission of sensation from the spinal cord. What we now designate the Brown-Séquard syndrome was disputed, and even ridiculed, at the time, but eventually accepted as accurate by a committee set up to investigate his claims.

In 1854, Brown-Séquard took up a professorship at the Institute of Medicine and Medical Jurisprudence in Richmond, Virginia, but the authorities disapproved of animal experimentation and the students complained about the unintelligibility of his French accent. Malicious rumours circulated, claiming that he had African blood.[17] He had already

delivered six lectures at the Royal College of Surgeons in London on the physiology and pathology of the central nervous system (between 1838 and 1858), and also lectured at St Bartholomew's Hospital and the Royal Society, where he met Charles Darwin and Thomas Huxley. Darwin kept in contact, later writing to Brown-Séquard in the hope that he might secure a favourable review for the *On the Origin of Species* in France, and praising his experiments which (wrongly) purported to show that spinal epilepsy induced in guinea pigs could be passed to their offspring. A year later, Brown-Séquard delivered a further series of 12 lectures in Edinburgh and Glasgow on the physiology and pathology of the central nervous system in front of large and enthusiastic audiences, before lecturing in Dublin. Shortly after this second tour of the British Isles, he wrote to James Arnott, president of the Royal College of Surgeons (6 December 1859): 'My dear Sir, You

---

[17] Given the attitudes of Victorian Britain, it is worth noting that Brown-Séquard was one of three physicians appointed at Queen Square in the nineteenth century who was of mixed race. Brown-Séquard was the son of an American sea captain and a Creole French mother; his maternal great-grandmother was of Indian origin. Pierre Victor Lanougarède Bazire, appointed as assistant physician in 1864, was also a native of Mauritius. His death aged 32 was by all accounts a tragedy for Queen Square and for medicine and, as his obituarist noted, 'he had barely indicated the rarity and richness of his promise when death stepped in. Words can only coarsely outline the large grief of so great a loss.' He was a lifelong friend of Brown-Séquard, who stayed in his house in Woburn Square on visits to London; and he also published on paralysis of the diaphragm and spinal cord disease. John Samuel Risien Russell was born in Demerara (now British Guyana) where his Scottish father was the owner of a sugar plantation and one of the island's richest men. Risien (as he was often called) attended the Dollar Academy and then graduated in medicine in Edinburgh (1886). He worked at St Thomas' Hospital, in Nottingham, at the London Metropolitan Hospital as pathologist, and was appointed resident medical

officer at the National Hospital (1888), pathologist (1895–7), assistant physician (1898), physician to the outpatients (1899) and full physician (1909–28). In the 1890s, he was appointed professor of medical jurisprudence and subsequently professor of medicine at University College. He was president of the neurology section of the Royal Society of Medicine, and appointed to the Board of Management of the National Hospital. He served as a captain in the First World War, based in London, and was especially interested in the treatment of shell-shock. He was a very popular teacher and sociable person, sporting a chauffeur-driven Rolls Royce and hosting dinner parties at which a small string orchestra played. He had an enormous private practice, and was said to specialise particularly in the treatment of psychotic and psychoneurotic patients, who appreciated his charm and understanding. Critchley includes him among the pioneer neurologists in the *Ventricle of Memory* (1990), reporting that he exuded great charm and friendliness and was elegant with excellent taste. He wrote: 'as House Physician, I would wait in the front hall of the hospital for his arrival. His Rolls-Royce car drove up and the chauffeur alighted to open the door for him. Risien bounded up the stairs two or three at a time, his movements being as quick as those of an athlete. As he made his way round the wards, he had a kind word of praise, or even flattery, for each patient. Each one felt buoyed up after the remarks he made smilingly, even though he never carried out a physical examination ... Today, Risien Russell is forgotten. In his time, he was one of the most important and colourful figures within the medical profession of Great Britain. He was a sincere friend and wise counsellor, and I mourn his passing.' He was renowned for unmatched dedication to his patients and, worn out by work, he died in his consulting room in Wimpole Street and is buried in Highgate cemetery (Windrush Foundation).

treated me with so much kindness when I had the honour of seeing you in London eighteen months ago that I feel authorised to ask you to help me obtain the appointment at a hospital for paralytics and epileptics soon to be established in your metropolis.'[18]

Brown-Séquard's application, sent from Paris to the Board of Management at the National Hospital (December 1859), was endorsed by several eminent British physicians and surgeons, including Arnott and James Paget. All those who considered his application agreed that Brown-Séquard was a man of great personal integrity and humanity whose physiological research had helped significantly to advance understanding of the nervous system. During his short time at Queen Square, Brown-Séquard attracted much interest in, and publicity for, the hospital. He held regular clinical demonstrations in the Board room on the ground floor of 23 Queen Square on Monday afternoons, and lectured in the hospital, contributions that also contributed greatly to its rising reputation.

Brown-Séquard resigned from the hospital in July 1863, claiming that his burgeoning and highly lucrative private practice was exhausting and interfering with his ability to continue research. An apocryphal story runs that he looked out one day from the window of his house and saw the whole of the square outside filled with the carriages of people who had come to consult him. The deteriorating health and homesickness of his American wife Ellen may also have been a decisive factor in his decision to leave London. It is clear that the Board was sympathetic to his request and, in gratitude for his services to the new hospital, he was appointed honorary physician and later honorary life governor.

During the American Civil War, Brown-Séquard was offered a new chair in the physiology and pathology of the nervous system at Harvard Medical School (1864). After resigning on three occasions from that post, he eventually returned to Paris (1867), and became professor at the École de Médecine before the Franco-Prussian War forced him, once again, to flee abroad, only to return briefly to Paris once

hostilities had ceased. He applied unsuccessfully for the professorship of experimental medicine vacated by Magendie, when Claude Bernard was elected. Despite this setback, Brown-Séquard had now established himself in France as a well-respected clinician scientist. The Académie des Sciences awarded him a bursary equivalent to £1,000 for his experimental work on epilepsy, and shortly afterwards he received the Montyon Prize for experimental physiology. Back in New York for another three years, he returned to Britain in a depressed state and was offered a chair at the University of Glasgow, which he declined (in 1864) because of the inclement Scottish weather. After further peregrinations, and now aged 61, he eventually realised his life's ambition and succeeded Claude Bernard in the prestigious chair of experimental medicine at the Collège de France in Paris (in 1873).

Despite holding positions of great scientific prestige in several countries, Brown-Séquard's career was troubled and at times he seemed unable to cope with success. Some of his achievements were dismissed as those of an out-of-date crank who performed inhumane experiments on animals[19] and besmirched his reputation through work on testicular extracts. An alternative view is that he profoundly changed medicine as a pioneer of endocrinology and hormone replacement therapy. His ideas on the function of the nervous system proved in some respects to be ahead of their time, but in others to be quite mistaken. He was an intuitive and imaginative observer with the ability to conceptualise, but his reasoning was sometimes convoluted and lacking in clarity.

In its first 50 years, other members of the medical staff at the National Hospital conducted influential experimental work, notably Bastian, Ferrier and Horsley. Amongst others, Horsley worked with Tooth, Beevor, Semon, Ballance and Risien Russell, and, although their work was not carried out on the

---

[18] L-C. Celestin, *Charles-Edouard Brown-Séquard: The Biography of a Tormented Genius* (Heidelberg: Springer, 2014), p. 107. Brown-Séquard has attracted the attention of several other biographers. See also J. Olmsted, *Charles-Edouard Brown-Séquard: A Nineteenth Century Neurologist and Endocrinologist* (Baltimore: Johns Hopkins University Press, 1946); and M. J. Aminoff, *Brown-Séquard: An Improbable Genius who Transformed Medicine* (Oxford University Press, 2011).

[19] It has been suggested (initially by Victor Horsley) that Brown-Séquard was the model for Robert Louis Stevenson's Dr Jekyll. Ian McDonald noted that, in line with Brown-Séquard's ideas on the brain, the persona embodying Jekyll's 'evil side' is less developed because it is underused; Hyde represents the atrophied, stunted right hemisphere struggling to break free of the controls imposed by the dominant left brain. Horsley also reported to Sir Arthur Salusbury MacNalty that Brown-Séquard's personality was perceived by some as containing contradictory elements which resulted in alarming behaviour, and this may have attracted Stevenson's attention.

premises, due to the lack of any laboratory or animal facilities, each contributed significantly to the hospital's visibility. This was still the era of gifted amateurs whose work was driven largely by intellectual curiosity. As with the work of Brown-Séquard, to the modern eye the experiments were remarkable for lack of governance and institutional engagement. The rapid translation of experimental findings into clinical practice, notably at Queen Square, is testimony to the quality and ingenuity of the staff in this period. However, the emerging reputation of the hospital as a centre of excellence in neurology was also becoming apparent in more conventional ways.

Other Physicians at the National Hospital

Note here is made of seven other physicians at Queen Square who helped in their different ways to raise the reputation of the hospital in its first 50 years, and who made significant clinical and academic contributions to the emerging specialty of neurology. The careers of the four most celebrated doctors at the hospital (Jackson, Ferrier, Gowers and Horsley) are described elsewhere. However, the work in neurology was consolidated and a system of care and clinical science established, within the limits of methods and knowledge of the day, by these seven others who left fine reputations in fields for which Queen Square became famous: epilepsy (Sieveking, Reynolds and Aldren Turner), influence and administration (Reynolds again), paralysis and aphasia (Bastian), clinical lectures on diverse topics (Buzzard), and the description of new diseases (Batten and Tooth).

Of the first generation, the most senior was Sir Edward Henry Sieveking. He was born in London into an eminent and influential Habsburg family, and studied medicine in Berlin, Bonn, University College London and the University of Edinburgh. After qualification in 1841, he was appointed physician to the London Lock Hospital, assistant physician to St Mary's Hospital in 1851, and to the honorary medical staff at the National Hospital between 1864 and 1868. Sieveking was interested in social aspects of medicine and medical advocacy on behalf of the poor, and contributed to many of the social debates of the time, denouncing, for instance, the philosophy of harsh deterrence that had been written into the Poor Laws of the 1830s. Early in his career, Sieveking published a book on the importance of ventilation in

healthy housing. He was personally involved in the training of nurses and wrote *Training Institutions for Nurses in Workhouses* (1849). He translated Romberg's famous *Manual of Nervous Diseases in Man* into English (1853); published a series of student notes, which were immensely popular; and co-authored a *Manual of Pathological Anatomy* (1854) illustrated with his own watercolours. Despite his proto-socialism, he was appointed physician to Queen Victoria (1888) and, later, King Edward VII. He was censor and then vice-president of the Royal College of Physicians (1888), gave the Croonian Lecture in 1866 and was the Harveian Orator in 1877. He was made a Knight of Grace of the Order of St John of Jerusalem (1886) and knighted by Queen Victoria in the same year.

Sir John Russell Reynolds was another renowned early physician at the hospital. He was born in Romsey, the son of a distinguished non-conformist minister and grandson of an eminent physician who had attended King George III. He was excluded from entry to Oxford or Cambridge on grounds of faith, but trained in medicine at University College London where he won three gold medals (1852). Due to financial uncertainties, he worked first in Leeds, but moved back to London and became the protégé of Marshall Hall. He was appointed professor of clinical medicine at University College Hospital (1862), physician at the National Hospital (1864) and elected FRS (1869) for his studies of the reflex functions of the spinal cord. He succeeded Jenner as professor of the practice of medicine a few years later. He was a major figure in British medicine at the time, appointed physician to the royal household in 1878, president of the Royal College of Physicians in 1893 and of the British Medical Association (1896), and made a baronet (1895). He delivered the Lumleian lecture (1867) and the Harveian Oration (1884). His interests were eclectic: he wrote on epilepsy, hemianaesthesia, meningitis, wasting palsy, poliomyelitis, paralysis agitans, marijuana in medicine, lunacy and criminal lunacy, and diagnosis in neurology. His lectures on 'Paralysis and other disorders of motion and sensation dependent on idea' (1869) were acknowledged by Charcot as influential on his own school's later work on hysteria. Reynolds was an important influence on Gowers in his early years, and promoted the career of his younger colleague. Reynolds wrote extensively, and perhaps his greatest achievement was the section on neurological disease in the *System of Medicine*

(5 volumes: 1866–79), which he largely wrote himself, with assistance from Hughlings Jackson, Ramskill, Gee, Gull, Anstie, Radcliffe and Buzzard. This is arguably the first modern comprehensive and detailed account of disorders of the nervous system in English.

Sieveking's junior by 19 years was Thomas Buzzard, who exemplified the style of a sound and practical physician that established the National Hospital as a centre for clinical excellence and teaching. He had an exotic and colourful early career, starting in 1855, when, as part of the medical team despatched to the Ottoman Army under Omar Pasha, he was present at the siege of Sebastopol and acted as special correspondent in the Crimea for the *Daily News*. He received the Crimean Medal with clasp, the Order of the Medjidie, and the Turkish war medal. Late in life, Buzzard published *With the Turkish Army in the Crimea and Asia Minor* (1915), an important source of information on this period. After the declaration of peace (1856), he continued to serve as a volunteer with the Queen's Westminster Rifles (1860–7). Buzzard was elected assistant physician at the National Hospital (1867) and consulting physician (1896). He wrote *Clinical Lectures on Diseases of the Nervous System* (1882), *Clinical Aspects of Syphilitic Nervous Affections* (1874), *Paralysis from Peripheral Neuritis* (1886) and *The Simulation of Hysteria by Organic Disease* (1891). He is remembered for Buzzard's symptom: 'the sudden giving way of legs in locomotor ataxy (tabes dorsalis)'. Buzzard continued in practice until aged 79, and he relaxed through sea travel and as a skilled water-colourist. His last contribution to the National Hospital was the appointment to its staff of his son, Sir Edward Farquhar Buzzard, of whom more later.

Following in the footsteps of Brown-Séquard was another scientist of repute, Henry Charlton Bastian. He was born in Truro, trained at University College, and worked first at the State Asylum for Criminal Lunatics at Broadmoor (1860), St Mary's Hospital (as lecturer), and then as the eleventh assistant physician appointed to the National Hospital in 1868. He was later appointed professor of medicine at University College Hospital and physician at St Mary's Hospital. He was an authority on nematodes, and named over 100 new species in his book on the *Anguillulidae*, and for this work was elected FRS in 1868 (at the age of only 31 years). After early work on insanity and the specific gravity of the brain, Bastian developed a more general interest in the nervous system, culminating in the publication of *The Brain as an Organ of Mind* (1880), an extensive treatise on the comparative anatomy of animal brains, written for lay readership, and which is a fine exposition of advanced contemporary knowledge. His work on aphasia which, adopting strict disconnectionist models, included original work on alexia and agraphia and receptive aphasia, was highly regarded and the subject of his Lumleian lectures (1897), later expanded and published as *A Treatise on Aphasia and Other Speech Defects* (1898). In the context of paralysis, Bastian's name is attached to the Bastian–Bruns sign, the loss of tone and tendon reflexes due to acute transection of the spinal cord. He wrote on the 'kinaesthetic cortex', in which he demonstrated that sensation is necessary for the brain to coordinate movement, and in which he criticised Ferrier for his insistence on separate motor and sensory cortical representation. Against this background, Bastian gave a series of eight lectures at University College Hospital, published in extended form as *On Paralysis from Brain Disease* (1875); later he wrote *Paralyses: Cerebral, Bulbar and Spinal* (1886), and *Various Forms of Hysterical or Functional Paralysis* (London, 1893). These books show just how far the neurology of paralysis had advanced in the preceding decades. He was a quiet and reserved man, considered one of the most intellectual physicians of his day, although reluctant to lecture or teach on ward rounds. In his later life, he canvassed some notoriety by advocating abiogenesis, the creation of living matter from non-living material, and heterogenesis, the transformation of one type of living matter into another. From the 1860s onwards, he had devoted many years of his life to experimentation in this field, thinking that he had observed the spontaneous generation of living organisms out of non-living matter (from a 'primordial soup'). His experiments were initially supported by Darwin, Huxley, Spencer and their colleagues, but were finally disowned by them. His support of abiogenesis resulted in heated and sometimes acrimonious argument, notably with Huxley and Pasteur. His book on this topic, *The Beginnings of Life: Being Some Account of the Nature, Modes of Origin and Transformation of Lower Organisms* (1872), was initially highly commended, and this was followed by later monographs including *The Evolution of Life* (1907) and *Remarks on Further Experiments Concerning the Origin of Life* (1912). Bastian, in his time, was considered a formidable intellectual and had a high reputation as a scientist and philosopher and helped embed science into the fabric of Queen Square.

We now turn to three neurologists of the next generation at the hospital. Henry Tooth was born in Hove, educated at Rugby School and trained in medicine from Cambridge, and then completed his clinical training at St Bartholomew's Hospital, where he was appointed assistant physician (1895) and full physician (1907) and as physician to the London Metropolitan Hospital (1887). He was appointed as assistant physician at Queen Square in 1887 and as physician in 1907. He served in the Boer War and in the First World War, and was created CMG in 1901 and CB in 1918, but is said not to have regained his full health after the anxieties of the war. He gave a renowned set of Goulstonian lectures in 1889 on secondary degeneration of the spinal cord, and was later appointed censor at the college. He is remembered today mainly for the description of hereditary peroneal muscular atrophy, based on his Cambridge doctoral thesis (1886), still designated Charcot–Marie–Tooth disease. He was a multi-talented man but it is said that he never fulfilled his early promise. He died aged 69 of a cerebral haemorrhage.[20]

A stalwart of the hospital was William Aldren Turner. The son of Sir William Turner, principal of Edinburgh University, he was born in Edinburgh, educated at Fettes and graduated in medicine in Edinburgh in 1887. After house physician posts in Edinburgh, he studied in Berlin and St Bartholomew's Hospital in London. His interest in neurology began with appointment as assistant to David Ferrier (publishing with him on cerebellar and sensory cortical connnections, and acting as his literary executor) in the neuropathology laboratory at King's College Hospital (1892), where he subsequently became physician in charge of neurological cases (1908) after being appointed physician at the National Hospital (1900–25). Turner published, jointly with Grainger Stewart, a *Textbook of Nervous Diseases* (1910). Aged 50 years at the outbreak of the First World War, he was sent to the front in France (1914), appointed neurologist to the forces at home (1915–19); to the War Office Medical Board (1919–40); as a member of the War Office Committee on Shell Shock (1920–1); to the Army nursing board; and as consultant adviser to the Ministry of Pensions (1930–43). His Bradshaw lecture at the Royal College of Physicians was on 'Neuroses and psychoses of war' (1918) and he seems not to have been

impressed by the treatment approach of Yealland at the National Hospital.

Finally, mention must be made of Frederick Eustace Batten. He was born in Plymouth, the son of a Queen's Counsel, and trained at St Bartholomew's Hospital. After a period of study in Berlin, he was elected a member of the Physiological Society and appointed 'pathologist' at the National Hospital in 1899, then physician in 1900 and dean of the medical school in 1908. He also held an appointment at the Hospital for Sick Children, Great Ormond Street, and worked at both hospitals until his untimely death at the age of 52 years, following an operation on his prostate. He published significant papers on muscle spindles, dystrophia myotonica, subacute combined degeneration of the cord, and contributed considerably to knowledge and management of poliomyelitis (the subject of his Lumleian lectures in 1916), but is now perhaps best remembered for his description of neuronal ceroid lipofuscinosis (Batten's disease) and his outstanding contributions to paediatric neurology, and not least for his renowned textbook, co-authored with Garrod and Thursfield, *Diseases of Children* (the first edition of which was published in 1913). He has been called the father of paediatric neurology and, in recognition of his work on polio, the respiratory unit at Queen Square was named the Batten Unit.

The Style of Medical Practice at the National Hospital

The eminence of these and other members of the consultant staff attracted clinical trainees who had to compete for positions. As early as 1880, the resident house physicians at Queen Square were relatively senior, having already completed internships in general medicine. After a few years 'on the house', aspiring neurologists usually proceeded to an assistant physician post in neurology. A vivid picture of the life of the junior medical staff at the National Hospital in the 1890s is provided by Purves-Stewart. He was appointed junior house physician (1896–8) when the hospital was 'at the summit of its fame'. The junior medical staff consisted of one senior and one junior house physician only. Each was assigned to individual visiting physicians, the selection of whom they should serve being made by the senior house physician. Purves-Stewart described how, on the ward rounds, the consultants treated their junior doctors:

---

[20] See J. Pearce, 'Howard Henry Tooth (1856–1925)', *Journal of Neurology* **247** (2000): 3–4.

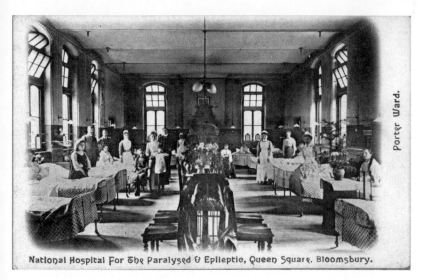

Porter Ward.

National Hospital For The Paralysed & Epileptic, Queen Square. Bloomsbury.

Figure 3.3 George Porter ward.

Different chiefs varied in their reaction … some listened placidly and without comment to the house-physicians' notes read out at the bedside … others corrected them kindly or sarcastically as the case might … some addressed the sufferer impersonally; others treated him with courtesy and kindliness; a few were impatient, rude and even domineering striving for dramatic effect.[21]

Wards were not allocated to individual physicians and, in this way, the National Hospital differed from most other hospitals. The ward rounds were forbidding experiences, with the juniors scurrying around the consultants like worker ants. One can imagine the tension when, as Purves-Stewart remarked, 'two physicians might happen to visit a ward at the same time, each of them attended by his satellite house-physician, clinical clerks and post-graduate visitors'.[22] The house physicians' duties were confined entirely to inpatients and they were not allowed to attend clinics. These posts were no sinecure, and they tested a young doctor's resolve and stamina. The house physicians were male (until the First World War), resident, permanently on-call, forbidden to leave the hospital without permission and must be unmarried. In addition to pandering to the requirements of the consultant physicians, they were responsible for taking histories, conducting physical examinations and keeping patients' notes. They were required to see the patients twice daily; supervise treatment and dispense drugs; organise the removal of patients showing mania, imbecility or feeble-mindedness; oversee the equipment and food and ventilation; and conduct post-mortem examinations. Despite the privations, house-physician posts at Queen Square were greatly prized and, after a few years, most applied for the post of assistant physician,[23] the junior house physician being promoted into his place.

---

[21] See J. Purves-Stewart, *The Sands of Time* (London: Hutchinson & Co., 1939). Sir James Purves-Stewart was subsequently physician at the Westminster Hospital and the West End Hospital for Nervous Diseases. His obituary in the *Lancet* (**253** (1949): 1122), which is unusually critical, records that 'he may not have been a great neurologist'. He was, however, intrepid and adventurous, a linguist and a patriot, and a man who loved travel, revelling in his military career during the First World War. He was knighted in 1918. Purves-Stewart became mired in a controversy over his claims for an infective origin, and the production of a vaccine, for multiple sclerosis. This was investigated by Carmichael and famously rubbished by Walshe, and as a result Purves-Stewart retired prematurely from the Westminster Hospital (in 1931). His country house, the Belle Toute lighthouse on Beachy Head, became another *cause célèbre*. Despite his disparagement by the Queen Square establishment, the autobiography records his early years at the hospital with great affection.

---

[22] Similarly tense stand-offs during ward rounds were later recorded between Gordon Holmes and Kinnier Wilson, and Lyndsay Symon and Roger Gilliatt. No doubt there were many other examples.

[23] In those days, initially at another London teaching hospital before applying to return as assistant physician at the National Hospital. A few gilded individuals were appointed as assistant physician directly from a junior position at the National Hospital.

There were no separate neurology departments in any of the London teaching hospitals, and appointment to a training post at either of the other two specialist neurology hospitals was regarded as very much second-best. As Purves-Stewart records, 'It was deemed even then impossible for a neurologist to attain more than a scanty foothold outside the sacred walls of the National Hospital, the staff of which, up till then, deservedly possessed almost a monopoly in this class of work.'

In the first years of the hospital, the numbers of patients began rapidly to expand. In 1869, there were 319 discharges but, by the 1890s, that figure had risen to 850–950 patients annually. The range of diagnoses also broadened. In 1869, of the 319 discharged patients, 138 had a diagnosis of paralysis of various types, and 142 of epilepsy, with only 39 with other diseases listed (not specified, but probably mainly psychoneuroses). By 1899, a year in which there were 905 discharges, only 14.5 per cent had epilepsy and 11 per cent hemiplegia. There were 28 categories of other diseases which included disseminated sclerosis (7.5 per cent), intracranial tumour (7 per cent), infantile paralysis (poliomyelitis, 6 per cent), functional paralysis (6.4 per cent), neurosyphilis (various forms, 5 per cent) and myelitis (4 per cent).[24] The hospital had become, in effect, a tertiary centre and, as the annual report for 1894 explained:

A large and increasing proportion represent patients sent here at the recommendation of medical practitioners or from other hospitals for an authoritative diagnosis of obscure and difficult cases ... distinguished members of the profession ... have from time to time borne testimony to the value of the hospital as an institution where the patient will obtain 'an opinion beyond which there is no appeal ... he will be candidly told whether his ailment be curable or incurable, and, if curable, he will have the best means which science at the present day can afford towards his restoration to health'.

Despite complexity in the mix of activities, daily routine was said to proceed in every department with the smoothness of a well-oiled machine. Russell Reynolds had said that there must be 'treatment, treatment, treatment always treatment'. In *A Hospital in the Making*, Burford Rawlings provides a vivid picture of what was offered:

Patients were rubbed, stretched, smacked, kneaded, straightened, electrified, hung from tripods on the roof, swathed in bandages and steeped in sulphur baths. Their torpid muscles were roused by passive movements. They were cased in plaster jackets, weights were attached to their legs and occasionally they were hypnotised. If, after all this had been done, the stubborn malady would not go away, it was only because the result striven for lay beyond the reach of human powers.

Towards the end of the nineteenth century, Robert Brudenell Carter published an editorial in *The Times* enthusing about the extraordinary advances in therapeutics for nervous disorders of movement and sensation treated at the National Hospital, but not everyone agreed and his article was followed by a sarcastic and witty rebuttal, anonymous but probably by Dr Charles Mercier, an Irish neuropsychiatrist and great admirer of Hughlings Jackson, who had 'walked the wards' at Queen Square as a young man:

We cannot say that we were at all favourably impressed with the treatment and the results we saw and we have looked in vain for any published results, which might tend to modify our opinion. We were struck by the admirable knowledge of nervous anatomy and physiology and by the diagnostic acumen displayed by the staff and by the eager enthusiasm with which the cases were discussed as examples of this or that theory, but we were completely disappointed when the subject of treatment was approached. There was a general air of hopelessness then, a sort of silent confession, 'well you know, one must give something but really little improvement can be expected'. When once the eminent physician has made a diagnosis, the patient is relegated to the out-patient department, where the fortunate recipients of the best advice modern medicine can give are seen once a week by the assistant physician, and run through at the rate of three a minute, the prescriptions being marked, often week after week, 'rep Omnia' or in plain English 'go on as before'. We yield to no one in our admiration of the brilliant results of Dr Hughlings Jackson's investigations on epilepsy, but we are convinced that he would be the last to assert that he has discovered any scientific treatment of that disease. In the above out-patient department may be seen numbers of epileptics in whom the disease has been localised, forsooth, and then left to run its course. These unfortunates may be seen with their bottles, 'forty feeding like one', on bromide and paraldehyde and other drugs, which a hundred years hence will be looked upon as we look

---

[24] Data taken from the medical superintendent's and registrar's reports in the National Hospital annual reports for 1869 and 1899.

upon the filthy excretions and abominations which our fathers in medicine called drugs.[25]

Notwithstanding this polemic, it had become clear that, by 1900 and within only four decades of its foundation, the quality of the staff had made the National Hospital the 'Mount Olympus of neurology'. From within, that eminence has never since been doubted; and, despite some ups and downs in its fortunes and the development of healthy rivals in and outside London, no charitable outside observer would argue otherwise, either then or, indeed, at any time afterwards.

The Written Record of the National Hospital

The National Hospital Case Notes

Within three years of its opening, physicians with admission rights at the National Hospital started to archive their inpatient case notes. Most have survived and are an important primary source in the early history of neurology.[26] The first casebook (1863 to 1867) documents the history of each patient, a note of the physical signs, the diagnosis and a list of the prescribed medicines. By 1870, the scope had broadened to include other details: occupation, family history, past medical illnesses, symptoms and duration of the presenting complaint, physical signs,

response to therapy, admission and discharge dates, and name of the admitting consultant. Later the admitting house physician is identified. Continuation sheets list treatments; measurements of temperature, pulse, respiration and weight; urine analysis; fit charts; details of sensory and visual perimetry; outpatient visits; drawings and photographs; and post-mortem findings. Correspondence with the referring doctor before and after discharge is occasionally included. Descriptions of seizures witnessed by the nurses, including their assessments of pupil reactions and limb reflexes, are also provided. Within 20 years, a scheme of history taking and clinical examination was in place that has since become standard throughout the world. Taking into consideration the advances in neurology and increased range of investigations in recent times it is surprising how many diagnoses made in the first 50 years still conform to modern concepts of neurological disease.

The case notes also indicate the approach to treatment used in the hospital during its first 50 years. Physical therapy, 'a congeries of baths in every variety', massage, and galvanic and faradic stimulation were prominent. Indeed, it was expertise in this particular field that received greatest coverage in the national press. Counter-irritation was much used, and ice bags to the spine were a favoured treatment for paralysis. Physicians such as Charles Beevor, who had trained in Paris with Charcot, were also adept at hypnosis. Occasionally, doctors from elsewhere, such as the eminent mesmerist Charles Lloyd Tuckey,[27] were consulted. Among the drugs in much use by the end of the nineteenth century were potassium bromide, paraldehyde, cocaine, hyoscine, Indian hemp, morphine, chloral, belladonna tincture, serine (physostigmine), antipyrum and chloroform.

In addition to the hospital notes, it was not unusual for house physicians and other trainees to keep a notebook listing the cases thay had clerked. Organised alphabetically as in an address book, it seems that these were issued (or commercially available) since they had printed throughout schema for drawing the distribution of sensory and reflex changes. Later,

---

[25] Anon., *Mad Doctors, by One of Them. Being a Defence of Asylum Physicians Against Recent Aspersions … and an Examination into the Functions of the Lunacy Commission, Together with a Scheme of Lunacy Reform* (London: Swan Sonnenschein & Co., 1890).

[26] The best account of the case notes comes from the centenary celebrations of the National Hospital (1960); see R. A. Hunter and L. J. Hurwitz, 'The Case Notes of the National Hospital for the Paralysed and Epileptic, Queen Square, London, before 1900', *Journal of Neurology, Neurosurgery, and Psychiatry* 24 (1961): 187–94. These notes illustrate how precise and detailed observation of clinical facts contributed to the growing science of neurology. They include the original description of many famous cases, including Horsley's operations for focal epilepsy; Gowers' case of a 16-year-old girl with 'tetanoid chorea' from 1888, which was found to be an early case of hepatolenticular degeneration (Wilson's disease); the Worster–Drought family, now known to be due to the *BRI2* mutation; and an early example of semantic dementia described by Critchley in 1938 (see P. Witoonpanich, S. J. Crutch, J. D. Warren and M. N. Rossor, 'The Undiscovered Syndrome: Macdonald Critchley's Case of Semantic Dementia', *Neurocase* 21 (2015): 408–12).

[27] Tuckey was author of the celebrated book *Psychotherapeutics or Treatment by Hypnotism or Suggestion* (London: Balliere, Tindall and Cox, 1890). There used to be a tradition of performing hypnotism by the National Hospital physicians. Sir Charles Symonds was perhaps the last to use this routinely in his neurological practice.

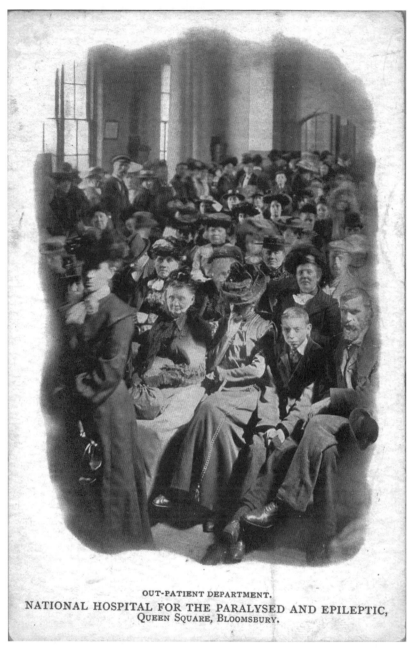

OUT-PATIENT DEPARTMENT.
NATIONAL HOSPITAL FOR THE PARALYSED AND EPILEPTIC,
QUEEN SQUARE, BLOOMSBURY.

Figure 3.4 The outpatients hall.

standardised admission forms were available as loose sheets for binding into the notes. One notebook survives (and no doubt others exist) that belonged to James Collier, and records several hundred cases seen by him from December 1894, with names, details of the history and examination findings.[28]

[28] This manuscript notebook was subsequently in the possession of Macdonald Critchley and purchased with various items from his library when this was sold at auction in 2016.

A representative example of information contained in the notes is the case of William Greenland Woodchester, aged 53, who worked as driver of a stationary engine near Stroud in Gloucestershire. He was admitted on 27 May 1877 and discharged at his own request 'in status quo' on 9 July. We learn that his father had died of a chill aged 34, and his mother at the age of 74 from old age. One of his two sisters had died of a haemorrhage and William had two surviving siblings. His past medical history was uneventful. The presenting illness had started two years before admission with tingling in the toes of his left foot, which spread slowly into his left arm. He then started to limp and could no longer fully elevate his left arm. Six months later, he developed a quivering of the left hand during rest. After four months, the trembling spread to the right arm. In the previous year, he had started to hold his head in a constrained position and felt a tendency to fall forwards or backwards when walking. He experienced flushing and a feeling of heat all over his body, with profuse perspiration even in cold weather. He was depressed and complained of insomnia. Feelings of uneasiness if sitting for any length of time forced him continually to adjust his position. He had recently experienced severe pain in the back of the neck. On examination, he was noted to be a tall, well-built man who looked somewhat younger than his stated age. He had a coarse intermittent lip and jaw tremor, aggravated by stress or talking and relieved by gently touching his chin. His hands had assumed the position of holding a pea, with flexion of the wrist and the forefinger firmly opposed to the thumb. There was a pronation–supination and flexion–extension tremor of the hands and forearms, and a mild trembling of the legs. The tremor disappeared during movement or exertion of the affected limb and was observed by the nurses to be absent during deep sleep. His neck was stiff and flexed, with marked restriction of head movement. When walking, he leaned forward and shuffled but did not break into a trot. The diagnosis of paralysis agitans (Parkinson's disease) was made.

Although the National Hospital did not develop a dedicated medical illustration service until the early 1950s, photographs can occasionally be found pasted into the case notes; and there is a manuscript entry by Henry Head, then the resident medical officer, to indicate that at least some were taken on the hospital wards using a handheld camera. Horsley illustrated the location of craniotomies with before and after pictures of the shaven skulls of his patients, the incisions marked out in ink. Even after the value of illustration as a concise objective record of medical conditions had been recognised, physicians remained reluctant to use photographs, and some, including Gowers, still preferred to sketch the physical signs encountered in their practices.

The following case, managed in 1885 by Buzzard (whose son, Edward Farquahar Buzzard, later described lymphocyte accumulations in the thymus and muscles of patients with myasthenia), includes the first photograph of a patient with myasthenia gravis:[29]

One morning in 1876 this 32 year old labourer from Thornton Le Fen, Lincoln woke with one eyelid half fallen (he could not recall which). There had been no ague in his neighbourhood. In 1881, he found one morning that his right hand was so weak that he couldn't lift or hold anything. In 1883 he couldn't walk very far and noticed that his legs would feel weaker after working. In 1885 he felt difficulty chewing his food, bad at times and better again; about the same time he would have difficulty with his speech. He was rather sleepy in appearance from drooping of the upper eyelids – only slight movement upwards was possible and there was very little power of movement of the eyes; the left moved a little inwards and upwards whereas the right scarcely at all. He was unable to close his eyes completely or chew well but he could swallow quite well. On laryngeal examination his cords move freely, closed well and opened fairly. His voice was a little nasal and after talking a little while he could scarcely get his words out. He could not get into the erect position when lying without catching hold of something above him. Sensation and reflexes were normal and he never had problems with his water or bowels. All upper and lower limb muscles acted very well to Faradism except the anterior extensor group of the right leg where a strong current was necessary to get a minimal contraction. He was discharged in status quo.

At the end of each year, the notes were bound in volumes (11 inches in height) by alphabetical order, with an index of patients' names and diagnoses included at the front. There were separate male and female sections, and notes for each consultant were bound separately. Depending on the caseload, an individual consultant might have several volumes covering any one year. In 1905, for example, there were details of 695 patients contained in 16 volumes.

---

29 Thomas Willis' description (1672) was largely forgotten. The first major contribution came a year after this patient developed ptosis, when Samuel Wilks reported a case. See S. Wilks, 'On Cerebritis, Hysteria and Bulbar Paralysis', *Guy's Hospital Reports* **22** (1877): 7–55.

During the First World War, the clinical assessment and examination were usually typewritten, whereas the rest of the file was in manuscript. The case notes continued to be archived up to formation of the National Health Service. Until the early 1980s, many were stored on shelves in consulting room C in the outpatients department, and others in the basement medical records department. When the outpatients department was relocated (1991), the notes were stored briefly in the Board room before being moved to a damp basement in Wakefield Street. Large steam pipes ran across the storeroom ceiling; the temperature was about 28°C and the outside wall was covered in black mould and leaked. When the Gowers library was temporarily moved to Guilford Street, new accommodation was found for the case notes in cool, dry, temperature-stable rooms. Here they remained after the Gowers library returned to hospital premises, being moved from one basement to another in Guilford Street as leases expired. Unfortunately, the nurses' residence was above the library and the volumes of case notes (and books for the patients) were threatened by flooding from overflowing taps. Eventually, the inevitable happened and water cascaded down one wall and damaged several shelves of books. These were rescued and transferred to the basement of 7 Queen Square in March 2007. In 2009, as part of an initiative to form a museum and archive for the hospital, the case notes were finally transferred to environmentally controlled conditions above the medical library on the fourth floor of 23 Queen Square. By this stage, several volumes had been borrowed and never returned.

A handwritten index, by condition, is available up to 1931 and each volume has been re-indexed at the front by patient's name and diagnosis. In 2017, volunteers are transcribing this onto a spreadsheet in order to improve searches, and a similar index for cases from 1932 onwards is planned. A first volume of case notes has been digitised and redacted, with plans for the rest to follow. These case notes are, by their very nature, a domestic record that speaks to the lives and times of ordinary people whose illnesses informed the description of neurological disease at the dawn of modern clinical neurology. But they serve another purpose, and that is to inform published accounts of knowledge on disorders affecting the brain, spinal cord and nerves that taught the world outside Queen Square the principles of neurology, as understood and practised at the National Hospital.

The Bible of Neurology

By 1880, the physicians at the National Hospital had published a number of books (at least 20) and these were at the time more influential than journal articles, being widely consulted and referred to as valuable sources of information. It was upon these books that the reputation of the hospital to an extent rested. Of these, one more than any other came to represent the Queen Square approach to clinical practice and became generally known as 'The Bible of Neurology'.

A Manual of the Diseases of the Nervous System, published in two volumes in 1886–8 by Sir William Gowers, is even now, 130 years later, still widely considered to be a crowning achievement. Volume I on diseases of the spinal cord and nerves contains 463 pages; volume II on diseases of the brain and cranial nerves, and general and functional diseases of the nervous system, runs to 975 pages. The two volumes of the second edition appeared in 1891 and 1893, respectively. Although lettering on the spines was unchanged, the subtitle of volume I was reversed to *Diseases of the Nerves and Spinal Cord*. Volume I of the third edition (1899), co-authored with James Taylor,[30] retained that arrangement and was

---

[30] James Taylor was a Scot who graduated from Edinburgh Medical School at the age of 30, after starting his adult professional life as a banker. He completed his house jobs at Edinburgh Royal Infirmary and did some postgraduate studies in Germany before taking up a house physician post at the National Hospital in 1889. He then served as senior assistant physician, outpatient physician and finally full physician (1893–1924), during which period he provided a link to Gowers and Jackson – filtering, translating and disseminating oral history and ideas to a new generation of British neurologists. He was a loyal disciple of both Hughlings Jackson and Gowers. Jackson would often turn up unannounced at Taylor's rooms and summon him even in the middle of a consultation without Taylor ever seeming to mind. When Taylor moved into his own home, Jackson presented him with a sofa and left him £500 in his will as a legacy of their longstanding friendship. He was a superb administrator, lucid teacher and kindly painstaking physician. Like Jackson and Gowers, he had a keen interest in neuro-ophthalmology, holding an appointment at Moorfields Eye Hospital for many years. His writings included the making of the distinction between tabetic optic neuritis and tabes dorsalis. He is now best recognised as the editor of the *Selected Writings of John Hughlings Jackson* (1931–2) and for the third edition of Gowers' *A Manual of Diseases of the Nervous System* (1899), but he also made significant contributions to neuro-ophthalmology and

expanded to 692 pages. Why volume II of the third edition never appeared remains something of a mystery. Gowers may have had in mind reducing the *Manual* to a single volume by omitting much of the anatomy and physiology contained in the first two editions. The work of producing the text and the illustrations for his major work had also, by the time of the third edition, caused Gowers' health to suffer. Critchley claimed to have seen a copy of volume II of the second edition marked up for the third, and he acquired page proofs for some or all of the final edition. But, of this preparatory material, all that survives are unmarked page proofs of the third edition, volume I, pp. 107–394 (as published); and, in line with Critchley's recollection, pages 142–213 and 299–301 of volume II from the second edition, of which pages 168–213 are indeed corrected in Gowers' hand. This work may not have been the first textbook of neurology, but the *Manual* is certainly the most renowned. Its two main characteristics, which reflect Gowers' own clear and concise prose style, were accurate clinical observation and logical organisation into a classification of neurological disease that has survived. Gowers created order out of chaos, placing the morass of different conditions within an overarching and logical nosology, and his analyses of symptoms and signs are still useful.

When the *Manual* appeared, Gowers had been working at the National Hospital for 14 years, largely in outpatients because he was not yet appointed as a full physician. His eye for detail and use of shorthand to document the clinical history allowed him to record accurately his findings in the clinic, better than many of his colleagues, and the book is rich in precise and pertinent observations. As Spillane wrote (*The Doctrine of Nerves*, 1981) the *Manual* was 'Free of those fustian lines and purple patches which characterized so much Victorian writing'. The style is economical and precise, uncluttered by speculation or idle hypothesis, and selective but fair in its references to other work. His writing exudes the authority of a man who knows his field and is prepared to sift evidence, apply statistical methods, and impart knowledge based on his own observations and interpretations.

At its launch, the book received an enthusiastic reception in the medical press. The *British Medical Journal* considered that 'no better manual on nervous

diseases had been presented to the medical profession'. Sir William Osler wrote that the *Manual* 'had placed the author at a comparative early age among the highest living authorities on all matters related to the nervous system'. But in *Brain*, after a copious and laudatory review, the editor Armand de Watteville concluded his appreciation with waspish criticism of Gowers' etymology.[31] As a great stylist and firm believer in plain words, this infuriated Gowers and he never forgave de Watteville. As a result, Gowers, alone amongst the academic physicians at Queen Square, did not submit papers to *Brain* while de Watteville was the editor; and he never served on the editorial board or as a guarantor of the journal.

The *Manual* is arranged as follows: I. General symptomatology, II. Diseases of the nerves, and III. Diseases of the spinal cord – all in volume I; and IV. Diseases of the brain, and V. General and functional diseases, in volume II. Each is extensively illustrated with Gowers' own careful and instructive line-drawings. His power of clinical observation is well illustrated by examples from the first section. Here he discusses defects of motion, sensation and coordination, and alteration in the tendon reflexes. He describes how paralysis of triceps prevents a person from raising his hat in the customary manner; and how weakness of infraspinatus can prevent movement along the lines when writing because of difficulty rotating the humerus. He advises that touch and pain sensation are tested separately because these may be differentially affected. Cricket balls containing various weights, and hot and cold spoons, are used as part of the sensory examination. The reflexes that Gowers tests are mainly cutaneous, such as plantar, gluteal, cremasteric and abdominal; but he makes a particular study of the patellar reflex, renaming it the knee jerk and commenting that it is 'probably never

---

paediatric neurology, writing *Paralysis and Other Diseases of the Nervous System in Children and Early Life* (1905) at the suggestion of Gowers. He retired from the Queen Square staff in 1924.

[31] De Watteville wrote: 'So in order not to derogate to the time-honoured tradition of reviewers always to find some fault with the work under notice, we shall attract Dr Gowers' attention to some verbal mistakes in the course of the book … We find that Dr Gowers adopts the absurd "pontine" for "pontal". Pontine is the name of marshes near Rome, but not the adjective derived from pons. Again, as the Greek "method" gives "methodic" so anŏd and kathŏd (usually misspelt and mispronounced anōde and cathōde) give anŏŏdic and kathŏdic, not anōdal and kathōdal. Again "faradaic" is not only pedantic but inexact; in forming an adjective from the name Faraday, the terminal diphthong *ay* should be replaced by the termination *ic*': *Brain* **11** (1888): 131–3.

absent in health'. He defines many diseases even if not specifically named (an example is what we know today as juvenile myoclonic epilepsy, which he clearly delineated).

Many sections of the *Manual* – such as those on epilepsy, headache, paralysis agitans and writer's cramp, and the clinical descriptions of disease – can still be read with benefit. Conditions such as Dubini's electric chorea have disappeared from current classifications, and the true nature of others such as saltatoric spasms remains obscure. Huntington's disease receives only a footnote in the first edition, whereas the frequency of writer's cramp among the army of clerks working in the city encouraged Gowers to wax lyrical in a detailed and thoughtful 20-page account. Sydenham's chorea, syphilis and diphtheria, all extensively covered, are now much less important causes of morbidity. His 40-page description of locomotor ataxia (tabes dorsalis) under diseases of the spinal cord received particularly favourable contemporary comment but is something of a period piece for the modern reader. Gowers eagerly embraced the new science of cellular pathology, which led to steady refinement of the term 'neurosis' for neurological conditions without a structural lesion. In interpreting the mechanisms of various neurological disorders, Gowers often invokes the work on mapping of cortical function by his colleagues Ferrier, Jackson and Horsley, and he also recognises that the emerging discoveries regarding heredity will radically change the classification of neurological disease.

Although he was a master nosologist, he finishes the *Manual* on a cautionary note, emphasising to his readers that many changes to the classification of nervous disease are to be expected: 'It is often better not to gratify the craving for nomenclature that is manifested by many patients, but rather to explain to them that to give their ailments a definite name would involve more error than truth.'

Paralysis at the National Hospital

The National Hospital was founded to provide care for people with paralysis and epilepsy. Paralysis was a feared and common affliction, often considered, up to this point, as a relatively unitary condition. One of the achievements of the early physicians at Queen Square was to develop a system for regional diagnosis, differentiating causes that were cerebral, spinal or peripheral – and also subdividing these categories

on a clinico-anatomical basis, and to an extent making aetiological diagnoses. Gowers was pre-eminent in this field, and his manual has superb sections concerned with the diagnosis and characterisation of paralysis in its various forms. In 1871, he listed the diagnosis of 168 inpatients at the hospital, of whom 30 had cerebral paralysis, 26 paraplegia due to spinal disease, three suffered from peripheral paralysis, five had disseminated paralysis, one had acquired diphtheria, and five were paralysed due to lead poisoning. Jackson also minutely dissected the symptoms and signs of paralysis, and this was one of the conditions that allowed him to formulate theories on the hierarchical structure of the nervous system.

Indeed, most physicians appointed to the hospital in its early years wrote on paralysis, but the definitive works were those of Bastian. He defined paralysis as the 'impeded conduction of motor stimuli to muscles owing to some morbid condition in or acting upon certain nerves, parts of the spinal cord or encephalon'. In contrast, convulsions are the result of 'an exalted transmission of stimuli to the muscles affected, owing to the existence of abnormal states of certain portions of the encephalon or spinal cord, but mostly of the former'. These two conditions coincide when their origins are in the encephalon, and, in this situation, the paralysis is almost invariably caused by morbid conditions that can be seen by visual or microscopic inspection, whereas convulsions usually result from invisible 'molecular disturbances'. Bastian describes the diagnostic approach to a case of paralysis as an initial regional or anatomical assessment and then offers a pathological diagnosis based on age, speed and mode of onset, and associated morbidities. No clearer exposition of the principles of clinical diagnosis is to be found, and the twofold diagnostic approach of 'where is' and 'what is' the lesion is still used, worldwide, as the basis for clinical analysis. Bastian considers the forms of paralysis due to encephalic, bulbar, cranial, spinal and peripheral origins – each based on regional and pathological diagnosis. His accounts are comprehensive in that he describes meticulously the vascular supply of various parts of the brain, mental symptoms, the crossed motor and sensory arrangements at different levels, and associated effects on vision, speech, reading and writing in the various cases of paralysis.

In relation to pathology, Bastian recognises thrombosis, haemorrhage, trauma, tumour, abscess, aneurysm, disseminated sclerosis, infections (especially cysticercosis), and the other causes, which include congenital forms, progressive muscular atrophy, Friedreich's disease and motor neurone disease. He discusses hysterical paralysis, a diagnosis that he recognises can only be made by exclusion, differentiating hysterical from functional weakness. The latter is dependent on an 'idea' in neurotic and impressionable people, and is a form of inhibition or reflex paralysis different from conscious simulation, i.e. hysteria.

As for treatment, Bastian's pragmatic ideas on management have lasted. Attention to general health and nutrition are vital for all patients. He emphasises that, after stroke, for example, improvement depends mainly on the natural history rather than any medical endeavour, and on age. Thrombosis might improve with amyl nitrite, perhaps through the formation of a collateral circulation. Skin care in paraplegia involves the use of warm dry bedclothes, free from rucks, or waterbeds. Daily baths, with the skin being thoroughly cleaned with soap and water and then dried, followed by rubbing with methylated spirits or eau de Cologne and dusting with talcum powder, should be regarded as standard nursing procedures. The feet must be separated in bed by a firm bolster and cushions placed under the Achilles tendon and the knees. Cradles are used to free the legs from the weight of bedclothes. Regular turning is essential to reduce the risk of pressure sores. These are treated with benzoin and glycerin emollients, and sometimes with eusol, aluminium acetate and dry gauze stimulants. Urinary retention is managed by aseptic catheterisation; and urinary infections treated by lavage with quinine sulphate, mercury oxycyanide or boric acid for infections producing alkaline urine, and silver nitrate or normal saline for those resulting in acidity. Profuse reflex sweating requires atropine liquor, and muscular spasms are helped by avoidance of triggers such as contact from bed clothes, the use of a warm bath and treatment with sedatives.

The fact is that no medicine was then available which had even the remotest effect on the mechanisms of paralysis. If there was anything useful to be done by way of intervention, this lay in the mysterious realms of electrical therapy and massage. After Bastian, no further monographs were published on the topic of paralysis by physicians at the National Hospital until

recent times – in marked contrast, for instance, to those on epilepsy. Bastian's work is comprehensive and definitive, and perhaps nothing more could be said. The topic as a whole seems to have attracted diminishing interest in the final decade of the nineteenth century.

Epilepsy at the National Hospital

Epilepsy, recognised since antiquity and mired in superstition and traditional beliefs, was the other condition specified in the name of the hospital. Early in the nineteenth century, epilepsy was aligned with insanity. Asylums were built to house epileptics, or wards set aside for their care in lunatic asylums. Outside Britain, these included the Heil und Pflegeanstalt für Schwachsinnige und Epileptische (1849) and Bethel (1867) in Germany; the Epileptic and Paralytic Hospitals on Blackwell's Island, New York (1867); and wards in the Bicêtre in Paris. The National Hospital was, however, the first to be opened specifically for inpatient and outpatient medical care – as opposed to asylum – of people with epilepsy. The inclusion of epilepsy in the hospital purpose seems to have been rather an afterthought at its foundation, but it soon became absolutely central to the work.

Several of the first 20 doctors appointed to the hospital had a major interest in the condition. Ramskill was much concerned with treatment, and Gordon Holmes indicates that 'almost every week [Ramskill] brought a specimen of a new drug, always hopeful that he had found in it a cure for epilepsy'. Ramskill reported the first use of bromides at the National Hospital and helped to popularise this new therapy that was to have such an important influence on the hospital's reputation.[32] Radcliffe (1858), Sieveking (1858), Reynolds (1861) and Echeverria (1870, after he had moved to Blackwell's Island Hospital in New York) each wrote monographs on epilepsy.

Radcliffe[33] had already written *Epilepsy and Other Convulsive Affections: Their Pathology and Treatment*

---

[32] J. S. Ramskill, 'Epilepsy Treated by the Bromide of Potassium', *Medical Times Gazette* **29** (1863): 221.

[33] Charles Radcliffe was born in Lincolnshire, graduated from London University in 1845 as gold medallist, and was appointed physician to the Westminster Hospital in 1857 and to the National Hospital in 1863. Radcliffe wrote on *The Philosophy of Vital Motion* (1851) and *Dynamics of Nerve and Muscle* (1871). His ideas were a 'blend of empiricism and theology' and, as Critchley put it, 'his obsequies asserted

(1858) at the time of his appointment, and given his Goulstonian lectures on this topic (1860). His concepts were idiosyncratic. Based on studies of *rigor mortis*, Radcliffe considered that muscle rigidity is due to the absence of nervous input, and that nervous supply is responsible for muscle relaxation not contraction. Epilepsy was, in Radcliffe's opinion, a state of the brain that is 'the very opposite of over-activity' – an enfeebled state where nervous energy is reduced due to a diminution of blood supply, rather than increased irritability. In these lectures, he discusses therapy in some detail, providing a glimpse into the rationale of contemporary treatments. He emphasises the avoidance of over-eating but also argues that 'unquestionable good will result from a proper allowance of sherry, weak brandy-and-water, or better still, of claret'. He argues for the avoidance of constipation with 'accumulation of effete matters in the bowels' and stresses the importance of exercise.[34] Radcliffe's chief claim to long-lasting recognition in the field of epilepsy relates not to his wholly inaccurate theorising on the physiology of the condition, but rather to his advocacy of bromides. In 1863, he wrote that he had used the drug first in hysterical epilepsy but, recognising its efficacy, then started to use it in all other forms of epilepsy. He realised that this did not act by 'calming the erotic disposition', as claimed by Locock, but that the drug might act to purify the blood of compounds analogous to uric acid.

Sir John Russell Reynolds published *Epilepsy: Its Symptoms, Treatment, and Relation to Other Chronic Convulsive Diseases* in 1861. He anticipated Jackson's views on positive and negative symptoms in neurology and advanced reflex theories of neurological disease, including the existence of a convulsive centre in the medulla. All his work showed the influence of his mentor Marshall Hall and of Brown-Séquard, who, for example, described spinal epilepsy in guinea pigs. Of more lasting interest was the first aetiological classification in which Reynolds divided epilepsy into idiopathic, eccentric, diathetic and symptomatic categories. His concept of idiopathic epilepsy, in particular, was to dominate thinking over the next 50 years, and his subcategories of symptomatic epilepsy also helped define the fields. Reynolds' clinical descriptions were excellent and his writing concise and thoughtful. He was a scholarly and influential physician and greatly respected by his contemporaries. It was he who helped Gowers obtain his appointment at Queen Square, and he remained an important intellectual influence on Gowers' work. Gowers acknowledged the debt by dedicating *Epilepsy and Other Convulsive Disorders* (1881) to Reynolds, 'whose example stimulated and whose friendship encouraged the work contained in the following pages'.

Sir Edward Henry Sieveking was a major figure in mid-Victorian medicine but today is mainly remembered for *On Epilepsy and Epileptiform Seizures: Their Causes, Pathology, and Treatment* (1858). This snapshot of orthodox opinion of the time was a popular work, as Sieveking noted in the preface:

> The labours of Bell, Marshall Hall, Flourens, Magendie, Müller and Brown-Séquard have illumined a field which before the beginning of the present century was enveloped in darkness ... the history of epilepsy, more than of other affections of the nervous system, until the most recent periods has been the history of one of the weakest sides of medical science.

For us, Sieveking's book is erudite and comprehensive, but backward looking. It provides a snapshot of orthodox opinion of the time and an extensive survey of the existing continental and British literature. However, it presents a view of epilepsy which was rapidly rendered obsolete by work over the next three decades, and not least that from the National Hospital which played a major role in advancing knowledge on the fundamental nature and clinical management of the condition. His chapters on treatment give an excellent overview of therapy before the introduction of bromides. Therein lies his cynical observation that 'there is scarcely a substance in the world, capable of passing through the gullet of man, that has not at one time or other enjoyed a reputation of being an anti-epileptic'. There is much on symptoms and clinical course. On causation, he places particular emphasis on sexual derangements:

> In a person guilty of masturbation we generally notice a peculiar hang-dog expression; an unwillingness to

---

that his mind ascended as by nature into the higher regions of philosophical mysticism'. He died on the day he retired, and was buried in Highgate cemetery.

[34] C. B. Radcliffe, 'Goulstonian Lectures 1860: On The Theory and Therapeutics of Convulsive Disease Especially Epilepsy', *Lancet* **75** (1860): 237–9, 287–90, 339–41, 461–3, 512–15, 564–7, 614–18. See also C. B. Radcliffe, 'A Course of Lectures on Certain Disorders of the Brain and Nervous System with Special Reference to Changes in Opinion and Practice which Result from Recent Researches in Physiology and Pathology', *Lancet* **81** (1863): 167–9, 227–30, 320–2, 406–9, 546–8, 572–3, 626–8, 685–7; **82**: 59–61.

meet the speaker eye to eye; a large sluggish pupil; a pale, livid hue and languid circulation of the surface, a general nervousness of demeanour … [was evident in] nine [cases] in whom the sexual system was in a state of great excitement owing to recent or former mastur-bation amongst a series of twenty-nine male epileptics.[35]

When Sieveking lectured at the Royal Medical and Chirurgical Society describing his own series of 52 patients with epilepsy on 12 May 1857, Sir Charles Locock – royal obstetrician and a fashionable doctor, but certainly no neurologist – was in the chair. In the discussion after Sieveking's lecture, Locock empha-sised the importance of onanism and then stated that there was a form of hysterical epilepsy associated with the menstrual period which was difficult to treat. He had observed positive benefits from bromide in hysteria unaccompanied by seizures and tried the remedy in what he considered hysterical seizures. It proved remarkably effective and 'out of fourteen or fifteen cases treated by this medicine, only one had remained uncured'. This is the first published record of genuine therapeutic efficacy in epilepsy and, as a result what was essentially an off-the-cuff anecdote, bromide was soon used worldwide. Sieveking's con-tributions are now largely forgotten, whereas Locock's chance and inaccurate observation became a land-mark in the history of neurology.

These physicians advanced knowledge on epi-lepsy, and placed the condition at the centre of med-ical attention. But it was Jackson and Gowers, and Ferrier and Horsley (whose work is described in later chapters), the quadrumvirate that made Queen Square pre-eminent in the world of neurology, who contributed most to the field of epilepsy. Jackson towered above all others of his time. His work laid the foundations for many current concepts in epi-lepsy, but it was the nature of seizures, their clinical manifestations, and implications for understanding evolution and dissolution in the nervous system, rather than treatment, that captured his interest.

Jackson conceived that an epileptic seizure is a dis-charge, chemical rather than electrical, and he was the first to identify that the origins of the discharge are in the cerebral cortex. He formulated the classic defini-tion of a convulsion as an occasional, excessive and disorderly discharge of nerve tissue on muscles; and of epilepsy as the name for occasional, sudden, excessive, rapid and local discharges of grey matter. These defi-nitions are still not bettered and were remarkable insights that transformed the concepts of epilepsy.

Jackson followed Reynolds in considering that the proximate cause of epilepsy, nutritive abnorm-alities of the nervous system, is the same in all cases. As Jackson wrote later, borrowing the ana-logy from Sieveking, a convulsion is 'a physiologi-cal fulminate … similar to the gunpowder in a cannon; and, just as gunpowder can store energy that is liberated when firing the gun, so the energy stored in nerve cells can be explosively liberated in an epileptic discharge'. He held that the abnormal levels of stored energy are due to deranged nutri-tion, and that this in turn usually results from congestion of the small blood vessels. He equated 'cause' with 'causal mechanism' and was in general not particularly interested in the question of aetiology in the sense that is currently used. His focus was on theories of physiology:

> The confusion of two things physiology and pathol-ogy under one [i.e. pathology] leads to confusion in considering causes. Thus, for example, we hear it epigrammatically said that chorea is only a symptom and may depend on many causes. This is possibly true of pathological causation; in other words it may be granted that various abnormal nutritive processes may lead to that functional change in grey matter which, when established, admits occasional excessive discharge. But physiologically, that is to say, from the point of view of function, there is but one cause of chorea – viz. instability of nerve tissue. Similarly in any epilepsy, there is but one cause physiologically speaking – viz. the instability of the grey matter, but an unknown number of causes if we mean patholo-gical processes leading to that instability.[36]

The discharge was, in Jackson's view, due to mor-bid nutrition, which is itself the result of various pathological processes. It causes cells to discharge

---

[35] Sieveking is following an ancient doctrine and one that had become a dominant aetiological theory during the pre-vious 50 years. Interestingly, the renewed interest in sexual causes of epilepsy was a rejection of the superstitious beliefs of possession and the occult. Tissot, the great French theo-retician of epilepsy, wrote on L'Onanisme, Dissertation sur le Maladies Produites par la Masturbation (1782), and almost all writers on the topic until the time of Sieveking focused on this physical cause of epilepsy.

[36] Published in 1874–6 in Medical Press and Circular; see Selected Writings of John Hughlings Jackson, ed. James Taylor, Gordon Holmes and F. M. R. Walshe (London: Hodder and Stoughton, 1931–2), Vol. I, pp. 162–273.

excessively – these having become a 'mad part' – and the discharge then spreads to neighbouring 'sane cells' which, in turn, are made to 'act madly'. Jackson did recognise that there are many possible contributing factors (remote causes) that might result in the nutritional disturbance which were at the heart of epilepsy, and those that he mentioned were tubercle, cicatrix, tumour, syphiloma, and haemorrhagic or ischaemic stroke. Jackson also realised that there is often no discernible cause.

Another remarkable contribution was Jackson's recognition that the symptoms of epilepsy depend on localisation of the excessive discharge. He defined the 'Jacksonian seizure' (a term coined by Charcot, who also noted that Louis Bravais had earlier described the same phenomenon), and this vindicated his view of somatotopic representation in the nervous system. Jackson realised that, although all parts of the body are represented in the corpus striatum, there exists a 'localisation of superiority … a localisation of specialty … certain parts of the motor centre specially superintending certain movements'. Thus, he recognised that features at onset of the fit reveal its site of origin: 'one of the most important questions we can ask an epileptic patient is how does the fit begin?' This revolutionary theory led directly to the introduction of neurosurgery based on clinical localisation.

Jackson first described temporal lobe seizures, the dreamy states that he considered to arise from the uncinate gyrus. One of his famous cases was that of Dr Z, whom Jackson treated in life and whose post-mortem examination he attended.[37] Jackson's

contribution was to define this seizure type and suggest its localisation to the temporal lobe. Finally, Jackson was interested in the postictal state and epileptic psychosis, as part of his wider consideration of the brain–mind debate. Jackson's epileptology was so novel and extraordinary that, perhaps unsurprisingly, not all of it has lasted. His classification of epilepsy, his attribution of some seizures to the corpus striatum, and his distinction between epilepsy and epileptoid seizures have not stood the test of time. Perhaps he had too heavy a reliance on Spencer's evolutionary physiology. Nevertheless, the claim on his behalf of being the 'father of epilepsy' is unassailable, and his concepts and theories are the foundation for modern understanding of epilepsy.

Sir William Gowers was neither a theoretician nor a philosopher; and he carried out little experimental work. His contributions to epilepsy lie in his clinical writings and teaching. His studies were focused, well organised and written in a lucid and elegant style, in marked contrast to Jackson's. Gowers wrote *Epilepsy and Other Chronic Convulsive Disorders*. In the first edition of 1881, a masterly 308-page description of all aspects of epilepsy, Gowers reported the findings of 1,450 cases observed during his years of practice at the National Hospital and, in the second edition (1901), added an additional 1,500 examples, together representing a prodigious clinical experience on which to draw in formulating his extraordinary work. These clinical descriptions are without parallel, and Gowers was undeniably the most important clinical teacher on epilepsy of all time. He was the first carefully to define the clinical course and factors resulting in causation, the role of heredity, and cessation of epilepsy. As with others of the period, he adopted the concept of the inherited neuropathic trait of which epilepsy was a part. Gowers also wrote *The Border-land of Epilepsy* (1907) concerned with conditions that are nowadays considered in the differential diagnosis of epilepsy.

Until the middle of the twentieth century, epilepsy was the only neurological condition for which there were effective specific pharmacological treatments. Even in 1881, Gowers was able to write more than 50 pages on therapy. An entire section is devoted to bromides, by then the standard treatment. He also provides an evaluation (not always positive) of the other substances then available, including digitalis,

---

[37] In a notable piece of medical detective work, Taylor and Marsh identified Dr Z as Hughlings Jackson's next-door neighbour in Manchester Square, Dr Arthur Thomas Myers (D. Taylor and S. Marsh, *Journal of Neurology, Neurosurgery, and Psychiatry* **43** (1980): 758–67). They reproduce Myers' obituary which shows a gifted young doctor with frequent temporal lobe seizures who, because of his epilepsy, slips down the social ladder. He was a brilliant student at Trinity College, Cambridge, and also a gifted cricketer. As the obituary continues: 'nature had, indeed, worthily designed him as one of those good "all round men" who are the glory of our public school education; but destiny thought fit to inflict upon him that terrible and inscrutable malady which occasionally harassed him in his early youth and with relentless tread, baffling the most devoted medical skill and ultimately involving a fine intellect in ruin and confusion. There can be no doubt but for this Myers would have obtained the highest medical distinction. His misfortune prevented his attaining to a post on the medical staff of a teaching hospital and this sad

disappointment, intolerable to most men, was borne by him with singular patience.'

belladonna, stramonium, cannabis, gelsemium, opium, zinc, iron, borax, mistletoe, turpentine, cocculus indica (source of picrotoxin – noting that this made fits more frequent!) and chloral, as well as the physical therapies of counter-irritation, trephining, castration and circumcision. As a result of the enthusiasm for bromide shown by Gowers and his colleagues, by 1899 2.5 tons of bromide compounds were being prescribed annually through the hospital pharmacy at Queen Square. In the second edition of *Epilepsy and Other Chronic Convulsive Disorders* Gowers placed even more emphasis on the role of bromides, with other drugs listed as adjuncts. Of these, borax was now prominent, along with digitalis, belladonna, gelsemium, zinc, nitroglycerine and cannabis, also mentioned as being helpful.

In the next generation it was William Aldren Turner who became the flag-bearer of epilepsy at Queen Square. His views are found in *Epilepsy – a Study of the Idiopathic Disease* in 1907 and in his Morison Lectures given before the University of Edinburgh in 1910. Turner was the first to apply statistical methods to the analysis of prognosis, reporting effects of age, response to early treatment, disease duration and heredity. He emphasised differences between new-onset and chronic epilepsy and proposed the division of epilepsy into four categories: organic, early, late and idiopathic epilepsy, a classification scheme which remains valid today. His study of over 1,000 patients treated with bromides and his observations on treatment, which occupy 56 pages of his book, are a classic statement of advanced treatment at the turn of the century. Bromides were described as the best first-line remedy, with remission obtained in more than 50 per cent of cases. In his series of 366 patients seen at onset, long-term remission was seen in 23 per cent, significant reduction in seizures in 29 per cent, and no effect in 48 per cent, but in chronic epilepsy bromide had 'relatively little value'. Bromide salts were formulated in various ways, and by 1914 there were at least 45 different combinations and preparations – many being quack remedies in Turner's opinion. He followed Gowers in taking the view that the sodium and potassium salts are more effective than strontium or lithium, but that intake should not generally exceed 45–60 grains per day (much higher doses were commonly employed at the time). To obscure the taste, syrup of Virginian prune could be added as a pleasant medium. Turner was particularly in favour of Gélineau's formulation, also advocated by Gowers. He recognised that high doses are associated with toxic effects:

This condition [bromism] is characterised by a blunting of the intellectual faculties, impairment of the memory, and the production of a dull and apathetic state. The speech is slow, the tongue tremulous and saliva may flow from the mouth. The gait is staggering, and the movements of the limbs feeble and infirm. The mucous membranes suffer, so that the palatal sensibility may be abolished, and nausea, flatulence, and diarrhoea supervene. The action of the heart is low and feeble, the respiration shallow and imperfect, and the extremities blue and cold. An eruption of acne frequently covers the skin of the face and back.

Turner did not mention the suppression of libido, the original reason for using bromides. Nor did he make clear whether he considered bromides to be responsible for the connective tissue changes in what he described as the 'epileptic face', but he did recognise that the cosmetic effects are appalling in some patients, for instance causing 'bromoderma'. The boils, pustules and weeping sores sometimes required surgical treatment. In chronic epilepsy, bromide had, in Turner's view, relatively little value. Other therapies he used, in addition to bromide, were belladonna, atropine (especially in reflex epilepsy), opium and strychnine, and zinc salts, which he considered to be occasionally successful, but evidently more so in the hands of French physicians. Another approach was calcium salts, a topic on which Turner advocates further study. Opium he pronounces to be helpful only in the early stages in young epileptics before or about puberty, and strychnine 'finds its most useful application in the treatment of nocturnal epilepsy'. Turner's miscellaneous methods of treatment include organotherapy (the administration of thyroid or thymus gland or cerebrin, the latter being a nitrogenous substance obtained from brain and nerve tissue), and serotherapy (the injection of blood serum from either another epileptic or the same epileptic). He is unimpressed by both.

Turner became physician to the Chalfont Centre for Epilepsy on its foundation, and was a strong advocate of institutional treatment in colonies for epileptics, championing the view that these institutions should be a hospital for the early cases as well as a refuge for confirmed cases; and that, with early treatment, cure was possible. He emphasises the benefits of proper care, nutrition and the minimisation of sedatives, and argues that medicinal therapy is only part of managing the person with epilepsy. For children:

No greater mistake is committed in the management of young epileptics, than withholding from them the advantages of the mental and physical exercises entailed by educational methods under special super-vision and direction ... In the last decade or two, the epileptic has received more general attention, particularly in relation to treatment in special institutions ... for no greater mistake can be made in the treatment of epilepsy than to rely solely on medicinal means, which so often fail to gain the desired end ... We have, therefore, in every case of epilepsy to treat the individual and not solely the disease.

Constipation much preoccupied epilepsy therapists of his day, and Turner recommended enemas, laxatives and (occasionally) even colectomy. Epileptics were 'notoriously big eaters, and being habitually subject to constipation, are prone to overload the digestive tracts and organs'. He was interested in the purine-free diet, and physical and mental hygiene. The physician should specify 'the proper allotment of work and rest, and the carrying out of those physical and mental exercises consistent with the malady'. Daily exercise in the open air, hot baths, spinal douches and massage are desirable. Alcohol should be avoided, and marriage discouraged. As for employment, 'an outdoor life is usually regarded as most suitable ... but there are many semi-sedentary forms of work suitable for the frailer epileptic such as drawing, modelling, and office work, book-keeping and the like.'

Turner was the major figure of his time in epi-lepsy. He represented Britain at the foundation in Budapest of the International League Against Epilepsy (ILAE: founded on 30 August 1909) and chaired the meeting of the organisation held in London (1913). He was instrumental in the founda-tion of *Epilepsia* and was a member of its 'comité de la redaction'.[38] He, perhaps more than any other of his generation, put epilepsy onto its modern course.

The National Society for the Employment of Epileptics and the Chalfont Centre for Epilepsy

An important initiative of physicians at Queen Square was the founding of the National Society for the Employment of Epileptics,[39] which used the Chalfont Centre for Epilepsy as its headquarters and colony. It is a story that typifies the late Victorian approach to social problems and is an example of the remarkable speed at which such initiatives were prosecuted. In July 1890, the Charity Organisation Society appointed a commis-sion 'to consider and report upon the public and charitable provisions made for the care and training of feeble-minded, epileptic, deformed and crippled persons'.[40] The commission, which included Ferrier and Buzzard as members, heard evidence that included a report by Ferrier of a visit made to the Bethel in Germany. Favourably impressed, the com-mittee recommended that a similar colony be estab-lished in Britain for 'sane and non-criminal epileptics'. With the aim of founding such a colony, Buzzard then called a meeting at his house (April 1892), at which were present several Queen Square medical staff – Buzzard, Ferrier, Hughlings Jackson, Gowers, Tooth, Ormerod and Coleman – members of the Ladies' Samaritan Society of the hospital, and representatives of the Charity Organisation Society. Jackson proposed 'to create a home for such epileptic persons as are capable of work but unable to obtain regular employment on account of their liability to fits'. Ferrier argued that 'it is expedient to establish in England an industrial colony for epileptics capable of work, on the same lines, so far as circumstances

---

[38] S. D. Shorvon, '*Epilepsia*', in S. D. Shorvon *et al.*, *International League Against Epilepsy 1909–2009: A Centenary History* (Oxford: Wiley Blackwell, 2009); S. D. Shorvon *et al.*, 'Notes on the Origins of *Epilepsia* and the International League Against Epilepsy', *Epilepsia* **50** (2009): 368–76.

[39] The Society's name was shortened to the National Society for Epilepsy in 1907, and in 2011 to the Epilepsy Society. Its history has been documented in J. Barclay, *A Caring Community: A Centenary History of the National Society for Epilepsy and the Chalfont Centre, 1892–1992* (London: National Society for Epilepsy, 1992); and W. Sander *et al.*, 'The Neurological Founding Fathers of the National Society for Epilepsy and of the Chalfont Centre for Epilepsy', *Journal of Neurology, Neurosurgery, and Psychiatry* **56** (1993): 599–604.

[40] The Special Committee on Epileptics of the Charity Organisation Society, *The Epileptic and Crippled Child and Adult* (London: Swan Sonnerschein, 1893). The charity was an important force in late Victorian society, and often in the front line of social care. It promoted self-help and the provision of assistance in a scientific manner, using 'scien-tific principles to root out scroungers and target relief where it was most needed'. The plight of sane epileptics, who were often destitute, was a particular focus of their work. The Charity Organisation Society also formed a separate 'Special Committee on the Care of Idiots, Imbeciles and Harmless Lunatics', which recommended that imbecile epileptics should be housed in asylums by the county councils.

should render advisable, as the colony near Bielefeld in Germany'. Further meetings took place at the National Hospital or David Ferrier's house, and the National Society for the Employment of Epileptics was founded.[41] An appeal was launched at the Mansion House, and the money required quickly raised. A farm was bought in Chalfont, 21 miles north-west of the centre of London, and buildings designed by the architect Claude Ferrier, David Ferrier's son.[42] The colony opened in 1894, with an address given by Thomas Buzzard. A committee of honorary medical staff was established, which included many of the Queen Square senior physicians. Turner and Colman[43] were appointed as visiting physicians, with Farquhar Buzzard taking over when Coleman resigned from Queen Square (1898). In 1896, the Medical Committee, based on their experience in the centre, issued guiding principles for the management and treatment of epileptics in colonies: removal of the epileptic from bad hygienic surroundings in towns to the pure air of the country; regular employment in the gardens, fields, orchards and workshop under the supervision of capable persons; a well-ordered and regular mode of life, with avoidance of any excitement and abstinence from alcoholic liquors; and abundance of nourishment of a simple nature. By the end of the first year, 16 men had been admitted. There was then rapid growth and, by 1899, 134 colonists were living at the centre. The men were carrying out farm and other manual work, and the women doing laundry and domestic work. Most took bromides. Thus, by the turn of the century, the Centre was established as a facility much admired in epilepsy circles internationally.

However, in 1908, a major clash occurred between the Queen Square physicians, who saw the priorities of the Centre as medical, and lay members who regarded it as a home providing refuge and social care. The argument arose over how best to use a large donation made by C. A. Tate, the sugar baron. The Medical Staff Committee of the Society proposed appointment of a resident medical superintendent to take charge of administrative and clinical affairs, and the building of a mortuary. The lay members of the Society's Executive Committee preferred to spend the money on providing a home for epileptic children. A bitter argument ensued, which resulted in the resignation of Turner and the entire honorary Medical Committee. Buzzard and Crichton-Browne also resigned from the charity's executive. The lay members then contracted a general practitioner to provide care, and links with the National Hospital were lost until the 1970s. There are interesting parallels with the row between physicians at the National Hospital and Burford Rawlings, a few years earlier. Both were symptomatic of the tensions that existed then between the perspectives of lay members of the governing bodies, reflecting the Victorian tradition of religious philanthropy, and the scientific priorities and ambition of the medical staff.

If a compromise had been reached, the Chalfont Centre might have developed into a fine medical and research facility, along the lines of the West Riding Lunatic Asylum, and perhaps this was in the minds of the honorary medical committee. As it was, the opportunity was lost and the colony became a medical backwater, and in effect a care home, for over 60 years. Had Burford Rawlings won his battle with the medical staff in 1901, a similar fate would very likely have awaited the National Hospital.

Physical Therapies at the National Hospital

Despite cynicism about the useless proliferation of substances for the treatment of epilepsy and paralysis, and in line with Russell Reynolds' urge to treat, patients at the National Hospital did have access to procedures generously dubbed as therapies.

Electrical Therapy at the National Hospital

Primary amongst these was electrical therapy, performed with an array of impressive technologies, of

---

[41] This committee included Horsley, Bastian and Beevor from Queen Square, as well as Joseph Lister, John Burdon Sanderson, William Broadbent, Andrew Clark, James Paget and James Crichton-Browne (the last interested in eugenics and keen to set up colonies so that epileptics did not marry).

[42] The Ferriers lived nearby. Claude Ferrier also designed their family house 'Hightrees' which was built with the assistance of labourers 'borrowed' from the colony. Lady Ferrier served on the colony's executive committee and took an interest in the colony, but relationships were soured because of her practice of commandeering colony nurses to perform massage at Hightrees.

[43] Walter Stacey Colman was assistant physician to the North-West London Hospital, the Hospital for Sick Children and the National Hospital, and then full physician at Queen Square (1896–8). He resigned to take charge of the children's department at St Thomas' Hospital. He was senior secretary of the Neurological Society of London and instituted the triennial Hughlings Jackson lecture established by the Society (1897).

a type which had often served to distinguish an ambitious hospital from its competitors, and so it was at Queen Square. The first medical electrical apparatus recorded in London was at the Middlesex Hospital (1767), and the first electrical department at St Thomas' Hospital (1799). Dr Cuthbert Golding Bird, a pioneer in electrical theory, opened, and became the physician in charge of, the famous electrifying room at Guy's (1836). However, there was widespread misuse, and electrical therapy was in many quarters regarded with great suspicion as a prime example of quackery.

Despite this background, the application of electricity at Queen Square for diagnosis and therapy, backed up by theory and experiment, was soon admired and considered a model of its kind. The electrical room was mentioned frequently by visitors and commentators, and electrical therapy contributed greatly to the hospital's reputation and esteem. A good starting point is *Lectures on the Clinical Uses of Electricity* (1871) by Sir John Russell Reynolds.[44] This served as a clear and authoritative practical manual for aspiring electro-clinicians. Contractility and sensibility in response to electrical current were compared in affected and unaffected muscles and used to differentiate cerebral, spinal and peripheral nerve disorders – as Bastian had done using clinical criteria. Beyond diagnosis, Reynolds claims a cure in some patients – particularly in hysterical illness. Used most commonly to ameliorate paralysis, and resulting in slow improvement in some cases (many of which no doubt exploited the natural history of disease), electricity was also applied to chorea, spasms, tics, dystonia, tremor, sensory disturbances, facial palsy and pain. It was used to treat epilepsy in asylum practice but not, it seems, at the National Hospital.

Three types of electrical machines were available. The first was the conventional electrical bath, which worked on the principle of franklinism. This was a glass-legged stool or sofa on which the patient was placed and completely insulated before being 'filled with static electricity' after connection of a brass chain to the machine. Static electricity was generated (for instance, by friction) using a van der Graaf generator. When the patient was used as the prime conductor

and connected via the chain to the machine, the hair stood on end but there was no discomfort. This was, without doubt, a strikingly theatrical performance. Reynolds reported that he had seen the successful removal of tics, sciatic pains, flutterings of the heart and many other 'odd and disagreeable sensations'. Sometimes, the patient was not filled with electricity but rather exposed to a spark from a generator applied to the offending part, for instance the throat in aphonia. Reynolds mentions in passing, largely to dismiss it, the use of shocks from Leyden jars, which he considered occasionally effective, but extremely unpleasant.

The second form of electricity was galvanism – a term used to describe the electricity produced by what was essentially a chemical battery. It produced a low-intensity continuous current. The diseased part was incorporated into the electrical circuit, which was used to treat spasms and pains, including headache. Weak currents produced no discomfort, but stronger bursts resulted in tingling, and sensations of burning, tension or tightness. The current could be interrupted, for instance by a vibrating wire as in Pulvemacher's interruptor. The patient sat with the feet in a saltwater bath, or with sponges applied to the relevant body part, so as to complete the circuit.

The third form of electricity was faradism. Pioneered by Duchenne, this produced a strong 'induced current'. As Reynolds wrote: 'It is made and broken very rapidly so that there are many pulses within a second of time in both directions.' The electricity was at 'high tension' and produced marked contractions of the muscles and a powerful action on the nerves of both motion and sensation. It was thought at the time that electricity applied as a treatment would activate a nerve or a muscle and revitalise the organ, in cases where either structure was underactive (paralysis or loss of sensation), and also reduce activity if this was excessive (for instance, in spasm). It was also used to revascularise and improve nutrition of skin or muscle – and thus, for instance, to reverse wasting. Electricity was considered to have been particularly useful in cases of Bell's palsy. The general view was that, although their therapeutic properties were rather different, faradism was superior to galvanism, especially when applications were repeated over a number of days.

Although Reynolds made perhaps the most important written contributions to the field, Charles Bland Radcliffe was the more active practitioner

---

[44] Based on three lectures given at University College Hospital in 1870. Reynolds did not keep his notes, but these were recorded verbatim by Gowers in shorthand and the transcript published in the *Lancet* (1870), and then revised as a book.

involved in electrical methods at the National Hospital. Radcliffe was later appointed chairman of the Royal Medical and Chirurgical Society's scientific committee No. 3, 'Of the Value of Electricity as a Remedial Agent', which met between October 1865 and January 1870 and was set up to explore the value of electrotherapy, not least because of widespread scepticism about its worth. Meetings took place at the National Hospital. Radcliffe was the first volunteer and found that his headache was immediately cured by an electrical charge from the positive pole. Dr Meryon[45] also found that it resolved his hip pain. Other physicians at Queen Square, notably Brown-Séquard, Gowers and Hughlings Jackson – were generally unconvinced about the use of electricity and, although Gowers referred many patients for electro-therapy and massage, he thought that they had little influence on the course of the symptoms. However, Radcliffe saw both as having positive psychological effects in stimulating the patient's faculties and helping to prevent chronic invalidism.

As medical superintendent at the National Hospital, Radcliffe's brother John Netten Radcliffe equipped, and was responsible for running, the electrical room. When this opened (1866), the *Medical Times and Gazette* singled out Netten Radcliffe and recorded that this was

> The first medical institution in which an electrical room, so fully representing the present state of medical electrisation has been set apart for treatment of poor patients ... and [one that] should act as a model for other large general hospitals ... [noting that] an important branch of medical therapeutics has been brought to bear on the treatment of a class of diseases which incapacitates an immense number of poor patients.[46]

Equipment included a Muirhead battery of 100 cells, with a novel rotating mechanism for including or excluding galvanism; an electrostatic generator with a 2-foot plate; an insulating stool, invented by Radcliffe; a Stöhrer's large Volta electric instrument; and Gaiffe's and Duchenne's magneto-electrical instruments for induced galvanism.

New methods of therapy for paralysis were announced in the annual reports, and the National Hospital seems rapidly to have become the centre for electrical therapy in London. A novel electrical bath was produced in which the patient lay immersed in warm water with metal plates at both ends, through which a current was passed. Within two years, over 4,000 treatments had been given, and the therapy was thought to be effective in the treatment of neuralgia, paralysis and atrophy, and especially in hysteria (100 per cent cure rate claimed in 1875) and chorea (94 per cent cure rate in 1875).

Three other neurologists were influential in London *électrisation*. Herbert Tibbits was medical superintendent at the National Hospital (between 1869 and 1875) but left to found the West End Hospital for Nervous Diseases (1878) which specialised in electrical treatment and neurotic disorders. Tibbits had a difficult personality and acquired many enemies, and his hospital became the subject of inquiry by a Parliamentary select committee.[47] Julius Althaus, who founded another competitor to the National Hospital, the London Infirmary for Epilepsy and Paralysis, Regents Park, in 1866, was also a prominent enthusiast of electrical therapy, and his hospital was equipped with an advanced electrical room. His *Treatise on Medical Electricity* (1859) went into several editions and was translated into French, German and Italian. Althaus considered that the therapy should be administered only by those experienced in its art: 'An application of the constant current to the brain ... is ... an artistic performance which requires

---

[45] Edward Meryon was a respected London physician at the London Infirmary for Epilepsy and Paralysis, another hospital with a prominent electrical room. It could be argued that both Radcliffe and Meryon had vested interests. Meryon described muscular dystrophy, although his precedence was overlooked when the condition was subsequently named after Duchenne (see A. Emery and M. Emery, *The History of a Genetic Disease, Duchenne Muscular Dystrophy* (Oxford University Press, 2011)).

[46] Anon., 'The National Hospital for the Epileptic and Paralysed, the Electrical Room', *Medical Times and Gazette* **2** (1866): 583.

[47] The reputation of many physicians depended at the time on their electrical skills, and a classic power struggle persisted, with the medical profession seeking to stop the treatment being used by unqualified people, and preventing medical electricians setting themselves up outside hospitals. The Select Committee on Metropolitan Hospitals of the House of Lords was set up in response to widespread unease about the number of specialised hospitals being founded in London. There was disquiet about the commercial nature and 'quackery' that tarnished the image of 'electrisation'. The National Hospital retained its reputation as a shining example of the benefits of specialisation. Tibbits was continually attacked by the medical and lay press, resulting in a lawsuit for slander that he lost.

not only knowledge but also much practice and some talent like a good musical performance … How often does one hear a sonata by Beethoven or a polonaise by Chopin actually murdered? The same applies to electrical treatment.'[48]

He concluded that franklinism was useless as a therapy, and galvanism also much less effective than faradism. His views became increasingly extreme and (at the age of 66 and the year before his death in 1899), Althaus declared that 'If old people receive about the sixtieth or sixty-fifth year … proper and faultlessly carried out electricity to the brain, either daily or every other day, for some time, they may keep their faculties fairly well until the age of eighty or ninety.'[49]

Armand de Watteville was another important figure appointed to the West End Hospital and the Regents Park Hospital, as well as St Mary's Hospital, where he was physician to the electrotherapeutical department. He was interested in the physics of electrical therapy and the quantification of dosage, and was frequently at loggerheads with others in the field, and published *A Practical Introduction to Medical Electricity* (1878). He was then appointed as the first single editor of *Brain* (1884), which published some of his writings on electricity. He was also instigator and a founding member of the Neurological Society of London (1887).

There was a widely held view in psychiatric practice that faradism stimulated and galvanism calmed nerves. To what extent electricity was in use at Queen Square for these refined purposes is unclear, but it was widely employed in mental asylums by the end of the century. Galvanic electricity applied directly to the head was used to treat hysteria, 'melancholia attonita', hallucinations and delusions, and dementia. Hysteria was widely treated by electrical therapy, although it was later recognised to be largely ineffective, at least in the longer term. Neurasthenia was also treated in this way, on the basis that it re-energised the circulation. Towards the end of the century, with the rise of hypnotism, it was being asked whether electrical therapy derived its benefits in psychiatric practice entirely through suggestion. Its effectiveness in melancholia is

interesting, given later work on electroconvulsive therapy (ECT) but, although it was known that if too strong a current was used, convulsions could occur, these were considered undesirable and to be avoided.

Massage at the National Hospital

The conviction amongst some members of the staff that electricity made its patients better was soon extended to exploiting the mystique of massage. Although by no means unique to the National Hospital, the extensive use of massage or medical rubbing as a mode of treatment, especially for paralytic patients, together with medical electricity for both diagnosis and therapy, was arguably the most distinctive feature of the therapeutic regime at Queen Square towards the end of the nineteenth century.[50] Medical rubbing was a labour-intensive process, requiring strength and stamina on the part of the operator. The first therapeutic use of massage probably dates from the National Hospital's earliest years and, according to Burford Rawlings, the surgeon William Adams had in the 1860s 'predicted that medical rubbing would take a foremost place someday among therapeutic resources'. However, until the 1880s, bodywork massage seems only to have been performed on an occasional basis by male and female nurses. Whereas there are many references to the electrical room and gymnastic equipment and exercise in the hospital records from 1863, it was not until 1881 that, at the instance of Gowers and Buzzard, the Medical Committee urged that 'steps be taken for the proper instruction for certain of the nurses in medical rubbing'.

A general massage lasted over one hour and a single limb treatment took 30 minutes. With 50 patients in a ward, and each male nurse not expected to pummel for more than two hours per day, very many nurses were required to learn the techniques. Massage had evidently become a routine part of the hospital's activities, and an increasingly important burden on the daily workload for both male and female nurses. In many respectable quarters of society, both massage and those who practised the

---

[48] J. Althaus, 'On the Treatment of Certain Forms of Paralysis by Galvanization and Faradization', *Lancet* **86** (1865): 258–60. A musical analogy is not surprising because Althaus was himself a fine musician and his wife a well-known opera singer and diva.

[49] J. Althaus, 'Treatment in Old Age', 'Old Age and Rejuvenescence', *Lancet* **183** (1899): 149–52.

[50] The beginnings of the modern Western (as distinct from Oriental) practice of remedial massage or 'medical rubbing' ('massotherapeutics') and its conception as a form of 'passive gymnastic movement' may be traced to the work of Per Henrik Ling in Sweden and Johann Metzger in the Netherlands during the first half of the nineteenth century, from whence it spread throughout much of Europe and the Americas.

technique were in danger of being misunderstood and indirectly tainted by association with brothels, and the National Hospital was taking quite a bold step in making massage an integral part of its therapeutic regime. That the Board was sensitive to the possible dangers is apparent from the adoption of a new bye-law (1894), formalising the order of the secretary-director which had been in force for some years, that 'massage shall not be carried out upon male patients by female nurses, nor upon female patients by male nurses'.

In 1894, the hospital offered three months' training for probationary nurses in massage and electricity at a cost of 13 guineas, and for day pupils at a cost of 5 guineas each for massage and electricity. Instruction in massage was by the assistant matron and a male nurse, who each received 13s from the fees for resident, and 15s for non-resident, pupils, in addition to their regular salaries. Certificates of competence were issued, but two years later this was restricted to fully trained nurses, and holders asked to refrain from advertising the fact in order to limit demand.

Just how important massage had become in the management of paralytic patients by the end of the century is clear from the evidence presented to the Fry Commission of Inquiry in 1901, in which the insufficient nursing staffing levels were blamed on the increasing demand for electrical treatment and massage ordered by the medical staff. No figures were presented but the claim was partially corroborated by the statement to the Commission of Wilfrid Harris, the then senior house physician, who stated that during his time at Queen Square treatments, especially massage, which had been ordered by the physicians were often either deferred, performed perfunctorily or not carried out at all, due to a chronic shortage of adequately trained and competent nurses. The Fry Commission agreed.

> There has been an increase in the hospital of paralytic as compared with epileptic patients, and … paralytic patients make larger demands on the strength of nurses than epileptic cases … the amount of massage now carried on in the hospital is very large, and makes a … heavy demand on the nursing staff … in recent times the amount of electrical treatment ordered both for in- and out-patients has increased; and … the staff of nurses now in the hospital is insufficient for the present demands upon it … some of the massage ordered has not been given; … the patients ordered to receive it daily have, now and then, received it only

on alternate days; … the time of treatment has sometimes been shortened.[51]

Some of these findings were disputed by Burford Rawlings but, at the suggestion of the Board of Management (in November 1892), the Medical Committee began to consider formal training and certification in the use of electricity and massage, and appointed yet another subcommittee to enquire into the issue of certificates for electricity and massage to nurses. The subcommittee duly reported and in 1904, a formal school of massage was opened.

Heredity at the National Hospital

Finally, a brief word on the contentious issue of heredity, and its impact on the practice of neurology at Queen Square. As mentioned earlier, the topic of heredity was a subject of much general public interest in the second half of the nineteenth century, and was highly relevant to epilepsy and many other neurological diseases seen at the National Hospital. Although theories of evolution and natural selection were first proposed in 1859, the mechanism of inheritance was then unknown, and Mendel's work (1865) largely overlooked until rediscovered by Bateson (1909). However, the manifestations of heredity were the subject of considerable statistical research, especially by Francis Galton and Karl Pearson at University College London. To understand what was implied by heredity in this period, the broader meaning of degeneration (*dégénérescence*) must be appreciated. This concept influenced thought in the humanities, sciences and arts, and was a predominant intellectual theory of the time. There were, as part of the rise of industrialisation, wide public concerns about social disintegration and the collapsing state of European culture, and fears that rapid population growth and urbanisation among the lower classes would sap national intelligence and morality. In medicine, the concept of inherited degeneration was widely applied to neurological and psychiatric disease, and this became an important focus of research, with clinical writings from Queen Square physicians proving influential in the field of neurology.

Various brain diseases were considered to result from the 'neurological (or neuropathic) trait'. This inherited taint was thought to result in progressive

---

[51] Report of the Committee of Enquiry [the Fry Commission], June 1901.

and worsening deterioration – physically, mentally and morally – over generations. According to this theory, many apparently disparate diseases were thought to be due to the same underlying inherited defects and mechanisms. The concept of the neuropathic family arose, divided into a psychopathological arm that included epilepsy and the major psychiatric disorders, and a neuropathological arm that manifested as chorea, migraine and paralysis agitans. According to these theories, the inherited endowment might, for instance, cause mild hysteria in one generation, then epilepsy in the next, and dementia or idiocy in a third. Epilepsy was the neurological condition upon which discussion about heredity was most focused. Sieveking, Russell Reynolds and Gowers, for instance, considered the topic in some detail, and, as Gowers wrote, 'there are few diseases in the production of which inheritance has more manifest influence'. Echeverria reported an inheritability rate in epilepsy of 25 per cent and Gowers of 42 per cent as one manifestation of the neurological trait, and three-quarters of those with inherited insanity also had epilepsy:

> 'It is well known that the "neuropathic tendency" does not always manifest itself in the same form, but it is not easy to discern the relation of its varieties … The chief morbid states (besides epilepsy itself) by which the same neuropathic tendency is manifested is insanity, and, to a much smaller degree, chorea, chronic hysteria, migraine, and some chronic forms of disease of the brain and of the spinal cord. Intemperance is probably also due, in many cases, to a neuropathic disposition' and because of the neuropathic trait, 'epilepsy and insanity were almost interchangeable terms'.[52]

Other diseases, mainly of muscle and nerve, were also recognised to have a familial tendency, although not as part of the neurological trait. Gowers, in particular, described extensively families and pedigrees with locomotor ataxia, chronic muscular atrophy, pseudohypertrophic muscular atrophy and spastic paraplegia.

A good overview of how heredity as a concept in neurology had evolved by the turn of the century can be seen from the Harveian Oration given by Ormerod on 'Heredity in Relation to Disease' (1908).[53] Ormerod

clearly recognised that inheritance (the 'continuity of the germ plasm') is mediated via chromosomes. He was aware of the controversy about inheritance of acquired characteristics, of Galton and Pearson's statistical work, and of the evolving science of eugenics. He cites Galton's law of ancestral inheritance and that of filial regression or correlation and mentions the rediscovery of Mendel's work by Bateson. Ormerod recognised the risks of consanguineous marriage as a way of bringing to light recessive characteristics and, in passing, noted that, in Wyoming, first-cousin marriages were banned in order to reduce the risk of disease. He also mentioned the term 'inborn error of metabolism' coined by Garrod a few months earlier in his Croonian lecture of 1908. In relation to neurological disease, Ormerod divides the inherited conditions into two categories. First are the neuroses, which include 'epilepsy, insanity, hysteria, neurasthenia, tics and alcoholism, etc. … characterised by perverted nervous action rather than by coarse structural disease'. Following his predecessors at Queen Square, Ormerod considered these conditions to be the expression of the neurological trait and 'varied and interchangeable *inter se*, of some one underlying nervous defect'. They are 'an ill-timed or inappropriate response of a nervous system which adapts itself badly to its surroundings'. The second group of diseases are those in which there is a clear family history of a related condition such as Friedreich's ataxia, Strumpell's spastic paralysis or periodic paralyses. In these diseases, Ormerod noted the remarkable precision in which features are reproduced through the generations. He also recognised the existence of sex-linked inheritance, for instance in peroneal muscular atrophy.

William Gowers incorporated the concept of the neurological trait in developing his own ideas on abiotrophy, a term coined to refer to diseases of the nervous system in which there is 'an essential defect of vital endurance, in consequence of which their life

---

[52] W. Gowers, *Epilepsy and Other Chronic Convulsive Disorders* (London: Churchill, 1881).

[53] Joseph Arderne Ormerod was born in Norfolk and educated at Rugby School and Oxford University. He came from a distinguished family of physicians and historians. He was appointed assistant physician (1880), physician

(1900) and consulting physician (1913) at the National Hospital. He also served as dean (see below). Ormerod wrote a *Student's Guide to Nervous Diseases* (1892). His presidential address to the neurological section of the Royal Society of Medicine (1910–11) dealt with 'Two theories of hysteria', those of Janet and Breuer and Freud. He was registrar at the Royal College of Physicians (1909–28), proving a shrewd and efficient administrator. He was described as 'a most considerate and unselfish colleague, entirely wanting in self-assertive dogmatism and extremely modest and reticent, an upright and kindly gentleman'. His Harveian Oration was published by Adland & Son, London (1908).

slowly fails'. Gowers presented his views on heredity to a meeting of the Royal Society of Medicine at which were present Bateson, Mott, Savage and Pearson, amongst others.[54] Here, Gowers recognised inheritance in three classes of disease: first, the early abiotrophies such as Friedreich's ataxia and various forms of myopathy; second, that class of disease which manifests after growth is over, such as Huntington's disease, myotonia congenita and Marie's heredoataxia; and, third, functional diseases such as epilepsy, insanity, hysteria and the neuroses, linked as part of the neuropathic trait and usually constitutional.[55]

Thus, neurology was heavily influenced by the concept of heredity in the 50 years after first publication of Darwin's monograph, as were many other medical disciplines and other areas of science and society. The understanding of inherited disease was at the time based almost entirely on clinical observation, and the mechanisms of inheritance were unknown. This was a major weakness, fully recognised at the time, and should have prevented the unjustified extrapolation of findings that was to occur in the next decades in the form of eugenics, a branch of science that was beginning to be accepted and applied to neurological disease, especially in the USA and in Germany, but sadly did not do so.

---

[54] The meeting was held in 1908, partly to commemorate Mendel's work, and was published; see W. S. Church *et al.*, *The Influence of Heredity on Disease, with Special Reference to Tuberculosis, Cancer and Diseases of the Nervous System: A Discussion* (London: Longmans, Green & Co., 1908).

[55] Although often linked, Gowers and later Turner (in 1907) recognised that the commonest manifestation of the trait in the family of someone with epilepsy is also epilepsy, and Gowers quotes a sermon by Jeremy Taylor, the sixteenth-century 'Shakespeare of the Divines': 'an epileptick son doth often come from an epileptick father'.

Chapter 4

National Hospital Quadrumvirate

Four people stand out as the towering figures in the first half-century of the hospital who played a dominant role in establishing the reputation of the National Hospital. Many others, already introduced, also made contributions, but no one of these quite matched the brilliance or influence of John Hughlings Jackson, David Ferrier, William Gowers and Victor Horsley.

John Hughlings Jackson

John Hughlings Jackson[1] dominated the development of new ideas on the nervous system in the second half of the nineteenth century. Dubbed the 'father of English neurology', Jackson perceived what the nervous system is for and how it has evolved. His ideas and concepts have influenced the work and understanding of all subsequent generations. Jackson used clinical observation as the basis for constructing dynamic models of brain function. He did no experimental work, but was happy to use such evidence in reaching his formulations. Jackson considered the nervous system to be 'an organ for the coordination of impressions and movements', driven by reflex

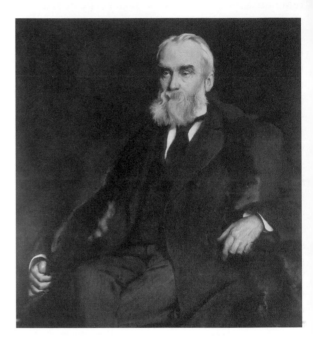

Figure 4.1 Oil painting of John Hughlings Jackson, by Lance Calkin, 1895.

activity, which adapts and integrates with its environment. He opposed the concept, originating from phrenology and endorsed by the work of Paul Broca, of abrupt geographical localisation in favour of hierarchical organisation within the brain and spinal cord. He argued that focal lesions are characterised by loss of the most evolved functions (producing negative symptoms) with release of subservient and more primitive activities normally suppressed in health (the positive symptoms). Thus, the entire nervous system contributes to the neurology of focal disease. Although essentially a materialist, Jackson finessed the relationship of mind and body, arguing that physical and psychical events occur independently but in parallel. Through his leadership, Jackson nurtured the identity of neurology as a specialty distinct from general medicine. Thus, the

---

[1] Throughout this book we refer interchangeably to Jackson and Hughlings Jackson. Whether or not Hughlings Jackson's name should be hyphenated has been the topic of much discussion. This has been intensively researched by Macdonald Critchley. A hyphen is to be found in volumes of *Brain* where Jackson is listed as founding editor; and, on 14 June 1871, he wrote to the house governor at the London Hospital asking to have a 'slight dash' inserted between his two names 'to individualise one's self'. At the same time, his National Hospital records show the unhyphenated style. Jackson never used the hyphen in any personal correspondence, and others (including David Ferrier) adopted both forms inconsistently in their writings. There was no hyphen on the brass plate of his home, in the signature of his Will, or on his gravestone. Critchley urges that 'it is to be hoped that the hyphenated name will not be introduced in the future in printed matter'. See also *Times Literary Supplement*, 23 October 2015, p. 6.

Neurological Society of London and *Brain*, a journal of neurology, were largely his initiatives. Jackson was a major influence on the school of neurology at the London Hospital but, because so many physicians and trainees attended Queen Square during the formative years after he was first appointed, the latter is the hospital with which Jackson is now primarily identified. Whilst some ephemera survive, there is no comprehensive archive relating to Jackson as he required his executor to burn all personal papers after his death in 1911.[2]

Jackson was born (4 April 1835) and first educated in Yorkshire. He was unimpressed by his schooling, taking the view that much of his later success would not have materialised had he gone to university, and that his teachers were 'not fit to sell penny pies on street corners'. Jackson was apprenticed (20 October 1850) to Dr William Anderson and his son Tempest, who practised as physicians in York. They were attached to the York Medical School where Jackson moved (1852) as one of ten students taught by a faculty that included Thomas Laycock, later professor of medicine in Edinburgh, who expounded the views of Marshall Hall on reflex activity of the nervous system. Jackson found his speculations brilliant and stimulating. Through interactions with Dr Daniel Tuke at the York Retreat, Jackson observed mental disease. Although unsympathetic to the work of alienists, the relationship of the mind to physical disorders of the brain and spinal cord influenced his subsequent formulations. The work in York involved attending lectures, outpatient clinics, operations and post-mortem examinations at various hospitals.[3] After attendance at the York County Hospital, Jackson was admitted as a licentiate of the

Worshipful Society of Apothecaries (10 April 1856). He became a member of the Royal College of Surgeons following a year at St Bartholomew's Hospital, London (1855–6), with instruction from James Paget. These qualifications allowed Jackson later to be examined for the MD degree of the University of St Andrews (1860). He returned to York (1856–8) in order to obtain further experience and qualify as a physician, working as resident medical officer at the York Dispensary and joining the York Medical Society.

Back in London, Jonathan Hutchinson enabled Jackson's appointment to the staff of the Metropolitan Free Hospital (1859). Later, he worked at the Islington Dispensary and the Royal London Ophthalmic Hospital (Moorfields Eye Hospital). On his appointment as assistant physician to the National Hospital (7 May 1862),[4] Jackson was required to 'visit the hospital twice a day and see the out-patients at their houses, for which extra services he will be allowed the remuneration of fifty pounds per annum'. This proved onerous and Jackson offered his resignation (16 July 1862), the managers agreeing that he should lose the £50 but retain the functions of assistant physician. Jackson was also appointed to the staff of the London Hospital (assistant physician, 1863; physician, 1874–94). Assuming that the appointment was secure, he failed to attend the interview until Hutchinson 'took a hansom cab and hunted him up'. By this time, Jackson (and Hutchinson) were employed by John Churchill (1801–75) as medical reporters for the *Medical Times and Gazette*, publishing a weekly column on 'Reports of hospital practice in medicine and surgery'. This role entitled Jackson and Hutchinson to attend other hospitals, where they were courted in their capacity as journalists. With a growing interest in cases of neurological disease, and much to Hutchinson's disappointment, Brown-Séquard steered Jackson's career towards neurology and influenced his ideas on physiology as the basis for understanding disease mechanisms. The timing was important since Jackson had become disillusioned with medicine and was planning to pursue a literary career, thinking that this would ensure a better income and provide more intellectual scope. Hutchinson had dissuaded him but wondered in

---

[2] The most informed biographies are: J. Hughlings Jackson, *Neurological Fragments* (Oxford University Press, 1925), with biographical contributions from James Taylor, Jonathan Hutchinson and Charles Mercier; Macdonald Critchley and Eileen A. Critchley, *John Hughlings Jackson: Father of English Neurology* (Oxford University Press, 1998), which is rich in detail of Jackson's genealogy, and the oral tradition of his work passed on by those who worked with him; and Kenneth Dewhurst, *Hughlings Jackson on Psychiatry* (Oxford: Sandford Publications, 2005).

[3] Jackson was supported over this period by a legacy of £2,000 from his maternal grandfather, John Hughlings. Jackson's father (Samuel Jackson) wrote urging him to be parsimonious, not to consort with the wrong company, to attend church, to maintain his activities in music, and to look after his books.

---

[4] Although appointed assistant physician in 1862, Jackson failed in his application for the post of full physician in 1864 when John Russell Reynolds and Edward Sieveking were preferred; Jackson then replaced Sieveking in 1867.

retrospect whether this had been wise, preventing mankind from benefitting to the full from Jackson's intellect and contributions to philosophy. Jackson was admitted as MRCP by examination (1860; and elected FRCP, 1868); and, with his reputation fully established, he was elected FRS (1878, aged 43). The eventual lack of a civil honour surprised and disappointed his colleagues.

Jackson was a poor communicator but held in great affection by those with whom he worked. He much preferred to discuss his thoughts in private to junior staff rather than to lecture. Charles Mercier, having assembled an example of isolated lesions of every cranial nerve except the eighth for a clinical demonstration by Jackson on paralysis, was told: 'there would have been as many [present] if you had put up a notice that Dr Jackson would kill a pig'. His nickname was 'the Sage'. Close acquaintances knew that he was being critical if Jackson referred to someone as 'a man I should be very polite to'. He hinted at the activities of a 'Mr Harris', a *diabolus ex machinâ* who haunted Jackson in order to hide items he was looking for, and when seeking explanation for something that had gone wrong.[5] Confronted by injustice, Jackson's advice was always 'the only thing to do is to say a great big damn, and have done with it'. He was absent-minded, had a poor memory for names, and often could not find his way around the hospital. He would re-read his own writings in order to remember what he thought about a particular topic. He might suddenly head off to another hospital to see an interesting case and there abandon his house physician to find his own way home. Kinnier Wilson liked to drive with Jackson in his open landau and make notes of what Jackson said to him (and, especially, what Wilson said to Jackson):

> I loved Jackson and more or less attached myself to him. I saw more of him than anyone of my generation, and I yielded to none in my appreciation and affection ... the neurologist's neurologist ... Jackson's genius consisted in combining ... detailed clinical observation with a philosophic breadth of thought and ... a gifted imagination ... his innate modesty never led to say more of his views than that they were theories and speculations and that someday he would be 'found out'.[6]

Thomas Buzzard considered that 'Jackson displayed characteristics which ... derive[d] from the nationality of each parent ... energetic, courageous, cautious in drawing conclusions ... on the other hand ... of a singularly tender and affectionate nature, far from impulsive in the acquisition of a new friendship, but ever staunch and firm in support of an old one.[7]

Farquhar Buzzard and his wife saw Jackson frequently at their home, where he befriended the children, having none of his own. The younger Buzzard wrote of Jackson:

> A kind-hearted but ... grave family friend or pseudo-uncle whose mind seemed to be in a state of constant conflict between his desire to give pleasure and his fear of being bored or bound ... [he] had no superior in the work of making detailed and accurate observations [and] no real rival in the art of generalisation or ... of integrating those observations so as to produce an harmonious design of the nervous system as a whole.[8]

Grateful for small kindnesses, Jackson was unforgiving of those who did not reciprocate his courtesy. He was meticulous in attributing the contributions of others to his ideas. Trainees in close contact with Jackson enjoyed his 'pawky' sense of humour. Keeping a straight face but with a twinkle in the eye, Jackson liked to warn a new house physician that he must never say anything which in any degree controverted Jackson's theories – only to be obviously discomforted when the young man took him seriously. He was careful to protect his trainees from blame or distress if they made a diagnostic mistake or contributed to poor management. His ward rounds were erratic in frequency and duration, and unpredictable in terms of which cases received most attention. Purves-Stewart remembered:

> His lofty, domed forehead and deep-set eyes. His white beard had a curious twist towards the left side of his chin. His voice and manner were gentle. During ward-rounds he spoke but little and limited himself to a few laconic remarks, every word of which was treasured by those privileged to hear them ... He used to drive about the streets of London in his open brougham, deep in thought, with his head sunk on his chest ... His conversation roamed over various

---

[5] 'Mr Harris' is borrowed from Charles Dickens' *Martin Chuzzlewit* (1844).
[6] S. A. K. Wilson, 'Hughlings Jackson Centenary', *Lancet* **225** (1935): 882–3.

[7] T. Buzzard, 'John Hughlings Jackson', *British Medical Journal* **2** (1911): 952–3.
[8] E. F. Buzzard, 'Hughlings Jackson and his Influence on Neurology', *Lancet* **224** (1934): 909–13.

by-ways of physiological psychology such as the origin and nature of laughter, the functions of the deeper parts of the brain, the sensations of hunger and thirst and so on.[9]

With patients, he could occasionally appear brusque through stating too exactly his opinion on their condition and its likely course. Jackson disliked being unable to offer help and would rather pass by the end of a bed than find himself caught in a sensitive clinical conversation. This difficulty in dealing emotionally with human suffering put him at a disadvantage in the highly competitive crucible of London private practice. Jackson attended ward rounds at the Bethlem Hospital with Sir George Savage, who noted that 'Jackson avoided close contact with chronic [patients] ... having a physical dread of the insane ... lacking sympathy ... regarding these cases as useless occupiers of beds in asylums.'[10]

Socially, Jackson was impatient and restless, disliked engagements and overseas travel, and hated to be kept waiting. He could rarely sit through the complete performance of a play. Jackson had married his first cousin, Elizabeth Dade Jackson in 1865, but tragedy was to follow, for she died (25 May 1876) of cerebral venous thrombosis presenting as 'Jacksonian' epilepsy. He never remarried and looked after himself in Manchester Square surrounded by pictures of cats and contemporary Japanese art. In later years, he became increasingly remote, perhaps due to deafness, and spent much of his time reading popular novels and thrillers of the day. Buying a 'yellow-back' at a railway station, he might tear off the covers and break the book in half placing the fragments in his coat pockets. Pages that interested him were torn out and sent to colleagues. At his death, the four volumes of the *London Hospital Reports* were found not to contain any papers that Jackson himself had contributed.

Jackson tried always to convey exact meaning in his words, chastising himself if he made an imprecise remark or description. But in this he failed for, although revered and highly respected, his writing left many confused and trailing in his intellectual wake.[11]

His handwriting was awful, and the printed text 'cluttered up with additions, elaborations, amendments, parentheses, qualifications, footnotes, after-thoughts, and asides'.[12] Hutchinson recalls Jackson confessing that his pet theories were likened to the love of God in that they passed all understanding. The Australian neurologist Alfred Walter Campbell, intending to lecture on Jackson's teachings, abandoned the idea on the basis that 'he might as well try and abstract the psalms of David'. Campbell had found Jackson no easier to understand in conversation when he attended Queen Square as a student, and failed to appreciate his greatness, being more readily influenced by Gowers, Buzzard, Bastian and Horsley.

A portrait commissioned by the London Hospital was painted by Mr Lance Calkin. At the presentation, James Paget explained that Jackson's work on the localisation of brain function 'had given lucidity to physiology and guidance to surgery'. Of course, slavish localisation is exactly what Jackson had not done. The portrait shows him with a bushy beard and moustache of the Victorian style, dressed in a buttoned-up frock coat. The original, bequeathed by Jackson, now hangs in the Royal College of Physicians with replicas at Queen Square and the London Hospital. A marble bust of Jackson by Herbert Hampton was commissioned by the staff, and presented by Gowers in a ceremony in the hallway of the National Hospital (1907), where it was duly placed. Purves-Stewart considered that 'it offered a stern expression which he never displayed to any of us'. Later the bust was stolen and offered for sale, as an unknown likeness, in an antiques shop in London.[13] Jackson retired from the

---

[9] J. Purves-Stewart, *The Sands of Time: Recollections of a Physician in Peace and War* (London: Hutchinson & Co. Ltd, 1939).

[10] G. Savage, 'Hughlings Jackson on Mental Disorder', *Journal of Mental Science* 63 (1917): 315–28.

[11] Hughlings Jackson was ahead of his times in other respects. In July 1876, only he and one other voted against the motion carried at the London Hospital that there should

be no change in the ruling that women were not admitted to the medical school; see Sir John Ellis, *LHMC 1785–1985* (London Hospital Medical Club, 1985), p. 43.

[12] One anonymous reviewer of the *West Riding Lunatic Asylum Reports* (Vol. **III**, 1873) noted 'why does Dr. Jackson deal so profusely in italics? No young lady in her teens writing to her dearest friend could be more liberal in underlining words and sentences. As an observer there is no one for whom we entertain a greater respect than for Dr. Jackson, but as a writer he drives us to despair; having done which he proceeds cruelly to pelt us with italics. We trust he will pardon us for laying down this as a literary canon: that a writer who has clearly conceived his ideas, and who has acquired the power of clearly expressing them, may presume the existence of sufficient intelligence in his readers to render it unnecessary for him ever to use italics.'

[13] The original was never recovered. Oral history relates that the identity of the thief was known but the individual never confronted with larceny. At the suggestion of Wilder

London Hospital on 1 October 1895 and from the National Hospital in 1906. He died from pneumonia on 7 October 1911, aged 76, and is buried in Highgate cemetery. In 1985, on behalf of the Association of British Neurologists, Peter Robinson attempted to have a plaque in memory of Jackson placed in Westminster Abbey but the request went unanswered.

Jackson was already celebrated in his lifetime. Walter Colman suggested that the Neurological Society of London should host a triennial Hughlings Jackson lecture; and Jackson delivered the first on 8 December 1897.[14] Shortly before it became the neurological section of the Royal Society of Medicine, the renamed Neurological Society of the United Kingdom dedicated the March 1907 issue of *Brain* 'as a tribute of respect and affection to JOHN HUGHLINGS JACKSON MD FRS in the 50th year of his medical practice'. The issue included the third Hughlings Jackson lecture in which Horsley paid tribute to Jackson:

> The lecture ... acknowledge[s] the great service he has done to humanity by his work ... the power of genius evinces itself by the happy use of analysis and synthesis, with, as a result, the discovery of principles ... no one rises from [Jackson's writings] ... without realizing that his conclusions are final without dogmatism ... and that his reader has learnt far more than can at once be simply and adequately expressed ... those of us who have enjoyed the inestimable privilege of being ... his pupils ... are indebt[ed] to him ... [for the] insistence on the necessity of correlating disturbances of function with the structural changes found after death.[15]

In 1901, William Osler wrote, at the request of Silas Weir Mitchell and James J. Putnam, asking whether Jackson would consider preparing a collection of his papers. The reply was that the old papers were not worthy and the new ones already antiquated and repetitive. However, he did agree to put together a volume, despite poor health, but this never materialised. Jackson told Wilfrid Harris that a book would allow his enemies 'to find him out'; and he wrote rarely in multi-authored textbooks.[16] His articles have proved not easy to identify, let alone locate.[17] Commenting on the *Selected Writings of John Hughlings Jackson*, edited by James Taylor (1931–2), Foster Kennedy refers to:

---

[15] V. Horsley, 'On Dr. Hughlings Jackson's Views of the Functions of the Cerebellum as Illustrated by Recent Research: The Hughlings Jackson Lecture, 1906', *Brain* **29** (1907): 446–66. The issue also contains a reprint, with comments added in 1906, of a 'case of tumour of the middle lobe of the cerebellum – cerebellar paralysis with rigidity (cerebellar attitude) – occasional tetanus-like seizures', first published by Hughlings Jackson in the *British Medical Journal* for 4 November 1871. The illustrations by Mr Stephen Mackenzie not originally printed are now included. Hughlings Jackson concedes: 'my own remarks preceding the narrative of the case and concluding the paper are old fashioned in the wording'. Ian McDonald considered this issue of *Brain* to be the finest ever produced and the epitome of everything to which the journal aspires (see *Brain* **134** (2011): 2158–76).

[16] He contributed chapters on 'Convulsions' and 'Apoplexy and Cerebral Haemorrhage', in J. Russell Reynolds, *A System of Medicine* (1868), Vol. **II**, pp. 217–50 and 504–43). Jackson adds a footnote displaying irritation that his manuscript has been reduced by a half, omitting the illustrative case material made available by various colleagues at the London Hospital.

[17] A list first appeared in the appreciation by Gustav Schorstein. Broadbent's Hughlings Jackson lecture contained a near complete bibliography to 1903. *Brain* published an issue devoted to a reprinting of Jackson's most important contributions on speech (**38** parts 1–2 (1915)), with an appreciation by Henry Head on 'Hughlings Jackson on Aphasia and Kindred Disorders of Speech', and a bibliography of Jackson's 36 publications on this topic (1864–93). *Neurological Fragments*, edited by James Taylor, contains a bibliography updating those prepared by Schorstein and Broadbent, which Taylor expanded and corrected in *Selected Writings of John Hughlings Jackson* (1931). Most recently, the scholarly and definitive *John Hughlings Jackson: A Catalogue Raisonnée* (2006), by George York and David Steinberg, identifies 537 articles, including 84 not previously known, published over a 50-year period (1861–1911), of which all but 18 were written by Hughlings Jackson alone.

Penfield, a replica had been made for the Montreal Neurological Institute (1932), a copy of which was then donated back to the National Hospital by Fred Andermann (1996), and received by David Marsden, dean of the Institute of Neurology, in a touching ceremony conducted with pomp and circumstance. The bust is now in the Rockefeller Library.

[14] For several years, it was customary to analyse Jackson's work rather than primarily to present the research and ideas of the speaker. In 1927, the lecturer Dr Charles Dana made a donation to support the lecture; and in 1931, at a meeting chaired by Mr Leslie Paton (ophthalmologist) a fund of £1,174 was established, allowing subsequent Hughlings Jackson lecturers to receive a gold medal (designed by Percy Metcalfe, weighing 4.5 ounces and made by the Royal Mint) and 100 guineas. Sadly, the most recent Hughlings Jackson lecturer has to report that neither gold nor guineas were received.

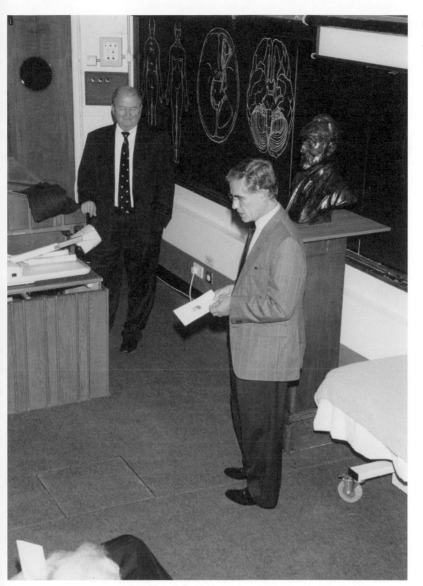

Figure 4.2 David Marsden receiving the replacement bust of Hughlings Jackson from Frederick Andermann of the Montreal Neurological Institute, in 1996.

A Periclean age in England in which great poets sang and great novelists wrote, in which natural law began to be understood … Darwin caused a new wind to blow through the murk of notions we had inherited from the middle ages. Of the same band of prophets is Hughlings Jackson who might be called the father of neurology … [his] guess was worth ten men's facts … in making the house of the physiology of the brain he was an adventurous engineer, he gathered materials … dug foundations – but even more was he a builder of flying buttresses.[18]

[18] F. Kennedy, 'John Hughlings Jackson', *Bulletin of the New York Academy of Medicine* **11** (1935): 479–80.

Taylor excuses Jackson's style on the basis that he was at pains never to overstate his case or go beyond the available evidence, thus accounting for the sense of under-statement in much of his work. Head considered Jackson to be the seed from which grew all subsequent contributions to neurology – avoiding the trap, into which others had fallen, of appearing exact by disregarding complexity, and expressing sympathy for the patient 'with a speech defect of cerebral origin stretched on the procrustean bed of some theoretical scheme … some diagrammatic conception that never has and never could have existed'. Head explains the perceived lack of full recognition by his contemporaries as due to Jackson's extreme personal modesty; his obscure style of writing 'peppered with explanatory phrases and footnotes'; his adherence to the psychological doctrines of Herbert Spencer; and the originality of ideas that were so far ahead of their time as to be incomprehensible to most contemporary readers.[19]

In analysing Jackson's legacy for neurology, it is important to remember his clinical methods and the cases that he preferred in order to formulate ideas on the nervous system in health and disease. Jackson studied focal seizures, chorea, hemiplegia, speech disorders and the mental state, but took a particular interest in epilepsy and aphasia. Above all else, he valued knowledge gained from pathology. He had introduced clinico-pathological conferences at the York Dispensary, and often travelled in order to obtain the brain of deceased patients – in one instance, upsetting nuns who had cared for a recently deceased child through his ill-contained enthusiasm for obtaining tissue. Walking at the weekend for relaxation with Hutchinson, Jackson steered a course to Farnham to see an old patient with ophthalmoplegia, who they found had just died. They arranged for autopsy and removal of the brain to London where Gowers examined the specimen.

As clinical assistant to Jonathan Hutchinson at Moorfields Eye Hospital, the early phase of Jackson's career focused on ophthalmic and ocular conditions. Through appointment to the Royal London Ophthalmic Hospital, Jackson routinely used the ophthalmoscope, and he always emphasised the importance for physicians of ophthalmology in the study and practice of medicine. In the first volume of the *Transactions of the Ophthalmological Society of the United Kingdom* (1881), Jackson writes on eye symptoms in tabes dorsalis observed in private practice, apologising for the fact that 'I am only a physician, not an ophthalmic surgeon.' The issue of *Brain* for December 1915 includes Taylor's presidential address to the neurological section of the Royal Society of Medicine (28 October 1915) summarising Jackson's contributions to ophthalmology. Taylor rehearses Jackson's assessment that, were he free to

study the physiology of movement, he would use as his laboratory the wards and outpatient clinics of a general hospital (hemiplegia, chorea and epilepsy); an ophthalmic hospital (paralysis of the cranial nerves and defects of sight); a special hospital (locomotor ataxy and certain epileptic seizures); an orthopaedic hospital (infantile paralysis and contractures); and back to the general hospital (speech and articulation, delirium, apoplexy, coma and laryngeal and throat disease). But, of these, it is especially the ophthalmological hospital that Jackson favours, not only for increasing knowledge of eye diseases but for illuminating different morbid conditions.

Jackson wrote on aphasia from 1864. Significant for the development of his ideas was the paper presented at the British Association for the Advancement of Science in Norwich in 1868, at which Jackson opened the discussion with Broca, arguing that there is no cerebral localisation, merely places in the brain where particular processes are most easily disrupted. He found incredible the concept that speech, being integral to thought, could conceivably be 'localised'. As he studied the topic, Jackson realised that affected individuals do not lack speech; rather, their language is reduced from a superior to an inferior level – sometimes confined to 'yes' and 'no', and not necessarily with appropriate use of either. From this, he argued the difference between propositional speech and emotional utterances. The unit of intellectual speech is the proposition not the word, although symbolic speech clearly does depend on selection and ordering of words. Imagination and the revival of images are distributed functions and therefore preserved – albeit 'lame' – even in the context of loss of speech.

Brown-Séquard had taught Hughlings Jackson the difference between speech, articulation and voice; and that the person with aphasia has lost the faculty of language, not just words. Later Jackson realised that speech and articulation can be distinguished by the examination of writing, and that patients with aphasia have normal mental functions but cannot translate their inner language into speech. Most of Jackson's colleagues at the National Hospital and elsewhere in the United Kingdom either were not much interested in, or failed adequately to understand, his work on aphasia. They accepted the doctrine of strict localisation. His strongest opponent was Bastian, who firmly believed in the role of centres and disconnectionist models of aphasia and related disorders. Broadbent gave Jackson 'Unanimously the first place among

[19] See Head, 'Hughlings Jackson on Aphasia and Kindred Affections of Speech', (*Brain* **38** (1915): 1–79). Later, Head wrote again on Jackson's contributions in *Aphasia and Kindred Disorders of Speech* (Cambridge University Press, 1926), Vol. **I**, pp. 30–53.

those who have contributed to neurology as a science ... [he] has not given us any complete theory of language, but I am not sure that he has not done more towards the elucidation of the problem of speech than those of us who have attempted its solution systematically.'[20]

Only in Sigmund Freud did Jackson find a reader who understood and appreciated his views. This intellectual lineage was extended by Arnold Pick and Henry Head, who each reiterated the distinction between physiological centres and the pivotal placement of lesions that result in symptoms and characteristic syndromes. Much later, Aleksandr Romanovich Luria explained that Jackson advanced principles in opposition to the strict idea of localisation – epitomised in the debate with Broca – that were distorted and not understood or accepted until the mid twentieth century, but which nevertheless played an important role in the subsequent development of neurological thinking.

Posterity has judged Jackson not to have had a sense of humour, mainly on the word of Sir Andrew Clark. But cleverness with words would cause Jackson to throw back his head and laugh with uncontrolled delight; and Thomas Buzzard, David Ferrier and James Taylor all found him witty and amusing. In his presidential address to the Medical Society of London (17 October 1887) on 'the psychology of joking', Jackson reminds his listeners that 'it requires a surgical operation to get a joke into the head of a Scotchman'. He tells us that he did once meet a medical man from Aberdeen who made a pun. Humour is hierarchical: punning is the most primitive form; wit is derived from punning; and humour evolves from wit. The pun is made when phonetics are identical but semantics differ: 'when is a little girl not a little girl? ... when she is a little hoarse'; and, rather painfully, he labours the joke by explaining 'hoarse (horse)'. Jackson expresses admiration for the primitive who rose above the intellectual demands of mere existence and coined the first pun, as an example of the aesthetic and intellectual advance in 'showing surplus mind for the greater ends of life'. Jackson suggests that people deficient in appreciation of jokes are also likely to be limited in their scientific imagination and ability to derive hypotheses.

Jackson avoided the term 'voluntary' with respect to movement, instead referring to actions as 'most' and 'least' automatic when considering spinal and cerebral representation. This steered a course between the extremes of strict localisation and the view that all movements are represented equally throughout the cortex. Jackson argued that those parts which move most – face, hand and foot – have the greatest representation, the cortex being concerned with movement not muscles: 'the speculation is that, although each movement is everywhere represented, there are points where particular movements are specially represented'. Somatopic representation occurred at multiple evolutionary levels, each subsuming the organisation of its subsidiary, and differing in its weighting for individual parts. These overlapped: 'every part of the body is represented in every part of the brain'. This weighting is dynamic and, in the context of disease, a lower system in the hierarchy or surviving parts of the affected area can adapt and resume some functions approximating to normality. In primitive terms, this 'principle of compensation' was a prescient account of plasticity accounting for recovery of function over time.

Jackson's main contribution was to set the manifestations of neurological disease in the context of interacting hierarchies. Each layer added complexity in rearranging the properties of a lower evolutionary system. The more primitive layers were subservient but brutish, restless and liable to erupt in mutiny; higher ones were tolerant, civilised and acting as specialists and governors. With evolution came differentiation of form and function, and integration of levels. With dissolution, the most differentiated and integrated suffered first, leading to deficits and releasing the lower levels. At first, Jackson defined three main levels: the lowest comprised the dorsal root entry zone and anterior spinal roots; the next involved the basal ganglia and motor cortex; and the highest depended upon the prefrontal motor cortex. But in the first Hughlings Jackson lecture (8 December 1897), Jackson refined his ideas on evolution and dissolution, assigning automated vegetative functions to the lowest level (tuber cinerum to the conus medullaris); 'chiefly motor and chiefly sensory' to the middle (cerebral cortex); and the anatomical basis of 'consciousness ... mental states ... and the physical basis of mind' to the highest (premotor frontal cortex).[21]

---

[20] W. Hughlings Broadbent, 'Jackson as Pioneer in Nervous Physiology and Pathology', *Brain* **26** (1903): 305–66. Jackson attended the lecture but told his brother that he had heard not a word, because of deafness.

[21] J. H. Jackson, 'Hughlings Jackson Lecture – Remarks on the Relations of Different Divisions of the Central Nervous System to One Another and to Parts of the Body', *Lancet* **151** (1898): 79–87.

Jackson admitted that his views on hierarchies were considered by others to be those of a 'Bedlamite theorist'. He wrestled with the relationship of mind and body, avoiding the need to declare himself either a materialist or a dualist through the concept of concomitance and parallelism in which each physical event has its own psychical counterpart: 'the idea is a faint percept, the perception a vivid idea. The image had in ideation is a faint copy of that had in perception.' On the topic of neuropsychiatry, Jackson argued that 'if there be such a thing as a disease of the mind, we can do nothing for it'. But, in that he regarded psychiatry as part of neurology, Jackson was ahead of the game in requiring the same rigours of biological analysis as in any other branch of medicine. Although Jackson saw the nervous system of man as a machine, and regarded Cartesian dualism as 'scientific blasphemy', he developed the concept of physical and mental properties existing in parallel through 'concomitance', a term borrowed from Gottfried Wilhelm Leibniz and in use amongst Victorian philosophers and psychologists. Mind was hierarchical: the highest level was consciousness; and it followed that all lower states were unconscious. Jackson joked that automatic activities of mind forming the 'unitary concept of unconscious cerebration' explained the rapid flow of ideas to Wilson, his last house physician. Over time, Jackson became increasingly uncomfortable with the concept of unconscious mental states, eventually declaring this to be a contradiction in terms. To some extent, this merger of the physical and psychical subsumed his doctrine of parallelism into a more overtly materialist formulation on body and mind. Mercier, a psychiatrist, considered that Jackson's 'Speculations on the ultimate nature of mental processes and their connexion with brain [function] are the most consistent and explanatory that have ever been attained; and they will undoubtedly form the foundation of a future system of psychology yet to be elaborated.'[22]

Gordon Holmes knew Jackson during the period 1900–10, but struggled with his writings. Although not sympathetic to speculation or philosophy, Holmes acknowledged that perseverance with Jackson's papers overcame the difficulties and obscure style, revealing a relevance to modern neurology that should persuade even the most critical and go beyond mere ancestor worship. In *The National Hospital* (1954), Holmes acknowledges that Jackson's writings were the product

'Not of large statistical reviews of a large material but the close study of a relatively small material ... We can salute his genius without believing that all he said is final and forever adequate to generalize the great additions to knowledge which have accrued since his day.'

Whilst ranking Jackson alongside Willis, Harvey and Hunter, Critchley remained uncertain whether, in time, 'the sage of Manchester Square' would still be remembered, given the advance of technical and scientific knowledge that has simplified much of the practice of neurology: 'Perhaps our neurological successors will not retain the same affection for our "father" that even beyond Queen Square – where we are sometimes still accused of ancestor worship – is felt today. Hazlitt said that no one is truly great who is great only in his lifetime, the test of greatness is the page of history.' [23]

Copies exist of a parody of the Athanasian Creed containing the essentials of Hughlings Jackson's principles of organisation within the central nervous system, written in the late 1880s by members of the Neurological Society of London. A copy was sent to Head by Armand de Watteville and then passed to Sherrington (8 October 1925), in which Head refers to a *jeux d'esprit*:

Quincunque Vult

WHOSOEVER will be saved, before all things it is necessary that he hold the Neurological faith, which faith except everyone do keep whole and undefiled, without doubt he shall perish everlastingly.

And the neurological faith is this: that Unity in the Nervous System, and the Nervous System in Unity, is to be recognized. Neither confounding the function, nor dividing the Structure. For there is one portion of the Brain, another of the Cord; and another of the Sympathetic.

But the structure of the Brain, of the Cord, and of the Sympathetic is all one; the cells similar and the fibre identical.

So likewise the Brain action is reflex, the Cord action reflex; and the Sympathetic action reflex.

And yet there are not three reflex actions; but one reflex action.

The Cord is made of none; neither made, nor designed.

[22] C. Mercier, 'The Late Dr Hughlings-Jackson', *British Medical Journal* **1** (1912): 85–6, reproduced in Hughlings Jackson, *Neurological Fragments*, pp. 40–6.

[23] Macdonald and Eileen Critchley end their biography of Hughlings Jackson with this analysis. The annotated typescript of their book survives and indicates that their original title was 'The Sage of Manchester Square' but presumably this was altered during copy-editing: M. Critchley and E. Critchley, *John Hughlings Jackson, Father of English Neurology* (Oxford University Press, 1998).

The Brain is of the Cord alone; not made, nor created, nor designed but evolved.

So that in all things, as aforesaid, Unity in the Nervous System, and the Nervous System in Unity, is to be recognized.

He, therefore, who will be saved; must thus think of the Nervous system.

Furthermore, it is necessary to Everlasting Salvation; that he also believe rightly the doctrine of Dissolution.

For the right faith is that we believe and confess; that the Special fails before the general, and the Voluntary before the Automatic.

This is the NEUROLOGICAL FAITH; which unless a man believe faithfully. He cannot be saved.

Glory be to the Brain, and to the cord, and to the Sympathetic.

As they were discharging, are now, and ever will be, reflex without end. Amen.

Sir David Ferrier

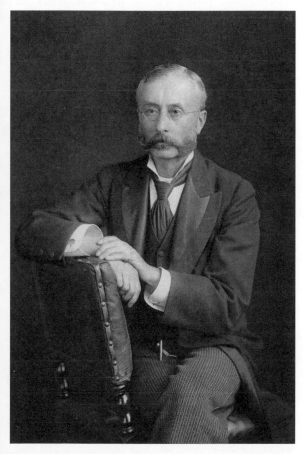

Figure 4.3 Sir David Ferrier.

David Ferrier was born (13 January 1843) and educated in Aberdeen.[24] He first studied logic, philosophy and psychology (1863) but then took up medical studies at the University of Edinburgh, from where he graduated (1868). His first medical post was as assistant to a general practitioner in Bury St Edmunds. According to Sherrington, Ferrier spent most of this assistantship pursuing research on comparative anatomy, carried out in the peace of the doctor's large garden. This formed the basis for Ferrier's MD thesis on the corpora quadrigemina of animals (1870). He decided on a career in physiology and was appointed lecturer at the Middlesex Hospital (1870), moving to King's College, initially as demonstrator in physiology (1871), then as professor of forensic medicine (1872) and, later, of neuropathology (1889). Appointed physician to the Hospital for Epilepsy and Paralysis at Portland Terrace, Regents Park (1872), his subsequent post on the consultant staff of the National Hospital (1880–1908) was conditional on resignation from the rival Hospital for Epilepsy and Paralysis. Ferrier was involved in a variety of medical and social developments in London, including establishment of the National Society for the Employment of Epileptics. He was elected FRS (1876) and received the Society's Royal Medal (1890); became a founding editor of *Brain* (1878) and of the Neurological Society of London (1886); was recognised by the Royal College of Physicians (Baly Medal, 1887; Moxon Medal, 1912); and received a knighthood (1911). Ferrier married Constance Waterlow, sister of the artist Ernest Waterlow,[25] who drew many of the illustrations to his published works. They had two sons,

[24] There is no extended biography of Ferrier. But see C. S. Sherrington, 'Sir David Ferrier, 1843–1928', *Proceedings of the Royal Society of London* **103B** (1928): viii–xvi; J. D. Spillane, 'A Memorable Decade in the History of Neurology 1874–1884', *British Medical Journal* 4 (1974): 701–5; Anon., 'Obituary', *British Medical Journal* 1 (1928): 525–6; S. A. K. Wilson, *British Medical Journal* 1 (1928): 526; R. Crawfurd, 'Obituary', *British Medical Journal* 1 (1928): 526; Anon., 'Obituary: The Late Sir David Ferrier', *British Medical Journal* 1 (1928): 574; and W. A. Turner, 'Obituary: The Late Sir David Ferrier', *British Medical Journal* 1 (1928): 574–5. Much of the information presented here is from these works.

[25] Ernest Waterlow was a landscape painter who had won the Gold Medal at the Royal Academy Schools in 1873. He was later elected associate of the Royal Academy and Royal Watercolour Society and was knighted in 1902. It has been suggested that he is not acknowledged as the artist in Ferrier's publications due to the risk of being identified to the anti-vivisection movement.

one of whom, Claude Ferrier, became a distinguished architect and designed the Ferriers' country house near the Chalfont Centre. Ferrier inspired loyalty amongst his friends and colleagues, and he was well liked. He was the last of the physicians at Queen Square to wear a top hat during ward rounds. According to Purves-Stewart, Ferrier was notably Scottish and 'brought with him into the wards a bracing and sunny atmosphere of enthusiasm. He was a dapper little man, scrupulously well dressed and groomed, spick and span, with singularly elegant hands and feet. He walked with a characteristic springy gait. His clear-cut features and piercing hawk-like glance made him conspicuous in any assembly.'[26]

For Sir Charles Ballance, 'as Hughlings Jackson is the Socrates of neurology, so Ferrier may be described as the John Hunter of neurology'. Turner described him in vivid terms:

> He was a man of action, forceful in purpose and tenacious of his opinions; yet withal a man of affectionate and kindly nature, and imbued with much human sympathy. His physical and mental make-up showed the character of the man. A short and spare figure, a strong nose and chin, and sharp features, combined with great alertness of mind and manner, and an inquiring disposition, denoted the energetic and successful seeker after information. He thought clearly, wrote clearly, and spoke clearly, his speech having a slight accent, denoting his Scottish origin.

At an early stage in his career, Ferrier had come under the influence of Jackson, whom he considered to be his main teacher and with whom he maintained a close and lifelong friendship. Wilson recalled Ferrier remarking, as they walked away from Jackson's funeral: 'Well, when I cease to take an interest in things it will be time for me to go'; and he was 'one whose life illustrated in perfection the meaning of the love of knowledge for its own sake, and who carried undimmed to the end the torch of science put into his hands sixty years before'.

Ferrier's advancement in the early 1870s was rapid. Soon after their first meeting, Sir James Crichton-Browne, who directed the West Riding Lunatic Asylum between 1866 and 1875,[27] invited Ferrier to Wakefield where laboratories were equipped and research encouraged, to develop the work of Fritsch and Hitzig using galvanic stimulation directly applied to the canine cortex. Jackson was also a visitor to Wakefield,[28] and Ferrier was heavily influenced by his theories of the cortex as a sensorimotor machine and Jackson's views on localisation of function. Provided with a 'liberal supply of pigeons, fowls, guinea pigs, rabbits, cats and dogs for the purposes of research', Ferrier started work in the spring of 1873.[29] He called his early paper on localisation of function in the *West Riding Lunatic Asylum Medical Reports* (1873), describing the method of low-intensity faradic stimulation of the cerebral cortex in anaesthetised animals, a 'preliminary statement', indicating that its primary purpose was to provide experimental proof of the views of Jackson on the cerebral localisation of symptoms in epilepsy. In fact, Jackson took a distributed rather than strictly localisationist view, although postulated that the symptoms of a seizure did localise the cortical focus. Ferrier concluded

---

in accusations of persistent abuse. In the wake of this scandal, the Wakefield Asylum was opened (1818) to care for the insane poor, following The County Asylums Act 1808. It was administered by magistrates at quarter sessions until 1889 when it was taken over, first by the county council, and then by the county boroughs. In 1948, it was renamed the Stanley Royd Hospital and came under the control of the local health authority. The hospital closed in 1995. See A. L. Ashworth, *Stanley Royd Hospital, Wakefield, One Hundred and Fifty Years, a History* (1975).

[28] In *Victorian Jottings* (Wakefield: Stanley Royd Hospital, 1926), Crichton-Browne recalls how Sir Wemyss Reid fell into conversation with a fellow guest – 'a man of great ability and culture' – at the Black Horse Hotel in Clapham, Yorkshire, and confided that he had returned to the place of his honeymoon on the anniversary of the wedding to his late wife, whereupon his chance companion, Hughlings Jackson, exclaimed: 'Incredible. Your case is mine! I spent my honeymoon here many years ago. I married young; I married my cousin; it was a very happy marriage. She is dead and gone. This is not the anniversary of our wedding but I have come here out of the stress and anxiety of professional life in London to stir up some dormant emotions.'

[29] Sherrington recalls having dinner with Ballance and Ferrier in December 1921, after which he wrote to Harvey Cushing: 'dear old Ferrier was there ... I got an interesting account ... of his original brain expts, that started modern physiology of the cortex. He was so modest about all that first-rate work, done in a little private room in a Yorkshire Asylum, by himself with very little to guide or help him; and the results so clearly and simply set forth in those early papers.' Ballance wrote later to Sherrington: 'It was Ferrier, not any surgeon, who was the originator and founder of modern cerebral surgery.'

---

[26] Purves-Stewart, *The Sands of Time* (1939).

[27] The West Riding Lunatic Asylum has an interesting history. The first Yorkshire asylum was the Lunatic Asylum in York founded by William Tuke (1774), considered the model of a modern asylum but, by 1813, embroiled

that Hughlings Jackson's theory that 'unilateral epilepsies are caused by discharging cortical lesions' was correct, as demonstrated by his 'artificial reproduction of the clinical experiments performed by disease'.

Ferrier's focus was on motor responses. He identified localised areas of the brain (centres), stimulation of which in a variety of species resulted in independent movements of many parts of the head and neck, fore-limbs, hind-limbs and tail. His most detailed work using stimulation and lesioning was in the macaque monkey; and he found that the longer the stimulation was applied, the more complex the movements became. Ferrier observed that, in general, a body part involved in movement produced by stimulation became paralysed or its movement impaired following a lesion of the same area. He argued that the cerebral cortex is organised so as to facilitate complex coordinated movement rather than simple muscle action; and that the combination of movements differs between, and is adapted appropriately to, individual species. In monkeys, Ferrier delineated areas responsible for walking, arm retraction, flexion and extension of the wrists, tongue protrusion, opening of the mouth and sneering expressions. He realised that the frontal areas determine changes of behaviour without affecting intellect or motor function. Ferrier corresponded with Bigelow on Phineas Gage, the famous 'American Crow-bar case', whose severe frontal lobe injury resulted in a complete change in personality without much affecting his intelligence or motor abilities and in whom at post-mortem the exact anatomical areas of damage were defined.[30] Ferrier carried out detailed stimulation and lesioning of the temporal, parietal and occipital cortex. He identified areas for taste and smell; found that total deafness results from bilateral lesions of the superior temporo-sphenoidal convolutions; and reported blindness following destruction of the angular gyrus.

Crichton-Browne wrote to Darwin in April 1873 that Ferrier 'has discovered that every convolution of the brain is in direct relation with certain groups of muscles, and controls their actions', and that the results will 'constitute the most important advances yet made in cerebral physiology'. Darwin replied: 'I have been profoundly interested ... it seems clear that the physiology of the brain will soon be largely understood. What a step it is. You have reason to be very proud of the volume.'[31]

Ferrier's experiments were far more sophisticated than the earlier work of Hitzig and Fritsch. They had applied high-intensity galvanic stimulation and induced twitches and jerks, whereas Ferrier used faradic stimulation which produced more sustained and complex movements. Furthermore, Ferrier varied duration and intensity of the stimulus and found that these were important in determining whether the result was a twitch and spasm or a more complex movement. Sherrington noted that, after the publication of Ferrier's first paper, 'The next decade saw a flowing tide of research setting toward localisation ... a vogue [which] reigned for nearly a quarter of a century and became in due course tedious and relatively infertile. But the importance of the work which ushered it in cannot be forgotten.'[32]

The initial experiments were concerned with various lower vertebrates but, with a grant from the Royal Society, Ferrier was then able to carry out work on primates (at King's College Hospital in 1874), and continue his research on other species. He was the first to recognise that cortical representation was similar in all species but that some parts of the body have larger representations in the cortex in different species – variations that he believed depended on the 'habits of the animals'. On the basis of this work, and although not yet elected FRS, Ferrier was invited to give the Croonian lecture to the Royal Society in February 1874 and, again, in 1875, on his further discoveries. Although the research, carried out over a very short period of time, excited great interest and established his reputation, publication of the 1874 Croonian lecture sparked the first controversy with which Ferrier became embroiled. In the introduction, he acknowledged the influence of Jackson and mentioned that his findings confirmed and extended the researches of Fritsch and Hitzig. However, he was accused by the two referees (Michael Foster and George Rolleston) of not acknowledging Fritsch and Hitzig sufficiently; and a third referee, T. H. Huxley, was asked to ascertain whether 'Dr Ferrier has or has

---

[30] Copies of their correspondence with Dr Bigelow, the American physician who reported the case, are in the National Hospital archives.

[31] Crichton-Browne had sent Darwin a copy of the *West Riding Lunatic Asylum Medical Reports* which contained the article by Ferrier (D. Ferrier, 'Experimental Researches in Cerebral Physiology and Pathology', *West Riding Lunatic Asylum Medical Reports* III (1873): 30–96).
[32] Sherrington C. David Ferrier, *Proceedings of the Royal Society of London*, Series B, **103** (1928): viii–xvi.

not done sufficient mention of the labour of his predecessors in the same field of investigation'. Huxley upheld the complaint and Ferrier was asked to revise the paper accordingly, which he did, but his referees still considered that 'the acknowledgement of Hitzig's claim to priority was so slight … that its publication would be … unfortunate to English Science'. Rather than make the changes requested by the referees, Ferrier then went ahead and published his experimental work on the macaque monkey, but omitting the studies on dogs and other animals. As Hitzig and Fritsch had not worked on monkeys, this was then accepted. The episode resulted in much publicity and vehement complaints by Fritsch and Hitzig. In retrospect, it seems to us that Ferrier's work extended the findings of Fritsch and Hitzig to such a degree that greater acknowledgement was unnecessary and, furthermore, his methodology and findings differed. Much later, when speaking to the Edinburgh College, Ferrier acknowledged that 'the whole aspect of cerebral physiology and pathology was revolutionised by the discovery, first made by Fritsch and Hitzig, that certain definite movements could be excited by the direct application of electrical stimulation to definite regions of the cortex cerebri in dogs.'[33]

These advances on previous work and Ferrier's new discoveries were summarised in a monograph, *The Functions of the Brain* (1876; second edition, extensively revised, 1886). He describes experiments on ascidians, fish, frogs and amphibians, pigeons, cats, dogs, rabbits, rats and jackals; and on the functions of the mesencephalon and cerebellum, optic lobes and corpora quadrigemina, medulla and spinal cord, as well as that of the cerebrum. Ferrier produced woodcuts (drawn, as mentioned above, by his brother-in-law Ernest Waterlow) that transposed findings in the macaque monkey onto outlines taken from Ecker's *On the Convolutions of the Human Brain* (1873). Ecker had written that 'The cortex … is not a single organ, which is brought into play as a whole in the exercise of each and every psychical function, but consists rather of a multitude of organs, each of which is subservient to definite mental processes.'

---

[33] D. Ferrier, *The Croonian Lectures on Cerebral Localisation Delivered before the Royal College of Physicians, June 1890* (London: Smith, Elder, 1890), p. 17 – however, in the lectures, Ferrier does go on critically to appraise their findings and makes it clear that his own findings greatly extended their work.

Ferrier predicted a 'science of the localisation of the mental functions' and considered this 'one of the most important problems for the anatomy and physiology of the next century, the solution of which will work no small transformation in psychology'. This was prescient. Ferrier's work was different from that of Fritsch and Hitzig in that he used long-duration faradic stimulation which allowed complex movements to be observed (not just spasm) and he examined much larger areas of cortex with greater degrees of sophistication. Ferrier's cortical maps became the basis for all subsequent work in this field; they are the (equally unacknowledged) precursor for Penfield's more famous homunculus. Ferrier identified association areas as well as motor and sensory centres and, adopting the Jacksonian view of hierarchies, coined the term 'noetiko-kinetic' to designate activity under the control of hemispheres involving consciousness, subdivided into 'ana-noetiko-kinetic' to describe actions conditioned by 'revived or ideal impressions', and 'syn-noetiko-kinetic' for 'compound associations'. He discussed homologies between the simian and human brain and also psychological functions of the cortex. Later, Ferrier also demonstrated sensory function and the control of eye movements by electrical stimulation of the cerebellum. He distinguished voluntary and reflex movements in decerebrate animals, and found that ablation of the hemispheres in lower animals (frogs, fishes and birds) results in complete loss of spontaneous activity but preservation of equilibrium and the ability to perform perfectly co-ordinated movements such as jumping, swimming, flying and walking. In higher animals, these properties are lost, together with the ability to maintain equilibrium or progression. The book is dedicated: 'To Dr Hughlings Jackson, who from the clinical and pathological standpoint anticipated many of the more important results of recent experimental investigation into the functions of the cerebral hemispheres, this book is dedicated as a mark of the author's esteem and admiration.'

Sherrington decided to follow a career in physiology after hearing Ferrier's Croonian lecture at the Royal Society; and he dedicated his classic Silliman lectures, published as *The Integrative Action of the Nervous System* (1906), to Ferrier in appreciation of that pioneering work.

Ferrier's subsequent work was encapsulated in the published versions of his Gulstonian (*The Localisation of Cerebral Disease*, 1878, dedicated to Charcot) and

Croonian lectures (*On Cerebral Localisation*, 1890) delivered to the Royal College of Physicians. Here, he extended his observations and, notwithstanding transposition of the earlier findings in the macaque onto a human brain atlas, acknowledged that 'there exist in different animals great differences in the degree of organisation ... and an exact correspondence (of hemispheric function) can scarcely be supposed to exist'. In line with the work of Jackson, Ferrier cautioned against exaggerated claims regarding cortical localisation being made by others based on his original work, and pointed out that interconnections and communication between separate areas of the brain are rendered invalid through over-simplistic views of cerebral localisation. He took a sophisticated view beyond simple anatomical localisation and fully recognised that, as Jackson had postulated, the functions of the cerebrum are sensorimotor and that ideation is also important: 'From the complexity of mental phenomena and the participation in them of both motor and sensory substrata, any system of localization of mental faculties which does not take both factors into account must be radically false.'

Nevertheless, Ferrier recognised that there are parts of the cortex to which discrete function could be assigned, and that lesions in these areas result in either 'irritative or destructive effects ... the two classes into which all may be theoretically reduced'.

Controversy continued to stalk Ferrier and this culminated in the notorious confrontation with Friedrich Leopold Goltz, professor of physiology in Strasburg, at the 1881 Seventh International Medical Congress held in London.[34] On the morning of 4 August 1881, as part of the programme on physiology and with Michael Foster in the chair, Goltz set out in German his views on equipotentiality. In support of his position, Goltz paraded a dog which he claimed had been subjected to wide bilateral decorticectomy, but without causing paralysis, and offered to sacrifice the animal in order to examine its brain. Ferrier then described his experiments on monkeys, supported by photographs and slides of brain preparations. He offered to present a hemiplegic monkey which, seven months previously, had undergone localised unilateral ablation of the motor cortex. In the afternoon, members of the section adjourned to King's College Hospital where Goltz' dog and Ferrier's monkey were demonstrated. Virchow and Charcot were both present and Charcot was so impressed by the hemiplegic monkey that, according to Ballance who was also in the audience, he exclaimed 'c'est un malade!' Ferrier also showed a second macaque in which bilateral resection of the superior temporal region had rendered the animal totally deaf so that it ignored a pistol shot fired close to the head. Ferrier considered that Goltz' experimental technique was flawed as he obliterated brain using a jet of water, rather than by careful excision, an imprecise method which made it impossible to know exactly which structures had been damaged. As one observer commented: 'What conclusions, it will be asked, are to be drawn from these singularly discordant experiments of Professors Goltz and Ferrier? ... Fortunately the two eminent experimenters whose graphic accounts of their work had been listened to with marked interest by the section determined upon a line of conduct destined to throw great light upon their experimental procedures.'

Both consented to examination of the two animals' brains and the section president organised examination by an independent committee (comprising Gowers, E. Klein, E. A. Schäfer and J. N. Langley). A preliminary report was issued on the last day of the Congress (9 August 1881). The committee reported that the brain lesions in Goltz' dog were not as extensive as claimed, with portions of the motor and sensory areas preserved; whereas Ferrier's monkey had, as predicted, a complete circumscribed lesion in the motor

---

[34] This was a truly remarkable meeting in many ways, and is well described in contemporary diaries and newspapers: 3,181 delegates attended and included, among many others, Hughlings Jackson, Semon, Ferrier, Lister, Hutchinson, Wilkes, Gull, Huxley, Pasteur, Virchow, Kaposi, Koch, Charcot, Austin Flint and Osler. Sir James Paget was president and the Prince of Wales, the future King Edward VII, attended. At the farewell dinner at the Crystal Palace, large firework portraits of Charcot and Sir James Paget illuminated the sky. Private parties were held in the London houses of Paget, Spencer-Wells and Langdon Down. The meeting was based at St James' Hall (an extraordinary composite group photograph exists of 684 delegates), with other venues including the National Hospital. Receptions were held at the South Kensington museums, the Albert Hall, the Society of Apothecaries Hall and the College of Physicians. A famous garden party was arranged by Lady Burdett-Coutts, which is illustrated in a large portrait by Archibald Tilt hanging in the Wellcome

Trust, in which, among others, Hughlings Jackson, Wilks, Argyll Robertson, Hutchinson, Allbutt, Paget and Charcot appear and represent the neurological interest (see A. Sakula, 'Baroness Burdett-Coutts' Garden Party: The International Medical Congress, London, 1881', *Medical History* 36 (1982): 183–90).

area. This conclusion was widely publicised and proved an enormous boost to the localisationalist school.[35]

But the whole episode was a step too far in the eyes of the powerful anti-vivisection movement and, in a furious assault, Ferrier was accused under the Cruelty to Animals Act (1876) of performing 'frightful and shocking experiments on monkeys for which he did not have a licence'. He was summoned to appear at Bow Street police court. Ferrier had previously been the subject of similar attacks by anti-vivisectionists, notably by Francis Cobbe who later had a very public and acrimonious row with Victor Horsley. The prosecution excited passion and worldwide interest and Jackson, Lister, Burdon-Sanderson and Charcot were among those who attended the hearing (November 1881). The British Medical Association provided legal support and published the proceedings in the *British Medical Journal.* The opening address of counsel was thought by an American journal to be 'the prosiest and poorest twaddle that could have been tolerated in the support of the feeblest case'; and the charge was thrown out – albeit on the technicality that it was Ferrier's collaborator Gerald Yeo who performed the operation and he did hold a licence – to the relief of scientific medicine worldwide. Samuel Wilks wrote an excoriating letter in the *Lancet*, warning against the dangers of the anti-vivisectionists, and the proceedings were deemed by the *Boston Medical and Surgical Journal* to have been a 'dishonour to the English nation in the eyes of the world'. Wilson wrote later: 'Only a few of his friends are aware of the personal abuse which this line of investigation brought [Ferrier] or of the extremes to which his opponents went in their endeavour to discredit his achievement.'[36]

The publications of Ferrier's papers and books were landmark events in the history of neuroscience; and they mark the beginning of a revolution in the scientific understanding of brain function. Ferrier had become a renowned international figure. He emphasised that exactitude is needed in defining the anatomy and topography of the cortex, as function may be localised in very small areas of the brain. His work, of course, led the way to brain surgery targeted on features of clinical semiology such as focal convulsions or paralysis. In his Marshall Hall oration (1883), Ferrier suggested that surgeons should 'venture to operate upon the brain, the dura being perhaps no more inviolable than the peritoneum had recently proved to be'. Horsley and Rickman Godlee were both in the audience at his demonstration to the International Medical Conference; and, in turn, Ferrier personally attended their first pioneering operations. Throughout his career, Ferrier took a very keen interest in human neurosurgery, which he felt was the ultimate clinical dividend of his work, and a vindication of research carried out in the face of the intense personal criticism from anti-vivisectionists.[37] In a paper read before the Neurological Society on 20 December 1888,[38] he reviewed the 48 cases of resective surgery of the cerebral cortex of which he was aware, diagnosed using cerebral localisation. He was pleased to note that many were successful and there was a mortality rate of only 15 per cent, which was rather less than that seen following what he called 'generally recognised legitimate operations' such as amputation or laparotomy. Ferrier withdrew gradually from experimental work in animals, but kept a close interest in the laboratory work of his successors. In the 1890s, he developed a

---

[35] The final reports were published several years later: E. A. Schäfer, 'Report on the Lesions, Primary and Secondary, in the Brain and Spinal Cord of the Macaque Monkey Exhibited by Professors Ferrier and Yeo', *Journal of Physiology* 4 (1884): 316–26; J. N. Langley, 'Report on the Parts Destroyed on the Right Side of the Brain of the Dog Operated on by Prof. Goltz', *Journal of Physiology* 4 (1884): 286–309; E. Klein, 'Report on the Parts Destroyed on the Left Side of the Brain of the Dog Operated on by Prof. Goltz', *Journal of Physiology* 4 (1884): 310–15. As an interesting aside, Sherrington's first published paper was a study on the Wallerian degeneration of Goltz' dog: J. N. Langley and C. S. Sherrington, 'Secondary Degeneration of Nerve Tracts Following Removal of the Cortex of the Cerebrum in the Dog', *Journal of Physiology* 5 (1885): 49–65.

[36] S. A. K. Wilson and David Ferrier, *British Medical Journal* 1 (24 March 1928): 526.

[37] A bizarre early application of his stimulation method was used in the case of Mary Rafferty, who developed a skull defect due to cancerous ulcer. The American physician Dr Roberts Bartholow applied faradic stimulation to her exposed brain and demonstrated that Ferrier's observations in the macaque could be reproduced in the human (1874). Stronger faradic stimulation caused convulsions and coma and the patient died. Bartholow was censured and forced to leave Cincinnati, and an editorial in the *British Medical Journal* stated that he had 'gone a step beyond Dr Ferrier, and in a direction in which Dr Ferrier is never likely to follow'. See J. P. Morgan, 'The First Reported Case of Electrical Stimulation of the Human Brain', *Journal of the History of Medicine and Allied Sciences* 37 (1982): 51–64. The claim that this was the first case of electrical stimulation is incorrect as Horsley had used the technique in 1881.

[38] D. Ferrier, 'Cerebral Localisation in its Practical Relations', *Brain* 12 issue 1–2 (1889): 36–58.

large consulting practice, and Aldren Turner commented on his enormous work schedule:

> For a period of about thirty years his working day began at 8.30 in the morning and rarely terminated before midnight … although his days were fully occupied by hospital duties and the heavy burden of an increasing practice, he found time to visit the laboratory [the neuro-pathological laboratory at King's College] most afternoons and to assist in experiments from time to time. One of the most remarkable features of his career was that throughout his professional life he combined the pursuit of science with the practice of his profession.

That said, Ferrier was not considered to be a physician in the class of Jackson or Gowers and, for Critchley, 'he did not excel as a clinician'. In *The National Hospital*, Holmes wrote (largely basing this appreciation on the obituary by Aldren Turner):

> For several years he had a large private practice, but to many he gave the impression of remaining a physiologist rather than of being a clinician; he lacked the faculty of patient and painstaking clinical examination both in the out-patient department and in the wards. He made few serious contributions to clinical neurology, and though clear and incisive in the statement of his opinions, he was not such a popular teacher as Gowers and other of his colleagues. His visits to the Hospital were usually short, and his examination of patients rarely comprehensive, unless their symptoms raised physiological problems that interested him, but his acute intelligence and extensive experience obviated risks of serious errors in diagnosis and treatment.

Ferrier suffered ill-health for several years before his death, and a close friend, Dr Raymond Crawfurd, wrote of 'the indomitable determination with which, for the last two years of his life, he faced and fought physical disability, engendered by a very grave illness, such as most men would have accepted as a sentence of complete and final disability'. On his death, a memorial fund was set up by Aldren Turner, Ballance, Purves-Stewart, St Clair Thomson and William Bulloch; and this funded the Ferrier lecture and medal awarded triennially by the Royal Society. Wilson wrote a thoughtful and affectionate tribute:

Sir David Ferrier was the last of the small and choice company of pioneers through whose labours the scientific neurology of to-day has come into being. Nearly sixty years have passed since he commenced researches on the functions of the central nervous system that brought him world-wide distinction and made his name familiar wherever neurology was taught. With those of Hughlings Jackson, Horsley, and Gowers, it will ever take that honoured position in the memorials of neurological science … The commonplaces of neural doctrine to-day were the discoveries of his early manhood, and we of a succeeding generation can appreciate but faintly the new world then revealed by the objective methods of precise cerebral experimentation.[39]

Sir William Richard Gowers

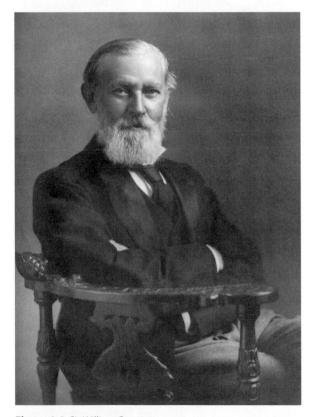

Figure 4.4 Sir William Gowers.

[39] S. A. K. Wilson, Sir David Ferrier, *British Medical Journal* **1** (28 March 1928): 526.

Sir William Osler dedicated his monograph *On Chorea and Choreiform Affections* (1894) to William Gowers: 'To the profession of the United States and Canada you stand as the most brilliant exponent of the complex science of neurology.'

Half a century later, Critchley suggested that Gowers was arguably the greatest clinical neurologist who ever lived. More than 100 years after Gowers' death, neurologists still remember him for the *Manual of Diseases of the Nervous System* (1886–8), widely considered to be the most authoritative textbook of neurology ever written.

William Richard Gowers was born (20 March 1845) and educated, initially, in the east end of London; but, when his father died, the family moved to Oxford.[40] On leaving school (aged 15 years), Gowers had no clear ambitions but was encouraged to try his hand at farming.[41] In 1861, he visited relatives in Essex where chance introduction to Dr Thomas Simpson resulted in Gowers being offered work as the family physician's 'inside' apprentice. After some thought, he accepted this opportunity for children from families with limited means to embark on a career in medicine. Apart from Simpson, Gowers was influenced by two congregationalist ministers in Coggeshall (Brian Dale and Alfred Philps). Nature walks helped Gowers to sharpen his powers of observation and grasp the importance of orderly classification in science. He was obliged to study botany as part of the preliminary scientific examination, and maintained a scientific interest in mosses throughout his lifetime. His subsequent clinical methods owed much to that of the great Victorian naturalists. After 1858, medical apprenticeships were phased out, but Gowers' son Ernest later recalled his father saying that the time with Dr Simpson had been of lasting value. Gowers married Mary Baines, the daughter of a prominent Yorkshire businessman and the owner of the Liberal-leaning *Leeds Mercury*. They had two sons and two daughters and Gowers was 'peculiarly happy in his married life and a devoted husband and father'. He wrote an extraordinary illustrated diary for his children's entertainment, and took them on regular visits to the zoo and Royal Botanical Gardens in Regent's Park. Gowers also had a number of friends outside medicine, including Rudyard Kipling and Leander Starr Jameson; and he was an accomplished draughtsman, some of his landscape drawings and etchings being exhibited at the Royal Academy of Arts.[42]

Philps introduced Gowers to William Jenner, professor of medicine at University College Hospital, who provided tuition during Gowers' studies for entry to that college, where, on arrival, Jenner used Gowers as his amanuensis. Jenner also came from humble origins and his sponsorship encouraged the young Gowers to raise his expectations and consider a career in hospital medicine. Following an undergraduate career in which he applied himself to the demanding course with great distinction, Gowers was appointed clinical assistant to Jenner, and for the next few years worked between University College Hospital and Jenner's consulting rooms (63 Brook Street). Gowers learned a great deal from Jenner but it was a younger member of the medical staff at University College Hospital, Russell Reynolds, who first stimulated his interest in the nervous system and encouraged Gowers to apply successfully for the newly created registrar post at the National Hospital.

In his first year at Queen Square, Gowers drew up an inventory of the diagnoses of all inpatients, listing 65 epileptics, 26 paraplegics and 28 hemiplegics. There were five cases of chorea, five of lead palsy, four of locomotor ataxia and four patients with brain tumour. He also reported on the treatment

---

[40] Born in Hackney, East London, Gowers was the only surviving child of William Gowers, a shoemaker, and his wife Ann Venables. He attended Hackney Free and Parochial School, a small endowed Church of England school affectionately referred to by the local cockneys as the 'Eton of the East End'. Following his father's death in 1852, his mother sold the cobbler's shop in Church Street and moved to live with her brother, a gun maker in Headington, Oxford. Gowers was able to secure a scholarship to attend Christ Church College School, Oxford, a school catering primarily for the Cathedral's choristers. It is likely that the young Gowers, as a non-conformist, may have found this experience difficult. He reminisced later that his only friend during the unhappy Oxford days was his pet dog. Not long after the move to Oxfordshire, Ann had been forced to return to Yorkshire to look after her ailing mother, leaving the young Jackson under the guardianship of her brother.

[41] See the two biographies of William Gowers: M. Critchley, *Sir William Gowers, 1845–1915: A Biographical Appreciation* (London: Heinemann, 1949), and A. Scott *et al.*, *William Richard Gowers, 1845–1915: Exploring the Victorian Brain: A Biography* (Oxford University Press, 2012).

[42] A copy of his illustrated diaries and examples of his draughtsmanship are to be found in the Queen Square archives.

outcomes of 500 patients seen during 1870. This industry was soon rewarded by appointment as honorary assistant physician (1872), following the resignation of Charles Elam. Nevertheless, Gowers was warned by Burford Rawlings that such rapid promotion would not give him precedence should a vacancy become available on the consultant staff as full physician in the foreseeable future. However, Burford Rawlings later underlined the importance of Gowers' appointment:

> Lacking proper channels for its dissemination much of the valuable knowledge obtained in the wards and out-patients rooms was running to waste, and the suggestion of the medical authorities that a registrar should be appointed was at once agreed to. The creation of this office was noteworthy. It was the first step towards investing the hospital with the great reputation as a teacher it long since attained, and the historical importance of the event was enhanced by the appointment to the post of Dr W.R. Gowers who has delighted to call himself a child of the hospital and whose active association with it has ceased only recently.[43]

At first, Gowers' responsibilities at the National Hospital were only for outpatients. The facilities were cramped, shared with a colleague, and ill-equipped. Gowers had an exceptional eye for detail and his use of shorthand to record clinical details rapidly and accurately gave him an edge over the other younger physicians.[44] Gowers argued that there was no evidence for use of shorthand damaging retentive memory and he enunciated his own *modus operandi*: 'in the present state of my ignorance it seems more useful to gather facts than formulate hypotheses'. Addressing the Society of Medical Phonographers as their president on 'The art of writing in relation to medical and scientific work', Gowers emphasised the absolute necessity for written records in science, extolling the simplicity of shorthand, which he claimed to be three times quicker and three times less difficult technically than longhand and therefore ideal for the rapid recording of transitory phenomena. He explained that longhand requires five different hand movements to symbolise each element of speech, the sounds of which have traditionally been presented as symbols that had undergone no alteration since the days of Caxton; and that shorthand can be used as final copy, and even transcribed with accuracy by the typewriter. Gowers expressed his enthusiasm: 'If a man habitually observes more fully, more precisely and more carefully he must become a better observer, able to perceive more accurately, more minutely more adequately and to attain precision more readily. This influence, moreover, whatever its degree must be progressive. We might take as our motto the words "writing maketh an exact man".'[45]

The enthusiasm for shorthand did not wane. Much later, his student Ernest Jones wrote:

> Gowers had a peculiar personality and was reported to suffer from attacks of megalomania; a priceless saying attributed – *ben trovato* – to him in one of these was that every day he conceived an infinite number of original ideas, any one of which would make the reputation of an infinite number of neurologists. But his real interest appeared to be in Pitman's phonographic system, a knowledge of which, so he seemed to think, would be the greatest imaginable asset to the medical profession; to this end he founded, edited, and largely wrote a medical periodical in Pitman's shorthand. At one time he induced Lord Lister and a few other enthusiasts to petition the General Medical Council to include a knowledge of Pitman as a compulsory subject in the entrance examination to the medical profession, but needless to say the deputation met with no success. When I was interviewed by him on the occasion of appointment at the National Hospital he somehow became aware of my acquaintance with the system, probably through seeing me read his periodical in the waiting room, and at once adopted such an intelligent person as a protégé; of course, all our correspondence had to be conducted in shorthand.[46]

---

[43] B. Burford Rawlings, *A Hospital in the Making* (London: Sir Isaac Pitman and Sons, 1913).

[44] Gowers had learned the art of shorthand during his time in Coggeshall and it became his 'secret weapon'. In 1894, he published two issues of a small shorthand periodical, the *Phonographic Record of Clinical Teaching*, with contributions from William Osler and Marcus Gunn, and later that year formed the Society of Medical Phonographers. Some of his original research and lectures were only published in the Society's journal, the *Phonographic Record of Clinical Teaching and Medical Science*. Throughout his life, Gowers maintained belief in the merits of using shorthand in medical research and insisted his juniors learn the technique.

[45] W. R. Gowers, 'The Inaugural Address on the Art of Writing in Relation to Medical and Scientific Work: Delivered Before the Society of Medical Phonographers', *British Medical Journal* 2 (1895): 817–19.

[46] E. Jones, *Free Associations: Memories of a Psycho-analyst* (New York: Basic Books, 1959).

Medicine for Gowers was a science that must be applied to human need, and for which the only sound method was clinical experience. He realised that long hours spent working alone in outpatients would offer a new materialist doctrine of the nerves. In his daily work, he searched for commonalities and exceptions that allowed deductions about where and why a particular area of the nervous system had become dysfunctional. After the patient's death, his enquiry would continue through pathological examination of the brain and spinal cord. In his lectures to the medical students at University College, he continually emphasised the importance of the natural sciences as the foundation of medicine:

> You cannot properly understand the higher forms of organic life without some knowledge of the lower, in which the problems are simpler and can be more readily comprehended, even if they cannot be solved. Moreover the very lowest forms of life have been lately found to have the closest connexion with our work. Nature is always surprising us by the union of extremes.[47]

More than 2,000 new cases were then being seen each year at the National, including a large number of children. Gowers felt that they provided information that few of his colleagues took the time to observe. His photographic memory, methodical system of case recording and openness to the use of new instruments for diagnosis contributed in no small way to his growing reputation as an exceptional clinician.

Although not yet affiliated to the University of London, the Board of Management recognised the importance of teaching at Queen Square and, from 1879, encouraged formal Thursday afternoon lectures. Gowers may also have started the long tradition of outpatient postgraduate teaching at the National Hospital. He brought enthusiastic medical students from University College to see cases in outpatients. Holmes relates how one of his patients, an aged doctor, had passed by Queen Square as a young man and was invited into the outpatient room by Gowers who discussed enthusiastically the symptoms of a case he had just seen; on leaving, Gowers invited the young man to come again and bring some colleagues.[48]

Word spread that those who attended Gowers' outpatient teaching would not be disappointed and his small room was soon crowded with doctors. Gowers taught without prior knowledge of the case. Although often aware of the diagnosis as soon as the patient entered the room, he disliked taking shortcuts in his evaluation of cases. He would start by asking the patient to relate the story of their illness, then clarify relevant points, and finally examine the patient. The history gave him the aetiology while the examination confirmed the suspected site of damage. He would then discuss the differential diagnosis and prognosis in what came over to his attentive audience as a sophisticated example of how to think aloud. His substantial and rapidly acquired clinical experience, combined with knowledge of the existing literature, allowed him to detect inconsistencies and appreciate their significance.

Forensic medicine was another emerging science in the late nineteenth century. As with neurology, this discipline sought to derive meaning from narrative, respected logic, and depended on powers of observation and deduction. The painstaking assembly of seemingly disconnected clues that often appeared insignificant to the lay person were decoded and used to 'solve the crime' and make a diagnosis. It is possible that, during his time working as an eye specialist, or later on his trips to the meeting rooms of the Spiritualist Alliance at 5 Queen Square, Sir Arthur Conan Doyle, a physician who wrote his thesis on syphilis of the nervous system, attended some of Gowers' teaching sessions. Many of Gowers' aphorisms transmitted to his pupils could have been used with advantage by detectives:

> Certain symptoms are very frequent in a given disease. Their presence may make that disease certain. But their absence does not prove that the disease does not exist. Neglect of this rule is one of the most fertile sources of error ... Whenever you find yourself in the presence of a case that is not at once and completely familiar to you in all its details, forget for the time all your types and all your names. Deal with the case as one that has never been seen before, and work it out as a new problem. Observe each symptom and consider its significance, then put all the symptoms together and consider their meaning.[49]

---

[47] W. R. Gowers, *Lectures on the Diagnosis of Diseases of the Brain. Delivered at University College Hospital* (London: J. & A. Churchill, 1885).

[48] G. S. Holmes, 'Sir William Gowers at the National Hospital', *British Medical Journal* **2** (1951): 1397.

[49] See W. R. Gowers, 'General Principles of the Diagnosis of the Diseases of the Nervous System', *Lancet* **139** (1892): 403–5.

As the attendance increased, Gowers was using the operating room in the Powis pavilion which doubled up as a clinical theatre. Between 1887 and 1896, 2,500 students and practitioners had attended clinical demonstrations given to around ten attendees on several days each week. With the appointment of Charles Beevor as the first dean of the newly formed medical school, the university agreed that the National Hospital could formally take fifth-year medical students from University College Hospital for elective clerkships. Qualified doctors might expect to see more neurology in a week at Queen Square than in a decade of hospital and private practice. As the National Hospital became recognised as one of the best places in the world for clinical instruction in the diagnosis and treatment of nervous diseases, Gowers emerged as its most illustrious instructor. Command of English and clarity of thought enriched his lectures. A measured but slightly harsh and high-pitched voice, and skill in making the occasional well-timed dramatic point, commanded the attention of his audience. Many of his lectures appeared in the weekly journals (and as published volumes); although now rarely read, their message has been transmitted by word of mouth through subsequent generations of neurologists and, silently, they still inform the neurological consultation.

Gowers' advice was pragmatic, aiming to reflect experience and observation rather than concept or theory:

> When I say you cannot have too much of diagnostic method I mean that the power you will hereafter need, the power of discerning the nature of disease, can only be gained by constant exercise … It is only by thoughtful perception of the reasoning, which varies in detail in every case that you can gain the ability to deal in like manner with cases that are unfamiliar … I need hardly remind you that between what we term 'theory' and 'fact' the transition is gradual; that much of which we regard as fact is only fact to our thought. Observation alone is certain observation pure and simple.[50]

He emphasised the need to apply judgement and common sense in the face of uncertainty and, if necessary, to think again.

> We must always remember it is the balance of evidence that determines diagnosis. The sciences concerned with disease deal largely with probabilities, almost wholly so in internal medicine. The probability varies in degree but usually falls far short of certainty. We must learn to take probability as our guide. We have to act. To act we must decide, and to decide we must weigh the evidence, and deal with the probable as if it were certain … and I would urge you to cultivate the habit of viewing a chronic case afresh from time to time; ignore what you have thought of it; put yourself in the face of a fresh observer and try and see if it thus bears a fresh aspect.[51]

And in this same lecture, Gowers sought to enthuse his listeners, remind students that there is more to the practice of neurology than accurate diagnosis, and stress the pastoral aspects of medicine:

> Gentlemen: many of those present, I doubt not, have just effected the transition to the Hospital, which constitutes the mid-point of the student's career. Others see, not far away, the gate of exit, beyond which lies an unknown future. To those who are beginning their clinical work and to those who are near its end, the case I have chosen as my subject presents much that should instruct and also much that can hardly fail to interest. It presents pathological features of great rarity and yet sufficiently related to that which is common to be useful. It constitutes moreover, a good example of diagnostic method and of this you cannot have too much. It also shows how important and direct is the relation to the sciences some of you have just mastered to the work on which you are now entered … Strive to acquire the habit of entering into the feelings of the sick, and into their modes of thought, to such a degree as to ensure considerate tenderness in dealing with them. Never forget that a 'patient' means one who suffers and that you come in contact with the tenderest parts of human nature.

To Gowers, diagnosis was a matter of probability based on rational deduction that occasionally, as a result of accurate observation, became a certainty. Wherever inference was involved, there was a corridor of uncertainty. However, Gowers knew that he was not infallible:

> Gentlemen: It is always pleasant to be right, but it is generally a much more useful thing to be wrong. If you are right, all that you do, as a rule, is to confirm your previous opinion, your previous habits of

---

[50] W. R. S. Gowers, *The Dynamics of Life. An address*, delivered before the Medical Society of Manchester. October 3rd 1894. (London: J. & A. Churchill, 1894).

[51] W. R. Gowers, 'A Clinical Lecture on a Metastatic Mystery', *Lancet* **166** (1905): 1593–6.

reasoning and your previous self-esteem. But if you are wrong you generally gain in knowledge and gain perception of the way in which your method of diagnosis needs improvement, and the influence on self-esteem is not likely to do you harm.[52]

Parallels can be drawn here between Jean-Martin Charcot and Gowers, in that both were outstanding teachers of neurology. However, there were differences: Charcot played to an audience whereas Gowers instructed his class.

Gowers was finally given admission rights to the hospital (1883), allowing him to admit patients without being obliged to have them under the care of Jackson. Less time was spent demonstrating cases in outpatients and Gowers concentrated on inpatient care and his large private practice. He attended his cases at least three times each week on Chandler, Bentinck and Albany wards – more frequently than many of his contemporaries. Seated at the bedside and dressed in his long frock coat, Gowers would read carefully the case notes prepared by his assistant. He would then go over points of uncertainty in the history, making notes in shorthand. His own examination, full and detailed but without the obsessional slowness of some others, followed. He noted the condition of the optic discs, reactions of the pupils, and the various cutaneous and tendon reflexes. He tested power by assessing voluntary movement of individual muscles, sometimes with the help of Erb's electrical stimulation. Simple tests such as drawing a straight line on a piece of paper, and finger–nose testing, were used to assess coordination. Light touch was assessed with the feather of a quill pen; and the other end used for pain. Test-tubes containing warm and cold water allowed him to evaluate temperature sensation. Sieveking's aesthesiometer, consisting of a graduated bar with two points, one moveable and the other fixed, was used for two-point discrimination. Weights were employed to assess what was known as muscular sense. A tug on the pubic hair was the recognised technique to expose hysterical coma. Investigations consisted of a few blood tests and examination of the urine. This was supplemented (from 1890) by lumbar puncture to obtain cerebrospinal fluid, but Gowers was said not to be an enthusiast for this procedure.[53]

He remained aware of deficiencies in the clinical investigation of nervous disease and embraced technical advances that would help to improve diagnostic accuracy. Like Jackson, he became a skilled opthalmoscopist. He also adapted the Duchenne–Charrière dynamometer for recording grip strength, and invented a magnifying lens which, like his other gadgets, was produced by the family firm of Hawksleys. However, Gowers always emphasised that these ancillary tools were no replacement for systematic clinical methods.

We get a flavour of Gowers' methods from case notes in the bound archival volumes. Some are in Gowers' handwriting, with occasional shorthand, detailed and with comments on histories clerked by his house physician. A few are illustrated: a 22-year-old female outpatient complained of headaches and inability to walk; Gowers diagnosed a cerebellar tumour; the patient died and the notes show Gowers' own drawings at autopsy of an upper mid-brain tumour pressing on the left side of the cerebellum. Further insights into his bedside technique can be gleaned from *The Border-land of Epilepsy* (1907):

> For many years I have kept a special list of all cases which seemed to be in the borderland of epilepsy – near it, but not of it. Many were so placed by their features and character; others because they had given rise to an erroneous diagnosis. When these cases were collected and classified, their comparison and study revealed a large number of unfamiliar facts and many instructive lessons, throwing light on the nature of the affections, on their relation to epilepsy, and on questions of practical diagnosis ... For the most part, they will be found to have a wider importance than their mere relation to epilepsy would suggest.

Here, Gowers records the histories of patients with episodic disorders such as migraine, fainting, vertigo and parasomnias, as well as epilepsy, and then attempts to answer the questions their stories pose

---

[52] W. R. Gowers, 'A Post-graduate Lecture on Mistaken Diagnosis: Delivered in the National Hospital for the Paralysed and Epileptic', *British Medical Journal* **2** (1894): 1–3.
[53] The first lumbar puncture was performed in 1889 by Dr Walter Essex Wynter, then a registrar at the Middlesex

Hospital. He reported the technique as a treatment of four children with advanced tuberculous meningitis and raised intracranial pressure – all died. His technique was to make a small incision at the level of the second vertebra near the midline and cut down through the intervertebral space to reach the dura, through which he introduced a Southey's tube to which a rubber cannula was attached. Gowers' opposition to the procedure prevented its introduction into clinical practice in other London hospitals. After Gowers' retirement, lumbar puncture became routine at Queen Square and proved particularly helpful in cases of meningitis and suspected active neurosyphilis.

in his own mind. For example, he concludes that although people frequently lose consciousness at the sight of blood, they never do so if it is merely portrayed.

By 1887, Gowers had collected more than 20,000 shorthand notes recorded from the study of nearly 5,000 patients. These were transcribed and used to derive descriptive statistics, which provided him with evidence on which to support or disprove observations made by himself and others in individual cases. Later in his career, when a clinical point or an unusual sign attracted his attention, he would check details in the *Manual of Diseases of the Nervous System*. If there was something new of note, he would then produce his small black pocket book and jot down a shorthand memorandum, amplified and indexed for later reference when he got home to Queen Anne Street.

Gowers was aware of the need for emergency surgery in cases of headache due to raised intracranial pressure, the importance of diagnosing 'optic neuritis' by ophthalmoscopy, and the relevance of focal signs in localising the site of lesions. In 1887, Gowers attended Captain G, who had already sought treatment in Shanghai, Aix-les-Bains and Constantinople for chronic intercostal neuralgia, unresponsive even to morphia. By the time he saw Gowers, he had asymmetrical weakness of the legs, a distended bladder and complete sensory loss below the sternum. Gowers diagnosed a slowly growing extramedullary tumour at mid-thoracic level and asked Victor Horsley to perform the famous first procedure to remove a spinal tumour (described more fully in our account of Horsley). Gowers' letters to Horsley give some indication of their close working relationship. When asking Horsley's opinion on surgery, Gowers was always cautious in stating the likely precision of his localisation. He would visit Horsley at home, and write and telegram his colleague asking him to operate on his ward cases, expressing impatience if Horsley did not respond promptly. Generally, their exchanges were rather formal and always polite.

> I consider it is for a physician to ask a surgeon as a last resort and for the surgeon then to ask the physician for his opinion as to doubtful points both relating to the question of an operation being performed – ie merely information to help him in forming an opinion, not to determine it, and perhaps also as to what.

If in this last the case comes up I have an idea but I would rather let it come after yours is formed.[54]

During his apprenticeship, Gowers had been expected to roll pills, prepare unctions and mix potions in Winchester bottles. These menial chores had not prevented an interest in the use of medicines and, in 1878, he applied unsuccessfully for the professorship of materia medica at University College. Gowers wrote several papers on medical therapeutics and used bromides, arsenic, belladonna, eserine, chloroform, opium, chloral and paraldehyde in his everyday practice. In common with Russell Reynolds, Gowers was also a strong advocate of Indian hemp for several nervous disorders. He used a cocktail of compounds that included nitroglycerine in alcohol, which later became known as Gowers' mixture, to treat headaches. He advocated borax for epilepsy and aluminium for locomotor ataxia: for pseudoseizures, Gowers recommended apomorphine, and he treated paralysis agitans with opium and cocaine, but considered these to be of little benefit. He also advocated sulphur and needle baths, ice bags to the spine, galvanic and faradic currents, and counter-irritation. But he was not above self-doubt and the need for evidence of efficacy in using these potions:

> Strive by every method you can think of to gain the utmost certainty attainable, in whatever it may be, whether the diagnosis of a disease or the action of a drug; or, at least, relentlessly expose, and candidly admit to yourselves, the degree of uncertainty.[55]

These personal observations allowed Gowers to be amongst the first to describe many neurological diseases, including ataxic paraplegia, Schilder's disease, vasovagal syncope, paramyoclonus multiplex, musicogenic epilepsy and distal myopathy. He also described the myasthenic smile, palatal tremor, sleep paralysis and fixation spasm. He studied his own severe lumbago and became very interested in a related cause of back pain, which he termed fibrositis, occurring in 'ladies of blameless habits and abstemious clergymen'. The patients were exhausted, unable to sleep and with pain so bad 'it would make a strong man cry out'. He considered manipulation of the painful areas and the use of cocaine rather than the

[54] J. B. Lyons, 'Correspondence Between Sir William Gowers and Sir Victor Horsley', *Medical History* 9 (1965): 260–7.
[55] W. R. Gowers. 'Introductory Lecture Delivered at University College London', *Lancet* 123 (1884): 582–6.

newly synthesised aspirin as most likely to provide relief.

Gowers was elected professor of medicine at University College Hospital (1888) but resigned a year later to devote the rest of his working life to teaching and the practice of neurology at Queen Square. Although his medical focus narrowed, loyalty to University College, which had accepted him for tuition at a time when Oxford and Cambridge were barred, never dimmed; and Gowers continued to teach at University College London. Education of the young was a responsibility he took seriously and one that he did not neglect even after his reputation soared. And Gowers was loyal to the hospital that had taught him medicine and nurtured his early postgraduate training, taking the rather personal view:

> Of your choice of place of study I need say little. For more than half a century UCH has shown other schools how medicine should be taught. Almost every step in medical education has first been taken by her. Thanks to her example she now has many rivals but remains surpassed by none and equalled by few, whether the test of comparison be that of method or quality of results. No department of science in which there is so much imperfect observation, hasty generalisation and fallacious reasoning than there is in medicine.[56]

Increasingly, his teaching focused on two or three formal lectures each term given to packed and increasingly sophisticated audiences. These were interactive. In speaking on tabes dorsalis (at the National Hospital, 1905), Gowers began by emphasising how little was known about the mechanisms of nerve damage in that disease. He then opened the presentation up to the assembled audience by asking their opinion on the presence of in-coordination of the legs and the absent knee jerks. When asked whether they believed that locomotor ataxia was a disease of the spinal cord, about half put their hands up in the affirmative while the rest vacillated. Gowers attributed this hesitation to the assumption that they feared a trap had been laid but did compliment the more reticent students on their wisdom in hesitating.[57]

Gowers also encapsulated his clinical wisdom more formally. His Gulstonian lectures at the Royal College of Physicians on epilepsy (1882) were based on 1,400 patients seen personally at the National Hospital; and he drew on cases from the hospital in his Lettsomian lecture on syphilis and the nervous system (1889), the Bradshaw lecture on the subjective sensations of sight and sound (1896) and the Hughlings Jackson lecture on special sense discharges from organic disease (1909). For these prestigious occasions, careful preparation was required and, once the topic was chosen, Gowers would write out the text in full, then revise and polish it for later publication. He never read from notes but memorised the content and, like great political orators, gave the impression of effortless improvisation.

Gowers had an astonishing publication record but, as Holmes observed, this did not spring from a compulsion to write but from the desire to communicate his considered opinions in the hope of advancing medical knowledge. He published mainly in the *Lancet*, *British Medical Journal, Medical Times and Gazette*, *Medico-Chirurgical Transactions, Transactions of the Clinical Society, Transactions of the Pathological Society, The Clinical Journal* and, with a few papers, in *Nature* and the *Proceedings of the Royal Society* and *Review of Neurological Psychology*.[58] He also published many papers in shorthand in the *Phonographic Record of Clinical Teaching* and *Medical Science,* and was a frequent correspondent with the editors of the *Lancet* and *British Medical Journal*. Despite his enthusiasm for writing up new findings, Gowers cautioned one of his house physicians on the pitfalls of publishing isolated case reports: 'It is a mistake to publish single cases. Far better to work up single points or publish … comparatively. Nothing pays except that which gives some new suggestion. The great thing is to create a feeling in the reader … "I must note anything else this man says."'[59]

---

[56] Foster Kennedy, Sir William Richard Gowers, in *The Founders of Neurology,* ed. Webb Haymaker (Springfield: Charles C. Thomas, 1953), pp. 292–5.

[57] W. R. Gowers, 'A Lecture on the Nature of Tabes: Delivered at the National Hospital for the Paralysed and Epileptic', *British Medical Journal* 1 (January 7 1905): **i:** 57–61.

[58] After publishing in the first few volumes, Gowers did not publish again in *Brain* for 20 years as a result of his dislike for Armand de Watteville (see Chapter 4). With a new editor in place, he finally agreed for his Hughlings Jackson lecture to be published in *Brain*. This shunning of *Brain* emphasises the impression that Gowers was not a man to accept criticism graciously, especially if it came from a loathed source.

[59] Note to a house physician, cited in Macdonald Critchley, *Sir William Gowers 1845–1915: A Biographical Appreciation* (London: William Heinemann, 1949).

The written work reflects Gowers' insight that 'words have a strong tendency to cause opacity if they be numerous', and contrasts sharply with Jackson's discursive style. To the modern reader, his writing is a paragon of clarity, as if he has directly transcribed his thoughts on to the page in an economical but enjoyable style. When he has nothing more of interest or importance to say, he stops, without hyperbole or speculative discussion.

Despite Gowers' pre-eminence in the history of British neurology, few eponyms survive that bear his name. 'Gowers' sign' is seen in children with proximal weakness in the legs. To Gowers, it seemed as if, on trying to get up from the floor, boys with Duchenne muscular dystrophy use their arms to climb their own thighs and trunk. Gowers described a bundle of nerve fibres in the spinal cord, the ventral spinocerebellar tract, which Bechterew later named 'Gowers tract'. Not by nature an individual in search of self–aggrandisement or lasting posterity, Gowers disliked eponyms.

> There are very few observations in medicine regarding which it is not obvious that they would speedily have been made by someone other than the actual observer; that it is very much of an accident that they were made by certain individuals. Scientific nomenclature should be itself scientific, not founded upon accidents. However anxious we may be to honour individuals, we have no right to do so at the expense of the convenience of all future generations of learners.[60]

Gowers had lectured to the Medical Society of Wolverhampton (October 1879) on the spinal cord, and his name is still remembered in dermatological practice for his description of a skin lesion seen in a young woman, also from Wolverhampton, whom he had first seen in 1885 with patches of morphoea and the disappearance of subcutaneous tissue on her face, shoulder and back. Following the presentation of a second case at the Clinical Society by Dr Harry Campbell (1902), and with the help of his house officer, Stanley Barnes, Gowers traced and contacted the first patient, writing up the condition still known as local panatrophy of Gowers (1903).

More important than these accreditations are his seminal contributions to the diagnostic process. He introduced the concept of upper and lower motor neurone lesions, a robust synecdoche that has stood the test of time and the starting point for determining broad classification of neurological disease. He realised early that the lower motor neurone makes the ultimate connection with muscle and wrote in the first edition of his *Manual of Diseases of the Nervous System*:

> The whole motor path, from the cortex of the brain to the muscles ... is composed of two segments, an upper and a lower. Each consists of a ganglion cell above, a nerve fibre, and the terminal ramification of the latter. The upper cerebrospinal segment consists of the cortical ganglion and its dendrons and the "pyramidal" axon which proceeds from the cell, passes through the brain and cord, and ends in the grey substance by division and terminal interlacement with several nerve-cells. The lower "spino-muscular" neuron consists of the spinal motor cell with its dendrons and the axon proceeding from it, which passes through the anterior root and nerve-trunk to the muscle. where it divides and ramifies on the muscular fibre ... It will be found that this conception of the motor path conduces to clearer ideas of many phenomena of disease.

Gowers presented experimental work on tendon reflexes and ankle clonus to the Medical and Chirurgical Society of London (1879). He had used a writing pen and revolving carbon drum attached to the patient's foot to record the movement resulting from a hammer tap on the knee. This allowed Gowers to determine that the latency between contact of the hammer with the patellar tendon and the ensuing quadriceps contraction ranged between 0.09 and 0.15 seconds; and this delay supported his contention that the knee jerk is a spinal reflex. The fifth volunteer in this research was a 44-year-old man admitted to Queen Square with a progressive history of severe asymmetrical paraparesis that had temporarily confined him to a chair. By the time of admission, he had begun to recover and could walk. Gowers noted that the left leg required 2 centimetres more of the secondary coil of Stöhrer's large battery to induce faradisation and contracted to two cells of the voltaic battery less than the right. There was left ankle clonus, a marked cutaneous reflex of the sole, a brisk right patellar reflex and an absent left patellar reflex. In a prescient observation that seems to predate current thoughts relating to spinal pattern generators, Gowers comments: 'These facts suggest that a reflex relation between muscular tension and contraction may play an important role in the mechanism by which often-repeated movements are co-ordinated.'[61]

---

[60] W. R. Gowers, *The Diagnosis of Diseases of the Spinal Cord* (London: Churchill, 1880).

[61] W. R. Gowers, 'A Study of the So-called Tendon-Reflex Phemomena', *Medico-Chirurgical Transactions* **62** (1879): 269–305.

It was these physiological studies, and work on sphincter innervation and eye movements, that led to his election as FRS (1887), at a time when individuals were increasingly admitted on the basis of their scientific contributions.

In 1896, the Board of Management at the National Hospital established a laboratory for microscopy. Gowers had attended Ramon y Cajal's Croonian lecture at the Royal Society (1895) and was an enthusiastic convert to what he considered the greatest discovery of his time, and one that would foster the 'new neurology' based on histological study of the brain using silver stains. Cajal's anatomical findings had confirmed that the brain is made up of a complex network of nerve cells whose processes are separated from each other by small gaps, named 'synapses' by Sherrington.

Gowers introduced the concept of loss of neuronal vitality as a cause for many cryptic neurological disorders (1902), apologising for coining a new term, 'abiotrophy', to describe this process, which he distinguished from the destructive proliferation of glial tissue with resultant fibrosis, and likened to the development of grey hair. He singled out paralysis agitans (Parkinson's disease) as an example of late-onset abiotrophy in which certain structures have an essential defect of vital endurance leading to slow but inexorable failure of function. This mechanism explained why no consistent signature of the disease could be found at postmortem. The study of heredity was still in its infancy but Gowers was aware of the constitutional susceptibility and the neurological trait in various disorders he had described as early-onset abiotrophies, such as Huntington's disease and the spinocerebellar ataxias.

Gowers had a slight physique and somewhat awkward comportment but was described as dignified and distinguished in appearance, with prematurely grey hair worn long and a distinctive square beard. His glacial blue eyes seemed to fix and then penetrate the mind of those with whom he came into contact. For Foster Kennedy, 'No picture of Gowers could be appreciated without at the same time having in the mind's eye his look of being a combination of one of the Wise Men of the East and the Ancient Mariner, and hearing too his harsh loud staccato voice speaking in sardonic humorous invective against the errors of the world.'

Even when incapacitated by illness in later life he was never idle, continuing to see patients and teach and stand up for his beliefs. Although his rigour and intellectual honesty were understood, some found him unapproachable, intolerant and fastidious. In

Free Associations: Memories of a Psychoanalyst (1959), Ernest Jones describes how Gowers suggested that Jones should carry out research on hemiplegic stroke in order to document the relative frequency of various accompanying clinical features that might help physicians make the distinction between cerebral haemorrhage and thrombosis. Gowers instructed him first to read the entire English and French literature on the subject, and then go through the casebooks of University College Hospital from its foundation (1834) and ascertain yet more cases by visiting the local borough infirmaries. This piece of research led Jones to comment how ignorant in general the medical profession was at the time on the theory of probability and the use of statistics; but it turned him from neurology to psychoanalysis. That Gowers had an acerbic sense of humour is illustrated by his son Ernest, recalling an American postgraduate student who spent a three-month elective period at the National Hospital. When the visitor left for a month of further study in Vienna, he told Gowers that he planned to study disseminated sclerosis. Gowers responded that this topic was of personal interest to him as he had been studying it for 35 years, and he would be grateful if the young man would send him a postcard with news of all he had discovered!

In later years, Gowers was said to have had a rather dogmatic style of lecturing and was intolerant of comment from the floor during his demonstrations, particularly if it came from people for whom he had little respect. He also felt uncomfortable with female doctors and disliked their presence on his ward rounds. Here he differed from Jackson, but not for almost 100 years was a woman finally appointed as a consultant neurologist at Queen Square. Those who knew Gowers considered his remote exterior to be a façade, concealing sensitivity and kindness and used to protect him from the intrusion of lesser minds.

Gowers and his wife both developed pneumonia in 1914: Lady Gowers soon died but Sir William lingered in failing health until 4 May 1915. His obituary in *The Times* (5 May 1915) described a famous nerve specialist praised for the way in which pathological anatomy and clinical symptomatology were brought into relation and laid down as the essential foundations of neurological practice. His many writings were all 'merely excrescences of the great work' the *Manual of Diseases of the Nervous System*, which Gowers constantly reconstructed and updated with case material based on new scientific discoveries, which made the book ever fresh and a pleasure for neurologists to read. Sir William Osler described Gowers as 'that brilliant ornament of British Neurology', but eventually he became an institution and arguably the greatest ever British neurologist. In November 1956, Sir Francis Walshe gave the first Gowers memorial lecture at Queen Square on 'The nature and dimensions of nosography in modern medicine'. The man and his hospital, which appointed him as its first medical registrar, and to which he devoted 40 extraordinarily productive years, were praised: 'And if, as we rightly do, we look upon Gowers' superb clinical writings as his monument, they are also the monument of the special hospital in which he laboured, and without which he could never have attained the rich achievement by which his name will live wherever neurological medicine is studied.'[62]

Sir Victor Alexander Haden Horsley

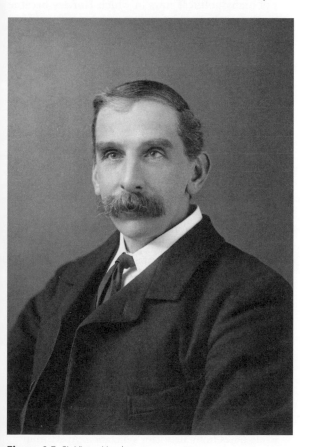

Figure 4.5 Sir Victor Horsley.

Surgeon, scientist, politician, social campaigner and soldier, Sir Victor Horsley was the epitome of a great Victorian – a man of extraordinary energy, versatility and intellectual brilliance. When he died in 1916, serving his country, the National Hospital lost one of its greatest figures; and the world lost its most significant founder of neurosurgery.

Horsley was born (14 April 1857) into a wealthy and talented family. His father John Callcott Horsley was a well-known Royal Academician,[63] Isambard Brunel was an uncle by marriage, and his godmother was Queen Victoria, who asked that the infant Horsley be named after her. Horsley studied anatomy and physiology at University College London, and then medicine.[64] Before qualification, he clerked at University College Hospital for Bastian, providing two drawings for Bastian's book *The Brain as an Organ of Mind* (1880), and illustrations for a paper in *Brain* published whilst he was a student, jointly with Bastian, entitled 'Arrest of Development in the Left Upper Limb, in Association with an Extremely Small Right Ascending Parietal Convolution' (1880). When he qualified in 1881, the 24-year-old Dr Horsley seemed set for an outstanding career, and he did not disappoint. His extraordinary talent was recognised early by his teachers, notably Marcus Beck, who 'held the firm conviction that Horsley was a genius and would have a brilliant future'.

Horsley was appointed surgical registrar at UCH (1882–4), professor-superintendent to the Brown Institution (1884–90), professor of pathology (1887–96) and of clinical surgery (1899–1902) at University College London, and elected FRS (1886)

---

[63] John Callcott Horsley RA was a famous painter whose works include frescos in the House of Lords. As rector of the Royal Academy, he protested against the fashion for nude painting and was nicknamed J C(lothes) Horsley (a pun on the clothes horse). He was a remarkable innovator and it was he who designed the first Christmas card and also the Horsley envelope, a pre-paid envelope which was the precursor of the postage stamp.

[64] Although a scientist by training and inclination, Horsley was also deeply interested in the arts, unsurprisingly in view of his family traditions, and was himself a skilful draughtsman. At University College, he obtained first-class passes in anatomy and physiology and was awarded the gold medal for anatomy and a university scholarship. His was a remarkable year at the medical school, for in his class were a number of brilliant students, who remained his close friends, including Francis Gotch, who married Horsley's sister; Frederick Mott; Bilton Pollard; Dawson Williams; C. J. Bond; and C. E. Beevor.

---

[62] F. Walshe, 'The Nature and Dimensions of Nosography in Modern Medicine', *Lancet* **271** (1956): 1059–63.

at the age of 29, where he delivered the Croonian lecture (1891) and received the Royal Medal (1894). He served as Fullerian professor at the Royal Institution (1891–3) and was knighted in 1902 for services with the Mediterranean Expeditionary Force. He married Eldred Bramwell, the daughter of Sir Frederick Bramwell, in 1887 and they had three children, Siward, Oswald and Pamela. Horsley was a devoted family man who wrote tender, loving and sensitive letters to his wife and family, and delighted in family holidays and gatherings. He died in 1916 whilst serving with the British Army in Mesopotamia.[65] A triennial memorial lecture in his name was first given by his teacher and colleague Edward Sharpey-Schäfer in October 1923, on the relationship of physiology and surgery.[66]

Horsley made his first important contributions to medical science at the Brown Institute, to which he was appointed through the patronage of Schäfer and Burdon Sanderson. Apart from studies on cerebral localisation – of which, more later – Horsley discovered that myxoedema can be caused by thyroid excision, and treated by thyroid extract. He recommended the successful transplantation of sheep thyroid in patients with myxoedema; his contribution seems to us no less important than that of his friend and colleague Emil Theodore Kocher, who later won the

Nobel Prize for similar findings. Horsley studied rabies, adding to scientific understanding of the disease and persuading government to take action to limit its effects. He identified and studied an outbreak of the disease amongst the deer in Richmond Park (1886/7), and in other animals brought to the Brown Institution, and became an outspoken advocate of moves to prevent the spread of the disease in Britain. As a result, Horsley was appointed secretary to a government commission to study anti-rabies vaccine (1886), and worked closely with Pasteur on inoculation. Later he proposed that the government should muzzle all dogs and introduce quarantine for animals imported to Britain (1889), a step that proved highly effective. Inevitably, Horsley clashed violently with the Dog Owner Protection Association and the anti-vivisectionists who upheld that rabies could 'come of itself'; and these exchanges proved to be merely the first of many political rows in which Horsley became embroiled and in which he responded with typical resolve.

Horsley's work on cerebral localisation is one of the landmarks of nineteenth-century neuroscience. He studied various species, including Barbary apes and the orangutan. It is recorded by Paget that, on one occasion, Horsley gave up a morning consultation to visit London Zoo to dissect the brain of a recently deceased walrus. Schäfer recognised Horsley's skills in antiseptic surgery, of which he himself had no experience, and together they embarked on a series of researches at University College on the simian brain, with a view to extending the work of Ferrier and Yeo. They mapped function in 4 mm^2 areas using a very weak current and electrodes placed 2 mm apart. Surgery was carried out with very strict antisepsis, and under anaesthesia with chloroform or ether and morphia, after which the animal was killed and the brain examined. Arthur MacNalty who worked with Horsley described how:

> Sir Victor set aside Thursday afternoons and Saturday mornings for experimental work. He sat at one end of the experimental table, arrayed in a long white coat and wearing a head mirror, which directed reflected light on to the exposed brain of the animal. Opposite him sat the anaesthetist, while I usually wrote notes from Sir Victor's dictation. Apart from these stated hours, at odd moments Sir Victor would appear in the laboratory, often in the early morning, and cut sections for about half an hour. I think the mere mechanical work of using the microtome rested him. At such times he would talk to one on all sorts of

---

[65] Horsley has been the subject of two substantial biographies: J. B. Lyons, *The Citizen Surgeon: A Life of Sir Victor Horsley* (London: Downey, 1966); and S. Paget, *Sir Victor Horsley: A Study of his Life and Work* (London: Constable and Company, 1919), the latter based on access to his family papers provided to the author by Horsley's daughter. There are also several informative biographical articles: E. Sachs, 'Victor Horsley', *Journal of Neurosurgery* **15** (1958): 240–4; G. Jefferson, 'Sir Victor Horsley, 1857–1916, Centenary Lecture', *British Medical Journal* **1** (1957): 903–10; A. MacNulty, 'Sir Victor Horsley: His Life and Work', *British Medical Journal* **1** (1957): 910–16; M. Powell, 'Sir Victor Horsley – an Inspiration', *British Medical Journal* **333** (2006): 1317–19; T.-C. Tim and P. Black, 'Victor Horsley (1857–1915): Pioneer of Neurological Surgery', *Neurosurgery* **50**. 3 (2002): 607–12; W. C. Hanigan, 'Obstinate Valour: The Military Service and Death of Sir Victor Horsley', *British Journal of Neurosurgery* **8** (1994): 279–88; and P. J. Parker, 'In Search of Victor Horsley', *Journal of the Royal Army Medical Corps* **152** (2006): 128–31.
[66] Edward Sharpey-Schäfer had changed his name from Edward Schäfer in 1918 in memory of his eldest son, John Sharpey, who was killed in the war, and also to perpetuate the name of his own teacher, William Sharpey. He was himself an outstanding physiologist, considered the father of endocrinology, and it was he who coined the terms 'endocrine' and 'insulin'.

subjects, and at intervals whistle tunes out of the Gilbert and Sullivan operas.[67]

MacNulty describes Horsley's workshop at 25 Cavendish Square:

The large sky-lighted room at the back of the ground floor was Sir Victor's workshop. It had been built as an anatomical theatre in the days when surgeons held private classes in anatomy, and Horsley said it was taken by RL Stevenson for his description of Dr Jekyll's chemical laboratory in *The strange case of Dr Jekyll and Mr Hyde* with which indeed, it closely corresponded. Here in any spare time Horsley worked with tools, microscope, and camera, dissecting, cutting sections, photographing and developing, making drawings and diagrams ... Shelves lined the walls of the workshop; they were stacked with lecture diagrams, photographs and negatives, lantern slides, trays of microscopical slides, and notes and papers.[68]

Horsley and his colleagues published eight celebrated articles in the *Transactions of the Royal Society*, amounting to 525 pages with 33 pages of plates (1884–91). These papers included studies with Schäfer on functions of the cortex, motor regions in the monkey brain and the internal capsule, and the various movements produced by electrical stimulation of the motor areas. They illustrate Horsley's methods using faradic current at minimal strength and ablating small areas of cortex. Studies of the mesial and lateral surfaces of the cerebral cortex provided the first detailed cortical maps of the central gyri, complemented by functional studies of the occipital and temporal lobes. In agreement with Yeo and Ferrier, but contradicting the work of others, Horsley showed that the prefrontal areas are not 'motor centres' and there is no effect on movement either from stimulation or ablation. In extending Ferrier's work, Horsley recognised that complex movements have large areas of representation and he devised a sophisticated theory of 'primary' and 'secondary' movement. He also described the topographical relationship of fibres in the simian internal capsule. With Burdon-Sanderson and Francis Gotch, Horsley showed that current descends to the spinal cord after excitation of the cerebral cortex with muscular contractions in the lower limb that are first persistent, then rhythmic, corresponding to tonic and clonic contractions and to convulsions.

Many other physicians turned to Horsley for help with their studies. Horsley worked with Beevor at the Brown Institute on a detailed analysis of cerebral localisation and the projection of cerebral neurones to the spinal cord in monkeys. Felix Semon and Horsley carried out work on central motor innervation of the larynx, and found the cortical centre for adduction at the lower end of the ascending frontal convolution in the monkey. Horsley studied the posterior roots and columns of the spinal cord with Mott and Howard Tooth, and the cerebellum with Schäfer, Risien Russell, and R. H. Clarke. Horsley's unsurpassed knowledge of comparative mammalian cerebral anatomy informed his subsequent approach to surgery of the human brain; and the similarity of his system for mapping and cortical stimulation to that now used in neurosurgery makes clear that much of the methodology introduced by Horsley has passed into routine practice.

The work of Horsley and Ferrier was closely related. As colleagues, it is not clear who was the intellectual leader. History favours Ferrier, but the quality of Horsley's work and the care with which his observations were made are so impressive that he possibly had the edge in terms of creativity and discovery. Neither was a crude localisationist and their concepts have a level of sophistication that inspired much of Sherrington's subsequent work. Horsley's own research was always directed towards finding ways of treating human disease, and there can scarcely be a more remarkable example of the translation of experimental into clinical work.

Horsley was always practical in his research. In 1894, whilst a rifle volunteer, he undertook a series of experiments on the physiological and clinical consequences of gunshot wounds to the brain. These were to prove of great importance for neurosurgical treatment of soldiers in the First World War. Horsley modelled the trajectory of bullets using clay, which had the consistency of brain, and then filled the cavity with plaster-of-Paris to create casts.[69] This showed that the explosive effect is directly proportional to the sectional area of the bullet, its velocity and the fluidity of the target

---

[67] A. S. MacNalty, 'Sir Victor Horsley: His Life and Work', *British Medical Journal* **1** (1957): 910–16. Sir Arthur Salusbury MacNalty was a physiologist, public health physician, authority on infectious diseases and endocrine disorders, medical historian and prolific author and editor. He was the eighth Chief Medical Officer of the United Kingdom.

[68] The connection between Stevenson's *Dr Jekyll and Mr Hyde* and Queen Square was twofold: Brown-Séquard inspiring the character and Horsley's laboratory, the setting.

[69] These are held in the museum of the Royal College of Surgeons.

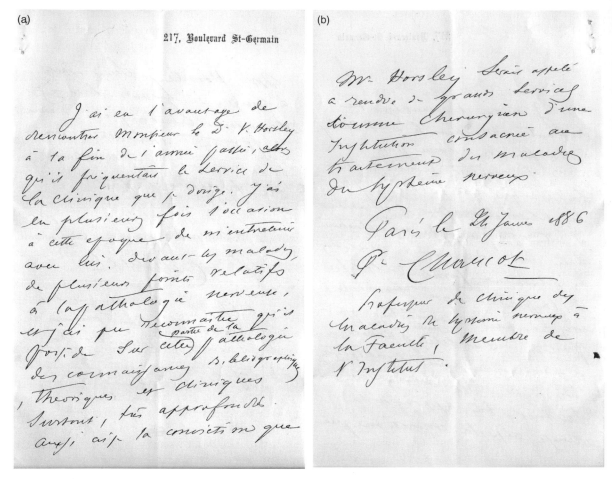

Figure 4.6a,b Jean-Martin Charcot's letter in support for the application of Victor Horsley to join the Queen Square staff, June 1886.

tissue. Horsley demonstrated that the forces of disruption are at an angle to the axis of flight of the bullet and its spin results in a larger aperture for exit than entry of the missile. He discovered that, in anaesthetised animals, death due to gunshot is preceded by a rapid rise in systemic and intracranial pressure and cessation of respiration, rather than cardiac arrest as had been the current orthodoxy. Horsley recognised the problems of brain herniation, which was usually fatal, and for this reason recommended leaving the wound open, to allow decompression. On the basis of his experimental studies, he made recommendations for battlefield resuscitation and management to include complete debridement of the wound and removal of bone fragments even if driven deep into the brain. As he wrote:

> [Sepsis is the result of] incomplete disinfection of the original wound and also to the fatal and detestable

practice of 'leaving head cases alone' which, being the outcome of ignorance, both of the functions of the brain and of the principles of antiseptic surgery, led many surgeons of the old school (some of whom apparently still survive) to leave a patient to steadily die rather than perform the duty of attempting to save him.[70]

The appointment of Horsley as assistant surgeon (1886), with a letter of recommendation from Charcot,[71] marks the beginning of neurosurgery at the National Hospital. Operating on the brain in life

---

[70] S. Paget, *Sir Victor Horsley: A Study of his Life and Work* (London: Constable and Company, 1919).

[71] Sent from 217 Boulevard Saint-Germain, in June 1886. 'Professor Charcot, professor to the clinic of diseases of the nervous system in the Faculty of Medicine and member of the Institute etc.' wrote (translated): 'At the end of last year, I had the advantage of making the acquaintance of Mr V.

had become feasible because of three recent discoveries: the principles of antisepsis pioneered by Lister; the introduction of anaesthesia with chloroform and oro-tracheal intubation by the Scottish surgeons James Simpson and William Macewen, and by Horsley himself; and the translation into clinical practice of the findings from the animal experimentation in cerebral localisation pioneered by Ferrier, Jackson and Horsley.[72] Horsley used the Harcourt regulator to administer chloroform, which he had previously used on animals and in experiments on himself. Vernon Harcourt[73] built a compressed oxygen cylinder according to Horsley's design, so that the chloroform percentage did not exceed 2 per cent. Horsley declined to give ether, which was then in common usage, because of effects on blood pressure, post-operative headache, vomiting and increased blood 'venosity', supposedly causing haemorrhages. This sanction of the use of chloroform by Horsley greatly raised the profile of this form of anaesthesia. The famous photograph of Horsley in his operating theatre (1906), prepared for an address of the combined meeting of the British and Canadian Medical Associations in Toronto, shows the Queen Square anaesthetist Llewelyn Powell administering chloroform, and Horsley on the left, with a bulky gown concealing sterile dressings worn, it is said, as a

prelude to an appendectomy he underwent next day. On his right is Emil Theodore Kocher, and facing him are the young Kinnier Wilson and Carmalt Jones.

Horsley's first intracranial operations were for epilepsy, and these had a profound effect on the subsequent treatment paradigm of this condition.[74] His first patient was a 22-year-old Scotsman, admitted under Jackson, who had sustained head trauma 15 years earlier, causing a depressed fracture of the skull. By 1885, he was having many seizures (2,870 were recorded in the first 13 days in hospital) and was in status epilepticus for several days. The seizures 'occurred in batches, with a well-defined "march" which started in the right leg and spread to involve the right arm and face with turning of the head and eyes to the right'. In discussion with Jackson and Ferrier, Horsley predicted the site of the epileptic focus on the basis of his experimental studies on cortical localisation. He opened the skull and dura over the central cortex of the left hemisphere (25 May 1886), with Jackson and Ferrier present, using scrupulous Listerian antisepsis, and found a highly vascular scar in the exact location predicted to be the cause of the symptoms. Excision of the focus and surrounding brain substance to a depth of just over 2 cm resulted in complete resolution of seizures.

The second operation (26 June 1886) was perhaps even more daring in that there was no depressed fracture to provide ancillary information about localisation. The patient was a 20-year-old man who had developed epilepsy five years earlier and had had frequent daily seizures:

> The character of the fits was almost always the same. They began by clonic spasmodic opposition of the thumb and forefinger (left), the wrist next, and then the elbow and shoulder were flexed clonically, then the face twitched, and the patient lost consciousness. The hand and eyes then turned to the left, and the left lower limb was drawn up. The right lower limb was next attacked, and finally, the right upper limbs. Paralysis of the left upper limb frequently followed a fit … Dr. Beevor and myself have shown that the

---

Horsley when he attended the practice in my clinical wards. On several occasions I have had the opportunity of conversing with him on various points concerning the pathology of the nervous system and it is evident to me that he possessed a very extensive bibliographical and theoretical knowledge but above all clinical experience in this branch of medical science. Furthermore, I am convinced that Mr Horsley if appointed would render valuable service as a surgeon to an institution devoted to diseases of the nervous system.'

[72] Lister was a key figure in the development of neurosurgery. Horsley consulted Lister and was fanatical in his adherence to Listerian methods of antisepsis. William Macewen, appointed to Glasgow Royal Infirmary (1877) aged 29, performed what were probably the first modern resective neurosurgical operations, between 1881 and 1888 when he published seven cases of surgery on cerebral abscess and meningioma).

[73] Augustus George Vernon Harcourt FRS was a famous British chemist who was a pioneer in the field of chemical kinetics. The first anaesthetist at the National Hospital was Mr J. F. Silk, a surgeon whose favoured apparatus was said to be the Clover's ether inhaler. Llewelyn Powell was a successor, working at the National Hospital for many years, and he was the Honorary Secretary of the section of anaesthetics at the Royal Society of Medicine and later its president. By 1919, there were two anaesthetists, Powell and Dr Zebulon Mennell.

[74] M. G. Echevarria is also known to have operated by trephination under ether anaesthesia on three patients with epilepsy, the first in February 1868. One had epilepsy from a scarred left occipital 'conical indentation'; and, in another with a fracture of the skull (1869), he 'trephined the site of injury and removed an old standing clot with immediate recovery of intellectual faculties'. See M. G. Echeverria, *On Epilepsy: Anatomo-pathological and Clinical Notes* (New York: Wood & Co., 1870).

movement of opposition of the thumb and finger can be elicited by minimal stimulation of the ascending frontal and parietal convolutions at the line of junction of their lower and middle thirds. Dr. Hughlings-Jackson witnessed one of our experiments demonstrating this fact, and expressed his belief that this patient was suffering from an irritative lesion of unknown nature, situated in the part of the brain thus indicated.[75]

Having predicted the focus on the basis of symptoms and his studies of functional anatomy, Horsley operated and found a tuberculoma in the expected position. He used an induction current, effectively carrying out the first case of electrical cortical mapping, and completely removed the lesion.

Horsley presented the results of his first three cases at the annual meeting of the British Medical Association in Brighton (1886), describing the clinical features of the patients' seizures; pre-operative preparation; the anaesthetic and antisepsis; the line of incision, treatment of the dura mater, and methods of brain resection; prevention of brain herniation and how bleeding was stemmed; wound closure and drainage; and post-operative care. He then described the clinical semiology of the three cases and details of the operations carried out. It can be said that modern neurosurgery was effectively born at this meeting, and Charcot, who was present, praised Horsley with the words: 'British surgery was to be highly congratulated on the recent advances made in the surgery of the nervous system ... Not only had English surgeons cut out tumours of the brain, but here was a case in which it was probable that epilepsy had been cured by operative measures.'[76]

A fourth operation was carried out on a patient with left hemiplegia and severe fits, who was semi-comatose for ten days before the procedure (23 September 1886). Horsley's pre-operative diagnosis was of a 'tumour of the cortex involving the upper part of the arm-centre in the right hemisphere'. A glioma weighing 4½ ounces was removed, the patient regained consciousness, the fits stopped, and he was able to walk with assistance. It was considered a brilliant result, but the patient died of recurrence six months later.

By the end of 1886, Horsley had completed ten operations for epilepsy, of which nine were deemed successful. He continued to operate on epilepsy throughout his active career. One patient was his own son, Siward, who developed convulsions as a teenager. Horsley, 'convinced that none of his colleagues had his own extensive experience of the treatment of convulsive attacks', decided to carry out the operation himself. Siward survived the operation, but the seizures recurred and he remained unwell for the rest of his life.

Another extraordinary landmark was Horsley's operation to remove a tumour from the spinal cord (9 June 1887). The patient was a captain in the Army with a three-year history of severe spinal pain, worse on movement. This progressed to total paraplegia with clonus and spasms, sensory loss below the level of the ensiform cartilage (the xiphoid process), root pain around the chest, and retention of urine which was chronically infected. He consulted William Gowers and William Jenner. Horsley agreed to operate; but despite having worked out a surgical technique for spinal operations from experimental surgery on animals, the operation was conducted in an atmosphere of much anxiety. Gowers and Kidd were present, and Ballance assisted. Laminectomy was performed at three levels but no abnormality was seen. Ballance urged Horsley to extend the laminectomy upwards, and there was exposed the small fibro-myxoma causing cord compression which Horsley excised. For two weeks following the operation, there was severe pain and leakage of cerebrospinal fluid but this was followed by remarkable and progressive recovery of sensory, motor and sphincter function. The patient was sent for rest and convalescence by the sea and within six months was pain free and able to walk three miles. After one year, he was working for 16 hours each day. The captain remained in good health until he died 20 years later from an unrelated cause. In reviewing this and 57 other published cases of spinal tumour in the world literature, almost all of whom died without undergoing surgery, Horsley opened a new chapter in the history of neurosurgery.[77]

Horsley was technically proficient, operating at great speed but with dexterity and accuracy. By 1900, he had experience of 44 operations for glioma, the earliest pituitary operations, procedures on spinal tumours and a process for managing malignant brain swelling. He had developed the semilunar bone flap, carotid ligation for cerebral aneurysm, the transcranial

---

[75] V. Horsley, 'Brain Surgery', *British Medical Journal* 2 (9 October 1886): 670.

[76] The comment by J-M. Charcot was added to the end of Horsley's paper cited in the previous footnote.

[77] W. G. Gowers and V. Horsley. 'A Case of Tumour of the Spinal cord. Removal; Recovery', *Transactions of the Royal Medical and Chirurgical Society* 53 (1888): 377–428.

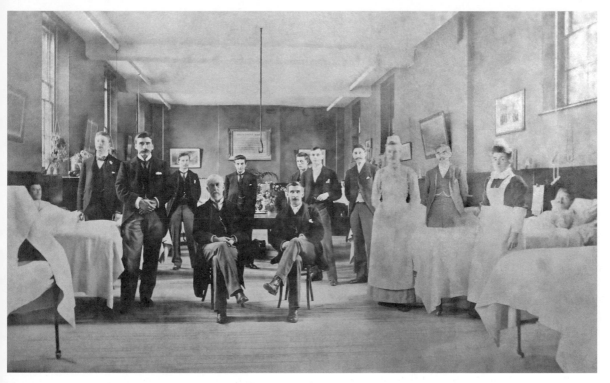

Figure 4.7 Victor Horsley (right) with William Trotter (left) in a ward of University College Hospital, 1900.

approach to pituitary surgery and intradural section of the trigeminal nerve root for trigeminal neuralgia. One of his specialities was gasserectomy, often performed in the patient's own house.[78]

According to Purves-Stewart:

> To watch Horsley operate on a brain was a stimulating experience. It took him only a few minutes to make a window in the skull, amid a shower of bony splinters.

Once within the cranium he was swift yet cautious. The very speed of his operations spared his patients a considerable degree of surgical shock which, in those days, sometimes followed the work of slower operations.[79]

Geoffrey Jefferson concludes that Horsley was an extraordinarily gentle, skilful and knowledgeable surgeon, who carried out a whole range of operations and was considered by his assistants as having exceptional surgical skills: 'It should be very plain that no neurological surgeon has ever turned his hand to the practical therapeutics of nervous diseases so well prepared by laboratory experimental work. And none has, as yet, continued, as he did all through his life, to spend so much time in devising and conducting new experiments.'[80]

Until 1890, Horsley operated in the day room of Margaret Gibbens ward but the stable block of Queen Square House was then procured and a somewhat unsatisfactory surgical theatre built. Mr Douglas Singer reported to the Fry Commission of Inquiry (1901):

---

[78] Horsley presented the results of 149 operations on Gasserian ganglion resection. He had a high success rate, and a mortality of 7 per cent, with death only in patients over the age of 50 years. He considered that the main risk factor was arteriosclerosis. It was the speed of his gasserectomy that upset Cushing who, brought up in the tradition of Halsted, interpreted this as carelessness and lack of skill. Michael Powell described their interaction: 'in 1900 Cushing accompanied Horsley to a private house, where Horsley both anaesthetized and operated on a patient's trigeminal ganglion, all within the hour. The astonished Cushing claimed to have seen nothing but blood and swabs and wrote that "there was nothing of modern neurosurgery that he could learn from Horsley". The two were chalk and cheese: it's hard to see the patrician, teetotal, non-smoker Horsley getting on with the forceful, brash, chain-smoking American.' See Powell, 'Sir Victor Horsley – an inspiration', 1317.

[79] Purves-Stewart, *The Sands of Time* (1939).
[80] G. Jefferson, 'Sir Victor Horsley 1857–1916: Centenary Lecture'.

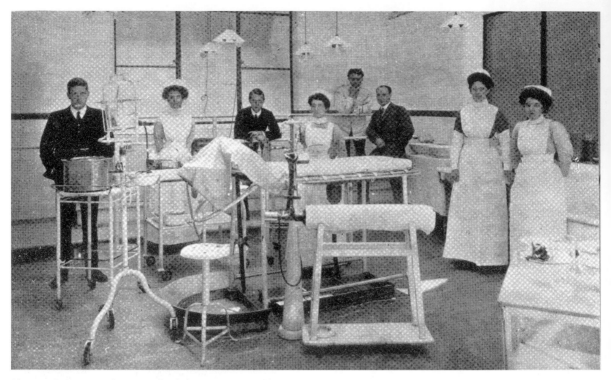

Figure 4.8 Operating theatre at Queen Square, *c.* 1900.

It is impossible to keep [the room] free of dust which collects on the rough wooden benches and the distempered walls and what looks like particles of paint of smuts which fall from the skylight (too high to reach) right upon the operating table! The theatre is heated by two large stoves and the process of heating in the winter takes at least 12–24 hours and is not efficient and emergency surgery is therefore made difficult. The lighting by gas is not good. Some of the dust and smuts arise from stoking the fires to warm the theatres which invariably occurs when the fires are first lit. Some possibly get in through the window panes several of which were badly cracked. The floor is laid in such a way as to not drain water, so there are great pools. The apparatus for sterilising dressings does not look sufficiently large. The stock of surgical instruments should be improved. In conclusion I may add that in my opinion it is hardly possible to alter the present theatre in any way to bring it up to modern standards.[81]

In 1904, the theatre was decommissioned and replaced by an equally inadequate room, designed by Langton Cole. This doubled up as a lecture theatre and had tiers of wooden seats which added to the work of cleaning. Despite these dreadful conditions, Horsley carried out a prodigious number of operations, and his fame as a neurosurgeon spread quickly.

Like Gowers, Horsley was fascinated by gadgets. He made important contributions to the design and use of a number of neurosurgical instruments and materials, including the invention of antiseptic bone wax, bone rongeurs and the use of an electrical stimulator of the cortex. His most remarkable innovation was the stereotactic frame developed with Robert Henry Clarke.[82] The principles of stereotaxy

---

[81] Queen Square archives, 14 May 1901, NHNN/A/35/1.

[82] The Horsley–Clarke stereotactic apparatus is in the museum of University College London. Robert Henry Clarke was a doctor and a physiologist, working in Cambridge and St George's Hospital. He applied mathematics to neuroanatomy and then worked with Horsley at the Brown Institute and at University College. According to Jefferson, Horsley's involvement in the design was minimal but the apparatus has all the hallmarks of Horsley's creativity and it was he who applied it to neurosurgery.

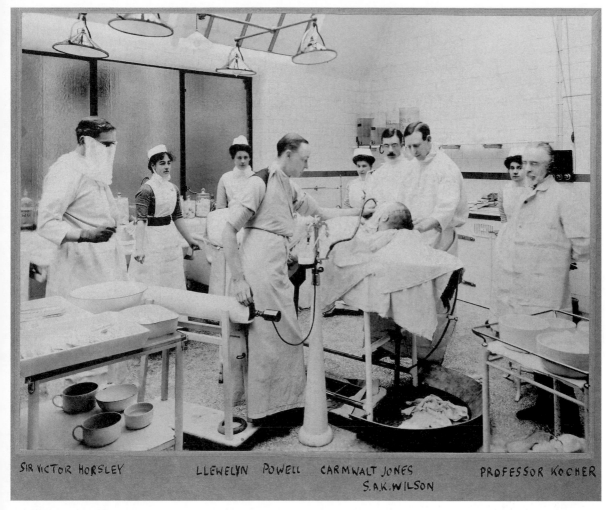

SIR VICTOR HORSLEY   LLEWELYN POWELL   CARMWALT JONES   PROFESSOR KOCHER
S.A.K. WILSON

Figure 4.9 Victor Horsley gowned up in his operating theatre in 1906, with S. A. K. Wilson assisting, Professor Kocher observing, and Llewelyn Powell giving the anaesthetic.

introduced by Horsley are the basis of all modern stereotactic methods and future developments in functional neurosurgery.

After 1900, Horsley did no further experimental work but continued to operate. Now he turned his energies towards national affairs. Horsley believed that, even in small quantities, alcohol damaged the brain and was a root cause of many social ills. He equated its evils to those of opium and considered alcohol to be responsible for crime, poverty, premature death of breadwinners and a source of huge financial loss to the nation. He became an ardent campaigner for its abolition, was elected vice-president of the National Temperance League (1892) and president (1913), and also president of the British Medical Temperance Association (1896). With Mary

Sturge, a general practitioner in Birmingham, he wrote a polemic entitled *Alcohol in the Human Body* (1908). Horsley became involved in numerous public debates including a libellous onslaught against Karl Pearson who had published studies of the effects of alcoholism from the point of view of heredity. Horsley and Sturge attacked Pearson's work, triggering an editorial in *The Times* (13 January 1911) advising the public to avoid the 'din of controversy'. Major Greenwood wrote to Pearson:

> Although Horsley's extravagant rudeness weakens his effect, his direct charges of falsification seem to tell. I suggest it would be desirable to concentrate on that point in your refutation ... I have very little doubt but that Horsley is on the brink of utter scientific ruin ... He has directly and plainly accused you

of forgery, pin him down to that, and the matter is at an end.[83]

The affair smouldered for several months, but luckily for Horsley did not end up in court. Horsley was also an ardent supporter of female suffrage, a subject on which his public utterances excited heated debate. He and his wife stood on many platforms advocating votes for women, strongly condemned the Temporary Discharge of Prisoners Act (1913), and denounced the forced feeding of militant suffragettes. His support of female suffrage lost him many friends and a seat in Parliament.

Horsley led the campaign against the anti-vivisectionists, becoming involved in a series of vicious arguments with members of the movement, which was at the time extremely active and backed by many in the government and Church. Typical of his approach was an address at the Church Congress (1892). Horsley took a typically uncompromising position, at one point denouncing *The Nine Circles* (1892) by Miss Francis Cobbe, a well-known religious figure from a family of archbishops and an active anti-vivisectionist who had already proved a thorn in the flesh of Ferrier. She countered accusing Horsley of torturing animals by experimenting without anaesthetic. This was untrue, and Horsley retorted by describing the saintly Miss Cobbe as 'one of the rankest imposters that had for many years defaced English literature', arguing that 'evidence of her persistent deceit and untruth stands in print, and has done so for many years'. She replied in a letter to *The Times* (8 October 1892) and a furious correspondence followed, with at one point the question raised of resorting to the courts. Huxley – writing from the Athenaeum – and Sherrington offered to support Horsley's costs, but the affair petered out. *Punch* had great fun at the expense of the protagonist with their cartoon entitled 'ANIMIS CŒLESTIBIS IRÆ: A modern scientific discussion'.[84]

After this, repeated attacks were made on Horsley by the other anti-vivisectionists, and, when Steven Bayliss, another UCL researcher, sued Stephen Coleridge, secretary of the Anti-Vivisection Society, for libel concerning his own experiments, Horsley was called as a witness. Under cross-examination, Horsley announced, to the amusement of the court and to the annoyance of the judge, 'There is no limit to the destruction of animals for food. Why should there be any for education?' Bayliss won, and the damages were used to set up a fund which *Punch* suggested should be called the 'Stephen Coleridge Vivisection Fund'. Horsley crossed swords again with Coleridge in giving evidence to the Royal Commission on Vivisection (1907) but his angry views, incautiously expressed, probably worked against him on that occasion, and the Commission sided with Coleridge on a number of important issues.

Coleridge had also tried to portray Horsley's surgery as inhumane. He circulated a surgical instrument maker's catalogue and wrote that Horsley was 'somewhat singular in using on his patients head-holders made of the strongest material and gags with steel bars passed through the mouth behind the teeth which are clenched upon it immovably with steel chains'. A patient of Horsley jumped to his defence in the correspondence column of *The Times*:

> [Victor Horsley] has operated on me twice – on the last occasion in the mouth … I felt no pain whatsoever either during or after either operation. In the second operation I lay on an uncanny looking table and Mr Horsley left behind him a pail full of iron-mongery, which I am sure would have made Mr Coleridge's clients shudder had he produced it for them from his German catalogue. It was all, I have no doubt, of the strongest made and of the best materials. What Mr Horsley may or may not have put in my mouth, after the insertion of the initial 'gag' to prevent me from choking during the anaesthetic, I do not know and do not care. But I hope that if ever again I have to undergo the knife Mr Horsley may hold it; for then I shall feel assured that I shall meet with all the care that science and skill can inspire and with all the gentleness and consideration that comes from a most kindly and straightforward nature.[85]

---

[83] Cited in S. M. Stigler, *Statistics on the Table: The History of Statistical Concepts and Methods* (Boston, MA: Harvard University Press, 2002), p. 45.

[84] The title translated is 'Anger in the minds of Gods' and is a quote from the *Aeneid*. The text in the cartoon reads: 'Miss Fanny (a gentle and most veracious child): "Yah! You cruel coward! You and your friends skinned a live frog." / Mister Victor (an industrious but touchy boy): "You're a liar! The frog was dead, and you know it!" / Miss Fanny: "Boo Hoo! Whether it was dead or not, you've no right to call me names: 'Cos I'm a girl, and can't punch your head!" / Mister Victor: "It's just because you're a girl that I can't

punch yours!. You should have thought of that before you called me a coward!"'

[85] Cited in J. B. Lyons, 'Sir Victor Horsley', *Medical History* **11** (1967): 361–73.

Horsley also became very active in medical politics. He was at his best defending medicine and doctors. He was elected president of the Medical Defence Union (MDU), and fulfilled his role with surprising diplomacy. He resigned this position to take up a place on the General Medical Council, which he held for ten years, during which he was a thorn in the flesh of the establishment and instrumental in a variety of reforms. He also served in many positions for the British Medical Association (BMA). Other causes he supported were sex-education as a way of avoiding venereal disease, which he considered the 'great national injury'; the use of sterile milk deliveries; alleviation of slum dwellings; social reform in health, housing and poverty; and a lifelong campaign against smoking. Horsley was fiercely principled, an egalitarian, and dogged in his championship of the many causes he espoused. His leanings were increasingly socialist, and this often brought him into conflict. His worst moment was the mass meeting at the Queens Hall where, speaking in favour of Lloyd George's National Insurance Act (1911), he was hissed at and shouted down by the angry and reactionary doctors.

It is perhaps not surprising that Horsley also tried on several occasions to gain a seat in Parliament, standing for the Liberal party. He did so believing it was a duty of citizenship:

> The Greeks called a man who refused to take an interest in the politics of his state an idiot, and meant thereby a man who is so profoundly selfish that it was nothing to him so long as he scraped together enough for his existence and to whom the welfare of others, and, above all, his colleagues and fellow-workers, was a matter of utter indifference.[86]

Horsley was adopted as candidate for London University (1911) but lost by a massive majority. It was said by his agent that failure to be elected resulted from his refusal to compromise; and because most medical men, who were the largest group in the constituency, reacted against his 'individuality and power of action making them nervous of some possible attack on their rights or privileges'. Later he was adopted by the North Islington Constituency but resigned, preferring nomination for the Leicestershire constituency of Market Harborough. However, his candidature there met with substantial opposition due to his strongly expressed views on suffrage, temperance, vivisection, prostitution, smoking, disease, sex-education, hygienic milk and slum dwelling; and in the end he was not adopted. At the time of his death, Horsley was on the verge of standing as candidate in the safe seat of Huddersfield, where his views were generally welcomed; and, had he lived, he would very likely have embarked on a new career as a Member of Parliament.

Horsley's personality and beliefs can be adduced from contemporary accounts. These paint a complex picture. He was universally recognised from his early student days as an intellectual. He had a deep knowledge of comparative anatomy and physiology; was an excellent clinician and scientist; maintained interests in the arts and architecture, and in archeology and history; and spoke several languages fluently. Horsley travelled extensively in Europe and was a connoisseur of European culture. Even whilst serving in France during the war, he visited churches and archeological sites. He shared with other well-educated persons of the late Victorian and Edwardian age supreme self-confidence; belief in the superiority of British culture, manners and mores; and loyalty to the rightfulness and principles of the British Empire. Yet, at the same time, Horsley was anti-establishment and a socialist. He was a generous and hospitable person, always surrounded by a coterie of loyal friends. Oliver Gotch, his nephew, records: 'His outstanding trait … was his magnetic personality. He seemed to light up a room instantly, on entering it, [exhibiting] a sort of radiant optimism without a trace of artificiality or self-manufactured make believe. He seemed to be completely without any of the pomposity or self-importance so common to most people of fame and distinction.'[87]

Horsley was energetic in any pursuit he decided to follow, hurrying here and there, taking on multiple tasks simultaneously, and working at a tremendous pace. After a long day, he would say that he must sleep a little while, do so for ten minutes, and wake refreshed and ready to continue work. At the Athenaeum, he would shock other members by running up the stairs. He designed his own rebus used in personal letters – a flying horse with V in position on the saddle, to convey restless energy. His thinking was logical and realistic; and he sallied forth on unwavering belief in his own ability.

---

[86] V. Horsley in *Quarterly Medical Review*, cited by J. B. Lyons, *The Citizen Surgeon: A Life of Sir Victor Horsley* (London: Peter Dawnay Ltd, 1966), p. 212.

[87] Lyons, *The Citizen Surgeon* (1966), p. 161.

However, his belligerence and inability to compromise proved handicaps. Horsley had an aggressive verbal manner to those with whom he disagreed, seemingly at odds with his kind and generous nature and sophisticated background. He seemed unable to accept that arguments often had two sides and refused to see virtue in views that opposed his own. This was born of belief in his own moral righteousness, and yet he was without a trace of arrogance. Horsley often hurtled into major and well-publicised rows, with little concern about the hostility his actions engendered. He could quite easily turn on friends and colleagues if he felt they were wrong. Behind his actions was the view that it was his duty as a citizen, and as a privileged person, to expound his views and change society. He was pugnacious and ferocious in public debate, where a more nuanced approach might better have served his causes. Horsley might have achieved more politically had he been capable of conciliation. Nonetheless, it is clear that Horsley was ahead of his time and most of his views are now vindicated. At Queen Square, he attracted the loyalty and respect of clinicians but, even in that stronghold of support, Horsley was capable of attacking colleagues such as Gowers and Brudenell Carter. He remained at loggerheads with Burford Rawlings, with whom he had several serious arguments and in whose downfall Horsley willingly – and, one suspects, gleefully – participated. His routine form of address to Godfrey Hamilton was 'My dear Idiot'. Eventually, Horsley fell out with Edward Schäfer, his teacher and erstwhile supporter at UCL.

By contrast, Horsley treated his patients with the utmost courtesy and respect, and many wrote affectionately of their experiences under his care. This kindness derived from a natural inclination to support the underdog or the persecuted, through his political views, and on the basis of strong moral humanism. As Dr Alfred Cox, medical secretary of the BMA, commented:

> The man who could be overbearing or even insolent to his equals and superiors was always most considerate to smaller men. Nothing in his character was more remarkable to me than the deferential way in which he would listen to the humble workers in the causes in which he was interested, and the way in which he would willingly give way on many occasions to personal experience in matters which he could only deal with theoretically.[88]

Horsley operated early in the morning on adult patients so as not to keep them waiting; and on children towards the evening, after their bedtime, allowing the mothers to settle the child in the hospital, so that he could administer the anaesthetic whilst they were asleep. One patient, a poor woman from East Dulwich, wrote:

> He was the only doctor who thoroughly understood my case and in whom I felt absolute confidence. He had the courage to say that my condition was due to my being injured by a quack, which no other doctor including specialists have done. I found him exceedingly gentle and full of sympathy, of which I had very little from other doctors. His great calm always impressed me.[89]

Horsley never charged fees to soldiers wounded on active service, or doctors and their relatives, and would travel great distances to see a case. Arriving in Ventnor, Isle of Wight, to operate on a doctor and offered a fee, Horsley replied: 'Dog does not eat dog!'[90]

When war was declared in 1914, Horsley's view on the situation was expressed in characteristic Horsleian prose: 'Until the officials are under the power of the whole people, men and women, this stupid, insane folly of war must go on … I can only hope that Socialism will get more strength and put an end to the arbitrary miseries, injuries and losses heaped on millions of people by their rulers.'[91]

Nevertheless, aged 57, he wanted to enlist, and when nothing materialised wrote directly to Sir Arthur Sloggett, Director General of the Army Medical Services: 'As I am extremely anxious to serve in the present War, is it not possible to transfer me to the Active Service List? … I may say I have my kit, and could leave at once.' Eventually, he was gazetted as temporary Major in the Royal Army Medical Corps (RAMC) and third-in-command of a unit to be sent to Alexandria. Before travelling to Egypt, Horsley was invited to the British General Hospital no. 23 in Wimereux, Normandy, directed by Sir Henry and Lady Norman, but found the set-up fatuous. On 20 May 1915, he set sail for Alexandria, which was then a staging post for the Dardenelles campaign. Promoted to Colonel and appointed director of surgery of the British Army Medical Service in Egypt, he visited

---

[88] A. Cox, *Among the Doctors* (London: Christopher Johnson, 1950).

[89] Cited by Lyons, *The Citizen Surgeon* (1967), p. 153.
[90] Paget, *Sir Victor Horsley* (1919), p. 269.
[91] Paget, *Sir Victor Horsley* (1919), p. 285.

Gallipoli and, in December, was posted to Western Egypt. The front was relatively quiet and Horsley was impatient. In May 1916, he spent several weeks in India and then volunteered for field duty in Mesopotamia in view of public disquiet about the shortcomings and mismanagement of the military medical facilities, which he intended to investigate and improve. He travelled from Bombay to Basra on 9 April 1916, and was appalled by what he saw. He bombarded Sir Alfred Keogh, director-general of the Army Medical Services, with a litany of complaints. On 7 June 1916, Horsley reported: 'When I was going through the cholera camps I discovered that the Indian Field Ambulances had no anti cholera outfits (Leonard Rogers's infusion apparatus, etc.) … I found a medical officer infusing a patient by pouring saline out of his own teapot into the patient's vein – all due to financial terrorism in times of peace.'[92]

After ten days in Basra, Horsley left for Amarah, where he found equally appalling conditions. The assault on Baghdad had been a military disaster and the British Army surrendered in Kut-al-Amarah (April 2016); 23,000 soldiers died, and 8,000 were captured, of whom half also died in Turkish forced-labour camps. Illness was rife in the remaining army and Horsley was contemptuous about the lack of organisation. Dr Robert Campbell Begg, a regimental medical officer, noted that the lifespan of an officer was six weeks. Horsley's death in Amarah was described by Begg:

> He was a man of decided opinions, and ardent teeto-taller, convinced that it was the use of alcohol which predisposed to heat-stroke, and that the power of the sun for harm had been greatly exaggerated. To illustrate his point, he was accustomed to go about his duties often bare-headed, while others cowered in their tents and shelters. He paid for these experiments with his life. One evening he was admitted to hospital with one of these incredible temperatures beyond the recoding range of any clinical thermometer and was dead before morning. Even amidst the universal holocaust, England paused for a moment to mourn one of her greatest sons.[93]

There has been debate about whether Horsley died of heat stroke or paratyphoid, which was epidemic at the time. On 15 July 1916, he had walked several miles to attend an injured colleague in extremely high temperatures and on his return to base complained of headache and then developed extreme hyperpyrexia. A temperature of over 107 degrees Fahrenheit was recorded. He was transferred to the No. 2 British General Hospital, where there were no antipyretics and only minimal amounts of ice. Horsley died on 16 July 1916. Heat stroke was recorded in the notes; and he was buried in the British cemetery at Amarah,[94] where 'Eighty officers attended his funeral. He had a coffin. Wood was precious in Amarah. There were some other bodies sewn up in blankets. A long, dusty march of a mile to the cemetery, a shallow earth grave, a brief ceremony, the same for all, and a weary tramp home in the sun that was the final picture.'[95]

Had the hospital been better equipped for heat-stroke victims – as Horsley had been advocating and later it was – his death might have been avoided. Lyons reports that there was 'a single block of dirty brownish ice' to lower his temperature. The idea that he died of paratyphoid A was revived by Lyons, who had spoken to Anthony Feiling who was a junior officer in the RAMC in the hospital at the time (and later physician at Maida Vale), although there was no confirmatory serology or bacteriology. At the time of his death, much was made of the fact that Horsley took no alcohol, which was widely believed in the army to protect against heat stroke, that he ignored advice about exerting himself in the heat and that he did not wear his solar topee. The most detailed exploration of the circumstances of Horsley's death has been given by Toodayan,[96] who has cited most existing contemporary sources, and also documented

---

[94] There is an interesting description of the modern-day cemetery by Captain P. J. Parker who was serving in early 2003 in Iraq: 'We found the cemetery, with its high walls, off a side-road in the town. We rang the bell and were admitted by the grave keeper. His family had maintained the cemetery for three generations since the war. He had not been paid since 1991! He showed us the papers and register of graves. Of the headstones, there was no sign: they had been taken to Baghdad in 1937. The wall plinths were pristine. The grass in the cemetery, although tired and brown, was cut short and the grounds, even in the centre of this small Iraqi town, were well kept. We found Colonel Horsley's grave-plinth': P. J. Parker, 'In Search of Victor Horsley', *Journal of the Royal Army Medical Corps* 152 (2006): 128–31.

[95] Paget, *Sir Victor Horsley* (1919).

[96] N. Toodayan, 'The Death of Sir Victor Horsley (1857–1916) and his Burial in Amarah', *Journal of the History of the Neurosciences* (2017), doi.org/10.1080/0964704X.2017.1298560.

---

[92] Anon., 'Sir Victor Horsley CB FRS MB FRCS', *British Medical Journal* 2 (29 July 1916): 162–4.

[93] R. C. Begg, *Surgery on Trestles: A Saga of Suffering and Triumph* (Norwich: Jarrold & Sons, 1967).

the fate of the British Army cemetery, headstone and memorial wall on which Horsley's burial inscription is to be found. His death was international news, and was reported widely.[97] A fulsome obituary tribute was published by Osler in the *British Medical Journal*:

> Better than any man of his generation Victor Horsley upheld a great British tradition, for he combined the experimental physiologist and the practical surgeon in a degree unequalled since John Hunter. In his deft hands experiment reached a perfection not before known in the laboratory. To have re-charted (with his friends Beevor, Schafer, Mott, Gotch, and Semon) the cerebral cortex was a brilliant achievement. A technique of such perfection was reached that the surgery of the laboratory was a decade ahead of the clinic. There was a mind, too, behind the hands – resolute, keen, and fertile in suggestion. He had the true scientific spirit, open and free, without secrets or seclusion, and a fraternal kindliness that often gave to others the lion's share of credit ... It was with no small measure of gratification that I saw Victor Horsley become the greatest Hunterian surgeon of his day.[98]

Three years later, Osler still referred to Horsley as 'by far the most distinguished medical victim of the War, whether among our own troops or with those of the Allies ... the outstanding British surgeon of his generation'.[99]

---

[97] Toodayan cites newspaper obituaries in America, India and China – 'Of professional jealousy he had not an atom' , Peking Gazette 1916 – as well as in Europe. (Toodayan 2017).

[98] W. Osler, *British Medical Journal* **2** (19 July 1916): 165.

[99] W. Osler, 'Reviews (of Paget biography)', *The Oxford Magazine* **38** (1920): 175.

Chapter 5

Roller-coaster Ride and the National Hospital Rubs Along 1902–1945

The first challenge to the untroubled growth of the National Hospital was the result of internal dispute. The Fry Commission report, and the events leading up to it, rattled the whole administrative and medical fabric of the hospital. Had the report not come down on the side of the medical staff in its power struggle with the secretary-director, and against the style of management and ethos that he personified, and had it not resulted in his resignation, it is quite likely that the hospital would have closed within a few years or become the benevolent nursing home favoured by Burford Rawlings and predicted by Brudenell Carter. As it was, the report led to a major restructuring and the National Hospital was in effect re-launched.

Even after the internal tensions responsible for dissent were over, the decades that followed were to prove just as turbulent for the National Hospital as it came to terms with new forces of change, which this time were largely external. With an emerging emphasis on medical science, other institutions aspired to practise neurology and neurosurgery, new units arose, the organisation and provision of teaching became more formalised and centralised, there was increasing state intervention in the delivery of medical care, and benevolence and voluntary contributions were no longer sufficient as a means of ensuring financial security. The ideals and social values of the Victorian period were replaced by a less paternalistic ethos, and class structures became more fluid. Outside events, including two World Wars, repeated national financial crises and societal changes, combined with the hospital's slowness to recognise or to respond to change, threatened its existence, and on several occasions the National Hospital teetered close to bankruptcy and closure. As the chairman of the Board of Governors summarised matters towards the end of the Second World War, the National Hospital somehow just about managed to 'rub along'.

Hospital Life 1902–1914

The Board of Management and the Medical Committee

The early years of the century provided the opportunity for a fresh start. With the exception of the honorary president, the Earl of Dudley, the entire top level of hospital management was replaced and, between 1902 and 1905, this attrition was extended to almost every other significant office and function in or connected with the National Hospital. Even the solicitors, Bower & Bower, who had acted since the late 1870s, seemed too closely associated with the old regime and were replaced by Messrs Paine & Paine. Out went the auditors and the trustees of the Charity. Only the consultant architect, R. Langton Cole, retained his post.

One of the first acts of the new Board of Management was to appoint a subcommittee charged with re-drafting bye-laws that defined the powers and duties of the hospital secretary. After the resignation of Burford Rawlings, the salary was reduced by a third to £400 p.a. The tripartite spheres of authority exercised by the hospital secretary, senior house physician and lady superintendent of nursing were strictly defined, and each was made personally responsible to the chairman of the Board. Their freedom to act independently without prior approval was limited. In practice, Burford Rawlings' successors, Thomas Kirby (February to September 1902) and then Godfrey Heathcote Hamilton (September 1902 to December 1939) were content to wait upon the chairman and Board for instructions, rather than pursuing their own initiatives.

The effect of adding two honorary medical staff to the Board, the issue that had given rise to so much earlier heated argument, seems to have been something of an anti-climax. Burford Rawlings had not been the only prominent member of the old hospital management to express serious doubts as to the wisdom of allowing direct medical representation on the Board of Management, but his alarmist predictions that the medical staff would hijack the Charity and sacrifice the interests of patients to those of scientific medicine proved unfounded. In the event, the presence of Dr Joseph Arderne Ormerod and Sir Felix Semon made very little impact on the Board's stewardship of the hospital during the early years of the twentieth century. Free from the divisive presence of Burford Rawlings, and with the tripartite managerial arrangements in place, peaceful relationships between the doctors and administrators were quickly re-established, and most of the medical staff seem to have been happy to leave day-to-day hospital administration to the Board.

Despite the revised management style, lay men and women continued to play a large part in policy-making and philanthropic activities of the National Hospital during the first few decades of the twentieth century. The new members were drawn from much the same elite social milieu of business, the professions, royalty and the leisured upper classes as had been their Victorian predecessors. Monthly meetings were not always well attended and some had to be postponed through not being quorate. During the early years of the new century, active members included Sir John Paget (son of the surgeon-baronet Sir James Paget), who served as vice-chairman for many years; Coningsby Disraeli MP, nephew of the Victorian prime minister Benjamin Disraeli; the Honourable Lionel Holland, brother of Lord Knutsford; and Sir Carl Meyer and Sir Edgar Speyer, both businessmen of German-Jewish extraction who were particularly active in fund-raising during the Edwardian period. The first chairman of the new Board, the Revd Dr Henry Wace, left to become dean of Canterbury. His successor, J. Danvers Power, who had played such an important part in getting rid of the old regime in 1900–1, was appointed in June 1903, and resigned in early 1905 to take up the position of Honorary Secretary of the King Edward's Hospital Fund, and in 1905, the Board found a strong and effective chairman in the publisher Frederick Macmillan (1851–1936).[1] He and the new hospital

secretary, Heathcote Hamilton, each worked at the hospital for almost four decades. The shipping magnate and philanthropist Lord Strathcona and Mount Royal (1820–1914) served as president from 1908 to 1912, and he also proved a generous benefactor. Strathcona was succeeded by the first Earl of Athlone (1874–1957), husband of Princess Alice, who was herself a frequent visitor and keen supporter of the Ladies' Samaritan Society.

The new Board of Management was thus a conservative body and initially exclusively a male preserve. However, shortly before the outbreak of the First World War, the Hon. Marie Constance Adeane and Lady Mallet, a former maid of honour to Queen Victoria, were appointed. Lady Alice Hylton and the Hon. Mrs Richard Lyttleton became members in the 1920s. After the death of Lady Mallet and the resignation of Lady Hylton, in January 1936, Beryl Countess of Rothes, daughter-in-law of the *Titanic* survivor Lucy Noelle, was invited onto the Board. These appointments were not mere tokens. Both the Hon. Mrs Richard Lyttleton and the Countess of Rothes contributed to the important standing committees dealing with finance and buildings, and the Countess of Rothes was also appointed as the Board's lay representative on the Medical Committee. Beautiful and intelligent, she must have enlivened their proceedings. She was appointed vice-chairman of the Board for much of the early 1940s, twice stepping-up during the Second World War, being the first woman to hold a senior executive position in the hospital. Elsewhere, the philanthropic and fund-raising activities were promoted by upper-class female patrons, most notably the Duchess of Albany and her daughter Princess Alice, Countess of Athlone. The Ladies' Samaritan Society continued to be well supported and remained highly influential with the governors and subscribers.

Relations between the administrative officers and the medical staff improved greatly in the period before the First World War. For many years, the minutes of meetings of the Medical Committee had started with the formulaic expression: 'A letter was read from the secretary of the hospital stating that all the [Medical] Committee's recommendations from the last meeting had been approved by the Board of Management.' In

---

[1] Sir Frederick was head of the publishers, Macmillan & Co., and uncle of Harold Macmillan, the future Conservative prime minister. He was a remarkable figure, who rendered enormous service to science and medicine by nurturing the journal *Nature* (published by MacMillan),

despite its financial loss for the first 32 years of its existence, and also giving the editor total editorial freedom. His long service to the National Hospital and the Royal Literary Fund were amongst his activities for public and philanthropic organisations.

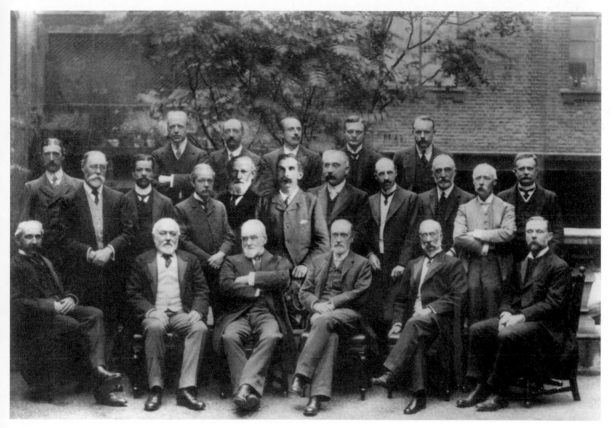

Figure 5.1 The senior medical and surgical staff of the National Hospital, 1906 (left to right: back row – Armour, Batten, Collier, Sargent, Buzzard (Farquhar); middle row – Tate, Beevor, Russell, Cumberbatch, Gowers, Horsley, Ballance, Turner, Taylor, Gunn, Tooth; front row – Semon, Buzzard (Thomas), Jackson, Bastian, Ferrier, Ormerod).

striking contrast to Burford Rawlings, Hamilton was sensitive to the medical tradition at the National Hospital, and deferential towards its medical staff. In fact, his main interests were in history and antiquities rather than institutional politics, and, as long as he remained secretary, neither the Board nor the medical staff were likely to face any serious challenge to their respective authorities.

As a symbol of the earlier power struggle between the medical staff and the Board, it is instructive to consider the venue for Medical Committee meetings. In the early 1890s, the Board refused repeatedly to allow use of the Board room.[2] As a result, from

around 1893, the Medical Committee met in the private consulting rooms of physicians in Harley, Wimpole or Welbeck Streets. After the departure of Burford Rawlings and establishment of the new regime in the hospital from January 1902, the Board hinted that perhaps the Medical Committee might 'have occasion to avail themselves of the boardroom'. However, in practice, meetings continued outside the hospital. In the summer of 1918, Heathcote Hamilton sought to take advantage of the sudden death of Batten, who had been secretary to the Medical Committee, in suggesting to James Taylor that: 'The time was ripe to improve the relations of the Medical Committee to the Board of

---

[2] See minutes of the Board of management, NHNN/A/4/4, 8 December 1891; the Board of Governors had prohibited the use of the Board room, but the minutes of 19 October 1892 document a discussion of how the Board should react to a meeting of the Medical Committee that had been held there in contravention of their ruling 'one evening after the secretary-director had left the hospital'. Burford Rawlings

also wrote a marginal note in the minutes for 9 February 1892, recording: 'The Board thought there was no need to communicate further as to the use of the boardroom their decision being final.' In 2015, the removal of the use of the Board room, temporary as it turned out, again became an issue dividing the administration from its medical staff.

Management, by having the Committee's minutes read at the Board and by the possible [appointment] of [Hamilton] as secretary to the Medical Committee.'

However, this was not well received and, at its meeting on 9 September 1918, the paragraph was deleted from the minutes. Instead, the hospital registrar, Percy Saunders, was invited to become secretary of the Medical Committee and nothing more was said about Hamilton's ill-judged proposal. Again, in 1921, the Medical Committee decided to continue meeting away from the hospital in Welbeck Street.

As a result of the Fry Commission report, the Medical Committee was able to wield greater power. Placed at the top of the hospital's hierarchies, its privileges were jealously guarded. Membership was restricted and self-appointed. With only eight persons often attending, a few active physicians exerted considerable influence. Prior to 1902, the appointment of senior medical staff was firmly in the hands of the Board. Thereafter, this most important function became the Medical Committee's responsibility, with their decisions almost always being rubber-stamped by the Board. As a result, the quality of newly appointed senior staff was indisputably high. Physicians taking up positions between 1900 and 1914 were William Aldren Turner and Frederick Batten (1900), James Collier (1902), Farquhar Buzzard (1905: the son of Thomas Buzzard, who retired from the staff in 1906, and so, for a short time, two Buzzards were on the staff – a unique familial feat), Thomas Grainger Stewart (1908), two Buzzards were Gordon Holmes (1909) and Conrad Hinds Howell[3] and Samuel Kinnier Wilson (1912). Two surgeons were appointed in 1906, Percy Sargent

and Donald Armour; and also Walter Tate (gynaecologist) and Sydney Scott (aural surgeon). Leslie Paton (appointed in 1907) had the unique distinction of being engaged by different hospitals as both an (ophthalmic) surgeon and physician. In practice, the Medical Committee also controlled bed numbers, the terms and conditions of employment for medical staff, the appointment of junior staff and all clinical policies. It oversaw the medical school. Physicians dominated the Committee's proceedings. The surgeons were regarded as essential but inferior, not granted admission rights and playing little part in the overall organisation of the hospital. Nurses, therapists and porters were answerable to the doctors. Patients were expected not to challenge or question medical authority. The Board of Governors took a subordinate and usually supportive role in medical affairs in the early 1900s, which was very different from that of the Victorian era, or indeed of the present day.

Hospital Life and Finances

The style of hospital life in the years between the Fry Commission and the First World War can be gleaned from contemporary sources, at least in broad terms. In many ways, with its genteel and homely atmosphere, Queen Square more closely resembled a venerable gentleman's club than a hospital. The walls displayed pictures and there was a good deal of coloured glass. The chaplain had an office, and services with playing of the organ took place in the chapel. The style of quiet elegance and traditional values was maintained until well after the Second World War, not least by the front-hall porter, Frank Wendon, who was an eccentric and well-known character. His distinguished appearance, in dark suit and immaculately polished shoes that would not have shamed the doorman at Claridge's, made him look like the archetypal consultant, and his manner exuded authority. He occupied that post for 40 years, retiring in 1971.[4] The domestic nature of the hospital, a feature of the early years, was preserved in the pre-war period and considered important to maintain. Homely touches included the Christmas tree to be found in the outpatients department, and the carol services, although festivities were perhaps dampened

---

[3] Conrad Meredyth Hinds Howell obtained first-class honours in physiology from Oxford and trained in medicine at St Bartholomew's Hospital. He was registrar and pathologist at the National Hospital, then assistant physician (1912) and full physician (from 1930 to 1942). He served as dean of the medical school, senior censor (1945) and treasurer (1942–5) of the Royal College of Physicians. He was president of the neurological section of the Royal Society of Medicine and the British branch of the International League Against Epilepsy, and a founder member of the Association of British Neurologists. He published little, but was known for his skill in Gasserian ganglion injection. Hinds Howell was a popular teacher 'concentrating on the basic principles rather than on the rare and the speculative'. He originally did not hyphenate his name, but adopted the hyphenated form after the Second World War.

[4] On one occasion, he remarked to Peter Gautier-Smith that 'I don't like the look of Dr Davies, sir, he is dragging his right leg', and he was proved correct as Hugh Davies died of a glioma some months later.

slightly by the Board's decree that puddings served on Christmas Day should no longer be flaming, since the practice was considered dangerous! Hospital life in that period was charmingly described by Matron Ling during the 1909 Jubilee appeal celebrations, and included Christmas parties,[5] concerts given by nurses and the junior house staff, and trips around the square for patients in the summer, including the use of bath-chairs and races for the children.

When Hamilton was appointed secretary in September 1902, he encountered what was still very much a Victorian institution, antiquated in its buildings, infrastructure and facilities, and badly in need of modernisation both in its medical and nursing organisation and practice:

> There were no fully trained nurses ... no telephones ... the hospital was lighted by incandescent gas-burners in the chief rooms and wards and fish-tail burners in the passages. There was no electric installation ... hence no X-Ray department. [Electric] treatment was given to patients chiefly by means of cell batteries. In the Office there were no type-writers ... There was no enquiry officer or almoner.[6]

One of the first acts of the new Board of Management was to install a telephone system and electric lighting throughout the hospital, at a cost of £1,175 4s 6d. Other modernising reforms followed swiftly and – in terms of infrastructure and day-to-day medical and nursing practice – the National Hospital slowly became a very different place from its nineteenth-century predecessor. Nonetheless, the physical constraints of its restricted urban site, the limitations of its fragile financial position and the conservative mentality of its lay philanthropic supporters did not disappear.

The yearly financial position and statistical details of the patients attending the hospital were given in annual reports of the period and those of the registrar.[7] As was the case in all voluntary hospitals, income was gathered initially by annual subscriptions,

special appeals and fund-raising events, legacies and donations. In the mid nineteenth century, public philanthropy had proved sufficient, but as time passed charitable income became less munificent. The Jubilee fund-raising appeal in 1909, made necessary to meet large debts incurred by changes demanded by the Fry Commission, had a disappointing response, and for the first time a major hospital appeal failed to reach its target. From the later years of the old century, better-off patients had been asked to contribute to their inpatient board and lodging, and costs of outpatient medication, and these charges were increasing – the issue of charging patients had been one factor in the rift between the Medical Committee and the Board but now it was accepted without demur.

In the early twentieth century, financial problems began to mount. The cause of this was, in Hamilton's view, that the old regime in the hospital had bequeathed a fundamental mismatch between available financial resources and the underlying cost of ongoing activities: 'Mr. Rawlings' Board sought to increase the number of beds whenever there was an opportunity and left their maintenance largely to chance. The administration that followed came to grief or preciously near it because it was forced into trying to manage a £40,000 a year hospital on a £35,000 income.'

Conversely, Burford Rawlings blamed the financial problems on the rupture of the hospital from its traditional and longstanding philanthropic supporters which was a consequence, as he saw it, of the conclusions of the Fry Commission. There is truth in both analyses. On coming into office in 1902, the new Board had intended to launch an immediate appeal for funds, but this had to be deferred due to the serious illness of Edward VII. As a result, the Board found itself compelled to raid £4,000 of capital funds to pay for changes required by the Fry Commission. They were also concerned by remedial works resulting from a 'thorough enquiry into the structural and sanitary state of the building' carried out immediately after taking office in January 1902. These resulted in an overall deficit of more than £2,260 for the year 1902, which had grown to more than £6,000 by the end of 1903. This was met by bank loans on the security of invested funds.

The annual income in the pre-First World War years ranged usually between around £10,000 and £20,000. Donations contributed 10–25 per cent of total income, and investments around 15 per cent.

---

[5] Right up to the 1980s, the medical staff used to dress up (usually as matron or a staff nurse) at Christmas, and tour the wards and carve the ward turkey.

[6] Godfrey Heathcote Hamilton, 'Tales of the National' (unpublished typescript, 1940; in the Queen Square archive).

[7] The registrars' reports, contained in the annual reports, provide interesting statistics on activity and diagnoses. They were started by Gowers, and continued by successive outpatient registrars. In the pre-war period, these were written by Wilson, Percy Saunders and Lewis Yealland.

Patients' contributions varied from around 20–30 per cent of total income, with the rest scraped together from a variety of other sources: around 10–15 per cent from subscriptions, 5–15 per cent from the King's Fund, 5–10 per cent from the National Hospital Sunday Fund[8] and around 2 per cent from the Saturday Fund. Despite cost-cutting measures and an increase in legacies and donations, the deficit was still more than £5,000 p.a. in 1905. This forced the Board to close the Finchley convalescent home to all but fee-paying patients, allowing Burford Rawlings to snipe from the sidelines that, under his stewardship, the Board had financial surpluses and actually planned to increase capacity at Finchley by 100 beds.

Prior to the First World War, the charge for contributing patients was £1 2s 3d per week. As with many voluntary hospitals, patients were screened on arrival by an inquiry officer or almoner to see whether they had adequate financial means, leaving free treatment only for those who were deemed to be impoverished. In practice, however, this type of means-testing resulted in most patients at Queen Square being treated without charge. The BMA disapproved of contributions on the grounds that they 'established a moral if not legal claim' to treatment.[9]

The National Insurance Act of 1911, the major social welfare achievement of the 1906–14 Liberal government, meant that, by 1913, 13 million workers had a form of health insurance.[10] Those in the scheme became eligible for treatment by a panel doctor. Tension ensued between these general practitioners and the hospital doctors over who should be responsible for care. Queen Square took a conciliatory position, and those coming to the hospital as non-emergency cases were now asked by a lay official whether or not they were insured. If not, and considered suitable for attention by a general practitioner, patients were advised by the medical officer to seek treatment outside the hospital. Despite predictions that this would prove counter-productive and reduce hospital activity, the chairman proudly announced in the annual report for 1912 that demand was as great as ever. Various other insurance schemes were run by friendly societies and welfare organisations, and some trades unions, and the hospital made efforts to obtain a contribution of 2s 6d per day for each insured patient. However, women, children and unemployed people generally were not covered by any scheme, and had to rely on the charity offered by the voluntary hospital. By juggling resources available through these arrangements, between 1,000 and 1,100 inpatients, and between 7,000 and 7,500 outpatients, together making 47,000–50,000 visits, were seen annually in the pre-First World War years. Occupancy of the 160 beds was usually about 95 per cent with an average stay of around 50–60 days. Plain X-ray was the main 'technological' investigation and, despite lack of utility in neurological practice, the number of examinations increased from 316 in 1910 to 667 in 1915. As a measure of the high level of disability of the patients, there was also constant demand for water-beds, which accounted for 28 out of the 180 hospital beds available.

The Diamond Jubilee Appeal 1909

The fiftieth birthday of the National Hospital in 1909 was seen both as an occasion for much celebration and as a much-needed opportunity for the hospital to replenish its account books. A public appeal was launched with the aim of raising £50,000. In many ways, this fund-raising appeal represented the last great hurrah of the hospital's traditional royal and aristocratic supporters. The Jubilee Committee included lords, ladies and baronets, and was presided over by HRH the Duchess of Albany, with Princess Alexander of Teck as vice-president and the Earl of Harrowby as treasurer. The form that the appeal campaign took and the way in which it was organised were largely the work of the Duchess of Albany herself, and the main thrust of the campaign was a 'collection of purses' from all over the UK and abroad, supplemented by special appeals to the City Corporation and Livery companies, and to the Lord Mayors, Mayors, Lords Lieutenant and clergy of other major cities and counties. A fund-raising dinner was held at the

---

[8] The Sunday Fund was a national organisation, set up in 1873, which raised money through church collections, and distributed the funds 'according to the needs and merits' of the National Hospital. The Saturday Fund was a workman's fund, in existence since the 1850s, with organised collections to support local hospitals. Its main aim was to 'collect small weekly subscriptions from the classes who cannot give considerable sums'.

[9] The typically self-interested BMA was, as always, concerned to protect the income of general practitioners, and thought the fund might encourage people to attend the outpatients department of a voluntary hospital.

[10] This required all those employed who earned under £160 a year to pay 4d per week, and this was matched by 3d from the employer and 2d from general taxation (Lloyd George called it the 'nine pence for four pence'). The payments were signified by the famous 'stamps'.

Mansion House in June 1909, and drawing-room meetings and concerts organised by society hostesses such as the Countess Grosvenor and Lady Durning-Lawrence. At the suggestion of Sir William Gowers, the appeal was further extended to the medical profession throughout the British Empire, and funds even solicited from wealthy Japanese. Donations were collected from more than 30 English and Scottish counties, as well as from the City of London and a number of charities, including the Annie Zunz fund and the Grand Lodge of Freemasons of England.

However, in the event, only £26,000 was raised, but these funds provided temporary respite from the spiralling cost of salaries, food, drugs and staff accommodation. They were also used for refurbishing and enlarging the outpatient hall, remodelling the dispensary, providing a small facility for the manufacture of tablets, establishing an exercise ward equipped with modern Zander apparatus,[11] and extending the massage and electrical departments. Perhaps these innovations made up for the termination, in 1914, of bath-chair exercises for inpatients – instigated originally by the Ladies' Samaritan Society – when it was discovered that the attendant had stopped taking the

patients for their prescribed perambulation and, by mutual agreement, was decamping with them to the local public house. The decision was also taken to commit a proportion of the monies raised to a reserve fund enabling the hospital 'to keep pace with the rapid advance of scientific discovery'. This represented a new departure for the Charity but, in the event, not enough was raised to support research.

On 9 October 1909, the Princess of Wales, soon to become Queen Mary, visited the hospital and was formally presented with the appeal purses. On Jubilee Day, 2 November 1909, a special service of thanksgiving was held in the chapel, presided over by Randall Thomas Davidson, Archbishop of Canterbury, and attended by the Duchess of Albany and Princess Alexander of Teck. Two days later, King Edward VII officially opened the new Jubilee extension buildings and, in the presence of a distinguished gathering, Frederick Macmillan, chairman of the Board of Management, was knighted on the premises. The patients and nursing and domestic staff were not forgotten. Special teas and entertainments were held at Queen Square and the Finchley convalescent home in December 1909, at both of which the Duchess of

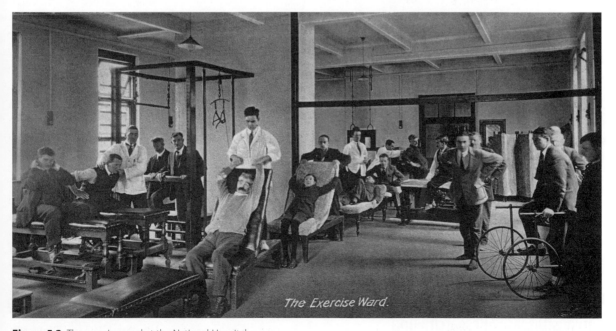

Figure 5.2 The exercise ward at the National Hospital.

[11] Well-regarded exercise machinery invented by the Swedish physician Jonas Gustav Zander.

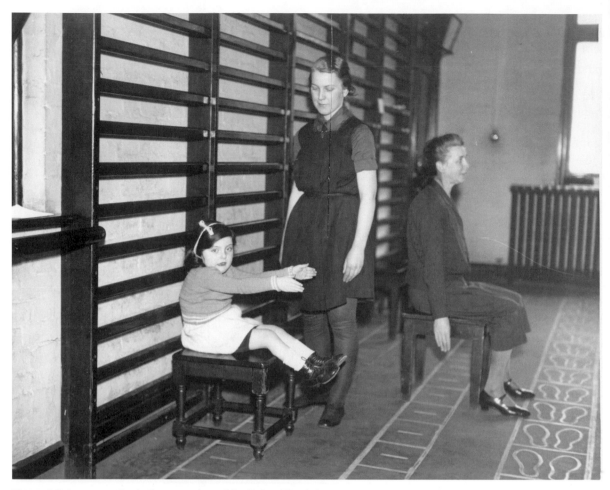

Figure 5.3 A young patient in the gymnasium of the National Hospital.

Albany was present. The show made by the Jubilee committee and the well-publicised activities of the royal and aristocratic supporters undoubtedly helped to restore public confidence in the National Hospital after all the unfavourable publicity attending the upheavals of 1900–1. However, although unfinished business from the time of the Fry Commission was now settled, in terms of resources for long-term growth and development, the hospital was doing little more than treading water.

Research and the Establishment of the Nervous Diseases Research Fund

Until the first decade of the twentieth century, there had been no question of the National Hospital financing research or of it becoming a regular recipient of funding for this purpose from outside bodies. The early clinical research was carried out by clinicians, in their own time, based on the hospital's clinical material and without specific funding. Neuropathological research was based in the clinical laboratories, but experimental research involving animals took place elsewhere, supported financially by other organisations. As time passed, however, research funding was to become a major source of income, both for capital investment and for meeting the running costs of the hospital. Indeed, as we shall see later, the 1938 Rockefeller grant predicated partly on research saved the hospital from closure and in the last decades of the twentieth century it was increasingly research activity that came to the rescue and protected the National Hospital during further rounds of scrutiny and austerity.

The first steps in the research funding history of the National Hospital were taken in 1903 when the Board declared 'that research into the origin of

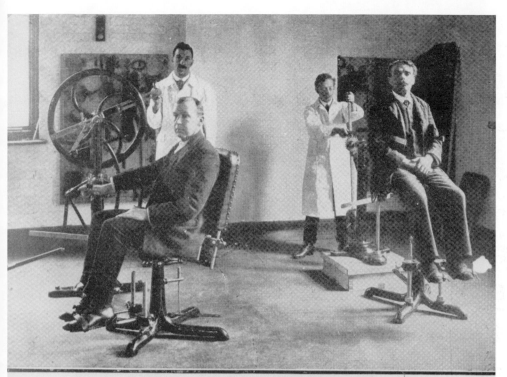

A CORNER OF THE EXERCISE WARD.

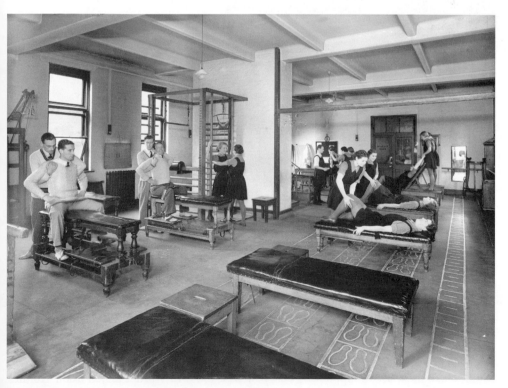

Figure 5.5 Remedial exercises at the National Hospital, 1937.

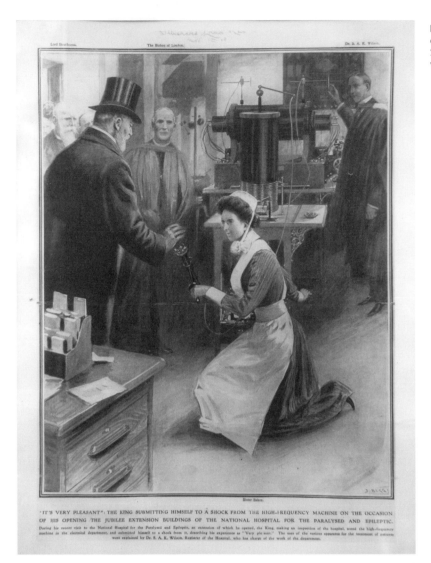

"IT'S VERY PLEASANT": THE KING SUBMITTING HIMSELF TO A SHOCK FROM THE HIGH-FREQUENCY MACHINE ON THE OCCASION OF HIS OPENING THE JUBILEE EXTENSION BUILDINGS OF THE NATIONAL HOSPITAL FOR THE PARALYSED AND EPILEPTIC.

Figure 5.6 The demonstration of electrical therapy to King Edward VII by S. A. K. Wilson. The King opines that 'it is very pleasant'.

nervous disease is one of the objects of the hospital'. A special appeal to raise funds for this purpose attracted donations from high-profile supporters including Lord Lister, Lord Avebury, Lord Strathcona and Mount Royal, the Bishop of London and Joseph Chamberlain MP, secretary of the Board of Trade. This encouraged the Board to establish a special Nervous Diseases Research Fund (NDRF) and to set up a small research laboratory within the hospital. From 1904 onwards, the NDRF became the subject of separate fund-raising appeals, activities and reports. Thus, in April 1904, Mrs Edgar Speyer, the wife of one of the wealthiest and most active supporters and member of the Board, and Mrs Derenberg,

another society hostess and philanthropist, organised a charity concert at the Aeolian Hall, London, in aid of the fund. This raised £263. In March 1905, Victor Horsley wrote to the Board offering to place £1,000 which had been entrusted to him by the executor of a Mrs Jessie Palmer 'to fund a table under the Nervous Diseases Research Fund', a donation which the Board duly accepted. In early May 1904, a committee consisting of four lay and three medical members was asked to administer the NDRF. Later the same year, the appointment of a pathologist as whole-time director of the NDRF was approved, at an initial annual salary of £250–300. In April 1905, Gordon Holmes resigned as resident medical officer and occupied the new post until June 1909. Under Holmes' direction, the pathology laboratory carried out neuroanatomical and neuropathological investigations into the origins of the pyramidal tracts, and the pathology of amyotrophic lateral sclerosis, myasthenia gravis and acute infantile paralysis. In May 1909, an appeal was launched specifically for contributions to the NDRF, but only £81 17s 6d was raised, and so, in November 1910, it was decided to wind up the fund and suspend the laboratory work.

This initiative did, however, establish an important precedent. In April–June 1914, at the suggestion of Frederick Batten, the hospital made its first request to the newly established Medical Research Committee and Advisory Council (which distributed funds raised under the 1911 National Insurance Act and became the Medical Research Council in 1919), to fund research to be conducted in the National Hospital laboratory. Later that year, a further application was made to cover general pathological laboratory work, an increase in the pathologist's salary, and funding for 'special work ... in the laboratory of the National Hospital by researchers appointed and assisted by the Medical Research Committee'. This was successful and, on the eve of the outbreak of the First World War, a grant of £200 p.a. was made to Greenfield for work on cerebrospinal fluid, although this was held over when he applied for a commission in the Royal Army Medical Corps. The Medical Research Committee clearly saw the National Hospital as playing an important role in its future plans and, in his report as dean to the Medical School Committee for 1914, Hinds Howell stated that:

> It seemed clear from conversation with Dr Fletcher [secretary to the Committee] that the Medical Research Committee was willing to recommend further grants in aid of research on nervous disease to be carried out in the laboratory of the National Hospital ... at the termination of the War it should be possible to build up a nervous disease research department at the hospital with adequate financial support for workers and materials.

In fact, war benefitted the hospital as far as research funding was concerned because, in February 1915, Fletcher wrote to Batten stating that 'the Medical Research Committee ... attach great importance to the prosecution of neurological enquiries in connection with the casualties of the present war' and offered a grant of £250 p.a. to Francis Walshe 'for part-time services in

collaboration with yourself and other members of the staff of the National Hospital for the proper study of neurological cases arising from the war'. This was eagerly accepted by the hospital which undertook to rearrange Walshe's duties, allowing him to carry out research but without limiting his hospital work. As it turned out, Walshe was not well suited to research and his contributions were confined to theoretical considerations and analyses of the literature published by others.

The National Hospital and the First World War

The National Hospital was not alone amongst hospitals in being largely unprepared when war broke out. In mid-August 1914, the Medical Committee concluded that it 'did not think that there is any immediate need to make an offer to the War Office of beds for service purposes'. As events proved, this relaxed attitude soon turned out to be misplaced. The number of casualties returning from the front line rapidly overwhelmed the existing medical facilities in London. Many civilian hospitals and large buildings were partly deployed as specialist, military, auxiliary, convalescent or private hospitals. Queen Square was designated as an Auxiliary Hospital, which gave some financial security, and a centre for the treatment of non-commissioned soldiers with organic and also functional illness. The number of military personnel treated initially was small but, at times between 1915 and 1919, nearly half of all male admissions were servicemen, and four wards, comprising up to 68 beds (about one third of the total number in the hospital), were assigned exclusively to War Office admissions. The most frequent diagnoses were traumatic injuries to the head and spine, and functional psychiatric disorders and, for instance, in 1917, of the 872 military and civilian patients discharged that year, the final diagnosis in 134 was that of traumatic injury (mainly gunshot wounds), and functional disorders in 123.

Staffing was problematic. Since many senior doctors were transferred to other wartime duties and could not attend regularly, the first of several wards had to be closed shortly after the outbreak of war due to lack of staff. By October 1914, Gordon Holmes and Percy Sargent were already in France, initially at the Astoria Hotel in Paris which had become the most important Red Cross Hospital with 500 beds, and later

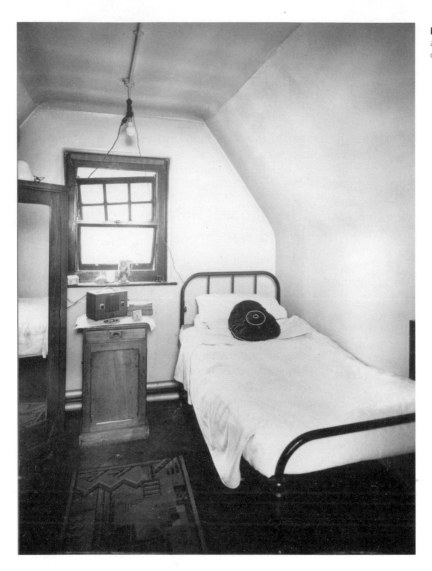

Figure 5.7 The female nurses' quarters – a typical bedroom in the early twentieth century.

that year in the Stationary Hospital no. 13 in Boulogne. Aldren Turner was also in Boulogne by January 1915, seconded there in the first months of the war to investigate the high incidence of mental breakdown among troops. After he returned to London a few months later, it was Turner who had the task of supervising the onward care of troops with mental disturbances withdrawn from combat duty, some of whom were transferred to the National Hospital. Howard Tooth was initially put in charge of the first London General Hospital, before being transferred to Malta and Italy in 1916. Farquhar Buzzard was made consultant to the London command. Grainger Stewart moved to the Ministry of Pensions Hospital in Hammersmith.

Risien Russell served in London as a captain with the Armed Forces. Victor Horsley was based in France, Egypt, India, the Dardanelles and then Mesopotamia where he died, the only casualty amongst the consultant staff of the National Hospital in the First World War.

It seems likely that Saunders (a Canadian, appointed to Queen Square in 1915), Collier, Hinds Howell, Taylor and Wilson were the only permanent physicians who remained at the National Hospital throughout the war. Neurosurgery, however, continued, with 134 operations performed in 1915, including 63 on the brain and 21 on the spine. With Percy Sargent away in France, the active surgeon was Donald Armour.

It became difficult to recruit junior staff to the National Hospital, and, of necessity, and despite the misgivings of some on the Board, female house officers from the only medical school in which women were admitted, the London (Royal Free Hospital) School of Medicine, were employed.[12] These robust ladies were Miss Violet Turner, Miss Helen Ingleby, Miss Elizabeth Ashby, and Miss Marjorie Blandy who also served in the Women's Army Corps under the former militant suffragists Flora Murray and Louisa Garrett Anderson. Blandy was one of the remarkable group of women doctors who successfully ran the famous hospital at Claridge's Hotel in Paris from September 1914.[13]

The public continued to donate funds between 1914 and 1918, and the War Office provided 28s per week for each of the 68 beds used for soldiers, 1s for a new outpatient and 6d for subsequent visits. Hamilton recalls that, in general, during the war years, the hospital was remarkably free from financial problems. However, the Board took a different view and complained that War Office payments did not even cover the costs of maintenance, let alone medical treatment, and the Medical Committee objected:

> The physicians and surgeons joining the staff of the Hospital supported by charity, implicitly and in some cases explicitly undertake to treat patients without remuneration. It can hardly be expected that such an understanding can embrace wounded or ill men for whom the state has been responsible.

The admission of large numbers of military casualties paid for by central government partly alleviated the funding problems of the hospital, but caused further pressure on beds. By 1917, the waiting list for civilian patients was higher than at any time in the history of the hospital. The number of inpatients in the war years varied from 840 to 1,113 per year, with an average length of stay rising from 56 to 78 days by 1918.[14] Drug costs also increased, a striking example being that of bromide, which cost 1s 6½d per lb in 1914, but over £1 per lb by 1918. By 1916, an additional £2,000 was being spent on drugs (chief amongst these were various bromide salts, belladonna, aspirin and phenacetin) and the physicians were being asked to consider ways of curtailing the bill.

In 1917, the Ministry of Pensions asked the National Hospital to take over the management of a convalescent home in Bray Court near Maidenhead for 50 sailors and soldiers suffering from neurasthenia, which it did until April 1920, and also another home for 25 soldiers at Lonsdale House, Clapham, south London. In 1918, two houses adjacent to the hospital ('the Annexe' – numbers 29–30 Queen Square) were converted for the use of 30 convalescent soldiers who were suffering from either paralysis or both paralysis and epilepsy. As was mentioned in the annual reports:

> At Lonsdale House, where the men are paralysed and mostly confined to bed, their chief occupations have been basket-making, embroidery and netting, by which means the patients have been, in many cases, able to supplement their pensions and make further provision for their families. At Bray Court, the patients are of an entirely different description, being those suffering from shell-shock and neurasthenia. Those of the patients who are under occupational treatment are employed in gardening, poultry and pig keeping, carpentry, fitting etc. … during the year a large gymnasium has been equipped and opened.[15]

---

[12] The London School of Medicine for Women, founded in 1874, was renamed in 1896 as the London (Royal Free Hospital) School of Medicine for Women when it entered into association with the London Free Hospital (previously named London General Institution for the Gratuitous Cure of Malignant Diseases), and later as the Royal Free Hospital School of Medicine.

[13] In the immediate postwar years, other female appointees at the hospital were Miss Eveleen Rivington and Miss Mary Barkas. For a biographic sketch of Majorie Blandy see S. LeFanu, 'Majorie Blandy', in Biddy Passmore, ed., *Breaking Bounds: Six Newnham Lives* (Cambridge: Newnham College, 2014).

[14] Patients were both soldiers and civilians, and their numbers reported in the annual reports. Thus, in the years 1915, 1916, 1917, 1918, there were, respectively: 1,113, 1,048, 1,034, 894 inpatients, and 952, 882, 872, 734 discharges; and 7,467, 7,961, 7,432, 7,602 patients made 48,044, 47,170, 31,829, 31,814 outpatient visits. In addition to these attendances, there were 15,853 visits for massage and electrical therapy in 1915; and 8,518 and 8,840 visits for massage and 7,826 and 7,383 visits for electrical treatment in 1917 and 1918, respectively.

[15] Lonsdale House continued to be managed by the hospital until its closure in 1936. By then it had only a few residents. Earlier attempts to close it had been made by the government, for instance in 1922 when there were still 37 exserviceman (half confined to bed) in residence. At that time, the hospital objected and appealed to the 'Not Forgotten Association' to keep it open. This appeal succeeded and the home remained open until 1936. Dr Saunders continued as the hospital's visiting physician and

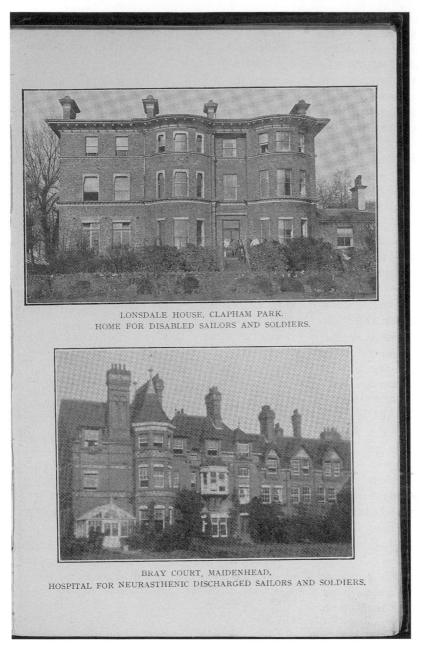

Figure 5.8 Lonsdale House and Bray Court.

LONSDALE HOUSE, CLAPHAM PARK.
HOME FOR DISABLED SAILORS AND SOLDIERS.

BRAY COURT, MAIDENHEAD.
HOSPITAL FOR NEURASTHENIC DISCHARGED SAILORS AND SOLDIERS.

By the end of the war, the finances were intact but fragile and the fabric decaying. Queen Square had survived but there were new uncertainties and

challenges to face in what proved to be the years between two World Wars.

Financial Crises, Near-Closure, a Name Change and Salvation 1919–1939

In the aftermath of the war, the poor state of health of the nation evidenced in the opinion of the public by the large numbers of those rejected from active service

later he was replaced by Adie. However, by 1936 when the lease expired, there were only a few patients remaining, and one senses from the minutes that the closure was accompanied by a sense of relief that the Board no longer had financial responsibility for the home.

on grounds of disability became an issue in its own right. Much intellectual debate turned to issues of welfare and public health. Rather remarkably, the Ministry of Health was put in charge of the house building programmes in the early 1920s, in a response to Lloyd George's promise of 'Homes fit for Heroes'. A new liberalism grew up, based on the work of a fresh generation of influential economists, concerned about how the free market could be managed so as to function better, to the advantage of the nation as a whole, as well as individuals. The concept of more fairness was not new, and had been signalled 100 years earlier by John Stuart Mill and by Bentham, but now the need for state intervention to assist the disadvantaged became political orthodoxy. The social surveys of Booth and Rowntree, and then Mass Observation, had demonstrated that poverty was often not 'deserved' but the result of circumstances outside the control of an individual. It was also clear that much talent and potential was lost through poverty and ill health, to the detriment of the country generally. The economists Pigou, Marshall and Keynes, and Beveridge (Director of the London School of Economics 1919–37) were advancing new theories of social welfare. The 'Poor Law hospitals' were now an anachronism, and their antagonistic relationship to the voluntaries a running sore. After the First World War, the Labour party proposed a health service for the whole nation, carrying the implication that doctors would become salaried employees, as in the Army Medical Services, and with the abolition of voluntary hospitals. A Ministry of Health working party was formed in 1919 to consider this suggestion but decided that formation of a National Health Service was a step too far. Nevertheless, the seeds of state control of medicine were sown.

The financial situation of the whole voluntary hospital sector in London then entered a new period of crisis, and Queen Square was badly affected. The hospitals clung to their freedoms as best they could, but, with the repeated financial crises, intervention was needed and the inevitability of state support and then control, eventually realised in 1948, grew ever more obvious. By 1920, there was public debate about the future of the voluntary hospitals and their financial crises. However, the calls for complete take-over of the hospital system with control ceded to local authorities produced an angry response and resistance in the medical bunkers: 'The voluntary hospitals will become the sport of parochial politics, into whose vortex they will have to plunge as the price of

continued existence. Their fate will be settled by chance aggregations of county councillors, profoundly ignorant for the most part of what hospitals do and what they need.'[16]

At the National Hospital, as the number of patients with war injuries fell and this source of income rapidly decreased, a severe financial crisis developed and closure of the hospital again had to be considered. At the end of 1919, the Board announced that, unless it could immediately raise £10,000, it would have to close the inpatient service. £1,600 was raised from charitable sources but this 'did not touch the fringe of the problem'. The hospital was effectively bankrupt, 'with no funds to meet tradesmen's bills and unable to raise a loan as all available securities were already pledged'. In June 1920, it was announced that the wards would close but outpatient activity continue together with the annexe for convalescent soldiers. The process of discharging all inpatients began and notices were displayed saying 'Help us to keep open'.

The impending closure caused widespread public dismay. The King Edward Fund, which had been given the responsibility for dispersing £250,000 of government funds, made an emergency grant of £8,000 to the National Hospital. This, and money raised by a further appeal to the public, saved the situation. The closure plan was reversed and the wards fully reopened in July 1920.[17] Patients were then also asked to make a greater contribution to the cost of their stay in the hospital (as they were in most London voluntaries thenceforward) 'after an enquiry into the patient's circumstances had been made by the Enquiry Officer'. As a result, at the end of this roller-coaster year, the hospital actually managed to end up in surplus, to the surprise of the Board, with yearly income exceeding expenditure by £8,668 9s 5d.[18]

---

[16] Anon. 'A National responsibility' (editorial) Hospital 68 (1920): 517.

[17] By the end of the year, there were 889 inpatient admissions at Queen Square (compared to 933 in 1919, in the 200 available beds – although the average bed occupancy in 1920 was only 173 due to the closures) and 7,917 outpatients made 56,052 attendances (compared to 7,764 and 53,086 in 1919). By then, in addition, 7,565 attendances were made to the electrical department and 7,587 for massage treatment. Discharged ex-servicemen accounted for 2,999 attendances. In that year, of 869 discharges, only 31 were for epilepsy and 108 for hysteria and neurasthenia (according to the registrar's report by Marjorie Blandy).

[18] Costs had risen markedly during the war and in the few years thereafter, but so too did income. The extent of this

The parlous financial state of the London voluntary hospitals was now the subject of much debate, the *Lancet* noting: 'it seems to be assumed widely that the day of the voluntary hospital is over'.[19] The King's Fund commissioned an influential report, in January 1921, which concluded that the voluntary hospitals were still the most effective and cheapest solution for providing best treatment and training, and advancing knowledge, and that a substantial part of their income should come from contributions. It recommended that state subsidies should supplement but not replace traditional modes of funding voluntary hospitals. The Board of the National Hospital had previously written to the King's Fund urging that it should administer any money from government since direct state support would compromise voluntary contributions.[20]. The government then established the Cave Committee[21] to consider the financial situation of the voluntary hospitals. Godfrey Heathcote Hamilton and Sir James Paget gave evidence on behalf of Queen Square, and when the Committee reported in May 1921, it concluded, as had the King's Fund, that it was in the public interest for the voluntary system to continue without permanent state funding, since that would change the ethos and nature of these hospitals. The Committee did, however, recommend an immediate state grant of £1 million, with further awards in the following year, to give hospitals time to reorganise their finances, and that the King's Fund should be tasked with distributing the money for London. In the event, the government provided £500,000 on the basis that the voluntary sector raised a matching amount, and the share to the National Hospital was £800. The various government grants, paid via the King's Fund, postponed the financial crisis for many of the voluntary hospitals, including Queen Square, but placed firmly in the public mind the notion that the government would eventually have to take responsibility for hospitals and their organisation. The slow process of moving to a National Health Service, with the absorption of the voluntary hospitals into state control, had been set in motion.

Another issue was the question of paying consultant staff. This practice had already begun in some provincial hospitals, and with support from the BMA. However, the Cave Committee also opposed that idea, having been told by two distinguished physicians that, if it was introduced, 'the bottom would drop out of the voluntary system'. The Cave Committee considered that 'Although the services of the staff are honorary, they obtain valuable return in the form of medical and surgical experience and the enhanced reputation which accrues to the members of the visiting staff of a great hospital',[22] a sentiment which clearly applied to the National Hospital staff.

By 1922, the hospital's finances had stabilised and, in its annual report of December 1923, the Board was able to announce that 'with much satisfaction ... the recent financial difficulties, which at one time involved the closing of wards, have to a large extent been overcome ... comparative freedom from anxiety as regards funds for the cost of maintenance has afforded the Board an opportunity of giving attention to some long wanted improvements'. A new operating theatre was opened, the substandard practice of using the minor injuries theatre as a waiting room for outpatients was discontinued, and new X-ray plant was installed. The annexe which had been used for discharged ex-servicemen was converted back for civilian use, and a new ward for contributing male patients created. The electrical department was also enlarged.

By 1924, many of the London voluntary hospitals, including the National Hospital, placed greater emphasis on providing separate arrangements for contributing patients (essentially, private patients), including their own X-ray facilities. This was violently opposed by the Labour party, which anticipated that hospitals were likely to prefer paying to non-paying patients. In fact,

---

change can be seen by the fact that the income of the hospital was £48,722 19s 5d in 1920, more than three times the amount for 1910. Expenditure in 1920 was £40,054 10s 0d.

[19] Anon., 'The Future of the Voluntary Hospitals', *Lancet* **195** (1920): 613–14.

[20] Letter of 9 March 1920 from the chairman of the Board of Governors.

[21] Chaired by George Cave, lawyer and Conservative MP, Home Secretary in Lloyd George's coalition government, and chancellor of Oxford University (from 1925). The Committee's beautifully written and concise report made a good case for continuing the voluntary hospital system. It noted that there were 952 voluntary hospitals in Britain in 1922. Of the 117 in London, 73 were in financial deficit. In addressing the question about whether the voluntary system was worth saving, the report commented: 'The voluntary hospital system, which is peculiar to the English-speaking peoples, is part of the heritage of our generation; and it would be lamentable if by our apathy or folly it were suffered to fall into ruin.'

[22] Cited in B. Abel-Smith, *The Hospitals 1800–1948* (London: Heinemann, 1964). The 'enhanced reputation' ensured a lucrative private practice.

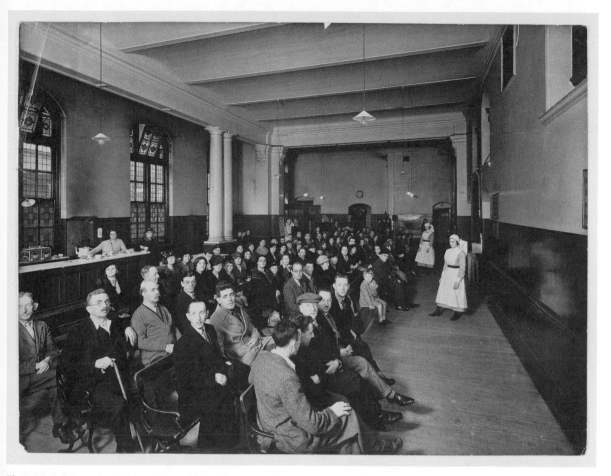

Figure 5.9 Outpatients hall (around 1920).

partly for financial reasons and also because of the rapidly advancing effectiveness of medicine, the type of patient using the voluntary hospitals was changing. Spending time in hospital wards, previously charitable facilities for the 'sick poor', was becoming acceptable for those who hitherto had distanced themselves from the voluntary hospital provision of medical care. The professional and middle classes – not just their servant girls, stable boys or cleaners – were now patients in all the London hospitals, including Queen Square. Paying patients provided 40 per cent of income, often through the various contributing schemes. The poor still received free treatment, and subscriptions accounted for less than 5 per cent of income.

In 1925, an enormous legacy of almost £45,961 from the estate of Mrs Roberts Smith[23] transformed

the balance sheet, exceeding the income of around £37,000 from all other sources that year. Also, thanks to deflation, the weekly cost of maintaining a bed remained stable throughout the 1920s at between £2 19s 9½d and £3 7s 11d. The hospital continued to hold fund-raising garden fêtes, matinées, musical concerts, soirées and recitals at Her Majesty's and the Criterion theatres by famous Drury Lane actors such as Sir Herbert Beerbohm Tree, Marion Terry and Charles Wyndham,[24] and the funds raised in these years roughly matched expenditure.

---

[23] This legacy is rather a mystery. We can find no record of the circumstances of the gift, nor seemingly was there

recognition through a permanent memorial, such as the naming of a ward – nor are we able to obtain any further details of Mrs Roberts Smith herself. This is very surprising, considering that the legacy doubled the income of the hospital in that year.

[24] Hamilton relates how the sister in the electrical department arranged a Christmas party. A patient with general paralysis of the insane pointed out that he much preferred

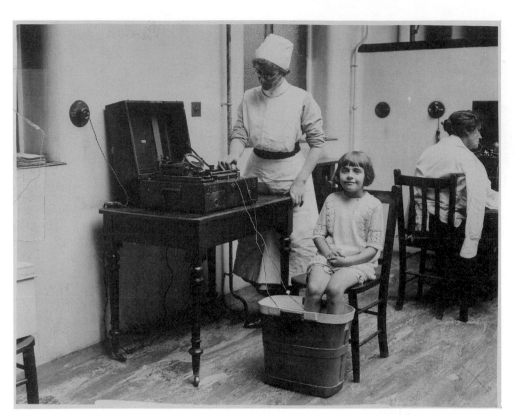

Figure 5.10 A child receiving galvanic electrical therapy in 1926.

An important outward change to the hospital's public profile took place in 1926. For the first time since its foundation, the name was changed from 'The National Hospital for the Paralysed and Epileptic' to 'The National Hospital, Queen Square, for the Relief and Cure of Diseases of the Nervous System, including Paralysis and Epilepsy' (usually abbreviated to 'The National Hospital, Queen Square'). This change, made following a petition by the hospital to the Privy Council in 1925, required a Supplementary Royal Charter, which was granted in 1926. It was based on the premise that 'For years past … the name … Hospital "for the Paralysed and Epileptic" has been a deterrent to the public coming to the hospital and that for this reason many of the honorary medical staff have always referred to … [it] as the National Hospital for Nervous Diseases'.[25]

With an increase in bed numbers to 190 in 1921, throughout the 1920s the activity on inpatients rose to around 1,200–1,400 per year, with an average bed occupancy of over 95 per cent. This increased to nearly 1,500 by 1935. Between 1920 and 1935, approximately 7,500–8,000 outpatients were seen, together making between 50,000 and 55,000 visits. These included 4,000–6,000 appointments for electrical treatment and 6,000–8,000 for massage. Annual income in the 1920s was usually around £35,000–40,000. This was a period of relative financial stability, and during this time the Board pressed on with plans for expansion and improvements at Queen Square.

In 1926, the freehold of Queen Square House was acquired for £32,000,[26] and the Board announced that

---

the traditional holly and mistletoe to coloured paper chains. Slogans such as 'the currents in our buns occur with high frequency' covered the walls. The resident medical officer sported white flannel trousers, evening coat and waistcoat, and a large white-and-blue spotted tie.

[25] A full account of the naming of the hospital is given in the preface. The change to the 'National Hospital for Nervous Diseases' was first brought up in the Medical

Committee in April 1917, but the suggestion was not adopted by the Board. The question of changing the name, with preference expressed for calling the hospital simply the 'National Hospital Queen Square' was again brought up in the Medical Committee in 2014, but by then decisions were in the hands of the UCLH Trust Board who showed little understanding of, or interest in, this point.

[26] This was possible as the previous owners, the Foundling Estate, moved out of London and sold its land. Queen Square House had long been coveted by the hospital. The

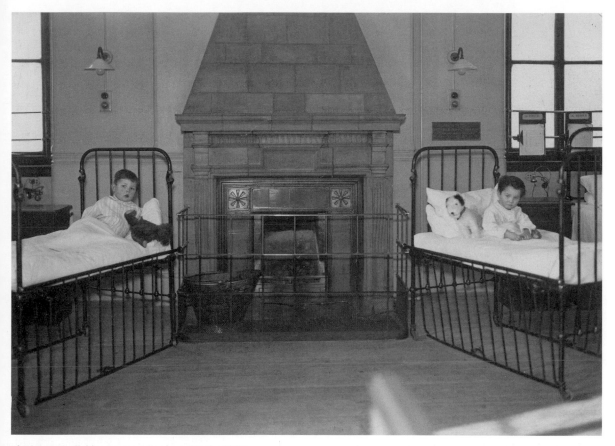

Figure 5.11 Child patients on Zunz ward in the 1930s.

the hospital now had sufficient freehold land for its immediate plans. In 1927, a small 'carefully chosen' committee was formed, with good medical and surgical representation, to define the priorities for further development. Two major schemes were identified. The first was to build a new pathology department (and mortuary) and surgical unit, still co-located on the site of the existing laboratory and surgical wing but increasing the number of surgical beds from 7 to 24, thereby avoiding the danger of premature transfer of post-surgical cases to the medical wards. The second was the provision of a new nurses' home on the site of 29–32 Queen Square, in place of the massage school, which was to be moved to Powis Place.

By the end of 1929, however, the financial situation again deteriorated, and the plans had to be modified so that the new surgical and pathology wing had

a home for male nurses built alongside, with its frontage opening onto Guildford Street on the site of the houses bought from the Foundling Hospital estate. A design for the building was commissioned from the architect A. H. Moberly RIBA. The plan for a nurses' home on the site of 29–32 Queen Square was abandoned, and the revised plan had no new provision for females. Nurse staffing was very problematic throughout the country, and the National Hospital levels were below establishment. It had been hoped that the provision of modern accommodation would enhance recruitment, and the failure to propose the building of a new nursing home was greatly regretted by the matron and Board, but it seems that the cost was simply too great. As frequently proved the case, the employment of nurses simply did not take priority over the medical requirements. In 1929, the hospital also announced that it could not meet the costs of remodelling the X-ray department, needed since the current equipment was inadequate (and

first abortive attempts to buy it were in the 1860s and 1870s but these were abandoned when the rising cost of the new build in the 1880s stretched hospital finances to the limit.

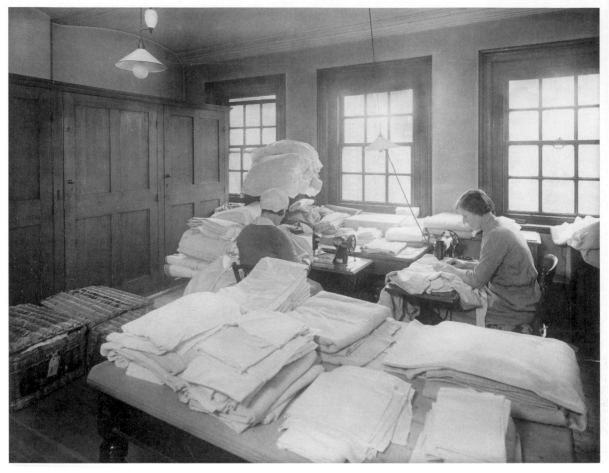

Figure 5.12 The hospital linen room, 1935.

some, indeed, was borrowed), with patients referred to other hospitals for treatment. In 1930 a special appeal was broadcast on the BBC for the provision of funds for the X-ray department.[27] By 1930, the Board was again expressing concern about the annual deficits, which now amounted to about 10 per cent of income. The estimated cost of the new surgical unit and pathology department had risen to £70,000 and it

was also hoped to endow the research and pathology work with a further £75,000, but no progress on raising funds or building work could be reported.

The situation was transformed in 1935 when, following an application by the medical staff, the Rockefeller Foundation agreed to award the National Hospital £120,000 (£60,000 for building and £60,000 for running costs). A new appeal was launched and the matching funds, required under the terms of the award, were quickly achieved. As part of the appeal, a newsletter, *The National Illustrated*, was produced, with remarkably sophisticated public relations. One particularly fulsome article was written by an ex-patient, James Douglas, who wrote:

> postgraduate lectures [are given] to students from around the world. The lecturers are living textbooks … The squalid little room in which these sacred debates are held made me blush with ashamed

---

[27] X-ray equipment was particularly expensive. In 1938, the hospital approved the installation of £2,357 of new equipment from the General Radiological Company, and in May 1939, the radiological subcommittee recommended that the 'radiological equipment on the surgical floor be brought into commission without delay, that the deep X ray therapy plant be modernized and that the diagnostic unit on the second floor near the outpatient department be brought up to date', commenting that 'until the deep X ray plant is working, the hospital is lacking in one of its essential services to humanity'.

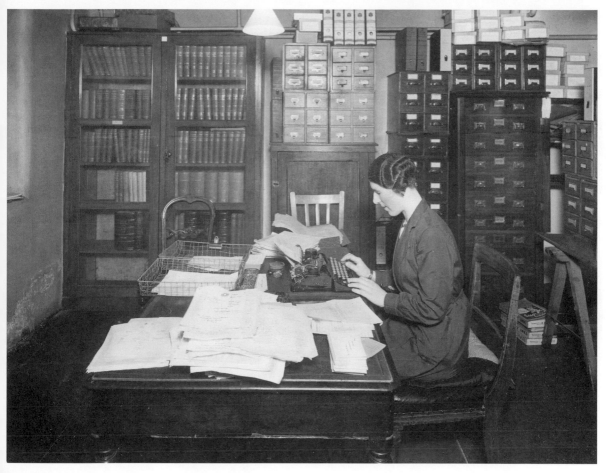

Figure 5.13 A medical secretary typing up notes, 1935.

wonder and wrath. It is a national scandal that all this advanced world research is carried out in a slum with miserably-improvised and makeshift apparatus patched together by the heroic staff ... It is a Heath Robinson hospital. They carry patients down old stone stairs to a cellar that is a nightmare ... I saw a fanstastic research contraption in which a music stand, a trench periscope, mirrors, discarded lenses, and an old door converted into an adjustable couch were added to modern apparatus. The sight made me want to laugh and cry and swear ... Think of it ! The Research Laboratories are housed in dingy basements and houses two hundred years old ... You would be horrified if you knew how little the great men who pursue research are paid, men who have no private practice, and whose holy toil is the pure love of pure science. If you saw the conditions under which they slave you would be shocked and ashamed ... I am sure the British people would have given this unadvertised and unpublicised [*sic*] hospital all the money

it needs, if they had not been anaesthetised by ignorance into apathy!

For good measure, Douglas also had a swipe at those urging the end of voluntary hospitals:

The old rich are poor and the new rich have not yet ripened into the full use of their opportunities of service and sacrifice. There is a deathrate of generosity, and the birthrate is caught in an inevitable timelag ... The voluntary system is dying hard, but I do not believe it is going to die, for it has bestowed upon us marvels of medical and surgical skill and miracles of selfless research which no country on earth can either equal or surpass. No state system can carry on this British triumph and conquest.

In 1936, the new King, George VI, had agreed to become patron to the hospital, as his father had been before, and this may also well have contributed to the success of the appeal. A string of advertisements and

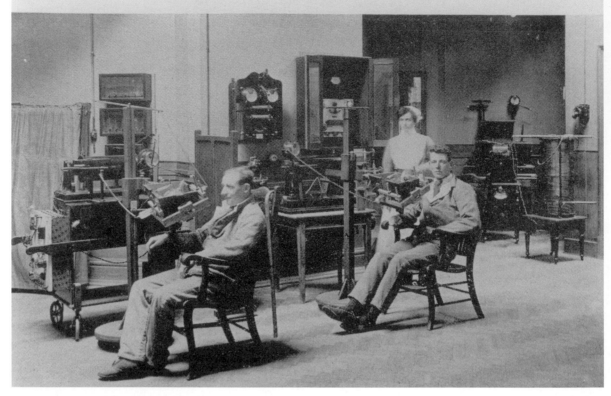

ELECTRICAL DEPARTMENT.

Figure 5.14 The electrical department.

articles about the hospital appeared in newspapers, including *The Times* (the appeal was sometimes said to be enabling the hospital 'to fulfill its destiny as the English Salpêtrière'!). Interestingly, much also was made of the hospital's work in the 'elucidation of psychological conditions, both healthy and morbid, in the light of ever increasing knowledge'. These it seems helped to attract funds. All this extravagant (and efficiently executed) publicity was effective, as the appeal rapidly hit its target.

On 19 July 1938, the new building was opened by Queen Mary, and named after her. This was one of the largest grants made by the Rockefeller Foundation,[28] and by far the largest single donation ever received by the National Hospital. It provided an enormous boost to the hospital's financial situation and reputation.

The Foundation's interest in the National Hospital had been facilitated by the establishment of an 'MRC research unit' in 1932, with a grant which provided for 20 beds in the annexe (31 and 32 Queen Square, previously used for convalescent servicemen) allocated for research purposes and also for laboratories and other facilities. The directorship of the unit was conferred on Arnold Carmichael, who had been appointed physician to outpatients in 1930. After the award of the grant, his full-time salary and those of his staff were paid by the MRC. This unit soon established itself as the most important facility for research in clinical neurology in Britain, and its work dominated British neurological research in the 1930s.[29]

---

[28] $298,650, as recorded in the 1938 annual report of the Rockefeller Foundation, and the largest donation that year to any institution except Yale University.

[29] At the early meetings of the recently established Association of British Neurologists, for instance, five members of Carmichael's group presented 23 of the first 136 papers.

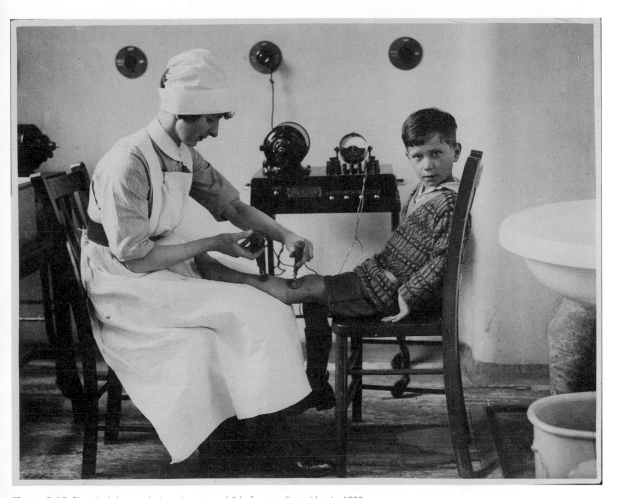

Figure 5.15 Electrical therapy being given to a child after a polio epidemic, 1928.

The Rockefeller award resulted not only from the very favourable impression Carmichael created on the Foundation's officers, but also from the desire to set up a surgical unit in Europe based on Cushing's methods. The Rockefeller Foundation had established an international office in Paris in 1923 as part of its effort to support public health globally. In 1930, Dr Alan Gregg, who had served in the British Army in the First World War and was then in charge of the Paris office, was appointed director of medical education at the Foundation, and Dr Daniel P. O'Brien took over the International Office. Gregg and O'Brien were interested in neurology and psychiatry, and both were frequent visitors to Queen Square. They were, according to Gordon Holmes, 'astonished at the conditions under which research was carried out ... and the few and primitive facilities afforded for it'. O'Brien was particularly impressed by Carmichael, as he wrote: 'he strikes me as a very high type and exactly the man for the place'.[30] In 1935, William Lennox also wrote to Alan Gregg that Carmichael's leadership had improved research at Queen Square and that, at the Association of Neurologists' meeting at Bath which he attended, there was none like him.

The MRC unit moved into the Queen Mary wing in 1938, and was renamed the Institute for the

[30] O'Brien was said to possess 'a great imaginative capacity, and a strangely sympathetic relation with shy and capable scholars': see E. Jones and S. Rahman, 'The Maudsley Hospital and the Rockefeller Foundation: The Impact of Philanthropy on Research and Training', *Journal of the History of Medicine and Allied Sciences* **64** (2009): 273–99; this may be part of the attraction of Carmichael. See also O'Brien's diary, 9 December 1933, cited by S. T. Casper, 'The Idioms of Practice: British Neurology 1860–1960' (PhD thesis, University College London, 2007), p. 317.

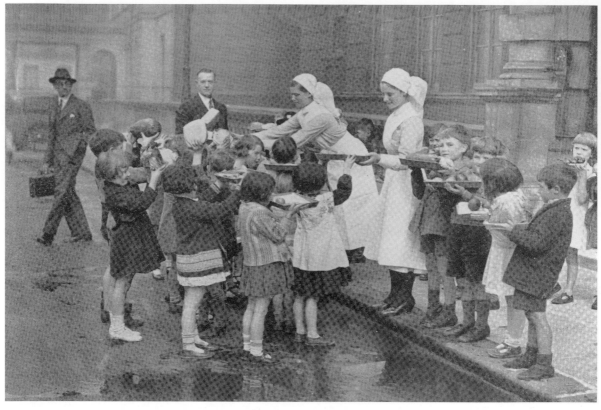

Figure 5.16 Children of the Infant's School of St George the Martyr bringing harvest gifts for the hospital.

Teaching and Study of Neurology. Laboratories and accommodation were provided for ten workers, along with facilities for physiological, biochemical, clinical and pathological investigation. Holmes reported that, by 1939, 11 people were engaged on research work in the building.[31] The

MRC and Rockefeller grants illustrate a striking new aspect of finances in the 1930s, which was the provision of very large sums for research. These supported hospital buildings, equipment and running costs, and this new source of income largely replaced philanthropy as the source of funds for new developments. As we shall see later, this stimulated the hospital to focus again on its academic portfolio.

The Rockefeller grant did not, however, come without its downside. The hospital accountants estimated that the new building would increase the annual maintenance budget by more than £6,000 per annum, in addition to increasing expenditure on nursing staff and technical support, and warned that there were insufficient funds. However, the Board recognised that the grant was essential for the National Hospital to retain its position as the flagship

---

[31] In the summer of 1939, arrangements for the autumn and winter courses at the Institute were made as normal. A highlight would have been the lecture by E. D. Adrian on the physiology of the nervous system (for an honorarium of 3 guineas), but the onset of war brought research activities to a halt. It is a matter of speculation what neurological research might have resulted from the initiative of the Rockefeller Foundation had war not intervened. It seems likely that Cairns would have moved his practice to Queen Square, supported by the Foundation, and would have greatly enhanced the position and role of neurosurgery at the National Hospital. As it was, almost all clinical neurological research immediately ceased, and the staff and facilities were redeployed. The laboratories were used by the Admiralty, the War Office and the RAF for medical

topics other than neurology, and the MRC located a Human Nutritional Research Unit on the site.

of British neurology, and it must therefore be secured.[32] In a letter to the King's Fund (July 1935), Hamilton continued to highlight the difficult position in which the hospital found itself. The distribution committee of the King's Fund largely shared Hamilton's view, and wrote to the Board in July 1935 indicating that they doubted the ability of the National Hospital to sustain the additional costs of the proposed expansion. However, the Second World War changed the hospital's situation and it avoided what seemed likely to be another financial crisis.

Deterioration in the financial position of the country in the 1930s had the added consequence of raising the spectre once again that the voluntary hospitals were insufficiently coordinated, too small and inward-looking – in short, an anachronism. The Sankey Commission was established, in 1937, to consider their position. Its report recognised that the freedom enjoyed by the voluntaries was 'an example of the dislike of over-control and bureaucracy which is inherent in the genius of our race'.[33] It also concluded that the rise of the public-authority hospitals and their small size rendered many non-viable. The Royal College of Surgeons advised the Commission that 'it was infinitely preferable for a general hospital to have specialist departments to numberless small special hospitals being set up independently as they were very often uneconomic and difficult to staff'. As a result, the Commission advised against the further establishment of special hospitals and recommended that the existing ones be grouped around a larger hospital. The Commission also stated there was a need for better accounting, hospitals to be supported partially by local authorities, and planning to be centralised.

In an attempt to defend their independence, 76 hospitals in London formed an Association of Special Hospitals, with the goal of mitigating the criticisms of the Sankey Commission. But, in reality, members of that Association were forced into a corner as local authorities and government exercised control of health matters. One by one, the smaller hospitals were sacrificed in the interests of saving their larger neighbours.[34] What happened to the Association of Special Hospitals is not recorded, but one suspects that inherent lack of coordination among the hospitals played a part in their failure to resist the greater social forces.

On 21 January 1938, the Board of the West End Hospital for Nervous Diseases approached the National Hospital with proposals for merger. The idea was met with some interest as the two hospitals were complementary – the West End Hospital had 76 beds (Queen Square at that time had 222 and Maida Vale 85) specialising in psychoneurosis, and also an excellent children's department, and the National Hospital dealt mainly with the neurology and neurosurgery of organic disease in adults. The Medical Committee initially concluded that the proposal should be accepted on the condition that (unspecified) 'medical difficulties' were overcome. However, a subcommittee considered that the amalgamation was not financially beneficial and that unification of the active medical staff of the two hospitals would raise 'difficulties too great to be overcome'. Therefore, in July 1938, it was decided not to proceed with the proposal. Once again, it seems that the consultant staff triumphed by parking the idea, appalled no doubt by the prospect of having the West End Hospital staff at Queen Square. This was a characteristically self-satisfied perspective since medical staff at the West End Hospital included such neurologists as Worster-Drought and Norman Hulbert who would have brought no disgrace to Queen Square nor ruffled its physicians' plumage.

The National Hospital and the Second World War

The Second World War had profound effects on the National Hospital. Clinical activity and staffing were severely reduced. Teaching and neurological research essentially trod water as the energies of the doctors and managers were focused on the survival of both the hospital and the country. The vulnerable financial position was re-exposed, and, once again, closure or

---

[32] Cairns was also lobbying the Foundation to attract the award to the London Hospital.

[33] British Hospitals Association (BHA), *Report of the Voluntary Hospitals Commission* (London: British Hospitals Association, 1937) (Sankey Commission).

[34] *Lancet* **232** (1938): 172. We also refer readers to 'Lost Hospitals of London', a useful website that describes the many small hospitals and buildings of London that have been demolished, some with their sites now rebuilt as housing estates, supermarkets or prisons; some lying vacant; and others that survive as community health care centres or nursing homes: see http://ezitis.myzen.co.uk.

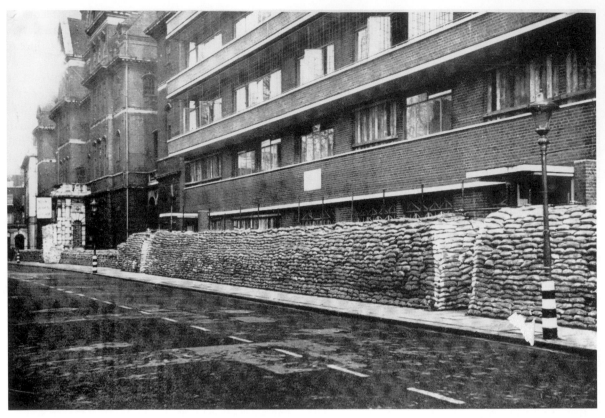

Figure 5.17 Sandbags at the main frontage of the National Hospital, *c.* 1940.

merger with other hospitals seemed a distinct possibility. The hospital struggled on, appearing, according to Matron Ling, as a cross between a mausoleum and a museum. But despite the many deprivations and difficulties, the hospital staff, and especially the nurses, were repeatedly commended for their stoicism and sense of duty during the Second World War. The hospital archives contain a unique collection of photographs and documents demonstrating the resilience of the staff at all levels during the war.

In contrast to the situation in 1914, central government had much more extensive plans in place for the organisation of civilian and military medical care in wartime.[35] The main perceived threat to London was the possibility of air raids. With uncharacteristic prescience, the Home Office had, in 1935, set up the

Air Raid Precaution Department, the responsibilities of which were partly to advise on the provision of emergency medical care for the victims of bombing. In 1936, the Goodwin Committee, constituted to examine civilian medical needs in the event of air raids, recommended that it would be necessary to clear 50 per cent of the beds in the London civilian hospitals within 48 hours of hostilities starting. In 1937, the McNulty Committee provided operational plans in support of this proposal. Since no accurate information was held centrally about the number of available beds, an early step was to survey all the London hospitals about their facilities, and Queen Square duly reported. The Munich crisis of 1938 stimulated further activity and more detailed plans were made, which were to prove their worth when war was declared. It had been predicted that within two weeks of the declaration of war, 100,000 bombs would be dropped over London, resulting in 320,000 casualties. Air-raid sirens were sounded on the day war was declared but no bombing occurred, and it soon became apparent that the initial impact of bombing

---

[35] For further details of the preparations for war and work of the Emergency Medical Service, see A. S. MacNalty, series ed., *History of the Second World War*, United Kingdom Medical Series (London: HMSO, 1952–66); and, especially, C. L. Dunn, ed., *The Emergency Medical Services*, Vol. **I**: *England and Wales* (London: HMSO, 1952).

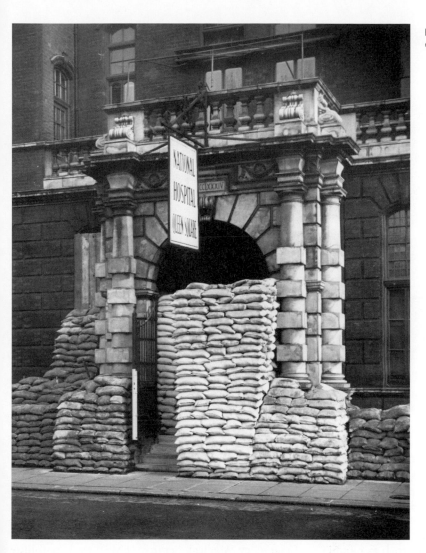

Figure 5.18 Sandbags at the main entrance of the National Hospital, *c.* 1940.

raids on London had been over-estimated. Conversely, what did become clear was that insufficient attention had been paid both to the routine medical problems of the population and to the number of wounded servicemen who would require specialist care. It was initially planned to treat servicemen in military hospitals but, as the war progressed, many ended up in civilian hospitals, including Queen Square, a fact which to some extent alleviated the financial crisis that the voluntary hospitals, including the National Hospital, faced.

In 1938, there were 146 voluntary hospitals in the London area – a number which, despite all the reservations, had increased over the previous decade – of which 64 were specialising in a limited area of medicine. As a body, they were deeply suspicious of interference in their governance and affairs and, fearful of the financial consequences, were generally unhelpful and uncooperative in relation to the government's wartime preparations. Relationships with the Ministry of Health were fraught, but the coming of war highlighted the precarious financial state of many small hospitals and this forced a more penitent and compliant approach. Furthermore, neither the public nor government were in the mood to resolve complaints which were perceived – accurately – as being focused largely on narrow self-interest.

It is an interesting reflection on human behaviour that, despite the imminent catastrophe which almost everyone anticipated, the immediate pre-war period

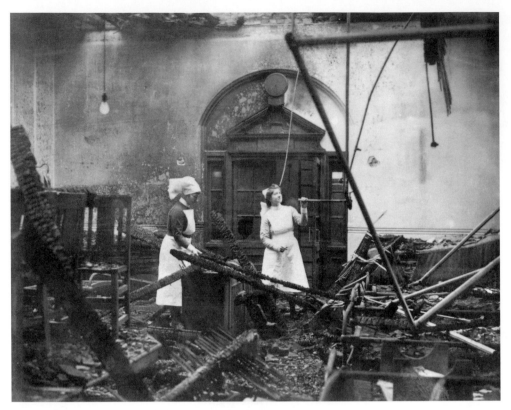

Figure 5.19 Bomb damage to Elizabeth Morgan ward, 1940.

at Queen Square, as elsewhere, was characterised by a general lack of urgency, and working patterns continued much as before. Business was conducted with no explicit advanced local emergency planning. The focus remained on domestic matters such as rebuilding and finances.[36] Indeed, in 1938, the administration actively resisted pre-war attempts by the Ministry of Health to make preparatory adaptations to the hospital services. When war did break out on 3 September 1939 and large-scale changes were immediately imposed by the authorities, these seemed to take the National Hospital by surprise. An Emergency Powers Act allowed the Ministry of Health to issue formal directions to all hospitals, including the

voluntary sector, and the hospital was, for the first time in its history, deluged with instructions from central government, who exerted firm control.

As soon as war was declared, the plans of the Emergency Medical Service (EMS) were put into operation, and a scheme for the reorganisation of hospitals enacted. The first order was evacuation of as many patients as possible away from inner London. The large mental institutions of the London County Council (and those which were previously part of the Metropolitan Asylum Board), such as Leavesden Hospital, were taken over by the EMS and recommissioned for medical and surgical purposes. Within a week, 56,000 patients had been moved out of central London, along with much medical and surgical equipment. Apart from 'a half dozen too ill to be moved', all patients at Queen Square were either discharged on 25 August 1939 or evacuated elsewhere. Much of the medical equipment was given out on loan. Many of the medical staff were moved into military medical roles. The neurosurgical staff and equipment were moved in their entirety to Hayward's Heath and to

---

[36] It seems remarkable how little the threat of war featured in the Board minutes, which conversely were full of trivial details (one that sticks in the mind was the discussion about whether the retiring secretary (Hamilton) could take the grandfather clock when he vacated his office; in the end it was allowed, as a permanent loan; another, later, in 1940, was a note that a butter-pat machine had been purchased for £8 10s 0d to allow butter to be correctly rationed).

Leavesden, where a head injury unit was established under the control of Wylie McKissock. No surgery was carried out thereafter at Queen Square until the return of the unit in 1945, and McKissock was appointed consultant surgeon at the hospital in 1946. Cumings moved his pathology services to Epsom and to Hurstwood Park to support surgical activities during the war, and he also was one of the first to return in 1945 and re-establish a laboratory in the Queen Mary wing.

The EMS scheme placed all of the London hospitals in ten sectors, and the National Hospital was 1 of 12 in sector IV, located in its inner zone. It was envisaged that the central hospital (University College Hospital for sector IV) would act as the immediate point of admission for patients, who were then moved elsewhere into outer-zone hospitals as soon as possible. Other class 1 (emergency) hospitals in the inner zone could also admit the sick and casualties in their locality, and would be paid for this work. A limited number of hospitals away from the centre were to act as 'advanced base hospitals' for the more serious cases, and to accommodate the full range of patients requiring surgery. The aim was to maintain as few beds as possible in central London, because of the perceived risk of air raids, and to expand hospitals in outer areas, including the large mental hospitals, which were converted into general medical and surgical facilities. George Riddoch played a vital role in the work of the EMS, and masterminded many of the local arrangements at Queen Square.

In their initial negotiations with the EMS, the primary concern of the Board had been to maintain the autonomy and special status of the National Hospital. When it was suggested that the hospital be designated a 'class I emergency hospital', the Board objected on the grounds that its physicians were not used to emergency medicine, there was little equipment, and only four surgeons were present – three of whom were not resident. Therefore, in 1939, the hospital was given class II status, with capacity for 79 patients, but not designated for emergency work or to admit casualties. The emptying of the hospital of its civilian patients resulted in a dramatic fall in income and the Board woke up to the fact that there would have been financial advantages in being designated as a casualty-receiving hospital, and, although Coutts agreed to extend the overdraft limit, it seemed that the hospital would have to rely on its investments as the only source of income. In a humiliating *volte-face*,

the chairman of the Board wrote to the EMS in October 1939 requesting reclassification as a class I hospital and making a further plea for financial assistance. Gordon Holmes wrote to Dr W. J. Pearson, the famed head of the EMS, stating that 'there were two new theatres with emergency lighting and air conditioning, and that new theatres could be built in the basement'. However, the appeal was turned down and, to rub salt into the wound, the Homoeopathic Hospital was designated as class I. Sector IV Headquarters wrote to Captain Styles, the chair of the Board, on 4 October 1939, graphically demonstrating the turmoil of the time:

> there is no chance of being reclassified as class I and to reserve casualty beds. It was a mistake to make the Homeopathic a casualty hospital and not the National, but now too late to change … I came out to Sector headquarters on September 1st and it has been a damnably disheartening job. By the same post we get contradictory instructions from different departments at the Ministry where there seems to be no proper central authority. The circulars they send out are like the utterances of the Roman sybil and they expect us at the sector office to know what they mean. We have a lot of class II hospitals in this sector and we have had to strip them and send their often new and magnificent equipment out to the workhouses, mental institutions, the Bonar Law College and such like which we have been turning into base hospitals … I do hope the National manages to pull through and I wish there was more I could do to help. I fear that I am only a small and shortly to be discarded cog in a first-class bureaucratic muddle.

Letters were also sent by the surgeons asking for the recommencement of surgery at the hospital, but, in November 1939, the War Emergency Committee wrote to the hospital asking it to stop making representations as they were doing their best to find a financial solution, and in December 1939 some payments were agreed, and the immediate threat of bankruptcy receded. As the war progressed new special neurological centres were established throughout the country and, at their meeting in May 1943, the Medical Committee urged that the National Hospital once again apply to receive similar recognition, but this status too was never achieved.

When, in May 1940, air raids over London did begin, the delay had allowed the EMS arrangements to take full effect and the redeployment of hospitals must have saved the lives of many patients. After 7

September 1940, when 320 bombers attacked London, raids became extremely heavy and remained so until May 1941, with an average of 200 enemy aircraft over London every night. Throughout the Blitz, a total of 46,518 bombs were dropped on London, 29,120 people were killed and 47,046 detained in hospital. Over this period, 360 bombs landed in Holborn and 277 people were killed, with 475 admitted to hospital. The heaviest raid was overnight on 10–11 May 1941, when 515 aircraft dropped more than 900 tons of bombs, killing 1,179 people and with 2,233 injured seriously enough to require hospital attention. About 2,000 people slept in air-raid shelters beneath Queen Square during the raids. The National Hospital had escaped relatively unscathed in the early period, although it did suffer a direct hit on 9 September 1940.

In October 1939, the Board wrote to the Ministry with a further plea for financial support: 'it is evident that the public had need of our usual services, and we have today 24 in-patients and an average of nine new and 60 old out-patients a day'. A minimum of 30 beds had been decided upon by the Board of Governors, in wards on the second and part of the third floors of the Queen Mary wing, and, in 1940, this was increased to an average of 45 beds. This compares with the 190 beds open in the pre-war years. The remainder of the third floor, the theatre floor and the entire sixth and seventh floors were handed over to the Ministry for their use. The wards in the old building were initially closed, but later Princess Christian ward was used for MRC-funded research into military medicine. There was a team investigating the optimal composition of flour on John Back ward, and the MRC Human Nutrition Unit was housed in the former surgical wing. Three floors of the Queen Mary wing were re-occupied by the hospital at the start of 1941, and the fourth in April, providing 37 beds, but then at the end of the year two floors had to be closed because of bombing. Morgan ward was destroyed by fire, following a direct hit by an incendiary bomb in January 1941 that also affected the sixth and seventh floors of the Queen Mary wing, resulting in repair costs estimated at £1,500. The alarm was raised by the matron at Great Ormond Street who smelled burning whilst engaged in dislodging an unexploded bomb from the lift shaft of her own hospital. Only 100 yards south in Old Gloucester Street, Boswell Street and Southampton Row, there was extensive damage and many buildings were totally destroyed. Several houses in Guilford Street were damaged and the row on the north side

of Queen Square House had to be cleared. A first-aid decontamination unit was then set up by the Ministry of Health at the hospital. The next serious direct strikes were on 14 March 1944 when 30 incendiaries fell on and around the hospital. One entered the chapel and another started a fire in one of the nursing sisters' bedrooms. The balcony of the Queen Mary wing was damaged by bombing. Finchley was leased during the war to the Middlesex County Council and, escaping bomb damage, acted as accommodation for elderly homeless people. Maida Vale Hospital was badly bombed in 1940 and two wards destroyed, with damage to the outpatients department and pharmacy. By the end of the war, there were only 33 inpatients in the hospital. One senses from the minutes and documents of the period that the feeling of crisis in London had somewhat abated by late 1942, or at least a routine had been re-established, and hospital activity began to increase – although, initially at least, to nothing like pre-war levels.[37]

At the outbreak of war, all hospitals in London were asked to take measures for their physical protection. The National Hospital installed sandbags and shutters, to secure the glass roofs, and moved the medical case notes into storage. A first-aid post for the Borough of Holborn was established on the ground and first floors of the Queen Mary wing (with no rent paid, as the Board observed to the Ministry). Geoffrey Robinson records that, on being offered the job of accountant at the hospital in 1945, he still had to negotiate the brick-built screen, erected at the top of the front steps to protect the doors against bomb blast.

---

[37] The total number of inpatients discharged in 1938 was 1,483, falling to 1,207 in the calendar year of 1939, 646 in 1940, and 502 in 1941, when only 37 beds were open. From 1942, inpatient numbers began to increase again to 709 in 1942, 736 in 1943, and 620 in 1944. The average length of stay for an inpatient in 1942 was 28 days in the 48 beds that remained open. Since there was a waiting list of 110 patients for admission, in 1943 it was agreed to increase the bed complement, although this did not prove possible until 1945 when the number had reached 78, including 30 still reserved for the EMS. By the end of 1946, the bed complement was 124, closer to pre-war levels. The outpatient clinics remained active throughout the war, with 16,007 visits made in 1940, 10,945 in 1941 (and 1,960 for massage and 2,493 for electrical therapy), and 15,315 in 1942 (and an additional 5,168 for massage or electrical treatment), compared with 34,695 in 1938 (and an additional 6,062 for massage or electrical treatment).

Although payment for the care of service personnel was relatively generous, it is no surprise that the finances of the National Hospital remained problematic during the Second World War. The accounts show income reduced from £46,121 in 1938 to £26,334 by 1941. This was due to a large reduction in donations and charitable support and also in income from contributing patients who, in 1942, paid 5 guineas for a curtained cubicle. It was said then that private wards at varying rates were in the course of preparation, but it is not clear whether any opened. The Ministry had initially refused to assist with requests for extra funding, but eventually a funding schedule was put in place, and at the annual general meeting on 24 March 1941, the acting chairman, Sir George Broadbridge, reported that:

> All voluntary hospitals in times of peace had a hard struggle to make ends meet. In wartime, the situation had grown very much worse since contributions by the generous public on which the hospitals relied so much had to a large extent been shut off. However, with the help of the King Edwards Hospital Fund and other voluntary contributors – particularly lately from the Bundles for Britain organization in America – the hospital had managed to rub along.[38]

The largest pressure was from salaries for nursing staff, which trebled in the early years of the war.[39] The

cost of maintaining a bed inflated from £5 9s 1d in 1938 to £19 5s 0d in 1946. The financial situation slowly improved from its nadir of 1943, when the accumulated debt of the hospital was over £55,000. The King's Fund continued to provide central support (£6,000 in most years during the war), without which the hospital would certainly have folded.

It was not long before the King's Fund, in 1940, again raised the proposal of amalgamating the National Hospital, Maida Vale and the West End Hospital. Each was in a precarious financial state. The National Hospital had, at the time, a £50,000 bank overdraft with Messrs Coutts and Company that could not be serviced, and it depended for survival on regular handouts from the King's Fund. Despite this, the idea of merging London's neurological hospitals was again met with opposition from the Board and Medical Committee. In part this was on academic grounds and, on 5 July 1940, the Board sent a report to the King's Fund stating that such a merger did not

> Discharge the responsibility facing the medical school committee of the National Hospital … [that] certain intellectual values have to be taken forward. Yet these intellectual values must take first place in the minds of those responsible for the maintenance and enhancement of British Neurological traditions and of the future of neurology in this country … [the] fatal flaw [was that] the position of all the staff in all three hospitals should not be prejudiced. Whilst this may not matter to a hospital where there is no systematic teaching or research, in the case of the medical school this is a matter of profound importance … A staff of some 70 persons predominantly middle aged men who are no longer engaged in active research or teaching would block the accession of young men which is a vital necessity in an advancing subject … the traditions of the medical school in particular, and of British Neurology in general, must inevitably perish beyond recall … the King Edward VII Fund was concerned only with the financial stability of the hospital, and does not concern itself with the welfare of the medical postgraduate school attached to the hospital. The Medical School committee of the hospital is unwilling to assent to a proposal that it believes to be profoundly detrimental to the future of neurology in this country.

No attempt was being made to conceal the attitude of superiority maintained by Queen Square, nor the undercurrent of contempt for the other two hospitals and, by implication, their staff. Nevertheless,

---

[38] National Hospital for Nervous Diseases, Queen Square, minutes of the annual general meeting, 24 March 1941 (Board of Management, January 1938–November 1945, p. 250). Bundles for Britain was a remarkable grassroots organisation that started as a 'knitting circle' in one New York location, but rapidly grew to have 975 branches and almost a million contributors. It delivered knitwear and clothing initially, but then also surgical instruments, medicines and medical paraphernalia. The total value of gifts to Britain exceeded $US2.5 million, and after the Second World War its founder Mrs Latham was awarded an OBE by the Queen.

[39] The nursing salaries were set by the government-appointed Rushcliffe Committee, which reported to the Minister between 1941 and 1948. It was the first national committee on salaries and emoluments for nurses. Pre-war salaries were very low – the Queen Square matron received £140 and male nurses £30, and although large increases were recommended, the salaries were still low. In 1943, for instance, the salary of a ward sister was only £130 per annum plus £70 living-out allowance. This was the topic of much critical comment in Parliament and elsewhere. It was not only nurses who had low salaries – in June 1941, the hospital porter H. Reynolds retired with a pension of £1 and 5s after 38 years' service.

negotiations did continue sporadically at the behest of the King's Fund. However, when representatives of the West End Hospital failed to attend a meeting in September 1942, the proposal was dropped and the rear-guard action of the National Hospital staff had, once again, succeeded. This small victory was merely a postponement, since forced merger with Maida Vale did take place in 1948, despite the repeated attempts of the National Hospital and its Medical Committee to prevent the amalgamation. At the same time, the attempt to maintain the independence of the medical school also failed, and it became incorporated into the British Postgraduate Medical Association in 1946.

The Practice of Neurology 1902–1945

In the early twentieth century, the medical profession referred deferentially to Queen Square as 'the temple of neurology'. Although not without its hierarchies, the hospital was largely free from the chauvinistic tribal spirit of the great London teaching hospitals. Its training and consultant staff were generally well qualified and carefully selected. After a thorough grounding in internal medicine, the novitiate was expected to serve an apprenticeship by endless clerking in outpatients and on the wards, and through acquisition of skills in medical electricity. Full neurological training, including a recommended year studying overseas, might take ten or more years. A physician at the National Hospital was expected to diagnose and care for the neurological sick, to teach undergraduate and postgraduate students, and to do some research – at its least, in the form of original clinical observation. But, without competence and a ritualised approach to clinical methods, no doctor could expect to work at Queen Square. The reputation for clinical practice there, encapsulated in the definitive account of the history and clinical examination by Gordon Holmes,[40] had its origins in the methods developed by physicians working at the National Hospital in the nineteenth century. Although no autocratic and highly personalised school of neurology dominated Queen Square in the nineteenth century (as it had at the Hôpital Salpêtrière in Paris under Charcot), Jackson and Gowers were revered and both highly influential in creating a system for assessment of patients. Their approach enabled symptoms and physical signs to be understood in terms of anatomy and physiology. By the start of the twentieth century, most doctors still considered neurology to be a difficult and complicated specialty. Eliciting abstruse signs allowed neurologists to perform diagnostic conjuring tricks that the rest of the medical profession could not match. Apart from an ophthalmoscope, their bag contained a torch, red-and-white hatpins, Snellen chart, tuning fork, patellar hammer and the mysterious two-point discriminator. At least for those based at Queen Square, neurology was seen as only for the most intelligent doctors.

This tradition of neurology at the National Hospital had evolved from clinico-pathological correlation. A thorough and ritualised examination was fundamental to the approach. When the patient died, post-mortem examination was essential and necessary training for the resident medical officers and house physicians. For the purposes of examination, Gowers had divided the motor pathway into an upper part comprising the motor centres in the brain and the pyramidal tracts terminating on the cranial nerve ganglia and anterior horn cells in the spinal cord. After 1878, cutaneous and deep tendon reflexes were being routinely elicited, but not until the late 1890s was the Babinski response added to Gowers' signs suggestive of an upper motor neurone lesion and routinely tested. The method and response varied but dorsiflexion or extension of the great toe, after the application of a mildly noxious stimulus to the sole of the foot, was considered by Francis Walshe to be the single, most important, sign. The lower motor neurone consisted of the anterior horn cell, nerve root, peripheral nerve and muscle. This distinction evolved steadily over 20 years, based on new advances in understanding the microscopic anatomy of the nervous system. Trainees learned that severe paralysis with flaccidity, wasting and absent stretch reflexes were due to a peripheral nervous lesion, whereas damage anywhere in the upper segment led to weakness, spasticity and clonus.

John Maddison Taylor, a neurologist from Philadelphia, had designed the first tendon hammer in 1888, specifically for assessing tendon reflexes – percussion hammers for examining the chest having previously been used. The tendon hammer had a triangular rubber head. The base was the same size as the striking surface of the ulnar border of the hand, and the rounded apex was designed to elicit the biceps jerk. A metal band connected to the handle encircled the head. This was the prototype of the reflex hammer

---

[40] G. Holmes, *Introduction to Clinical Neurology* (Edinburgh: E. and S. Livingstone, 1946).

still popular in the USA and many other parts of the world, and known disparagingly at Queen Square as 'the tomahawk'. It is claimed that the inventor of the Queen Square hammer was a nursing sister called Wintle, who went by the nicknames of 'Sister Electrical' or 'Buns'. In 1925, she hit upon the idea of fitting a ring pessary to a solid brass wheel and mounting it on a bamboo stick sharpened at the other end to elicit the plantar reflex. For many years, she made these herself and sold them to the doctors.[41] This hammer design made with plastic moulds rather than wood is still used in hospitals in Britain and many other parts of the world. A modified version with a telescopic metal wand allows the precious piece of apparatus to be carried in the pocket without the danger of impaling the user with the spiked end. Exactly when the tuning fork was first introduced at Queen Square is unclear, but it was certainly being widely used early in the twentieth century.

It was under the tutelage of Jackson and Gowers that Gordon Holmes gained the clinical skills that eventually led him to perfect the neurological examination. Holmes emphasised that Jackson's method was simple, and owed nothing to apparatus or instrumental techniques: 'the un-resting contemplation of facts of observation, scrupulously and untiringly acquired'. Combined with his deep knowledge of neuroanatomy, Holmes' method permitted accurate localisation and suggested the probable pathology. His understanding of physiology allowed him to speculate on the underlying mechanisms of neurological disease. Usually clear on the diagnosis after taking a careful history and observing the patient enter the consulting room, Holmes would nevertheless instruct his patient to undress for examination from top to toe. Sensation was assessed meticulously, with separate assessment of touch, pain and proprioception even in patients without any likelihood of sensory deficits. Holmes wryly commented that two types of people were unsuitable for sensory testing: those who rambled and vacillated and were unable to answer

'yes or no', and Scotsmen who suspected a catch in every question. Macdonald Critchley took the view that Holmes could coax physical signs out of a patient, like Paganini on the strings of a violin.

Curiously, in contrast to the rigorous examination technique used to diagnose neurological disorders, precision in assessment of the cognitive and mental state was still lacking. Along with most of his colleagues at Queen Square, Holmes disliked functional nervous disorders and lacked patience with those complaining of psychological symptoms. For many years, the examination of higher cerebral function – including memory and language – recorded in the case notes remained cursory. This, together with the rise of medical psychology and psychoanalysis, contributed to the schism that developed between neurology and psychiatry in the UK, which was in marked contrast to their closer relationship in continental Europe.

Much work in the hospital took place in the outpatients department in the Powis wing. Consultations were brief, with the time taken up in screening patients for their need and appropriateness for hospital investigation or simply in issuing repeat prescriptions. This could be counter-productive since, as Ernest Jones[42] reported, 'the physicians at Queen Square got their stimulation from morbid anatomy but their income from rich neurotics'. Large numbers of patients sat waiting tightly packed on hard wooden benches. Between 3 and 12 new cases were seen each day by physicians working in rooms A and B. Patients already known to the hospital were asked to attend in the afternoon and grouped into those with and without epilepsy, the two categories being requested to attend at different times. Cases scheduled for admission were asked to attend at 2.30 p.m. Patients were instructed on arrival to present their card to the hall porter, who would issue a numbered outpatient chit. The porters were also responsible for arranging the case notes and calling patients in the correct order. In 1935, a modified outpatient record system was devised, consisting of case notes with coloured discs to indicate the physician responsible for each case: Kinnier Wilson was red, Walshe blue and Symonds black. The treatment card had a similar disc. Letters were marked with one coloured disc and placed in the room where the patient was to be seen, whereas the

---

[41] This story appears in J. M. Pearce, *Fragments of Neurological History* (London: Imperial College Press, 2003). He mentions that the hammer used for percussing the chest was introduced by Dr Henry Vernon of the Great Northern Hospital in 1858 (i.e. before John Madison Taylor) and also that Gowers was quick to realise the value of using a hammer in the neurological examination. Pearce also attributes the use of the tuning fork to test vibration sense to Heinrich Rumpf, professor of medicine in Marburg, who published his method in 1898.

[42] Alfred Ernest Jones was an early English proponent of psychoanalysis and became Sigmund Freud's official biographer.

treatment card and its disc were handed to the patient. At the end of the clinic, the various letters and cards were collected from the three consulting rooms and the dispensary, and filed together in the individual case notes with the treatment card inside the letter.

In 1909, the outpatient hall in the Powis wing was enlarged and upgraded, but space continued to be a problem, so that in 1912 the classroom was converted into an additional consulting room with space for teaching (C-room). A-room contained tiered seating for about 30 students, and the A- and C-teaching rooms continued to be used in an unchanged form well into the 1980s. At the same time, the staff dining room was moved to the first floor to provide accommodation for the massage school. Despite an increasing number of referrals, some physicians continued to combine outpatient consultations with teaching, taking the history but abbreviating the examination and then, adopting the style of Gowers, discussing the differential diagnosis, probable cause, prognosis and options for therapy. The A-room clinic was staffed from Monday to Friday by the consultant in charge of outpatients, starting at 10 a.m. and with formal teaching for the first 90 minutes.

From the earliest days of the National Hospital, ward rounds had been a frightening experience for patients and intimidating for junior staff. This tradition lasted well into the second half of the twentieth century. Nurses of all grades played a subservient role, although some, such as Sister Varney, did exert a considerable degree of moral authority and were held in high regard by the doctors. Gordon Holmes' ward round took place behind locked doors. The loyal Nightingale nurses stood in awe and saw to it that the patients lay motionless on their beds clad in nightdress or underclothes. No one was permitted to read a newspaper lest the rustle prove distracting to the 'Great Man'. Only a jug of water with a glass was permitted on the locker top. In certain cases, a vomit bowl might be provided, but this was not to be touched except in dire circumstances. The use of a bedpan, however pressing, was not even to be contemplated. Patients, asked to describe the facts of their case to the entourage of doctors, were frequently chastised by Holmes for explaining symptoms in terms of the perceived cause rather than in an objective fashion. Any attempt to be other than passive during examination was another cause for irritation. As Francis Walshe later wrote, 'it is facts not amateur interpretations that are needed'.

Holmes had the habit of physically shaking his juniors if they failed to live up to his demanding standard. It was not uncommon for him to tear up the house physician's notes recording the history and examination if he felt these to be substandard. Occasionally when teaching, he would grasp a worried student by the lapels of his coat and gently rock him backwards and forwards in rhythm to his instruction. On other occasions, he might interrupt the ward round and gaze out of the window for several minutes. It was never clear whether this was to ease his troublesome dyspepsia or give time to think about a case. On one ward round, Holmes was confronted with a glamorous *Daily Mirror* beauty queen admitted with tension headaches. After the firm had moved to the next bed, Holmes told Critchley to 'get rid of her'. Perhaps, in order to maintain the interest of the junior staff, Critchley desisted. The following week, the young lady was hidden, unsuccessfully, from Holmes, who declared that either the patient or Critchley must leave the hospital.

There was particular animosity between Holmes and Wilson, and, when making their respective rounds at Queen Square, each with his own retinue of doctors of all ranks, and meeting in the passageways, neither of them would move aside for the other, so that lengthy blockages ensued. Critchley concluded

> Students who came to Queen Square found themselves in modern Verona, with the Montagues and Capulets at war. They had to align themselves either with the Kinnier Wilson clique or with the camarilla of Holmes. Never could they do both. Wilson was a vain and touchy man jealous of Holmes, and he would ostracize anyone who strayed into the other camp. Holmes, for his part, couldn't care less and simply ignored his colleague … many neurologists treasured the memories of their apprenticeship to one of the giants of neurology, and to a staunch, fundamentally warm-hearted counsellor and guide. In his profession, as in his garden, Holmes planted seeds for the profit and wonderment of generations to come.[43]

Critchley also records that James Collier, although an interesting and stimulating exponent at the bedside, used methods that caused alarm and consternation both to his juniors and to the nursing staff.[44]

---

[43] See J. M. S. Pearce, 'Sir Gordon Holmes (1876–1965)', *Journal of Neurology, Neurosurgery, and Psychiatry* 75 (2004): 1502–3.

[44] M. Critchley, 'James Collier, 1870–1935', in *The Black Hole and Other Essays* (London: Pitman Medical Publishing Co., 1964).

Collier's tactlessness was embarrassing and reminiscent of an earlier generation of physicians. He would proclaim loudly in front of other patients diagnoses such as syphilis, cancer and paralysis, and then announce to the whole ward that the unfortunate sufferer had a hopeless prognosis: 'the last patient I had with this complaint perished miserably and his brain is in the museum at St George's'. Collier seemed unable to grasp why his patients frequently burst into tears during the round. Arriving on Chandler ward, Collier sniffed the air insisting that 'there is a case of infantile paralysis on the ward' and explaining that the odour of poliomyelitis was characteristic. His conversation was punctuated by tics and mannerisms, including a hunch of his shoulders, a facial grimace and a sniff.

In 1911, a structure of medical firms was put in place, with each group of physicians having an admission day. Patients were expected to be discharged the day before their team was 'on take' because new cases were not allowed to be admitted into a bed assigned to another firm. The wards during this period were David Wire, Bentinck, Albany, Morgan, Annie Zunz, John Back, Princess Christian, Westminster, Chandler, George Charles Parker, Gibbens and the annexe.

The only consultant staff appointment made during the First World War was that of Percy Saunders,[45] a Canadian physician who made little impact on neurology. In the inter-war years, however, a number of physicians were newly appointed, many of whom became important figures in the growing specialty: Francis Walshe and William Adie in 1921, James Birley[46] in

1923, George Riddoch in 1924, James Purdon Martin in 1925, Charles Symonds in 1926, Macdonald Critchley in 1928, E. Arnold Carmichael in 1930, Derek Denny-Brown and Denis Brinton in 1935, and John St Clair Elkington in 1937. Julian Taylor in 1931, Hugh Cairns and Geoffrey Jefferson in 1933, and Harvey Jackson in 1935 were appointed as neurosurgeons. Those in other surgical specialties were Cuthbert Lockyer (gynaecologist) in 1920, Theodore Just and Terence Cawthorne (aural surgeons) in 1921 and 1936, Frederick Williamson-Noble and Keith Lyle (ophthalmic surgeons) in 1925 and 1937, George Perkins and Jackson Burrows (orthopaedic surgeons) in 1926 and 1933, and H. Lardwick (dental surgeon) in 1937. Two radiologists were appointed: Russell Reynolds in 1919 and Hugh Davies in 1931. Bernard Hart was appointed physician in psychological medicine in 1926. Many of these specialists became well known in their fields and in this inter-war period, as before, the National Hospital was staffed in many areas by leaders of the profession.

In the 1920s, the mixture of new cases and those under long-term follow-up for chronic conditions began to alter. Whereas multiple sclerosis (first known as insular, and then disseminated, sclerosis) had been a rare diagnosis for inpatients in the nineteenth century, it was now responsible for 10 per cent of admissions – much the same as neurosyphilis and brain tumour. Syphilis could still be acquired in the areas close to Queen Square, earning that condition the colloquial designation 'Covent Garden ague'. The catch-all label of functional nervous disorder was applied to about 15 per cent of admissions. One striking change was the fall in the number of patients with a primary diagnosis of epilepsy, from 35 per cent in 1880 to 4 per cent in 1929.

In the early 1920s, the dispensary issued typed annual reports to the Board of Governors which

[45] Percy Whittington Saunders graduated in medicine from Toronto University (1902), moved to England, and was resident medical officer (1909), pathologist, registrar and assistant physician (1916) to the National Hospital. He was also assistant physician to the Royal Free Hospital (1913), and full physician (1922). He was a conscientious and extremely hard-working physician, putting in enormously long hours in outpatients and in teaching. The *British Medical Journal* recalled him as: 'singularly shy and retiring, entirely lacking in the arts of self-advertisement and push-fullness … only too ready to sacrifice his own interests on behalf of others, and seemingly incapable of an unkind or ungenerous word or action. His death is a grievous loss to the hospitals he served so faithfully … and in the last five years he suffered severely from several attacks of influenza, and finally succumbed, after a long illness to an obscure form of malignant disease.'

[46] James Leatham Birley qualified at St Thomas' Hospital (1911) and was appointed resident medical officer at the

National Hospital (1912). With the outbreak of war, he served in France with the Royal Flying Corps and became its chief medical officer in France, for which he was appointed CBE (1919). Later, he was consulting physician to the Royal Air Force and a member of the War Office committee on shell-shock. He gave the Goulstonian lectures (1920) on the medical problems of flying and adaptability of the human organism to the stresses involved. He was appointed assistant physician to the National Hospital (1923) but resigned (1926) to take up the position of assistant physician and then full physician at St Thomas', where he succeeded Sir Farquhar Buzzard as director of the neurological department. He published little but showed, according to *Munk's Roll*, prowess on the cricket field and at the billiard table.

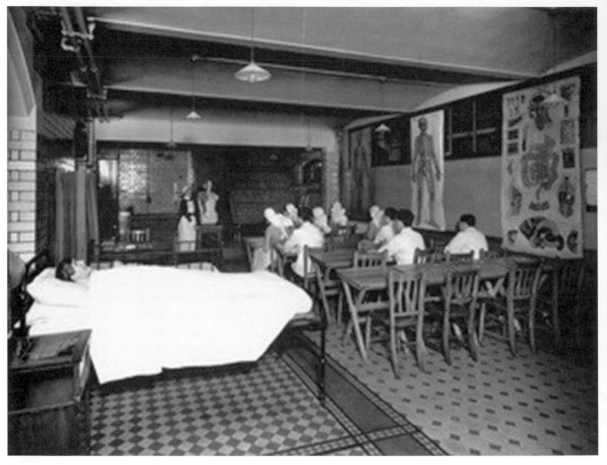

Figure 5.20 Nurse training school, 1935.

provide a snapshot of hospital prescribing. In 1920, for instance, bromides topped the list (costing £646), with other anti-epileptics such as iodine salts (£217), valerian (£35) and paraldehyde (£26) contributing to the great majority of the cost. By 1924, the prescription of drugs had doubled (and the amount of wine and spirits dispensed had also markedly increased). Although the price of bromides had fallen from its 1918 peak – due, it was thought, to the industrial situation in Germany – this was still the major source of pharmacy expenditure (the price of a pound of sodium bromide had fallen from 17 shillings in 1915–20 to ninepence in 1923). There was a suggestion that the pharmacy should open a laboratory making galenicals and tablets. There was then the first mention of an increasing outpatient prescription of the new anticonvulsant Luminal (phenobarbitone), which completely transformed the care of epilepsy (in 1922, its annual cost to the hospital was £63). Expenditure on phenacetin, belladonna and

aspirin had also risen. In 1922, there were 16,605 inpatient and 34,544 outpatient prescriptions handled by the pharmacy, and the physicians were asked to consider altering their prescribing habits in order to reduce expenditure.

In the 1920s, various other professional developments occurred. The General Nursing Council recognised the National Hospital as a training school for male and female nurses. Eye, ENT, psychiatry and post-operative surgical clinics were established, and physical therapy facilities were further expanded. Despite the fact that in 1920 the Ministry of Pensions discontinued funding for massage or electrical treatment for ex-servicemen (as they had arranged their own facilities), both the massage and electrical rooms were still heavily oversubscribed. In 1923, each treated around 4,000–8,000 patients annually, and more equipment was provided (at a cost of £3,525). The two departments separated in

1924 and a fourth house physician was hired in 1926 to cope with the increasing workload.

Junior staff appointments grew in the inter-war years and the first house surgeon was appointed in 1934. The registrar had responsibility for the upkeep and classification of case notes and records of patients who had been discharged, and provided statistics on patient numbers and diagnoses for each annual report. In those years, each member of the clinical staff received a slim pamphlet that contained the bye-laws and charter of the National Hospital and laid down the duties of trainees, as well as those of the matron, secretary and consultant staff. The first rule for a physician was that 'On reaching the age of 65 he shall retire.' For residents, one rule was: 'He shall not spend a night out of the hospital without the written permission of the chairman of the board of management.' Displayed in the doctors' mess was a list of all the medical officers who had worked at the hospital since its earliest days, and presumably obeyed this restriction. But in 1922 James Purdon Martin, who had recently been appointed as house physician, married Marjorie Blandy. The wedding was kept secret because only unmarried men and women were permitted to be employed in junior staff positions. Sometime later, Dr Blandy wrote to the Medical Committee:

> Dear Sir. I would like to draw to the attention of the medical committee 1. The hospital notes … 2. The warming pipes of the registrar room adorn the ceiling. They have contained a plentiful supply of cold water since I took over the room. At my personal request a gas stove was installed in the room and this stove 9 inches by 12 inches has been placed within two yards of the door which opens directly upon it. Only by seating oneself within less than one yard of the stove can one hope to keep ones right half warm ones left half has had fibrositis. The remainder of the room is so bitterly cold that to work in it has been and will be impossible during the winter. There is a considerable feeling about this amongst the resident staff and prospective registrars. I would be obliged if the Medical Committee would look into these matters.

No response is recorded, but soon afterwards Blandy was replaced. In reflections published 60 years after his appointment to the staff, Purdon Martin found that, despite a significant increase in medical staff at Queen Square during his time, the number of outpatients reduced, although the number of inpatient admissions doubled.[47] Purdon Martin attributed these changes in part to the disappearance of Sydenham's chorea, tabes dorsalis, postencephalitic Parkinsonism and general paralysis of the insane.

In some respects, the Victorian age seemed not to have faded. Even in the 1920s, Purdon Martin recalls seeing a beautiful carriage and pair of gleaming horses with footmen and coachmen in livery on the box waiting for the chairman. However, one postwar change was in the doctors' attire. The professional silk hat, formerly *de rigueur*, disappeared and, for some time, many consultants continued to wear military uniform. In 1930, the medical staff were grouped into four firms that reflected the organisation of outpatients, a concept which had not changed over the previous 30 years. Firm 1 comprised Drs Collier, Adie and Carmichael; firm II, Drs Grainger Stewart, Walshe and Purdon Martin; firm III, Drs Holmes, Riddoch and Symonds; and firm IV, Drs Hinds Howell, Kinnier Wilson and Critchley. Firm I was allotted 45 beds, firm II 53, firm III 47, and firm IV 45. The neurosurgical cases were admitted into the physicians' care pre- and post-surgery, and each firm had one male and one female ward, with Chandler and Bentinck set aside for contributing cases and to absorb any surplus from the other parts of the hospital. Thus, by the early 1930s, the medical staff had again settled into a traditional form of practice, and neither they, nor indeed the country, were expecting the renewed conflagration of the Second World War.

The number of consultant staff became seriously depleted after 1939. Not only were staff deployed to the military, but Scott, Reynolds, Stewart, Holmes and Hinds Howell retired or resigned their positions during or just before the war, and Hart and Danvers Bailey left at the end of the war. Cairns and Jefferson moved to consultant work elsewhere, and the decision by Denny-Brown, on 29 July 1941, to take up a professorship at Harvard was a further blow to the academic reputation of the hospital. Between 1938 and 1944, no new consultant staff were appointed other than Charles Hallpike, supported by the MRC, in 1944, as aural physician. The only physicians who were not commissioned and remained active at the hospital for the duration of the war were Walshe, Purdon Martin, Carmichael, Greenfield and Elkington.

---

[47] J. Purdon Martin, 'Recollections of Queen Square', *British Medical Journal* **283** (1981): 1640–2.

As it became clear that a victorious end to the Second World War was probable, thought turned again to the hospital's future configuration. The Medical Committee listed the requirements they considered to be needed: improved outpatient facilities; accommodation for a capacity of 350 beds – 220 for medical cases, 60–75 for surgical cases, and 60 for psychiatry; new building, and the probability in the future that every hospital would offer a private wing, with 100 beds, were suggested; and a 'chronic wing' of 200 beds for long-term care of those neurologically disabled patients. In January 1945, the Hospital Development Committee provided its own list of needs, noting that research and instruction were the primary purposes of the hospital: 300 beds, including 14 for private patients; 246 nurses, 58 resident domestic staff, 10 resident medical staff, 10 student doctors; a new building programme, starting with a nurses' hostel and a new block for outpatients and special departments; and a third block for inpatients (with Moberly again suggested as the architect, reflecting satisfaction with the structure and arrangements of the Queen Mary wing). These optimistic proposals were clearly made without any appreciation of how dire the financial position of the country was to be in the postwar years.

After the cessation of the war, activities gradually returned to normal. The EMS was formally disbanded and the 24 beds earmarked for their use were re-allocated to neurosurgery. The military vacated their requisitioned wards (David Wire, Princess Christian and John Back) in January 1946. Brinton, Riddoch and Symonds were demobilised. Jackson and McKissock returned to the hospital in August 1945 and very soon were operating regularly. In the following year, two resident neurosurgeons were appointed (Dr Hertz and Dr Swarzwald) and the number of procedures increased from 149 to 366 by 1946. There had been no deaths amongst the senior medical staff during the war, but a grievous loss for the hospital was that of George Riddoch, who died in 1947, aged only 58, from complications of abdominal surgery; his death was attributed to overwork during the war, and he was universally mourned.

Some Physicians of the War and Inter-war Years

The biographies of the dominant five physicians at Queen Square in this period (Holmes, Wilson, Walshe, Critchley, Symonds) are given in the next chapter, and of the surgeons in Chapter 9. These were the doctors who led their disciplines and played the greatest role in determining the course of the hospital, and of neurology. But, here, as a brief aside, we mention six other physicians who also played an important part in the hospital and/or in neurology in the early and mid twentieth century; they were supporting actors, but nevertheless stamped their mark on the hospital history. They were doggedly supportive of the work of the hospital and they contributed to its modest scientific output.

Four were born into the Victorian era, and make a vivid quartet. The first was Sir Edward Farquhar Buzzard, the eldest of Thomas Buzzard's four sons, who, like his father, became a leading physician at the National Hospital. He was educated at Charterhouse and won a scholarship to Oxford. His career there was largely on the playing fields, where he won a blue in football but only a fourth-class degree in natural sciences. His academic performance improved at St Thomas' Hospital, and, after qualification (1898), he became house physician to his father's close friend, Hughlings Jackson, and then was appointed as assistant physician at the National and the Royal Free Hospitals (1905). He gave the Goulstonian lectures in 1907 on 'Toxic and Infectious Diseases of the Nervous System' and forged an impressive reputation in these pre-war years. In 1910, he was appointed as visiting physician to St Thomas' Hospital and the Belgrave Hospital for Children. He was the classic Edwardian Englishman, and during the war had a distinguished record in the London command where he attained the rank of colonel and was an important figure in the shell-shock debates. At Queen Square, he held various posts, rising to the position of physician to the outpatients. He resigned prematurely from the hospital staff in 1921, presumably due to his other many commitments. His departure was a significant loss to the hospital not least as his career continued to flourish. He was appointed physician-extraordinary to King George V in 1923, and made a baronet in 1929, and in 1928 appointed Regius professor of medicine at Oxford. There he was instrumental in obtaining support and finance from his friend Lord Nuffield and was the key university figure in the setting up of the Nuffield department, and for which he was rewarded with the Osler Memorial Medal (1940). Highly effective in committee work, and as a medical politician, he was elected president of the Association of British Neurologists and the British Medical Association, and later as the first chairman of the Nuffield Provincial Hospitals Trust. He tried his hand at national politics, but was the unsuccessful Conservative candidate in the Oxford University seat in the 1937 by-election (losing to Arthur Salter, the Gladstone professor of political theory and institutions, and another leading academic figure of the period). As president of the BMA, he played a part in the creation of the National Health Service and was an important influence on various aspects of its development, especially promoting preventative and social medicine. He foresaw the end of the voluntary hospitals but helped their incorporation into the NHS. He was a eugenicist but made few original contributions to neurology, his chief contribution to the subject being perhaps his co-authorship with Greenfield of the textbook *Pathology of the Nervous System* (1921). *Munk's Roll* relates that 'students found him awe-inspiring and ponderous' but 'unusually silent, and his ward teaching was reduced to the essentials of diagnosis', a reticence due to shyness which 'contrasted with the polished fluency of his prepared public disquisitions'.

He must have been an interesting contrast to the fellow Conservative, Thomas Grainger Stewart, who was one of the longest-serving consultants on the staff of Queen Square, although one who left almost no neurological traces. His distinguished medical father must have thought highly enough of himself to give his son exactly the same name, and certainly the younger Stewart had a promising early career qualifying as a gold medallist in medicine in Edinburgh, he studied in Munich, and was then appointed house physician at the National Hospital (1902) and rose steadily through the ranks, as resident medical officer, assistant pathologist (1904), assistant physician (1908) and physician (1924–45, thus serving the hospital for over 40 years, including 34 on the consultant staff). However, his academic contributions were relatively slight, and he is best known for a now little-known textbook of neurology co-written with Aldren Turner, his work on cerebellar tumours with Gordon Holmes, and the eponymous Stewart–Holmes sign of inability to check a movement when passive resistance is suddenly released (the rebound phenomenon). He was apparently careful and seemed oblivious of time when examining patients on ward rounds and in outpatients. His obituarist in *Munk's Roll* paints a striking picture of a man with plentiful reddish hair, a solemn expression and with

his chin sunk onto his chest when contemplating a problem. He could be gruff, and apparently disconnected from his milieu, and, in contrast to his father, was a notoriously dull and oligo-syllabic lecturer. His initial friendship with Gordon Holmes cooled and deteriorated to the point of a fist fight with coats off in the hospital laboratory, after which the two men barely spoke and, despite his long association with the hospital, Holmes does not mention his name once in his own history of Queen Square (of 1954). Grainger Stewart had a prolonged period of unspecified illness in the early 1920s, with physical and psychological components, which restricted his private practice. He was shy and laconic and, perhaps surprisingly, was praised by Walshe,[48] who wrote that he was:

A high-principled and unselfish man, a considerate chief and colleague, a sound clinician of the old school, a conservative in the best sense of that abused word, and a man conscious in his later years of having lived into an age he liked less and less … haste was unknown to him, and slow in speech as in movement, his outpatient sessions and ward rounds were no brief events, but went on, regardless of the clock, until he had discharged his sense of duty to the task in hand. The weekly pattern of notional half-days that forms the chessboard upon which the modern consultant makes his permitted and allotted hospital movements could not have contained him, and had one, unkindly, explained it all to him and discussed its influence upon the life and thought of the physician of today, he would have been horrified.'

Of his leisure time, *Munk's Roll* records:

shooting and deer-stalking were his favourite sports. He was an expert with the shot gun and … an intrepid, tireless and skilful stalker … he had tales to tell of being held by the legs while leaning over a precipice to shoot a stag below … and he was never happier than when after a stag on the high tops.

It was not uncommon for him to stalk from early morning til mid-afternoon, catch the night train to London to see his patients the next day, then travel back to Aviemore the following night and do a full day's stalking. A deer track across a steep scree where few ever ventured is called the 'Doctor's Walk' after him.

A younger version of Grainger Stewart in many ways was James Purdon Martin. Born in County Antrim, he was educated at the Royal Belfast

---

[48] F.M.R. Walshe. 'Thomas Grainger Stewart'. Lancet **270** (1957): 693–4.

Academical Institution and trained at Queen's University Belfast, graduating with first-class honours in mathematics; but, considered unfit for service during the First World War, he then studied medicine, and qualified in 1920. His first house physician post was in Liverpool, but within a year he had been appointed to the National Hospital and, in 1925, became a consultant. He also held appointments at the Hammersmith Hospital and the Seaman's Hospital Greenwich. In 1946, he was elected the first dean of the newly con-stituted Institute of Neurology, on Greenfield's sudden resignation. For some years, he served as associate editor of *Neurology* and he gave the Lumleian lecture on 'Consciousness and its Disturbances' (1947). His most significant achievements in neurology relate to the basal ganglia, and in 1927 he described the association between hemiballismus and contralateral lesion in the subthalamic nucleus. Based on studies on post-encepha-litic Parkinson's disease carried out at the Highlands Hospital after retirement, he published *The Basal Ganglia and Posture* (1967). Considered slow and pon-derous by his critics and daunting by some of his juniors, Purdon Martin became seemingly fossilised as he aged, although Reginald Kelly thought that history might judge him one of the greatest clinical contributors of his day. Louis Sachs described him as:

> endlessly thoughtful and ingenious in designing a variety of mechanisms and methods that made it possible for even the most incapacitated patient with Parkinsonism to achieve an artifical normality in gait and posture; lines painted on the floor, coun-terweights in the belt, loudly ticking pacemakers to set the cadence for walking, and these he always learned from his patients to whom his great book is dedicated. He was indeed a great human pioneer, and understanding and collaboration were central to his medicine. Patient and physician were co-equals, on the same level, each learning from and helping the other and between them arriving at new insights.[49]

In his youth though, he was something of a Lothario, famous for what became known as 'Purdon's leap', a jump across a gap in the roof of the hospital which he was said to perform in pursuit of nurses, a form of athletic pursuit which he no doubt gave up in 1922 on the occasion of his secret marriage to Majorie Blandy. His over-riding passion outside work was ballroom dancing, and the porters at the National

Hospital kept the telephone address of the Hammersmith Palais as one of his contact numbers. After retirement, he took an apartment in Queen Square and, even in the 1980s, was occasionally asked to visit the hospital to give a clinical opinion, requiring the registrar to receive him on the hospital steps as he descended from his sumptuous motor car. He died in his ninetieth year, in the hospital he had served for most of his working life.

The fourth member of the late Victorian quartet was William John Adie. He came from an unconven-tional background, was born in Australia and left school at 13 when his father died, to work as an errand boy. Recognising his intelligence, the employer arranged for him to have evening classes and Adie passed the examinations necessary for university entrance. An uncle based in Massachusetts then paid for a one-way ticket to England where Adie obtained a scholarship to Edinburgh and graduated in medicine in 1911. He had picked up knowledge of German while in Australia and obtained a postgraduate scho-larship to visit Berlin, Munich, Vienna and Paris before returning to London. In the First World War, he served as a doctor in France and, away from the battle due to measles, was one of few survivors in the Northamptonshire Regiment's retreat at Mons. He transferred to the Leicestershire Regiment and was mentioned in dispatches for improvising a gas mask made of clothing soaked in urine. He was given med-ical charge of the 7th General Hospital and appointed consultant to the 2nd Army Centre for head wounds in 1916. After the war, Adie was appointed medical registrar and, in 1921, consultant to the Charing Cross Hospital, and assistant physician to the National Hospital and Moorfields, also working, for a while, as physician to the Royal Northern and Royal London Ophthalmic Hospitals and as neurologist to the Mount Vernon Hospital. His contributions to neurol-ogy were varied, but he remains best known for describing his eponymous pupil (with Holmes; based on a series of 19 patients) and for his descrip-tion of narcolepsy. He also wrote on pituitary tumours, head injury (described in Chapter 9) and multiple sclerosis, and, with Critchley, described 'force grasping and groping' in frontal lobe disease. He was a founding member of the Association of British Neurologists, and was present at the famous founding meeting on 28 July 1932 in Gordon Holmes' house in Wimpole Street. He was by all accounts an exceptional teacher, and described as having a

---

[49] Cited in his *Munk's Roll* obituary (Royal College of Physicians, Vol. VIII (1984–1988), p. 323).

personality 'that was not merely attractive but immediately lovable – modest, simple, and approachable – and [with] all the other qualities of character and training that go to make a great physician'. He was a keen ornithologist, and his obituary in *IBIS*, the journal of the British Ornithology Union, talks of his frequent Sunday visits to the causeway in Staines for the study of ducks. Adie retired early because of coronary artery disease, and died months later, aged 48.

The other two physicians were born in the first years of the twentieth century. Denis Hubert Brinton had an upbringing in striking contrast to Adie's. Educated at Eton, where his father was a classics master, he glided effortlessly to Oxford where he read classics (awarded a first) before turning to medicine at St Mary's Hospital Medical School. He was appointed first as registrar at the National Hospital and then as consultant at St Mary's and the National Hospital in 1935. *Munk's Roll* recalls his 'elegance, charm and excellent character. No one could doubt his altruism, lack of prejudice except for quality, and overt honesty. He had humour without malice.' He served in the RAF as a neuropsychiatrist, rising to the rank of air commodore, and also had a strong faith, being invited by Archbishop Fisher to serve as a member on the Commission on Divine Healing (1953–8). Ian McDonald, a pupil and close friend of Brinton, attested to his 'warmth, generosity, humour, sense of fun, and abiding interest in people made him beloved of those who knew him well'. Gautier-Smith remembers him as 'without doubt one of the nicest and kindest men on the staff during my nearly thirty years at Queen Square'. He was rather unworldly, and Gautier-Smith recalls an occasion, at a ceremony to mark the opening of the new student building at St Mary's, when he announced to the mirth of the audience that 'We have every reason to be proud of this magnificent erection', and the tabloid press had a field-day. The funeral address by Sir Richard Nelson encapsulated his qualities: 'careful objective compassionate, skillful, and bounding in common sense'.

Final mention goes to John St Clair Elkington. The son of a general practitioner in Shropshire, he excelled in his Newport Adam's grammar school and won a scholarship to Trinity College, Cambridge, studying medicine there and at St Thomas' Hospital (1928). He was elected E. G. Fearnsides Scholar of the University of Cambridge in 1932, the year in which he was also appointed consultant neurologist at St Thomas' Hospital, aged 28, on the premature death of James Birley. He joined the staff of the National Hospital in 1937 and gained the reputation as an excellent teacher and and stalwart of the Medical Committee. Elkington was a keen College man, being elected as Murchison Scholar (1930), fellow (1934), censor (1954) and then senior censor. He wrote the chapter on neurology in Price's *Textbook of Medicine,* and his special interest was in cerebrovascular disease, the topic of his Lumleian lectures (1958). He flourished in London as an aesthete and fastidious bachelor. His *Munk's Roll* obituarist describes him as a man who entertained with generosity, but with the formality of a perfectionist, surrounded by objects of beauty in his house in Montagu Square. When abroad on medical business, he preserved 'very carefully the elegant, precise, distantly courteous image of the accomplished London physician', but when on holiday preferred lone travel in rough clothes and with a rucksack, a 'voluntary scholar-gipsy'.

Contributions to the Medical Literature 1902–1939

It is a strange paradox that, after the spectacular achievements of the nineteenth century, and despite acknowledging the importance of advancing the science of neurology, further contributions by the hospital staff to the repository of knowledge on neurology and neurosurgery after 1900 were less dramatic. There were several reasons for this lapse. Most common neurological disorders had already been described and, before new disciplines and technologies began to influence the understanding of mechanisms of neurological disease, the possibilities for further original discovery were limited. Progress depended on individual brilliance and, taken together, the cadre of neurologists based at the National Hospital early in the twentieth century, always small in number, did not match that of the previous generation. Civilian practice was interrupted by the two World Wars which committed many consultants to matters of wider national priority. The rise of neurology elsewhere in the world and at a few rival centres in Britain reduced the hegemony of Queen Square. The changing patterns and regulation of British medical practice left less room for innovation. That said, both World Wars created neurological injuries on an unprecedented scale, enabling significant contributions from members of the consultant staff. The pandemics of influenza and encephalitis lethargica after

1918 also provided that generation of Queen Square neurologists with unexpected research opportunities. Although the National Hospital still remained in the vanguard of clinical neurology in these years, and the outstanding work of Horsley and Gowers spilled into the twentieth century, it is surprising how few Queen Square alumni were considered to have made contributions of lasting value. The exceptions in this period were Holmes, Wilson, Walshe and Symonds, whose work is described in the next chapter. For the rest of the staff, the enduring achievements appear somewhat meagre. Here we adopt the undeniably artificial approach to evaluating the role of the National Hospital academically by scrutinising the list of papers and books that appear in *Morton's Medical Biography: An Annotated Check-list of Texts Illustrating the History of Medicine.*[50]

In 1900, based on post-mortem findings in seven cases, Risien Russell, Batten and Collier described simultaneous involvement of several tracts, but sparing grey matter, due to subacute combined degeneration of the spinal cord. The posterior columns were most affected throughout the length of the cord, but also with involvement of the direct and crossed pyramidal tracts extending from the lumbar region to the medulla and pons. After considering vascular damage or inflammation, they concluded 'There only remains for our consideration the view that a toxic agent is jointly responsible for the changes in the spinal cord and for the anaemia in those cases in which this symptom exists; and to this view we strongly incline.'[51]

By 1900, Gowers had largely completed his contributions to clinical neurology. His monograph on the *Border-land of Epilepsy* remained to be published. But he had one more important concept to report. In his paper on myopathy (1902), reproducing a lecture given at Queen Square, he suggested that muscle disease arises from abiotrophy. Gowers developed a metaphor on the struggle for survival of muscle lacking nutrition revealed by the 'overgrowth of interstitial tissue'. On the pseudo-hypertrophic form of muscular dystrophy, Gowers recalled an engraving by Raphael of 'The Transfiguration', allegedly depicting an epileptic fit, which hung over the fireplace in the consulting room at Queen Square. Gowers told of a visit once paid to the hospital by Duchenne, who pointed to the angel's calves as an example of the disease named eponymously after him. But, apart from referring to his own monograph on Duchenne's disease,[52] Gowers' main purpose was to describe a new form of muscular dystrophy that exclusively affects the distal musculature. Medicines and electrical therapies were useless and all that Gowers could recommend as a means of delaying the otherwise inevitable decline in muscle strength was exercise: 'We should also do our best to try to save [patients] from efforts to obtain good from the many straws held out for hope to grasp at, which are magnified by promise into rods of rescue. Those who promise with assurance that which cannot be, always find too ready credence, as is often only found too late.'[53]

---

[50] Fielding H. Garrison produced *An Index Catalogue of the Library of the Surgeon-General's Office* 17 (1912): 89–178; later this was revised as *A List for Students Published as a Supplement to the Bulletin of the Johns Hopkins Hospital* 1 (1933): 333–434. Leslie Morton published the much-expanded *A Medical Bibliography* in 1943 (London: Grafton), pp. 412). Garrison and Morton has remained in print from that time, most recently updated in print by Jeremy Norman (Norman, ed., *Morton's Medical Bibliography* (Aldershot: Scolar Press, 1991), pp. 1241) and now available online: http://historyofmedicine.com. Apart from papers discussed in more detail below, the contributions from Queen Square were (in alphabetical order): C. A. Ballance, *Some Points on the Surgery of the Brain and its Membranes* (1907); C. A. Ballance, *Essays on Surgery of the Temporal Bone*, 2 vols. (London: Macmillan, 1919); C. A. Ballance and A. B. Duel, 'The Operative Treatment of Facial Palsy by the Introduction of Nerve Grafts into the Fallopian Canal and by Other Intratemporal Methods', *Archives of Otolaryngology (Chicago)* 15 (1932): 1–70; M. Critchley, *The Parietal Lobes* (London: Edward Arnold, 1953); W. R. Gowers, *The Borderland of Epilepsy: Faints, Vagal Attacks, Vertigo, Migraine, Sleep Symptoms, and their Treatment* (London: J. & A. Churchill, 1907); H. Head and G. M. Holmes, 'Sensory Disturbances from Cerebral Lesions', *Brain* 34 (1911): 102–254; G. M. Holmes, 'A Case of Virilism Associated with a Suprarenal Tumour: Recovery after its Removal', *Quarterly Journal of Medicine* 18 (1925): 143–52; V. A. H. Horsley, 'The Linacre Lecture on the Function of the So-called Motor Area of the Brain', *British Medical Journal* 2 (1909): 125–32; S. A. K. Wilson, 'Progressive Lenticular Degeneration: A Familial Nervous Disease Associated with Cirrhosis of the Liver', *Brain* 34 (1912): 295–509; S. A. K. Wilson, 'Pathological Laughter and Crying', *Journal of Neurology and Psychopathology* 4 (1924): 299–333; and S. A. K. Wilson, *Neurology*, ed. A. Ninian Bruce (London: Williams & Wilkins, 1940).

[51] J. S. Risien Russell *et al.*, 'Subacute Combined Degeneration of the Spinal Cord', *Brain* 23 (1900): 39–110.
[52] *Pseudo-hypertrophic Muscular Paralysis: A Clinical Lecture* (London: J. & A. Churchill, 1879), p. 66.
[53] W. R. Gowers, 'On Myopathy and a Distal Form', *British Medical Journal* 2 (1902): 89–92.

With a shared interest in gadgets, in 1908 Robert Clarke and Horsley described a stereotactic frame for making precise lesions in the brain. The following year, Horsley took as the subject for his Linacre lecture delivered to the Master and Fellows of St John's College, Cambridge, 'The Function of the So-called Motor Area of the Brain'. Horsley had been loosely caught up in a monumental drubbing aimed at Ferrier in a paper on the kinaesthetic sense in which Bastian argued forcibly that there is no motor cortex, all movement being sensation derived from the muscular and kinaesthetic sense.[54] On the occasion of this debate at the Neurological Society of London, on 16 December 1886, Horsley had pointed out that any emphasis Bastian placed on the cases Horsley had operated upon was misplaced since they were too few in number to add any weight to the matter. But Horsley was persuaded that the boundary between afferent and efferent activity occurs at a molecular level within the layers of the cortex and not in gross anatomical separations of sensory and motor centres. Returning to this topic nearly 20 years on, Horsley regretted that Bastian's term, 'kinaesthesia', had not gained acceptance. Working with Charles Beevor from 1885, Horsley showed that movement (of the arm) in response to electrical stimulation is most predictable when cortex in front of the Rolandic fissure is stimulated, especially in species higher up the evolutionary scale. Horsley had never elicited movement when stimulating the post-central gyrus. He concluded, on this basis: 'We may be certain, therefore, that the more essentially motor part of the kinaesthetic representation of the upper limb lies in the gyrus in front of the fissure of Rolando.'[55] Bevan Lewis had previously correlated the increased density of giant pyramidal cells of Betz to motor excitability of the pre-central gyrus. Yet, as Jackson had taught, all function is indivisibly 'sensori-motor', and it was not logical to designate any one part of the cortex as exclusively sensory or motor in its representation. It followed that strict cortical localisation was an awkward concept.

William Adie was newly appointed at Queen Square when, in 1926, he published a paper on sleep and falling with emotion. Adie favoured the term 'narcolepsy' for the sleepiness and 'cataplexy' for the falling attacks.

> The disease I am about to describe is characterised by … attacks of irresistible sleep without apparent cause, and curious attacks on emotion in which the muscles relax suddenly so that the victim sinks to the ground fully conscious but unable to move … two kinds of sudden attack occur, sleep … without cause and cataplexy on emotion … [such that] anyone possessing this knowledge would be able to recognise a typical case … narcolepsy-cataplexy is an endocrine-nervous, the crucial lesion being restricted to … the floor of the tween brain in and around the vegetative centres that form a part of the pituitary system … it is almost certain that hormones play a part … my study of narcolepsy has taught me that … nervous and endocrine organs work together as equivalent parts of an intimate system.

Not everyone was impressed. Within a year, Wilson, who later fell out with Adie, published his own account of the narcolepsies:

> Recent communications dealing with the subject are reduced in value by ignorance or neglect of previous work … hypotheses are evolved which suffer … fatally … from failure to take all the germane data into consideration … to describe … narcolepsy as a *morbus sui generis* is a nosological error, yet in the communication of … Adie … this regrettably occurs *passim* … experience should surely have convinced the neurologist that no good purpose is served by a hard-and-fast schematization of a clinical syndrome – which is all that narcolepsy can possibly be – to fit a conception based solely on an original description … I was able to observe an [emotional attack] from beginning to end and to examine the patient's neurological condition during it. Dr Macdonald Critchley, the present registrar at the National Hospital, was with me at the time … testing the knee-jerks I found them completely abolished and … Dr Critchley … obtained a slight but definite left extensor response … which I corroborated … just as we were finishing … the patient said 'I'm all right, sir' … testing his knee jerks again, I found them active.[56]

In his descriptions of narcolepsy, Wilson wrote of 'easy gradations from somnolence to sopor, sopor to stupor, and stupor to coma'. This was a reference to

---

[54] H. C. Bastian, 'The "Muscular Sense": Its Nature and Cortical Localisation', *Brain* **10** (1887): 1–137.

[55] V. A. H. Horsley and R. H. Clarke, 'The Structure and Functions of the Cerebellum Examined by a New Method', *Brain* **31** (1908): 45–124.

[56] W. J. Adie, 'Idiopathic Narcolepsy: A Disease Suis Generis; with Remarks on the Mechanism of Sleep', *Brain* **49** (1926): 257–306; S. A. Kinnier Wilson, 'The Narcolepsies', *Brain* **51** (1928): 63–109.

the mysterious 'sleepy sickness' that led eventually to half a million dead or disabled victims. Patients with acute encephalitis lethargica were admitted to Queen Square but, at first, the epidemic had far less impact on the case mix of the wards than had been seen in the preceding four years when admissions were dominated by the large number of cases of war neuroses.[57] Between 3 and 11 cases were admitted annually for each of six successive years from the end of the First World War. Purdon Martin, who had seen some of the first cases of encephalitis lethargica recorded in Britain during his medical post in Liverpool, wrote that, by the time he was appointed as house physician at the National Hospital in 1921, the pandemic appeared to be past its peak. Addressing the Medical Society of London on the ambulatory form of encephalitis lethargica, in which a relatively mild flu-like illness was followed by devastating sequelae, Farquhar Buzzard described the prevailing mood and concern among the medical profession:

> When I had the honour of addressing this society on the subject of lethargic or epidemic encephalitis in December 1918, our interest was aroused by the recent outbreak in our midst of a disease which we regarded as a stray-visitor, whose sojourn might not unreasonably be expected to be of short duration, and whose back we should not be sorry to see. Events have not justified this expectation, as our guest is still outstaying his welcome and shows as little inclination to take his departure as we can have of ability to expedite it. At the end of six years his role has changed from that of a casual unwelcome visitor to that of a resident pest providing a serious menace to the health of the community.[58]

Macdonald Critchley and Aldren Turner summarised the experience of clinical features seen in cases managed at Queen Square.[59] Starting in the early 1920s, a different clinical picture was starting to be recognised. Now admissions for the late sequelae of the illness were observed, with at least 30 suspected cases admitted each year from 1922 to 1931, peaking at 84 in 1926. The residual mental disturbances were so profound in many of the survivors that, in 1925, the Metropolitan Asylums Board established a unit at the Northern Hospital, Winchmore Hill (later to become known as Highlands Hospital) to take 100 of the most severe paediatric and young adult cases for residential care. Kinnier Wilson was appointed to the staff but is said to have visited only occasionally. He did, however, publish extensively on post-encephalitic Parkinsonism and the description of the pandemic in his textbook (*Neurology*, 1940) is important as a historical source of information. Charles Symonds took a particular interest in the neuropsychiatric sequelae of encephalitis lethargica following his appointment to the staff of Guy's Hospital:

> Of equal interest is the defect of moral sense resulting in children from encephalitis lethargica. Many examples were recorded at the time of the epidemic without recognizable impairment of intellectual function, and sometimes without any of the physical sequelae commonly observed after the illness. There can be no doubt of the organic basis of the defect, which is usually irreversible, though we have no clues in this instance for localization. What is most remarkable is that this sequel did not occur in adults, suggesting that whatever structures are involved are essential for learning to distinguish between right and wrong but not necessary for the preservation of such distinction, or, to put it in another way, if learning has continued long enough the process involved has produced physical changes in such a widespread net of neurones that local damage has not the same effect as it would have at an earlier stage of the process. Whatever the interpretation may be, we seem to be dealing with a kind of moral agnosia, and observe the mind deprived of this sense proceeding to the most ruthless extremes of antisocial conduct. In this there is reasoned direction, and often great skill in escaping detection and punishment.[60]

The unit at the Northern Hospital almost closed before it had a chance to prove itself useful because of a difficulty in recruiting nursing staff, but it managed to survive and later to expand, and, with strict discipline and occupational therapy, the children improved, although many developed a Parkinsonian syndrome. In the 1960s, these were amongst the first patients in the UK to receive levodopa, responding

---

[57] Neither Wilson's paper on narcolepsy nor any of the articles relating to encephalitis lethargica that follow are listed by Garrison and Morton as classics in the literature of neurology.

[58] E. Farquhar Buzzard, 'Encephalitis Lethargica', *British Medical Journal* (27 November 1924): 937–9.

[59] W. A. Turner and M. Critchley, 'Respiratory Disorders in Epidemic Encephalitis', *Brain* 48 (1925): 72–104.

[60] C. P. Symonds, 'Critical Review: Encephalitis Lethargica', *Quarterly Journal of Medicine* 14 (1921): 283–308.

spectacularly, but rapidly developing intolerable side-effects.[61]

The Schools of Massage and Electrical Therapy 1902–1945

As described earlier, massage and electrical therapy occupied a special place in the hospital in the nineteenth century. Both helped to differentiate Queen Square from other hospitals in London, and each had proved a significant factor in bringing the hospital to public attention and establishing its reputation. The electrical department, in particular, was frequently singled out for praise and commendation, and this despite the fact that an influential section of physicians considered both massage and electrical therapy as no better than elaborate mumbo jumbo. Cushing also wrote of 'the poverty of the therapeutic tripod of iodine, bromide and electricity'[62] in marked contrast to the place of neurosurgery. Gowers decried their lack of biological efficacy, but nevertheless prescribed both extensively for their 'psychological' (or placebo) effect.

By the end of the nineteenth century, it looked as if electrical therapy might become redundant but, bizarrely, with the advent of diagnostic radiology its use again began to flourish, since, illogically, the two were linked, at least in the minds of the public. In 1907, the Royal Society of Medicine founded a section of electrotherapy but this was closed in 1931. Before 1914, treatment in the electrical department at Queen Square remained a significant part of outpatient activity, and throughout the inter-war years around 10,000–15,000 treatments were given annually. The electrical room and the gymnasium and massage departments were re-equipped several times. Massage therapy was enhanced by the introduction of the Swedish method,[63] which proved popular with

soldiers, who must have appreciated the soothing hands of the therapists after the brutality of war.

Because of its prominence, it did not take long for there to be calls to improve teaching and instruction. Books were written by the physicians and informal teaching provided, but this was recognised to be insufficient, and the formalisation of teaching took an important step forward in 1903–4 when, as part of a widespread review of nursing education and training, the new Board of Management appointed a committee which included Risien Russell and Aldren Turner 'to enquire into and report upon the teaching of massage and electrical treatment in the National Hospital'. In December 1903, the committee presented its report, arguing that: the hospital should adopt the Swedish system of massage; that special non-resident instructors in massage be engaged to teach the Swedish system under the supervision of the resident medical officer, rather than that of the assistant matron; that a new system of examination and certification in massage and electricity be adopted; and that a dedicated School of Massage be established with an annual intake of at least 12 pupils. As for the curriculum, the committee insisted that:

> An elementary knowledge of anatomy and physiology is a necessary part of a medical rubber's education … the art of massage and a competent knowledge of electrical treatment cannot be acquired in less than three months … fairly close study … persons holding the National Hospital's certificate ought to be distinctly above the average and recognised to be so by the medical profession … [although] we do not consider that the teaching has hitherto been deficient … On the contrary, it has been careful and painstaking.

The report was a landmark in the history of therapy at the hospital, and its recommendations were accepted by the Board. A school of massage, under the direction of Madame Gripenwald, was duly opened in October 1904, with the first nine students soon enrolled. Certificates of efficiency were awarded to 28 students by the end of 1905. Described in annual reports as 'very successful', a further 38 students qualified in 1906, 31 in 1907, 42 in 1908, 36 in 1909 and 50 in 1910. James Collier told the Medical Committee in March 1908 that the teaching of massage in the hospital was

---

[61] The condition continued to attract attention. Robert De Niro and Robin Williams visited Highlands Hospital when making the film *Awakenings*, an adaptation of Oliver Sacks' book of the same name (London: Duckworth, 1972) about the effects of levodopa on post-encephalitic Parkinsonism. Cases of sporadic encephalitis lethargica continued to be seen at Queen Square and Maida Vale into the 1980s. Macdonald Critchley came out of retirement to see one of these patients and agreed that it was highly reminiscent of the cases he had studied in the 1920s.

[62] 'The Special Field of Neurological Surgery', *Bulletin of the Johns Hopkins Hospital* **16** (1905): 78.

[63] The Swedish method comprised long strokes (*effleurage*), muscle kneading and rolling (*petrissage*), friction and

---

rhythmical chopping and tapping (*tapotement*), friction and vibration, combined with joint movements. It was said to promote relaxation and reduce muscle tension.

'undoubtedly the most efficient in London at the present time'. However, he expressed concern about the steadily increasing demand, especially in the outpatients department, and a subcommittee appointed in May 1910 was critical of the administration and standards of practice for both massage and electrotherapy. It recommended wide-ranging reform of these practices and the adoption of an official scheme for exercise applied systematically throughout the hospital.

Facilities for physical treatment were greatly enhanced by implementation of these changes and the opening, in 1910, of a new gymnastic room and physical therapy department quite separate from massage. As wounded soldiers returned from the front during the First World War, the numbers of patients requiring therapy for paralysed limbs increased, and both inpatient and outpatient massage and electrical therapy were in great demand.

In response, the massage school and school for electrical treatment were merged in June 1917 into a new School of Massage and Electrical Treatment with a joint Committee of Management established by the National and University College Hospitals, chaired by Sir Frederick Macmillan, and housed in 29 and 30 Queen Square. Although the core course in medical electricity resembled that previously offered by the school at the National Hospital, the curriculum for massage and medical gymnastics was more intensive, included Swedish remedial exercises, and was extended to 24 weeks. It conformed to requirements of the Incorporated Society of Trained Masseuses (ISTM), the main body responsible for setting standards for training, examination and qualification in massage in the UK since 1895, and students who had successfully completed the National Hospital/UCH joint course were eligible as candidates for the ISTM professional examinations. In general, the new joint school offered a somewhat broader and more academic approach to training than its predecessor. In addition to student nurses from UCH and the National Hospital, who could enrol at half the standard fee of 15 guineas per course, individuals affiliated to the National Institute for the Blind were eligible for a specially designed eight-month course in medical massage and gymnastics at a fee of £25. In December 1917, it was decided to extend the instruction in electrotherapy instituted in 1910 to include Finsen light treatment,[64] use of radium and radioactivity, and diathermy treatment.

The new school ran into difficulties during its first year as there were few applications for the electrical courses, which therefore were reduced from four to two each year, and the instruction of male students, especially in Swedish remedial exercises, proved difficult to organise satisfactorily. In the first 18 months, almost all the nurses sent on the electrical and massage courses came from Queen Square rather than University College Hospital, although the small financial surplus achieved was divided between the two equally. The balance sheets for 1918 and 1919, the school's first two full years of operation, showed that nearly 80 per cent of income generated from fees came from the massage course. Later, the contribution from the electrical and Swedish remedial exercise courses grew more even. However, as the school became established, student numbers increased and, by the early 1920s, the medical electricity courses usually had between 40 and 60, and the massage and medical gymnastics courses 50–90 students. However, by the late 1920s, the school seems to have been thriving, the link between the National Hospital and UCH was working well, and the school was proud of the fact that it was the only one providing instruction in massage for male students. Throughout the 1920s, the school achieved a modest financial surplus, and in some ways this was its heyday. Initially, demand for treatment was high but this did not last, and a deficit of £37 5s for 1932 increased to £323 2s 4d by 1934, met by a levy on the participating hospitals. Following an increase in course fees from £30 to £40, student numbers fell significantly, so that the deficit soon reached £500. By 1936, senior staff were leaving and the school's finances proved a serious drain on the resources of both hospitals.

In November 1936, the school was forced, through construction of the new Queen Mary wing, to move into the basement of 48 Guilford Street, described as 'cold, stuffy, noisy and so cramped that … if more students enter the School it will be difficult to find room for them'. There was still considerable demand for the treatment and Matron Cecily Tafe's report to the Nursing Committee of 12 October 1937 noted that, apart from those undergoing treatment in the electrical department and the exercise room, the number of patients receiving daily massage varied from 60 to 80 on the wards and from 15 to 30 in the outpatients department. The massage staff consisted of one sister, three assistants and two instructresses. Conversely, Matron Tafe estimated that staffing in

---

[64] Niels Finsen, a Faroese-Danish physician who received the Nobel Prize for physiology or medicine (1903) for the introduction of phototherapy.

the electrical department was insufficient for the number of treatments being prescribed. She recommended merger of the massage and electrical departments with a joint staff complement of one nursing sister, four full-time senior assistants and ten half-time workers. In 1937, with the deficit now £895 8s 3d, it was decided 'not to enrol any more pupils ... and generally to arrange the closure of the School of Massage and Electrical Therapy as soon as possible'.

There was, at the time, a crisis in nursing recruitment (at Queen Square and, indeed, generally in London hospitals) and it is possible that the matron considered that running the massage school was simply not practicable. However, its loss was not much mourned. The importance of massage and electricity in the therapeutic work of the National Hospital had diminished by 1930, and there was general scepticism about the value of both therapies. In 1928, the neuropsychiatrist and former Army neurologist Thomas Ross, first director of the Cassel Hospital, had reiterated Gowers' opinion and described electrotherapy and massage as forms of 'concealed psychotherapy'.[65] In 1940, Hamilton regarded both therapies as ineffectual and offering nothing more than a placebo effect: 'Hospital physicians still prescribe these forms of treatment and the patients are in most cases obviously relieved in body and ... in mind because so many wonderful things are being done for them'. The last Queen Square doctor with any interest in electricity was Danvers Bailey who was not listed in annual reports in the period, and was effectively marginalised by his more influential colleagues. The electrical room at Queen Square was finally closed in the 1940s, without anyone really noticing. Massage, however, evolved into 'physiotherapy' which has since remained a core therapy in all hospitals.

---

[65] T. A. Ross, 'The Characteristics of a Psychogenic History', *Journal of Neurology and Psychopathology* **8** (1928): 287.

Five Dominant Physicians

There is an apocryphal story told of the perfect case at Queen Square in the 1930s: the history to be taken by Charles Symonds; the physical examination carried out by Gordon Holmes; the differential diagnosis discussed by Kinnier Wilson; and William Adie to speak to the relatives. The story may have originated from Macdonald Critchley.[1] Significantly there is no place here for Sir Francis Walshe, but between them, Holmes, Wilson, Symonds, Walshe and Critchley were those members of the consultant staff whose personalities and clinical activities dominated the practice of neurology at Queen Square over a period of five decades.

Gordon Morgan Holmes

Gordon Morgan Holmes was the leading figure in British neurology during the first half of the twentieth century.[2] He was born in Dublin on 22 February 1876. His mother, Kathleen Morgan, inherited land in County Louth that his father, also Gordon, farmed. A shy and solitary boy, Holmes learned about the flora of the Wicklow

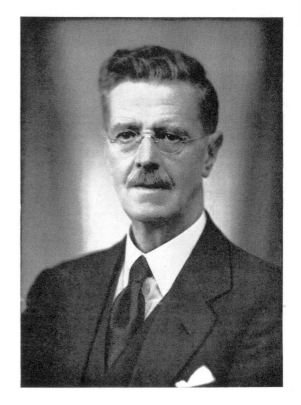

Figure 6.1 Gordon Holmes.

[1] Symonds himself describes Holmes and Wilson as 'great physicians ... Holmes a master of the discipline of physical examination; Wilson profound in thought. I recall Holmes twisting my arm to emphasise a fault in my clinical description; Wilson pacing up and down frustrated by his inability to solve a problem.' Symonds considered Holmes to have a warm and impulsive nature whereas Wilson was cold and calculating, although with a deeper mind.

[2] For a biographical account of Holmes, see F. M. R. Walshe, 'Gordon Morgan Holmes. 1876–1965', *Biographical Memoirs of the Fellows of the Royal Society* **12** (1966): 311–19. Outstandingly, the best biographical essay is by (Basil Gerald) Parsons-Smith: B. G. Parsons-Smith, 'Sir Gordon Holmes', in F. C. Rose and W. F. Bynum, eds., *Historical Aspects of the Neurosciences: A Festschrift for Macdonald Critchley* (New York: Raven Press, 1982), pp. 357–70. The various other essays, including our own, lean heavily on Parsons-Smith, who wrote from personal knowledge, and information provided by Kathleen Holmes, his daughter.

Hills and acquired skills in making wheels and carts from men on the farm. Largely self-taught, but encouraged by the village schoolmaster, Holmes eventually went to Trinity College Dublin, intending to study mathematics or classics but switching to natural sciences and then to medicine. He qualified with a BA (1897), MBBCh (1897) and MD (1903), obtaining several prizes as a student. After graduation, he worked in Dublin at the Sir Patrick Dunn Hospital and Richmond Lunatic Asylum.

Between 1898 and 1900, Holmes studied comparative neuroanatomy with Ludwig Edinger and Carl Weigert at the Anatomical Institute in Frankfurt, supported by a Stewart scholarship from Trinity College. Things did not start well. Edinger instructed Holmes to draw sections of the spinal cord, but after two days his efforts were deemed inadequate and torn up by Edinger.[3] Eventually, at the eighth attempt, Edinger was satisfied and, before long, Holmes was so highly regarded that Edinger assigned to him the precious specimen dating from 1892 when Friedrich Leopold Goltz removed the forebrain of a dog about which Edinger confessed 'I can't make anything of it.'[4] Later, Holmes was offered a post as assistant neurologist in Frankfurt, and might have stayed had it not been necessary for him to assume German nationality.

On his return from Germany, Holmes brought recommendations from Edinger addressed to Gowers and Horsley. He visited Gowers while he was at dinner who, with napkin in hand, told Holmes brusquely that he was not good enough for the National Hospital. With only an hour to pass before catching the boat back to Ireland, where he intended to stay, Holmes called later on Horsley, who was enthusiastic about the work in Germany and supported his application. At a Board of Management meeting of the National Hospital held on 22 July 1902, by the casting vote of the chairman, Holmes was appointed second assistant house physician.[5] It is said that Hughlings Jackson, aged 74 and deaf, was unable to hear discussions on the various candidates and asked his neighbour for whom he should vote: Taylor wrote on a scrap of paper 'Holmes'. In time, Holmes worked at the National Hospital as house physician, resident medical officer, pathologist, director of research (1906) and physician (1909–41). His consultant appointment was delayed and people younger than Holmes joined the consultant staff before him because, at that time, Holmes lacked the essential MCRP qualification.[6]

In 1904, Edinger published the seventh edition of his book on neuroanatomy, dealing with the nervous system of mammalia, especially humans, in advance of a second proposed volume covering comparative anatomy of the brains of lower vertebrates.[7] We learn something of their relationship and the influence that Edinger had on Holmes' activities in London from a letter on National Hospital notepaper dated 15 May 1904:

My dear Professor … [Congratulations] on the greatest possible improvement in [the] book … a volume which is far better than any I know on the anatomy of the nervous system. The portions in italics on topographical diagnosis are excellent … Many thanks for having sent me the paper by Bing. I have read it over very carefully but must say that I cannot at all agree with his views … as regards tabes he does not seem to understand the disease and has not raised any objections to the Ersatz-theorie that I could not easily answer. Of course I admit that your theory does not explain all, but this is only a negative argument against it and as such is much weaker than positive objections and neither he nor anyone else has raised such against the Ersatz-theorie which have not or cannot be answered. I have now examined a couple of hundred cases of tabes and am more than ever convinced of the value of your view. I have seen 30–40 cases (at present there are 6 cases in the hospital) … so I may be pardoned for assuming some knowledge of the condition. I may say that it has been observed here that the knee jerks may be absent in children of families so affected before they have begun to walk, and till then surely the child uses his arms more than his legs; and then too Bing assumes that the degeneration of the pyramidal tracts occurs in a late stage of the disease but I have found Babinski's sign present in the earliest cases I have seen and I believe it may sometimes be found before the loss of the knee jerks. No one has been more convinced than I of the value of your work, but its

---

[3] Edinger was himself something of a draughtsman and, when his portrait was being painted by Lovis Corinth, helped the artist to depict the brain that Edinger was dissecting as part of the image. See F. H. Lewey, 'Ludwig Edinger (1855–1918)', in W. Haymaker, ed., *The Founders of Neurology* (Springfield: Charles C. Thomas, 1953), pp. 27–31.

[4] G. Holmes, 'The Nervous System of the Dog Without a Forebrain', *Journal of Physiology* **27** (1901): 1–25.

[5] At the same meeting, Farquhar Buzzard was appointed pathologist in place of Collier, and Grainger Stewart appointed senior house physician.

[6] Grainger Stewart was appointed before Holmes. This may have contributed to their subsequent rift, although eponymous assignment of the rebound phenomenon in cerebellar disease to Grainger Stewart, not Holmes, may also have been a factor.

[7] L. Edinger, *Vorlesungen über den Bau der nervösen Zentralorgane des Menschen und der Tiere*, 7th edn, Vol. **I** (Leipzig: Vogel, 1904), p. 398. Holmes' notice appeared in *Review of Neurology and Psychiatry* but we have been unable to locate this.

application must have some limitation. I shall await with eagerness the appearance of the second volume of your book for as you know the comparative anatomy interests me very much, but I suppose it will be some time till you have it ready for publication. As you will see by the address I am still here [and] will probably remain nearly another year. I have not yet found time for any pathological or anatomical work but have as much clinical material as I can possibly use.

Shortly after qualification, Holmes worked his passage to New Zealand as a ship's doctor. On the return journey he stopped in South Africa, volunteered to work for the British, and was due to be interviewed by Cecil Rhodes but left hurriedly when his ship was ordered out of port at the outbreak of the Boer War in 1899. Holmes retained the spirit of adventure and applied to join the *Terra Nova* on Robert Falcon Scott's expedition to the South Pole. But, meanwhile, a ruptured Achilles tendon had allowed Holmes to prepare for the MRCP examination which, once passed (1908; FRCP 1914), made him eligible to apply for a vacancy on the staff at Queen Square when Charles Beevor died unexpectedly and he was appointed. So Holmes waved goodbye to the ill-fated expedition at the quayside when, in 1910, Scott and others left for the South Pole. Perhaps through the contact with Hughlings Jackson, who had introduced him to use of the ophthalmoscope, Holmes was also appointed to the consultant staff of Moorfields Eye Hospital (1914–27).

At the outbreak of war in August 1914, Holmes volunteered for service in the Royal Army Medical Corps but was rejected because of myopia. Occupation as a special constable did not suit his ambition and he went to France with Percy Sargent to work in a Red Cross Hospital. Sensing the enormous contribution Holmes could make to the war effort, his myopia was soon ignored and he was commissioned in the Royal Army Medical Corps and appointed consultant to the British Expeditionary Force in France, where he remained until 1918, at the front or based at Stationary Hospital No. 13. He was put in charge of medical services on the Western front, replacing Charles Myers, whose tolerance of shell-shock Holmes could not stomach, and thereafter he introduced a much more hostile approach to the condition.

Harvey Cushing met Holmes and Sargent in France on 3 May 1915 and was impressed by the extraordinary workload and opportunities that this presented for research on function through studying focal injuries of the brain and spinal cord. Holmes showed Cushing 12 cases of injury to the longitudinal cerebral sinus producing quadriparesis in the acute phase, but with recovery; and of cervical cord transection with paralysis and disturbed thermal regulation, for which there were notes of more than one case for each and every spinal segment. A few weeks later (24 May 1915), Cushing wrote to Holmes at Stationary Hospital No. 13, sending reprints of studies on cerebrospinal fluid that Holmes had requested:

I saw H[enry] H[ead] in London and had a very interesting evening with him and heard him tell his amusing and exciting experiences in Brittany at the outbreak of the war … I find a lot of activity over here [the USA] in regard to sending expeditionary units from this side. The Harvard group will be succeeded by a contingent from Philadelphia, led by a man named [James P.] Hutchinson. He was here yesterday and told me that [Joseph] McCarthy is going over with him and you may want to get in touch with him. The proposal from Keogh for a group from here to take a unit of 1040 beds has been accepted and I believe that they are planning to leave by the first of July. It is just possible that they may be at Etaples. One of my young assistants here who is an A-1 man, would I think like to go over very much and work with you and Sargent as a volunteer and take over some of the burdens of history taking and so forth. Would you care to have him and would it be possible for him to be taken on in this way?

But, evidently, Cushing found the hospital, staffed by only ten doctors with 900 acutely ill soldiers and a further 300 arriving daily, uncomfortable and with inadequate medical records. He wrote of the deplorable conditions of the patients with trench foot, demoralised by the effects of poison gas, infested with lice, maggots and scabies, and sick from contact with rats bloated with human flesh. Later, Cushing and Holmes disagreed on the management of cases:

Sargent … rushed in a poor Canadian … whom Nature had treated badly by giving him a cleft palate, and the Boche had added insult by a penetrating wound of the skull. One of the types of cases I fear Sargent and Holmes and I are going to disagree about, for they favour leaving them alone. At all events there was a stinking abscess in the temporal lobe and under local anaesthesia this was found and

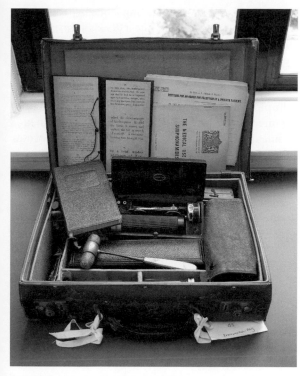

Figure 6.2 Gordon Holmes' medical bag.

opened, and the missile easily extracted with the magnet.[8]

Near the end of the war, on 29 June 1918, Cushing and Holmes attended a research committee in Paris:

Foster Kennedy – excellent! Gordon Holmes urges more neurology and in the afternoon we got it – three more papers by Frenchmen whom no one could understand as they undertook to read it in English. [André] Léri spoke and also Pierre Marie – nice old man! Later a meeting of the Committee with tea for the sake of the British, though afternoon tea is *défendu* nowadays in Paris.

Holmes had an impressive war record, attaining the rank of lieutenant-colonel, being twice mentioned in dispatches. During the war, Cushing had sent 'an excellent Kodak [photograph]' taken by him of Holmes and others, with copies for Lady George Makins, Lady Percy Sargent and Sir Cuthbert Wallace, 'for I am not sure whether or not you have wives. If you have not, you should

have and give them these prints as a gift from me.' In fact, Holmes had met Rosalie Jobson, daughter of Brigade Surgeon W. Jobson, in France, where she was working as a medical officer. Rosalie, an Oxford graduate who represented the university at three sports, was also a hockey international, and later became a paediatrician. He proposed while rowing on the Thames during leave from France. They married in 1918 and were demobilised after the armistice as Colonel G. M. Holmes CMG CBE and Captain R. Holmes. Introduced initially to boating by Beevor, after the war Holmes hosted an annual event in which he took three residents from the National Hospital, including Walshe, to Oxford, where a skiff was hired at Folly Bridge and the four rowed downriver to Staines, staying the night at Wallingford and Hurley. Holmes' two-month annual summer holiday was taken in Ireland, working on the farm, coaching the local team at tug-of-war and attending country house parties. Holmes and Rosalie lived in a large house at 9 Wimpole Street, with nine servants to look after the family.[9] He started each day with a cold bath and washed his thick hair, a habit acquired in France to remove lice, read *The Times*, walked to Queen Square or Charing Cross, and played golf every Wednesday and Sunday. In the evening, Holmes read Shakespeare or Thackeray, and the poetry of Tennyson and Francis Thompson, before going to bed. The family moved to Farnham, Surrey, during the Second World War when the bombing was intense and the house in Wimpole Street, now too large, was wanted by the American military.

After the First World War, Holmes returned to his appointments at the National Hospital, and also at Moorfields Eye Hospital from where he resigned in 1927, being replaced by William Adie with whom Holmes worked at Charing Cross (from 1920).[10]

---

[8] See H. Cushing, *From a Surgeon's Journal* (London: Constable & Co., 1936), p. 256; and see p. 388 for Cushing on the subsequent meeting in Paris.

[9] There were three daughters – Kathleen, Rosalie and Betty – each of whom joined the Women's Services during the Second World War.

[10] See G. M. Holmes, 'Partial Iridoplegia Associated with Symptoms of Other Diseases of the Nervous System', *Transactions of the Ophthalmological Society of the United Kingdom* **51** (1931): 209–24, and W. J. Adie 'Pseudo-Argyll Robertson Pupils with Absent Tendon Reflexes: A Benign Disorder Simulating Tabes Dorsalis', *British Medical Journal* **1** (1931): 928–30, for description of their eponymous pupillary abnormality. This had already been described by Morgan and Symonds: O. G. Morgan and C. P. Symonds, 'Internal Ophthalmoplegia with Absent Tendon Jerks', *Proceedings of the Royal Society of Medicine*,

Holmes also saw patients at the Seaman's Hospital in Greenwich. As a young consultant at Queen Square, Holmes earned his living in private practice working in New Cavendish Street and then at 58 Harley Street, London. Without time or funds designated for research, Walshe considered that the later generation of medical investigators owed people such as Holmes much respect because, although the pre-clinical and other sciences were well catered for, it was the voluntary effort of individual researchers that kept clinical science alive in the British Isles during the inter-war years. In 1939, Holmes again served as consultant to the Emergency Medical Service and, with George Riddoch, was largely responsible for setting up an adequate service in neurology during the Second World War.

Holmes was tall and imposing, with a hawk-like gaze and lowered eyebrows, and seemingly inexhaustible physical and mental energy. In the foreword to Holmes' history of *The National Hospital, Queen Square* (1954), Sir Ernest Gowers paid tribute to 'the robust strength which made possible his long hours of work, to his remarkable powers of observation and concentration, and to his talent for taking great pains and for accuracy in detail'.[11] These personality traits made Holmes an outstanding teacher of neurological medicine, characterised by lucidity uncontaminated by theatricality or rhetoric in bedside teaching, although he did not lecture well. He could be fierce. Challenged by a co-examiner who felt that he was being unduly severe on a candidate who appeared distressed, Holmes roared with laughter and explained that 'he was very good, very good, and I had already given him high marks when I found out

Section of Neurology **24** (1931): 867–9; but, as Symonds said later, 'I missed the tonic reaction so it doesn't designate.'

[11] On 15 March 1963, Jack (John Benignus) Lyons wrote to Holmes remembering a visit made 12 months earlier, in which Lyons had sought details of Sir Victor Horsley for his proposed biography, 'which has not made much progress since I have been busy with other matters' (J. B. Lyons, _The Citizen Surgeon: A Life of Sir Victor Horsley_ (London: Dawnay Ltd, 1966), p. 305), and saying how much he had enjoyed re-reading Holmes' history of _The National Hospital_, noting that 'nurses thought that Sir Victor's ghost haunted the place. I am also rather puzzled by the failure of the War Office to give Horsley employment in France. Perhaps he was too old for active service? On the whole it seemed rather odd that he was sent to the Middle East.' This letter is tucked within Holmes' copy of J. B. Lyons' 'The Advent of Neurophysiology', _Journal of the Irish Medical Association_ **52** (1963): 55–61.

he was Irish and we were having a blazing row about Dublin'. In *The Spice of Life* (1993), John Walton relates that Holmes and a brilliant female student in Newcastle were shouting at each other across the ward: 'we were all concerned lest he decided she was not fit to pass the examination, but when he came stumping along the ward in high dudgeon his only comment was "best student I have ever examined"'. Holmes had humour but no wit, did not tell anecdotes and fidgeted visibly during speeches after dinner, which he disliked. He had many friends among London doctors, including Leslie Paton, James Collier, Frederick Batten and James Taylor. Later he was especially close to Walshe and Symonds at Queen Square, and Lennox Broster at Charing Cross.

Between the wars, many trainees from the former Commonwealth and the USA came to work with Holmes as clinical clerks and, although they had to survive scrutiny not unlike recruitment to a Guards' regiment, survivors became his lifelong devotees and often close friends. Denny-Brown regarded a clerkship with Holmes as the 'most highly prized opportunity'. Holmes expected residents at the National Hospital to show initiative in developing a piece of research during the three years of their appointment. We can assume that it was Charles Aring who dubbed himself 'the American ambassador to the court of Saint Gordon' and who repeatedly watched Holmes spend time, despite a busy schedule, resolving difficult diagnoses, following the doctrine that 'more clinical puzzles are solved by taking a new history than by all the laboratory tests'. Holmes went further in arguing that 'the laboratory is useful when kept to heel'. Aring considered that 'Never the philosopher, [Holmes] tended to distrust speculative thinking and relied rather on the accurate recording of clinical observations and their correlation with pathologic data.'[12]

For Aring, Holmes was the ultimate exponent of the medical history. However, the anecdote with which this chapter opens acknowledges that Symonds took the art of history to a higher level, especially since he allowed the influence of emotional factors. After Holmes, his were the rounds most cherished by foreign students. Denny-Brown regarded perfection of the clinical examination as Holmes' greater skill, and considered this not to be well

[12] C. D. Aring and D. Denny-Brown, 'A Tribute to Sir Gordon Holmes: On the Occasion of his 90th Birthday, February 22nd 1966', _Journal of Nervous and Mental Disease_ **141** (1966): 497–504.

appreciated. Holmes expressed likes and dislikes without much diplomacy and made apparent his disdain for the careless or ineffective resident. Bad case reports were torn up – the trick learned from Edinger – in order to improve their quality. Holmes was critical of notes that were amended and with text rubbed out: 'I learned from Henry Head never to erase. You might later want to know what it was you wrote. It is better to cross out.' Aring, with others, formed 'The pants-down club', otherwise known as the 'Grand order of the braces', for those whose clinical opinions and methods had been corrected by Holmes and who had benefitted from his exacting discipline. Much later, Holmes was pleased to receive a 10-dollar gold piece from these former students in recognition of their admiration and affection.

As did all visitors at that time, Aring had noticed that Holmes shared an attitude to psychological illness that many of the visitors found awkward and poorly aligned with contemporary ideas in psychiatry. In fact, Holmes can be considered the person who most influenced attitudes to neuropsychiatry at Queen Square between the wars, and he was considered somewhat rough with these cases. As Critchley recalled on Holmes' attitude to men with shell-shock:

> He never liked these people ... and house physicians would hide patients thought to have an hysterical illness during Holmes's ward round partly, at least, to save their own skins Holmes having ordered that the patient be discharged.

That said, Holmes wrote:

> Even normal persons are suggestible; anyone can walk along a plank lying on firm ground, but may be unable to do so when it spans an abyss; and suggestion is useful in clinical neurology because it may be the basis of symptoms and it can be managed.[13]

Holmes always maintained that there is a lineage in the methods of medicine, as in all fields of scholarship. Edinger taught Holmes the functional significance of anatomical investigations. His own skills in taking the history and methodology also had their origins in the physiological philosophy of Hughlings Jackson and Henry Head, supported by the work of Ferrier, Sherrington and others. But for Denny-Brown, this preoccupation with clinical evaluation and anatomical and pathological detail, at the expense of an experimental neurology and understanding of disease mechanisms, was one of the failures of British neurology. Nonetheless, Denny-Brown excluded Holmes from criticism, arguing that his special and outstanding contribution was a series of classical investigations on the significance of physical signs of nervous system disease in man.[14] Denny-Brown makes the point that Holmes used pathological verification to validate his elucidation of physical signs. He was interested in the dynamic aspects of physical changes and their physiological significance. For Holmes, eliciting scientific data at the bedside required a discipline of methods as rigid as that of the laboratory, and this was the basis for the high standards he demanded of clerks and house physicians. Unlike the theatrical performance, ritual tests for labyrinthine and cerebellar function, 'obscure and devious reflexology', endless matching of innumerable eponymous syndromes and hagiographic mnemonics celebrating their inventors that characterised the style of neurology in continental Europe and gave the impression of knowledge without advancing understanding, Holmes taught 'the *how* of symptomatology' and ways of eliciting physical signs that gave them infallible significance. Furthermore, the doctrine of physical signs was not a poll in which enough boxes ticked ensured a diagnosis, but, rather, a process of deductive analysis at which Holmes was the undisputed master.

Holmes was elected to membership of the Neurological Society of London on 22 January 1903, and appointed on 15 October 1907 to the Committee of Management. He acted on behalf of the Guarantors at the meeting at which arrangements were put in place with Macmillan for publishing *Brain* under the editorship of Henry Head. Holmes attended 38 meetings of the Committee of Management or Guarantors between 15 October 1907 and 18 February 1953.[15] He was absent during the First World War, attending no

---

[13] See G. Holmes, *Introduction to Clinical Neurology* (Edinburgh: E. and S. Livingstone, 1946), p 176. In all his work, Holmes insisted on an anatomical substrate in support of mechanistic or physiological hypotheses.

[14] D. Denny-Brown, 'A Tribute to Sir Gordon Holmes', *Journal of Nervous and Mental Diseases* **141** (1966): 497–504.
[15] The archives of *Brain*, albeit very scant and deficient, retain two hard-bound notebooks containing manuscript entries and other material pasted-in, recording minutes of the Committee of Management and the Guarantors from 1 October 1907 to 7 February 1936 (volume 1) and 12 November 1936 to 6 April 1967 (volume 2).

meetings after 9 February 1914 until 16 December 1918. Holmes acknowledged that the high reputation of *Brain* in the medical and scientific literature was largely due to Head's editorship. In turn, Holmes was often singled out in the minutes for having given particular help to Head over many years. Holmes served as editor of *Brain* between 1922 and 1937. His name had been added to those appearing on the cover of each issue, from 26 January 1920. He was clearly exempt from the accusation made later that none of the cover names, 'who are supposed to assist the editor', did in fact do so. For Holmes, editorial work was onerous and, although discussions had periodically taken place regarding the need for an editor's assistant, on 24 October 1928 Holmes threatened to resign if the committee did not provide additional support. Therefore, Walshe and Greenfield were appointed as assistant editors in 1929. This settled matters for almost a decade but, on 5 November 1937, Holmes restated his intention to resign and this time he meant it. His resignation was accepted with 'the utmost regret' and, in 1938, he was succeeded as editor by Walshe.

At the Annual General Meeting of the Guarantors on 1 February 1927, Holmes agreed to write a history of *Brain* and its relationship to neurology but, scheduled for volume 50, this never appeared. The Guarantors returned to that suggestion on 23 January 1928, when it was proposed that Ferrier and Crichton-Browne should write a history to include photographs of the founders. Ferrier died later that year and Crichton-Browne was then aged 88. Again, nothing happened. Over this period, the finances of *Brain* improved and there were various suggestions for disposing of surplus income. In the event, rather few of Holmes' proposals were supported. But what did emerge was enthusiasm for publishing collected papers by distinguished neurologists and scientists. On 23 January 1929, the decision was taken to republish the writings of Hughlings Jackson under the editorship of Taylor. The two volumes of *Selected Writings of John Hughlings Jackson* duly appeared in 1931–2 and, despite not recouping their costs, the Guarantors soon committed to a second publishing venture during Holmes' editorship – the *Selected Writings of Sir Charles Sherrington*.[16]

Meanwhile, in the interests of scholarship and informing the modern reader, the Guarantors continued to honour their alumni by reprinting earlier publications. Working with Horsley from 1883 to 1887 on the 'minute representation of movements' in the cerebral cortex, Beevor had studied the impairment of action in muscles following cerebral palsy. This work formed the basis for his four Croonian lectures delivered to the Royal College of Physicians during June 1903, and published as *Muscular Movements and their Representation in the Central Nervous System* (1904). Holmes acknowledged the importance of this contribution to neurology, considering that 'It did much to clarify fundamental questions on the cortical localisation of motor functions which had become confused in the spate of publications that followed the original investigations of Hitzig and Ferrier.'

Such was Holmes' enthusiasm for the work that, on 7 March 1950, he advised the Guarantors to reprint Beevor's lectures. This was approved (500 copies at a cost of £192 10s 0d, plus 15 per cent for charges from Macmillan, to be sold at 5s). As with most of the books and other occasional material published by the Guarantors, this did not sell well and the reprint failed to cover its costs.

Notwithstanding their losses on these publishing ventures, the Guarantors of *Brain* did not neglect their former editor. Holmes was a clinician scientist who used the lessons of clinical neurology, and especially the medical experiences of the First World War, to advance ideas on the functional anatomy of the central nervous system. This is his great contribution to neurology. We are advantaged through having two collections of his selected papers, each containing a bibliography of Holmes' writings. Walshe selected ten representative papers in 1956 and Charles Phillips chose 24 in 1979.[17]

On 5 November 1954, Greenfield had proposed marking Holmes' eightieth birthday by reprinting 20

---

[16] Walshe wrote to Holmes: 'I believe the plan is to choose – or to let Sir Charles choose – a connected series of his papers showing the development of his work on, say, the coordination of movement ... would you care to approach him about it – or alternatively, tell me how to set about it'; and later: 'I

have composed – and enclose – a letter to Sherrington. If you agree with its tenour [*sic*], will you please send it to him with a covering letter of your own ... The Guarantors can put up £300 or £400 for publication ... [they] have £1100 of invested money that is of no use to anybody except for such purposes as this.'

[17] See *Selected Papers of Sir Gordon Holmes* (London: Macmillan, 1956), p. 262; and *Selected Papers of Gordon Holmes* (Oxford University Press, 1979). The Guarantors of *Brain* also established a lecture in honour of Holmes, given, to date, on 21 occasions – the first by Professor Günter Baumgartner on 5 November 1983.

of his papers. Various options were considered. The cost of the celebration was estimated at £1,754, plus a 15 per cent surcharge from the publishers, Macmillan & Co. Even with expected sales of up to 1,000, this budget was considered excessive and the scale of the project was therefore amended. A *livre jubilaire* could not be produced in time (and Holmes had not wanted one for his seventieth birthday), and a portrait would be difficult to arrange at short notice. Eventually a supplement of ten papers, published at a cost of £700–800, to be edited by Walshe, was approved. On 12 March 1956, Walshe reported that he had agreed with Holmes the selection of papers for inclusion, on vision and the cerebellum. Riding an old hobby-horse in his preface to the 1956 volume, Walshe writes:

> It may be timely here to remind the reader that all the work represented in the long and impressive bibliography with which this volume closes, has been the voluntary achievement of a physician, without university post or title, engaged in both the hospital and private practice of neurological medicine, in a special hospital and medical school that during all the relevant years had neither university recognition nor support. Here indeed is a striking example of sustained scientific endeavour that may serve as a salutary corrective to some widespread current illusions as to the administrative conditions under which alone, it is suggested, can fruitful research in medicine be carried out.

Walshe quotes extensively from Holmes' address at the opening of the Montreal Neurological Institute on 27 September 1934.

> If I was asked to select a motto, or a creed, for this new institute, I could do no better than copy out Francis Bacon's statement of his scientific attitude, written more than three hundred years ago. 'For myself I found I was fitted for nothing so well as for the study of Truth; as having a mind nimble and versatile enough to catch the resemblance of things (which is the chief point), and at the same time steady enough to fix and distinguish their subtler differences; as being gifted by nature with desire to seek, patience to doubt, fondness to meditate, slowness to assert, readiness to reconsider, carefulness to dispose and set in order; and as being a man that neither affects what is new or admires what is old, and that hates every kind of imposture.'

On 25 February 1957, Walshe wrote to Sam Nevin pointing out that, at a dinner held for Holmes at the College of Physicians, Arnold Carmichael had mentioned presenting a bound volume of his papers but regretted this was not possible at the time. Holmes, asking after the fate of the volume, was merely sent one of Walshe's paper-bound copies of the *livre jubilaire*. Walshe did nothing more on the basis that 'I felt that having produced that volume my task was ended and that the Guarantors would see to the rest.' At £1 10s 0d each, sales were poor, and on 12 July 1963 Macmillan & Co. returned 500 of the remaining 668 copies of the *Selected Papers of Sir Gordon Holmes* to be disposed of at the National Hospital for 10s each. On 2 February 1965, a further lunch was planned at the new Royal College of Physicians to mark Holmes' ninetieth birthday. But, on 7 June 1966, Lord Brain reported that Holmes had not been well enough to accept the invitation, and had in fact died before the birthday.

Eventually, in 1979, by which time publication of *Brain* had moved to Oxford University Press and the journal was on course for much greater financial stability than had existed under the Macmillan & Co. imprint, the Guarantors agreed to mark the centenary of Holmes' birth with a fuller volume of *Selected Papers of Sir Gordon Holmes* edited by Charles Phillips, containing 24 (from among his 174 papers, of which 37 were published in *Brain* between 1904 and 1939) on the cerebellum, vision, spinal cord, sensation, eye movements and a few miscellaneous topics. Phillips added further text from Holmes' address in Montréal from 1934:

> Can we then express in a few words what is required of the clinician who seeks knowledge and truth by the methods of science? In the first place, he must be trained to observe accurately, to see not merely what he is looking for, but to examine all phenomena connected with the question, and to neglect or discard no fact no matter how apparently trivial. In the second place, he must learn to describe observed facts accurately and completely, but simply and concisely. The practice of systematic description is doubly useful for the student, for in addition to placing observations on record, the routine of minute description by words or by drawings is certainly the best training in accurate observation. In the third place, the student must equip himself with that intellectual honesty and independence which refuse to submit to authority or to be controlled by preconceptions, and which are ready, when ascertained facts require it, to reject a theory or hypothesis which has perhaps been

hallowed by tradition or become an article of faith. Finally, he must learn to doubt conclusions too hastily or too easily reached; it has been truly said that 'suspended judgment is the greatest triumph of intellectual discipline'. But, on the other hand, the student must have the courage to formulate, when ready to do so, observations into hypotheses or rational generalisations, for, as Bacon has told us, 'truth can emerge sooner from error than from confusion'. These are the qualities in the observational sciences of natural history or biology, in which medicine may be included when it pursues knowledge by studying the processes of the body in health and disease.

The 1979 volume contains an analysis of Holmes' contributions to neurological anatomy by Alf Brodal. Brodal outlines Holmes' paper on Goltz' dog; the other major paper written from Edinger's laboratory on the comparative anatomy of the auditory nerve in a large number of species; and the work with Grainger Stewart on connections of the inferior olive and cerebellum,[18] in which Holmes articulates the general principle of topographical representation throughout the brain and to which he returned in his later work on vision. With Page May,[19] Holmes described the origin of the pyramidal tract from Betz cells in the fourth layer of the cerebral cortex within areas that excite the activity of the limbs and trunk. Brodal argues, however, that, over time, it became clear that this offered too narrow a view on connectivity of fibres occupying the pyramidal tract. In 1906, as pathologist and director of the research department at Queen Square, Holmes had used the staining techniques of Weigert and Bielschowsky to explain the discrepancy between clinical symptoms of cord and brain stem compression and degeneration of the long tracts, arguing that

> The presence of myeline [sic] sheaths is necessary for the functions of the tract fibres of the cord as conducting strands, and that when these are lost there may be physiological block in the fibres. This condition, from the point of view of function, is equivalent to a structural break in the fibres but differs in the fact that the anatomical integrity of the axis cylinder and its trophic cell remain unaffected.[20]

When others at Queen Square reasserted this truism, Walshe wrote: 'It should not be necessary at this date to pile Pelion on Ossa to establish that the secondary degeneration of spinal cord tracts, pyramidal or other, subject to focal lesions, is not an essential condition of physiological block, for demyelination alone may achieve this.'[21]

Nevertheless, the relative contribution of demyelination and axonal degeneration remained a recurring theme of research at Queen Square through to the 1980s. But Holmes also made the point that, since the axon is intact and the trophic cell survives, reparative processes remained possible, thus articulating the concept of remyelination.

Holmes had described a new form of familial degeneration of the cerebellum in 1907,[22] and this informed his later work on injuries of the cerebellum. The papers Holmes wrote on this subject during the war were brought together in his Croonian lectures delivered to the Royal College of Physicians (1922).[23] Holmes points out that the 70 cases reported in 1917 were incompletely documented. Later in the war, he was more systematic in his observations and followed up survivors into civilian life, adding 25 cases of cerebellar tumour seen since the war ended.

---

[18] See above, and G. Holmes, 'On the Comparative Anatomy of the Nervus Acousticus', *Transactions of the Royal Irish Academy* **32B** (1903): 101–44; G. Holmes and Grainger T. Stewart, 'On the Connection of the Inferior Olives with the Cerebellum in Man', *Brain* **31** (1908): 125–37.

[19] Page May held a junior post at the National Hospital and was then appointed pathologist to the City of London Hospital for Diseases of the Chest. Faced with ill health, he spent the winter in Egypt, where he developed a seasonal neurological practice at Helouan on the Nile; in the summer, he conducted physiological research at University College, where he was lecturer on the physiology of the nervous system. May discovered a tract of descending fibres in the posterior column of the cervical region of the spinal cord, known eponymously as 'May's tract'. Despite disability, he was a good golfer, fisherman and shot. He died in Brighton, his collapse caused by his anger at the sight of a carrier ill-treating a horse: see *Munk's Roll*, Vol. IV (Royal College of Physicians, 1955), p. 440.

[20] G. Holmes, 'On the Relation between Loss of Function and Structural Change in Focal Lesions of the Central Nervous System, with Special Reference to Secondary Degeneration', *Brain* **29** (1906): 514–23.

[21] Ian McDonald, 11th Gordon Holmes lecture: 'Gordon Holmes and the neurological heritage', *Brain*, **130** (2007): 288–98.

[22] G. Holmes, 'A Form of Familial Degeneration of the Cerebellum', *Brain* **30** (1907): 466–88.

[23] G. Holmes, 'The Symptoms of Acute Cerebellar Injuries Due to Gunshot Injuries', *Brain* **40** (1915): 461–535; G. Holmes, 'Clinical Symptoms of Cerebellar Disease and their Interpretation (Croonian Lectures)', *Lancet* **199** (1922): 1177–82, 1231–7; **2**: 59–65, 111–15.

Furthermore, by 1922, Holmes had been influenced by the writings of, among others, Sherrington and Walshe. Holmes described alterations in tone based on the novel definition of Sherrington that this is the resting state of muscle contraction needed to maintain posture. The clinical tests he devised to assess this aspect of movement included alterations in 'attitude', perturbations of the tendon reflexes, and the presence of 'associated movements'. Next, he characterised the tremor, incoordination (especially for complex movements), abnormality of speech and eye movements, and ataxia seen in cerebellar disease; the controversial issues of asthenia, fatigability and jerky muscular contraction during voluntary movement; and altered sensation in terms of the ability to judge weight. It is remarkable that, in the work carried out in France, working in the field and under impossible circumstances, Holmes had been able to make smoke-drum and light-box recordings of these alterations in movement.

For Holmes, the fundamental physiological defect in cerebellar disease is alteration in muscle tone, but this has two meanings: resistance to stretch and displacement, and the accurate combination and timing of the phasic and tonic elements of movement with ordered relaxation and contraction of agonists and antagonists. On localisation of cerebellar function, Holmes would only concede that the midline vermis is concerned with movements that simultaneously involve both sides, and the hemispheres with homolateral limb movement. Holmes returned to the cerebellum in his Hughlings Jackson lecture (1938), updating the work from 1917 to 1922 but covering the same manifestations of disease. He did not diverge in principle from the view that injury to the cerebellum results in postural hypotonia, asthenia and fatigability; abnormality in the rate, regularity and force of voluntary movement; and failure of certain associated movements. In rejecting the concept of a 'centre for coordination' rather than breakdown into more distributed aspects of motor control, Holmes advanced the Sherringtonian concept of the cerebellum as 'the head ganglion of the proprioceptive system'. He also argued that it reinforces or 'tunes up' the cerebral motor apparatus, including subcortical structures with motor functions, so that they respond promptly to volitional stimuli, and their impulses excite properly graded muscular contractions.

Although he had contributed to each in advance of the First World War, Holmes' work on the cerebellum and on vision depended much on the study of gunshot injuries. Holmes reworked this material in the 1930s, adding further details and insights, and adding papers on eye movements.[24] Everything was brought together in his Ferrier lecture to the Royal Society (1945), in which he paid tribute to those who wrote on vision in the nineteenth century, especially Ferrier, and his own work from 1914 to 1918. This allowed a definitive statement, modified somewhat from his earlier writings, on point-to-point projections from the retina to the occipital cortex and surrounding structures. Holmes wrote of his work on vision:

> My own work on the visual cortex ... has required the collection of a large number of observations, for while the physiologist can rely on experiments which he can select and control ... the clinician must depend upon the analysis of observations which are rarely so simple or clear cut ... the physiologist may be compared with the builder in ashlar or hewn stones which can easily be fitted together, the physician resembles the mason who has to use irregular rubble and therefore requires more time and labour to obtain his end. But in some branches of neurology the rubble collected and put together by the clinician is essential ... Observations on human subjects ... indicate that ... primary visual perception, including colour vision, relative localisation in space and perception of form, is subserved by the cortex of the striate area, and that though there is an exact geometric or point-to-point projection of the retina on this area its functional organisation is not rigidly determined by this point-to-point representation, but is to some extent plastic or modifiable. More highly differentiated visual functions, which are developed by the association of visual with other sensory impressions, on the other hand, depend on the integrity of the brain outside the striate area.[25]

---

[24] See G. Holmes, 'Observations on Ocular Palsies', *British Medical Journal* **2** (1936): 1165–7; G. Holmes, 'Looking and Seeing: Movements and Fixations of the Eyes. The Sixth John Mallet Purser Lecture Delivered at Trinity College, Dublin, June 4th 1936', *Irish Journal of the Medical Sciences* **129** (1936): 565–76; and G. Holmes, 'The Cerebral Integration of Ocular Movements: The Victor Horsley Memorial Lecture Delivered at University College Hospital Medical School on July 12, 1938', *British Medical Journal* **2** (1938): 107–12.

[25] See G. Holmes, 'The Ferrier Lecture: The Organisation of the Visual Cortex in Man', *Proceedings of the Royal Society Series B* **132** (1945): 348–61.

In reflecting on mechanisms of recovery, as with his earlier work on the spinal cord, Holmes had taken issue with Wilson's suggestion that 'temporary organic changes, as capillary haemorrhages, minute lacerations and disintegrations of the myelin' explain reversible visual loss following cerebral concussion. Holmes preferred the explanation that resolution of oedema is the principal explanation for recovery of visual function, although he did not articulate exactly how this might interfere with function on a temporary basis.

In his work on sensation, Holmes acknowledged the great originality of ideas developed by Henry Head, with whom he worked until 1914. But, in aligning with Head's views, Holmes was exposed to criticism, against which he defended himself in his writings. Holmes agreed that the optic thalamus is the centre of consciousness for certain elements of sensation and that cortical lesions modify but never abolish sensation. But he had to conclude that the lack of an anatomical basis for Head's research with Rivers, from which emerged the concept of protopathic and epicritic sensation, undermined the work, as Walshe was also only too happy to point out. Conversely, Walshe did admire Holmes' work with Head on cortical and thalamic sensation: 'As spectator and auditor of many of the sessions that went to make up this work at the National Hospital, many were the animated debates carried on over the patient's head during their course, and it was sometimes he [Holmes] who emerged the more exhausted.'[26]

Given his views on psychological illness, it is perhaps not surprising that Holmes considered hysteria to play an important part in the symptomatology of cerebral lesions apparently resulting in hemi-anaesthesia. The sensory disturbances of cortical origin could be classified as discriminative rather than crude appreciation of individual modalities. Information on localisation could be discerned from two-point discrimination of compass points and appreciation of weights (both generally distributed), sense of movement and joint position (localised to the postcentral gyrus), and the recognition of form (parietal cortex).

Holmes received many honours. He was made FRS (1933) and served on Council (1945–6). He was elected to foreign membership of academic and neurological societies in Germany, America, Estonia, France, Germany, the Netherlands, Romania and Sweden, and received honorary degrees from the Universities of Durham (1944), Edinburgh (1952) and Dublin (1933), and the National University of Ireland (1941). Holmes was twice mentioned in dispatches during the First World War, appointed CMG (1917) and Commander of the British Empire (1919) and knighted (1951).[27] His hobbies included woodwork and repair of furniture, and he had an interest in Gothic architecture and the construction of English cathedrals. In retirement, Holmes' main interest was gardening, especially the lighting of bonfires,[28] and golf, at which 'he was a powerful hitter but of less striking precision'. John Walton recalled that he was required to act as caddy when Holmes asked to play golf whilst examining in Newcastle. After several scuffed tee-shots and vain attempts to find his ball, Holmes threw down his clubs, tore out his false teeth and declared: 'never could play with these damn things!' Rick Tyler spent 1954–5 at Queen Square and, having worked with Denny-Brown and knowing how much he admired Holmes, wrote asking if he could visit. After meeting him and his wife at the station (in Farnham, Surrey), Lady Holmes drove the family round in their old car,[29] showing them the sights of Surrey. Holmes

---

[26] See F. M. R. Walshe, 'The Anatomy and Physiology of Cutaneous Sensibility: A Critical Review', *Brain* **65** (1942): 48–112.

[27] As with so many who receive civil honours, Holmes felt the need to be dismissive or falsely modest; and he had always genuinely disliked hearing his achievements discussed in public. He wrote to Sir Charles Dodds, Harveian librarian at the Royal College of Physicians, on receiving his knighthood: 'I have never been keen on honours, but my friends have overwhelmed me with congratulations and my family seem pleased.' In 1935, as president of the Second International Neurological Congress, he was invited to a reception at Buckingham Palace where King George V asked to speak to him, but Holmes had decided not to attend and some considered that this delayed the knighthood for many years. Holmes was equally diffident about having his portrait painted by Harold Knight on the occasion of his eightieth birthday.

[28] Mrs Eileen Critchley recalls that the collection for Holmes' portrait was sufficiently large for there to be surplus funds. Asked what he would like as an additional present, Holmes answered 'a flame-thrower' (McDonald archive: letter to Ian McDonald dated 27 November 2004).

[29] Holmes was a keen motorist and drove in motor trials: see B. G. Parsons-Smith, 'Sir Gordon Holmes', in F. C. Rose and W. F. Bynum, eds., *Historical Aspects of the*

had planted various items in his garden and he was making observations and conducting experiments on their variable number of petals. He had on his fireplace a model of the brain, which he had used to draw the lesions when evaluating visual field defects in the First World War. By then, he was aware of some loss of memory that prevented him writing serious neurological papers, but he was working on a biographical account of Edinger. Rosalie Holmes died from heart failure in 1963; Holmes continued to play golf and work in his garden, looked after by his daughter Kathleen, until a few days before he died at home in his sleep on the morning of 29 December 1965.

Samuel Alexander Kinnier Wilson

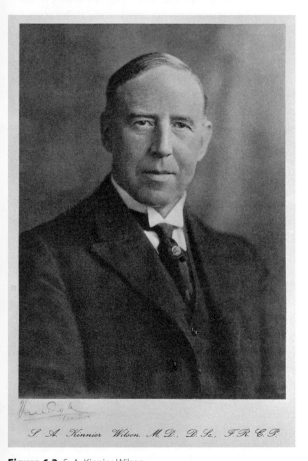

S. A. Kinnier Wilson. M.D., D.Sc., F.R.C.P.

Figure 6.3 S. A. Kinnier Wilson.

In the second and third decades of the twentieth century, Kinnier Wilson and Gordon Holmes, two men large both in physical and intellectual stature, reigned supreme in British clinical neurology. They were affectionately referred to by Macdonald Critchley as the Gog and Magog of Queen Square.[30]

Wilson was born in Cedarville, New Jersey (6 December 1878). After the death of his Irish father, the Revd James Kinnier Wilson, his bereaved mother brought Samuel across the Atlantic to her ancestral home in Edinburgh, where his formative years were spent. He graduated *cum laude* from Edinburgh University in 1902 and, after a house officer post working for Sir Byron Bramwell, professor of medicine at the Royal Infirmary, won a Carnegie Research Fellowship to study neurology in Paris with Pierre Marie and Joseph Babinski. During this *Wanderjahre*, he immersed himself not only in the advanced anatomo-clinical methods of the Salpêtrière but also in the richness of French culture. After this two-year stage in his neurological training, Wilson moved to Germany where he worked in Leipzig with Paul Fleschig. This influential part of his training allowed Wilson to keep abreast of the extensive German literature throughout the rest of his career. On his return to the British Isles in 1905, Wilson applied successfully for the post of resident medical officer at the National Hospital, where, like many others, he was much influenced by Hughlings Jackson, who had retired from the staff but continued to visit the hospital and ask the trainees to show him patients of interest. It is claimed that Wilson kept detailed notes of these encounters and retained a collection of Hughlings Jackson's papers bound in two volumes on his desk. In 1912, Wilson was appointed assistant physician at the Westminster Hospital, and a year later was promoted to assistant physician at the National Hospital. With a grant from the British Medical Association, he now embarked on a research project in Victor Horsley's laboratory examining the effect of lesions in the lenticular nucleus in monkeys. After the First World War, he was offered a post at King's College Hospital and a lectureship in neurology at King's Medical School, at which point he resigned from the Westminster Hospital. In 1921, Wilson was promoted physician to outpatients at the National Hospital, and a year later became a physician with admission rights. In

---

Neurosciences: A Festschrift for Macdonald Critchley (New York: Raven Press, 1982), p. 359.

[30] Macdonald Critchley, 'Remembering Kinnier Wilson', *Movement Disorders* **3** (1988): 2–6.

227

1927, he was appointed neurologist to King's College Hospital.

Perhaps in deference to and recognition of Hughlings Jackson, at the age of 30, in 1908, Wilson wrote 'A Contribution to the Study of Apraxia', with a scholarly review of the literature, and, in 1928, a short but highly praised monograph on aphasia.[31] But the study of higher cerebral function was not his main interest. In time, Wilson became the expert on disorders of the basal ganglia. After passing the MRCP examination, Wilson had translated Meige and Feindel's monograph *Les tics et leur traitement* (1902; English edition, 1907). A few years later, he defended his doctoral thesis at the University of Edinburgh entitled 'A Fatal Familial Nervous Disease Associated with Cirrhosis of the Liver' whilst working as a junior doctor carrying out post-mortem examinations at the National Hospital. In the dissertation, he described four children or young adults with a rapidly progressive neurological syndrome characterised by tremor, difficulty in swallowing and speaking, muscular weakness, spasticity and fixed dystonic contractures, which he named 'progressive lenticular degeneration'. This outstanding piece of work was awarded the Gold Medal by the university in 1911. A brief version appeared in the *Lancet*, but the following year Wilson published the definitive account in *Brain*, emphasising the clinical relevance of damage to the lenticular nucleus and the important coexistence of liver cirrhosis.[32] Wilson included an addendum relating to a patient already described by Völsch that he felt sure was an example of progressive lenticular degeneration, and he also unearthed a typical case in Friedrich Theodor von Frerichs' *Klinik der Leberkrankheiten* (1858–61).[33] Wilson also acknowledged the earlier reports by his senior colleagues at Queen Square.[34]

The 1912 paper rehearsed Gowers' previous case, with further details of another affected family member provided to Wilson by the index case's mother. Details of Ormerod's patient were supplemented by access to the case notes at Queen Square. Following the review of prior examples, Wilson then reported in detail on the four cases personally observed, of whom three came to autopsy. Wilson provided the most authoritative account of what later came to be recognised as the first treatable metabolic disorder of the brain, in this instance caused by a disorder of copper transport. The paper also offered a new approach to research on motor function of the basal ganglia and demonstrated conclusively that lesions of the lenticular nucleus result in abnormal involuntary movements. Quite when his Greco-Latin rubric lost favour and became 'Wilson's disease' is uncertain but the eponym was probably adopted by German neurologists who, along with the French, were the first to appreciate the importance of Wilson's work. In the UK, Greenfield and Denny-Brown were using the eponym by the mid-1930s and, in later life, Wilson was only too happy to refer to 'my disease'. He vehemently rejected von Strumpell and Westphal's claims to precedence, arguing that they had failed to emphasise the importance of hepatic pathology. However, Wilson did not like use of the term 'abdominal Wilson's disease' by liver specialists. What Wilson had missed, and continued to deny through most of his career, was the distinctive green ring of copper deposited on Descemet's membrane of the cornea, first described by Kaiser (1902) and by Fleischer (1903).

As a result of his pathological research, Wilson acquired a detailed knowledge of the anatomy and function of the 'old motor system' (the basal ganglia). He was described by Critchley as the 'Marco Polo' of the extrapyramidal system, a term that Wilson had, with typical self-aggrandisement, first used about himself. His Croonian lectures (1925) were on disorders of motility and muscle tone, in which Wilson speculated that the tremor of Parkinsonism must originate in the cerebral cortex through the influence of the striatum and pallidum. The presentation was illustrated with some of his own cinematographic films recorded in Queen Square. Wilson was among the first to demonstrate persistence of the glabellar tap, which for a while was known at Queen Square as 'Wilson's sign'. His

---

[31] S. A. Kinnier Wilson, *Aphasia* (London: Basic English Publishing Co., n.d.), p. 108.
[32] S. A. K. Wilson, 'Progressive Lenticular Degeneration: A Familial Nervous Disease Associated with Cirrhosis of the Liver', *Brain* **34** (1912): 295–509. At 214 pages, this occupied practically an entire issue of the journal for March 1912 (the only other article was a short paper on subacute combined degeneration of the spinal cord by Theodore Thompson).
[33] See M. Völsch, 'Beitrag zur Lehre von der Pseudosklerose (Westphal-Strumpell)', *Deutsche Zeitschrift für Nervenheilkunde* **42** (1911): 335–52; and footnote to the English translation of von Frerichs' treatise by Murchison published by the New Sydenham Society (1860).
[34] See W. R. Gowers, *Manual of Disease of the Nervous System* (London: J. & A. Churchill, 1888), Vol. 2, p. 656;

and J. A. Ormerod, 'Cirrhosis of the Liver in a Boy with Obscure and Fatal Nervous Symptoms', *St Bartholomew's Hospital Reports* **26** (1890): 57.

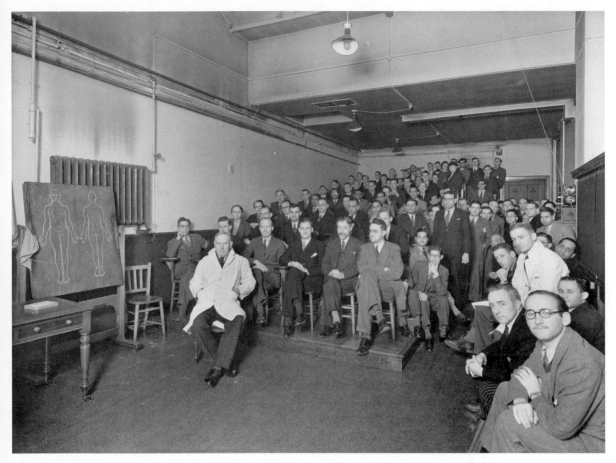

Figure 6.4 S. A. Kinnier Wilson holding a teaching session for 110 postgraduate doctors from 22 countries, c. 1930.

lasting interest in the 'basements of the brain' was also fuelled by his experience of the encephalitis lethargica pandemic, but Wilson objected that:

> Some writers now appear to envisage all motor symptoms through an encephalitic fog, arguing for a striatal localization of peculiarly elaborate movement-complexes because the virus of encephalitis has a striatal site in Parkinsonian cases! ... Assuming from the complexity of the movements that they are of cortical type, the inference would be that the corpus striatum is higher in the physiological hierarchy than the cortex itself, and that it controls the latter, so that when it is disordered cortical activity is 'let go'. This is contrary to all our conceptions of cerebral physiology.[35]

Wilson also conceived of akinesia as a reduction in the will to act and, although he did not speculate on the mechanism, felt that the cerebral cortex must be involved in some way.

Wilson's whole life was neurology, but his training as a classical scholar and his love of the arts greatly influenced his approach to medicine. He had a photographic memory and a penetrating eye and all his clinical endeavours were minutely detailed. He was a large man with rather coarse rustic features and ham-shaped hands. He was critical of many of his British colleagues, as recalled by Macdonald Critchley:

> On a ward round at Queen Square I enquired to Wilson how his BMA lecture had gone in Leeds. 'Terrible!' Wilson retorted. When I asked what went wrong he said 'I hate the North of England and if there is one city I particularly loathe its Leeds.' Pressed for more details he said 'I got there in the afternoon. It wasn't until nearly seven o clock that I was offered a sweet glass of sherry. Then at dinner I was seated next to a woman

---

[35] S. A. K. Wilson, *Modern Problems in Neurology* (London: Edward Arnold & Co., 1928), pp. 253–4.

who never stopped talking. Her sole topic was Bernard Shaw and if there is one person I detest it's George Bernard Shaw.' What about the lecture I asked? 'My subject was epilepsy, and you know the sort of material that intrigues me. What is the biological meaning, if any of the convulsive seizure? What does it represent? An abrupt release of inhibition? An excitatory phenomenon? Or chemically initiated? I hadn't been talking more than ten minutes when an oafish voice from the back shouted "speak up". I stopped, turned to the Chairman and said. "Mr Chairman I have been lecturing for twenty five years and never before have I been told my voice doesn't carry". At the end of my talk the Chairman invited questions. There was a long silence and then someone said I would like to ask the specialist from London what dose of bromide he recommends. My dear Critchley I ask you!'

Wilson was probably at his best seated in an armchair in outpatients, when his intellect, flashes of lateral thinking and persuasive enthusiasm enchanted the small coterie of admirers. He took his patients as themes for discourse and shared with his audience the enjoyment of performance. One of his mannerisms when demonstrating cases was to roll up the collar of his white coat, bringing the lapels together under his chin and folding his arms across his chest. The word most often on his lips when teaching was 'fascinating' and when presented with new facts by his junior colleagues he would always demand, 'why?'. Charles Symonds related an anecdote from when Hugh Garland, who later became a consultant neurologist at the Leeds General Infirmary, was Wilson's house physician. Garland flattered Wilson over tea with this reflection: 'Sir, your teaching this afternoon was wonderful.' To which Wilson replied: 'Yes, I know, Garland but say it again, I like to hear it!'[36] He had a well-known narcissistic personality, and with the craving for admiration went a difficulty in accepting criticism, which he took as a personal affront. His aloof and touchy nature resulted in some difficulties with his colleagues. Holmes, with whom he had a strained relationship, considered Wilson to be vain, whereas Denny-Brown complained about his pomposity. Symonds, however, considered that the power of his intellect outweighed these faults and stated that he was the most influential neurologist of his time. Insight into Wilson's bedside manner can be deduced from another anecdote. When making rounds with his former colleague and friend Foster

Kennedy, at the Bellevue Hospital, New York, Wilson spent over three hours examining a patient with lateral medullary syndrome. However, the signs were inconsistent with the anatomy. Eventually, Wilson turned to the patient and asked, 'Will you see to it that I get your brain when you die?' Another apocryphal story survives of an elderly woman who had been diagnosed by Wilson with multiple sclerosis in 1922. Some 60 years later, she related that he had told her 'It's tough luck, old girl. You'll be in a wheelchair in four years. That will be 5 guineas.' When relating the story, she delighted in pointing out that she had survived Wilson by 40 years. On her death at the age of 87, the post-mortem examination revealed a total of three demyelinated lesions.[37]

In 1920, Wilson founded the *Journal of Neurology and Psychopathology*, and editorial work consumed much of his limited time for leisure. The contents of the journal reflect Wilson's interest in psychiatry and medical psychology, perhaps stemming from his continental training. He read and spoke German and French fluently, travelled widely and had many influential friends in continental Europe and America, explaining why Wilson commanded a far greater reputation overseas than at home.

The other major achievement for which Wilson is remembered in Great Britain is his encyclopaedic two-volume 1,838-page textbook *Neurology* (1940) with its 276 illustrations and 16 plates. At his death from cancer at the age of 59, Wilson was still working on the book, for which he had gathered material over decades of clinical practice and reading. Over three-quarters of it was written, although he had wanted to revise some sections, and there was also a pile of rough notes on other topics not yet covered. It was left to his brother-in-law Ninian Bruce to edit the draft manuscript and complete this magnum opus which was eventually published posthumously. The book sold well and, despite its patchiness and inadequate subject index, was recognised as the greatest single-author work of reference on clinical neurology written in the twentieth century. It is not particularly useful to rank textbooks but, for us, *Neurology* is precious for the historical threads provided on each of the topics covered, and the extensive index of authors, even if the organisation is less balanced and comprehensive than Gowers' *Manual*. And it would be invidious not to mention Hermann Oppenheim's

---

[36] C. P. Symonds, *Studies in Neurology* (London: Oxford University Press, 1970), p. 3.

[37] T. J. Murray, *Multiple Sclerosis: The History of a Disease* (New York: Demos Medical Publications, 2005), p. 221.

Lehrbuch der Nervenkrankheiten (1908) as well, a work that was loosely connected to Wilson in that it had been translated into English by Alexander Bruce in 1911. In Kinnier Wilson's *Neurology*, diseases are grouped into sections according to presumed causation: toxi-infective disease; special forms of toxi-infection; special forms of toxicosis; degenerative or toxi-degenerative disorders; disease of vascular origin; tumours; metabolic and deficiency states; congenital anomalies and disease states; conditions of uncertain nature; and the neuroses.[38] Conditions of uncertain nature include the epilepsies, narcolepsies, familial periodic paralysis, migraine, myasthenia gravis and tetany. The final section labelled 'neuroses' covers motor neuroses, myospasms, rhythmias, torticollis, occupation neuroses, miner's nystagmus, lightning stroke, and sensory and reflex neuroses. Within are descriptions of Gilles de la Tourette's syndrome, myotonia and many craft palsies. Wilson wrote well, and always had a copy of Fowler's *A Dictionary of Modern English Usage* open on his desk. He is especially respectful of the German and French literature, each chapter beginning with a carefully researched historical synopsis.[39] The style is distinctive, flamboyant and polyglot – quite different from that of Gowers but nevertheless easy to read, despite the detail and discursions. Wilson allowed himself many amusing asides. His fertile imagination often shed light from an unusual angle on well-studied topics and bequeathed to the reader a litany of unforgettable adages. An example can be seen in the following aphorism relating to Sydenham's chorea: 'Someone has said that the choreic child is punished thrice ere his condition is recognised – once for general fidgetiness, once for breaking crockery and once for making faces at his grandmother.'

The anonymous reviewer in *Brain* praised the book as a valuable reference source and commended particularly the sections on affections of the extrapyramidal system, including the description of epidemic encephalitis lethargica and the motor neuroses, such as tics and torticollis. Only 18 pages are dedicated to paralysis agitans, compared with 25 for progressive lenticular degeneration. Conversely, the neurological complications of syphilis take up 114 pages, reflecting its continuing importance in the pre-antibiotic era. Unevenness was felt to be one shortcoming, along with the relative lack of pathological illustrations. Wilson's well-known use of neologisms and obsessive desire to revise current terminology also did not escape criticism. Hysteria was a surprising omission, and one needs to turn to Wilson's masterly review published in *Encyclopedia medica* (1919) to learn of his views. It seems likely that, had Wilson lived longer, he would have added a section on this topic. When Ninian Bruce edited the second edition (1954), the omission of any discussion of aphasia in the first edition was corrected by including a new chapter written by Russell Brain on aphasia, apraxia and agnosia; and the long account of neurosyphilis with discussion of treatment in the antibiotic era was re-written by Sam Nevin. For his Harveian Oration (1926), Wilson chose the subject of the epilepsies, a term he had introduced to emphasise the clinical conditions that he considered as motor, sensory and psychical types. In 1928, he published *Modern Problems in Neurology*, in which the first four chapters are devoted to the epilepsies and the next to narcolepsy, whereas the last three, illustrating his particular preoccupations at this time, concern pathological laughter and crying, the neural correlates of dysaesthesia, and the Argyll Robertson pupil.

Wilson served as secretary general at the second International Congress of Neurology held at University College in London in 1935. In 1932, Lord Adrian and Sir Charles Sherrington both proposed Wilson for election to the Royal Society, but despite other influential support, and carrying forward the proposal in successive years, Wilson died without having been elected. In 1934, he expressed an interest in the vacant chair of clinical medicine at Edinburgh but was advised not to apply. Macdonald Critchley, who was a great admirer of Wilson and described him as Olympian, concluded that his former teacher's petulant vanity, showmanship and touchiness contributed to his unpopularity with certain members of the National Hospital staff and, as a result, somewhat diminished his standing in British neurology.

In common with Hughlings Jackson, Wilson had no great passions outside his work. He was a genial host, enjoyed his garden, played golf (badly) and liked the light entertainment of music-halls. An obituary in the *Lancet* described Wilson as having no facile grace, but when he was in the mood he could be an excellent

---

[38] Wilson was one of the last neurologists to use the term 'neurosis' in its original neurological context, defined as a disorder of nervous system function without local pathology.
[39] Wilson's extensive medical library of more than 1,500 books and many reprints, including those he had been given by Hughlings Jackson, are now in the Royal College of Physicians' library in Edinburgh.

conversationalist. He had a Puckish sense of humour, wrote funny poems for his children and took them to the pantomime every Christmas.[40] A hangover from his time in Paris was his penchant for French liqueurs. He also remained faithful to his American roots, buying first a Palladium and then a Buick motor car. He became a friend of Charlie Chaplin, and on one of his many American trips was invited to Chaplin's Californian ranch where Wilson played tennis and went tunny fishing. This encounter may have also led to his early interest in the use of cinematography as an aid to the teaching of neurology.

Francis Martin Rouse Walshe

Francis Walshe was the dominant figure on the staff at Queen Square in the middle decades of the twentieth

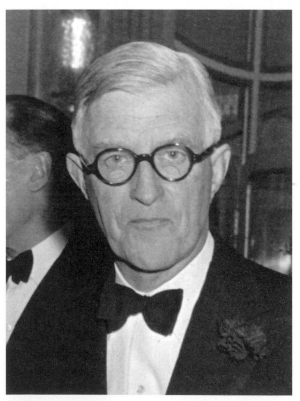

Figure 6.5 F. M. R. Walshe.

century. He was a remarkable and complex man, yet his contribution to the National Hospital as well as to British neurology is decidedly ambiguous. He remains, more than any other of the great Queen Square figures, on the periphery of world neurology and an enigmatic figure – an undoubted intellect but a poor judge, an orator whose lectures have not stood the test of time, a leader but inept politically, and a kind and honourable man but with an impulsive urge to criticise and humiliate, who could not resist an acid remark in the interests of witticism.

Francis Martin Rouse Walshe was born in London (19 September 1885), educated at Prior Park College near Bath and at University College School, London. His decision to enter medicine was made by his father, against the advice of his headmaster, and Walshe began that training with no scientific background. He studied medicine at University College Hospital, and, whilst doing his second MB, became interested in physiology, being supervised by W. M. Bayliss and E. H. Starling. He was much influenced by the work of Sir Charles Sherrington, and wrote in 1965:

> It was then that I first made the acquaintance of Sherrington's *Integrative action of the nervous system* … and that determined me to work in neurophysiology or clinical neurology in a then foreseeable future … It would be impossible for me to overemphasize the excitement of mind this book produced in me – and kept alive over many years. I owe to it more than to any other single inspiration … In detail, its study determined me to seek to analyse the very numerous so-called reflex reactions present in various diseased conditions of the nervous system in men (and hitherto empirically regarded as practical aids to localizing diagnosis only), and to carry over to man – if possible – the analysis of reflex reactions which was the work of Sherrington.[41]

Walshe was awarded first-class honours in the BSc (1908), and graduated in medicine in 1910. After a year at University College Hospital as a houseman, he was appointed to the National Hospital, 'where I remained as house physician and resident medical officer for close upon four precious and happy

---

[40] Wilson is remembered with affection and as a loving father by his son James Kinnier Wilson, an Assyriologist in the University of Cambridge (1955–89), whom we interviewed in 2016. Not surprisingly, other than as 'Dad', Wilson was known at home and to his close friends as 'Sak'.

[41] Many biographical and other details are taken from Charles Phillips, 'Francis Martin Rouse Walshe 1885–1973', *Memoirs of the Fellows of the Royal Society* **20** (1974): 456–81.

years'. During this time, Walshe was awarded his MD and passed the MRCP examination. In 1915, he joined the Royal Army Medical Corps and became consulting neurologist to the British forces in Egypt and the Middle East.

He was awarded the OBE for his war efforts, in 1919, and elected FRCP in 1920. He was appointed as physician to the National Hospital in 1921 and founded the neurology department at University College Hospital in 1924. In 1921, Walshe spent six months as Welch lecturer in clinical physiology at Oxford and carried out animal experiments. He had been encouraged by Henry Head, who gave him £100, but Walshe found himself not well suited to laboratory work. As he wrote: 'I realized, however, that the experimental physiology of animals was not for me, and that I must pursue my physiological curiosities in clinical neurology.' He never carried out any further experimental work, basing his future writings on observing the phenomena of clinical neurology and proving a formidable commentator on other people's research. He was editor of *Brain* (1937–53) and of *Epilepsia* (1959–61). Walshe was elected FRS in 1946 and knighted in 1953. He was president of the Association of British Neurologists (1950–1), the Royal Society of Medicine (1952–4) and the Royal Institute of Public Health and Hygiene (1962–4). He received many other honours, gave various prestigious lectures, and was feted internationally. Walshe was considered highly by his American colleagues, and was approached to consider applying for professorships of neurology at Johns Hopkins in 1925 and later in New York, as well as positions at Cambridge in 1935 and 1942. He turned down all these approaches, and continued his career at the National Hospital, for which he was a passionate advocate.

Walshe met his wife during the First World War, when she was a nursing sister in 17 General Hospital, Alexandria, where he was working as a physician. Walshe recalled that, to his great amusement, Horsley was there too, but held a lower rank. During his time in Alexandria, Walshe met T. E. Lawrence (of Arabia), whom he found to be rather insignificant. Lady Walshe died in the 1950s and Walshe then lived with his private secretary. John Walshe recalls a devoted father and family man, who spent hours assisting his dyslexic grand-daughter. His main hobby was fishing and he spent a month each year before the war, and two weeks annually thereafter, with his family on fishing holidays, often in County Mayo where his father had been born. He was an excellent host, passionate about books, and no doubt a popular member of the Athenaeum Club.

When he did eventually cease practice in his eighties, Walshe moved to the small village of Brampton, Cambridgeshire, where he enjoyed his garden. He died of a stroke in 1973, aged 88.

Walshe contributed an interesting but brief autobiographical preface to the special issue of *Brain*, comprising 200 pages, edited by William Gooddy and produced by the Guarantors at a cost of £1,000 as a Festschrift marking Walshe's eightieth birthday in 1965. Invitations, approved by Walshe, were sent to contributors,[42] and the issue contained a contemporary photographic portrait taken outside the National Hospital with Walshe smoking a small cigar.[43] The biographical note made clear that Walshe's lifelong interest in neurology preceded the influence of Sherrington: 'Familiar figures of my youth were Sir William Gowers and Dr Hughlings Jackson who lived within a few hundred yards of my home, whose work and scientific eminence were constantly impressed on me by my father – this determining in large measure a later leaning on my part to specialize in clinical neurology.'

The reference to Walshe's father – an authoritarian figure – may partly explain his own tendency to be critical and often personally wounding. As with others of his generation, Walshe's income derived from an extensive private practice and he received no scientific grants. As for an academic position: 'This was a fate … I had seen … happen and was forewarned … having avoided professorships on more than one occasion, I have retained a freedom of life and action that are essential to me.'[44]

---

[42] There was no paper by Walshe himself: the 23 contributors included Charles Aring, Lord Brain, Macdonald Critchley, William Gooddy, Derek Denny-Brown, Wilder Penfield and Georges Schaltenbrand (who later came in for criticism over his research on transmitting images about multiple sclerosis involving mentally defective institutionalised subjects who lacked the ability to give any form of consent, informed or otherwise).

[43] 'A Tribute to Sir Francis Martin Rouse Walshe on the Occasion of his Eightieth Birthday. Prepared by Direction of the Guarantors of *Brain* and Edited by William Gooddy', *Brain* **88** (1965): 653–854.

[44] Walshe's attitude to academic appointments, and his role in the saga of the professorship of neurology at Queen Square are described in detail in Chapter 12.

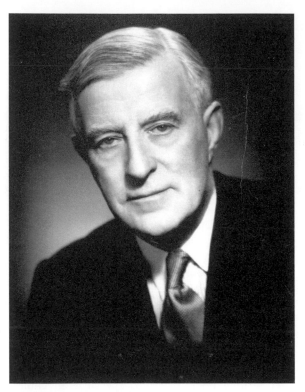

Figure 6.6 The photograph of F. M. R. Walshe which was displayed on Critchley's desk (collection of Alastair Compston).

Walshe's main academic contributions to neurology were observations of human reflexes, carried out in the 1920s at Queen Square and University College Hospital. He studied paraplegia-in-flexion, paraplegia-in-extension, spastic hemiplegia, nociceptive flexion reflex, the knee jerk, the tonic neck reflexes, the phasic ipsilateral flexor response and the extensor plantar response. Later, he worked on the functions of the cerebral cortex and awareness of pain. Charles Phillips wrote: 'To Walshe, also, belongs the credit for emphasizing the differences of physiological quality and anatomical distribution which distinguish spasticity from Parkinsonian rigidity; and for demonstrating Parkinsonian rigidity and tremor could not have a common physiological origin.

Interestingly, towards the end of his life, Walshe was critical of those, such as himself, who wasted time on anatomy and physiology, taking the view that the future lay in disciplines such as biochemistry, tissue culture and electron microscopy. On contributions to human physiology, he concluded that 'It was, however, not possible ultimately to forget

that such quests, however fascinating, did not contribute to the aetiology and pathogenesis of nervous diseases; surely the first responsibility of a neurological physician.'[45]

The interest in biochemistry may have been kindled by the work of his son, John Walshe, on the biochemical basis of Wilson's disease, of which he was justifiably proud. Nevertheless, however much he dismissed its importance later on, it was physiological work in patients that had established Walshe's reputation as a leader of clinical neurology in the 1920s. He did write on many other topics but usually as reports, commentaries or reviews: peripheral neuropathy, the effects of toxins on the nervous system, disseminated sclerosis, intracranial tumours, epilepsy, poliomyelitis, Wilson's disease, meningioma, carcinomatous meningitis and hysteria. Walshe published a short textbook of neurology which went into 11 editions (from 1940 to 1973, the year of his death).[46] None of these writings achieved enduring influence. Particularly after 1940, his lines of thought, as evidenced in the written work, became increasingly difficult to follow. In the later stages of his life, Walshe became interested in the question of consciousness and the mind–brain problem. Perhaps reflecting his strong Catholic faith, in 1965 he wrote:

> In old age the philosophical problems, and I deny that they are or can be purely physiological, involved in the mind–brain relationship engage me. This is a hazard of advancing years, yet it is only then that the need to widen and deepen one's range of thought becomes imperative, and then only can one openly question the omnicompetence of natural science to comprehend God and His Universe. Only the Peter Pans of science do not feel this urge, the very clever young men who never seem to grow up.[47]

Walsh was tall and handsome, and always elegantly dressed. These personal characteristics contributed to his success. He had a patrician air, as did Wilson and, to a lesser extent, Critchley, and all three gave the National Hospital, and indeed British neurology, a reputation for being highbrow, exclusive, elitist and

[45] F. M. R. Walshe, 'The Present and Future of Neurology', *Archives of Neurology* **2** (1960): 83–8.

[46] This rather idiosyncratic textbook was never as popular as Russell Brain's *Diseases of the Nervous System* (1933), now in its 12th edition (published in 2009).

[47] Cited in C. D. Aring and W. M. Landau, 'Francis Martin Rouse Walshe, 1885–1973', *Archives of Neurology* **29** (1973): 355–7.

difficult – a subject that ordinary doctors should not attempt. His detractors found him cold, aloof and arrogant, and an impression of self-righteousness and arrogance is certainly gained from his written polemics.[48] Critchley considered that Walshe's combination of 'banter with rebuke was apt to prove humiliating … Many scientists whose researches had been criticized by Walshe, bore a lifelong resentment.' It was not only colleagues who were the victims of his pen. On hysterical headache, Walshe wrote: 'it was not a pain at all … the patient remaining as rosy as an apple and as plump as a partridge'.[49] Brilliant as an orator, Walshe's lectures and prose were renowned for their wit, construction and savage power. He made exceptional use of an extensive vocabulary, elegant phraseology and metaphor. These verbal skills not only made it easy for Walshe to express his opinion, but also fuelled his tendency to be critical – and, at times, vicious. Some of his later writings were lacerating. Perhaps rather generously, Denny-Brown commented, about his friend, that Walshe's 'great forte was criticism, serving in medical science the important function of the literary critic in the realm of arts and letters'. Walshe recognised his tendency for trenchant attacks on those with whom he disagreed, but was unrepentant: 'As the years passed my writings became more predominantly critical and have so remained, though no plaudits greet the critic. The task is its own reward … [quoting Dingle] criticism can no more prevent the emergence of the good than that of the bad, but it can create an atmosphere in which the good flourishes and the bad withers.'

In Walshe's copy of *The Collected Papers of Wilfrid Trotter* (1941), the following passage is heavily underscored: 'The common tendency to regard destructive criticism as always easy and generally reprehensible is one that I do not share … At no time in the history of the intellect has the sanitary work of destructive criticism been more needful.'[50]

Walshe fully expected that digesting his selection of critical thoughts would make students of neurology 'more gourmets than gourmands'. On journals, he was especially clear – these being 'repositories of obsolete lumber indiscriminately and slavishly rehashed for the massive omnibus tomes that constitute the modern textbooks that no student should be asked to bear'. But this attitude did not prevent Walshe from serving as an editor himself. He had first published in *Brain*, aged 29,[51] and was made a Guarantor on 17 October 1923, pledging 2 guineas for a period of five years. He was appointed to the Committee of Management from 23 January 1924 and to the executive committee of the Guarantors from 5 December 1930. He served as assistant editor from 1929 to 1938. When Holmes resigned as editor, Walshe was one of four Guarantors forming the committee charged with appointing his successor and, in the event, Walshe was himself elected. Before resigning, Holmes had suggested that the Association of British Neurologists be invited to take over the ownership and management of *Brain*. Walshe quickly dismissed the suggestion, indicating that he would prefer to work with the existing Guarantors, and the committee agreed. Walshe appointed deputy editors: Greenfield from 1929 to 1953, and Macdonald Critchley from 1946 to 1953. Evidently, their work was not onerous. On 24 February 1944, Greenfield wrote to the Committee of Management indicating that he had done no editorial work at all for *Brain* in the previous year and could not accept the £25 annual honorarium. By comparison with the many classic papers published under the editorships of his predecessors, Head and Holmes, the period after 1938 was not the golden age of the journal and the issues were often thin, with a distinct shortage of copy – understandably, during and soon after the Second World

---

[48] Walshe once referred to medicine as being unchanged since someone had thrown a handful of foxgloves into a boiling cauldron, whereas neurology was based on science, and this infuriated his medical colleagues at University College Hospital who thereafter advised students not to go into neurology.

[49] Cited by Critchley in *The Ventricle of Memory: Personal Recollections of Some Neurologists* (New York: Lippincott Williams & Wilkins, 1989).

[50] *The Collected Papers of Wilfred Trotter* (Oxford Medical Publications, 1941). Walshe was prone to underscoring and

annotating books in his library. Wilfred Trotter FRS, director of surgery at University College Hospital, was a major figure in neurosurgery and also well known for his work on psychology. He proposed the concept of the 'herd instinct' and was an early advocate of the works of Freud. He was an original intellect and a major influence on Walshe's thought. Walshe's copy of the *Collected Papers* was subsequently in the possession of Macdonald Critchley and then Ian McDonald.

[51] S. A. Kinnier Wilson and F. M. R. Walshe, 'The Phenomenon of "Tonic Innervation" and its Relation to Motor Apraxia', *Brain* 37 (1914): 199–246; and F. M. R. Walshe, 'The Physiological Significance of the Reflex Phenomena in Spastic Paralysis of the Lower Limbs', *Brain* 37 (1914): 269–336.

War. On 20 March 1951, after 13 years as editor, Walshe asked to resign, but this was declined by the committee and he agreed to continue until the end of 1953. At that point, he and all members of the editorial board, other than Denny-Brown, did resign. Walshe received a long-service payment of £250. The minutes of the meeting for 29 July 1952 indicate that – Symonds having been preferred, but declining the invitation – Brain was appointed as Walshe's successor.

During his editorship of *Brain*, Walshe published a number of long papers, which were often of exceptional quality and masterful reviews of their subject, but he did also have a tendency to use the journal as a vehicle for criticism and to fly his colourful kites. As Phillips wrote:

> Walshe probably felt that it was the critic's business to hack away over-exuberant brushwood from the neurological jungle; his admirers saw it crackling briskly in the bright flame of his prose … his off-the-cuff comments on people and ideas with which he disagreed were pithily epigrammatic, and his victims must often have smarted under his attack. Michael Jefferson, who was his house physician at Queen Square in the late 1940s, felt that mean action was not in his nature and that one might view his lifelong function as a critic as devoted to rooting out what he saw as heresy of thought rather than aimed to cause personal hurt.

Such generosity is not evident in his typically pithy summary of neuropsychiatry, which 'like the mule, has neither pride of ancestry nor hope of progeny'.[52] Other victims of his Belloc-like pen included distinguished international neurologists and scientists such as Brodmann, Fulton, Penfield and Gastaut. Despite having asked him to contribute to the special issue of *Brain* (1965), Walshe's attacks on Penfield were particularly severe, and certainly overstepped the boundaries of courtesy.[53] He was a friend and admirer of Denny-Brown, but told his son that the latter (with

whom John Walshe worked as a Fulbright scholar in Boston) 'treated his monkeys like scrubbing brushes'. His excoriating pen was also wielded on home territory. His caricature of Head and Rivers' 'protopathic' animal, based on their theory of protopathic–epicritic sensation, is a typical example of stylish but ultimately cruel prose:

> The protopathic animal, in response to a stimulus which it cannot localise, which has but a single intensity and gives no information as to the nature of the stimulating object, makes a response which consists of profuse sweating, bladder evacuation, and powerful tonic flexion of the hind limbs, or squatting. The primitive animal thus endowed would be an organism utterly unfitted to cope with its environment. So helpless and bewildered a creature could not survive long enough to perpetuate its race, even if it could make an effective effort to do this, and with its appearance the process of evolution must almost inevitably have ceased … such a creature, even if it could take the steps necessary to propagate its bewildered kind, which appears doubtful, could have no survival value, for on receipt of a stimulus which it could not localise, from a stimulating agent whose nature it had no means of discovering, it could respond only by curling up and micturating. Yet this is the animal that Head and Rivers present to us as our common ancestor.[54]

Walshe was passionate about Queen Square, and admired greatly the clinical traditions of Jackson, Gowers and Horsley. He was very much against the fusion of the National Hospital with Maida Vale. But loyalty to the institution did not prevent him from commenting adversely on the staff. Walshe was a close friend of Critchley and enjoyed the company of McKissock. He wanted William Gooddy to be his successor on retirement from University College Hospital (which he was). However, he disliked Charles Symonds, had a low opinion of Denis Williams whom he thought 'lightweight', and Collier, Purves-

---

[52] Quoted by J. Walton, 'The Tardy Development of UK Neurology', *Brain* **137** (2014): 2868–70.

[53] Walshe criticised Penfield on many occasions in abusive terms, largely in relation to Penfield's 'Centrencephalic Integrating System'. J. M. Walshe remembers one family holiday in Rome, when by chance his father bumped into Penfield under the statue of Marcus Aurelius (rather appropriately, the last of the Roman emperors and a Stoic philosopher) and they had a very awkward time trying to be civil to each other. It must have been an interesting exchange under the baking Italian sun.

[54] F. M. R. Walshe, 'The Anatomy and Physiology of Cutaneous Sensibility: A Critical Review', *Brain* **65** (1942): 48–112; see also C. Phillips, 'Francis Martin Rouse Walshe 1885–1973', *Biographical Memoirs of Fellows of the Royal Society* **20** (1974): 456–81; and A. Compston, 'The Anatomy and Physiology of Cutaneous Sensibility: A Critical Review. By FMR Walshe', *Brain* **65** (1942): 48–112. Walshe wrote the review in 1921 and showed it to Trotter, who advised against publication whilst Head was living. As editor, Walshe did not wait long after Head's death to publish this in *Brain* at a time when copy was in short supply.

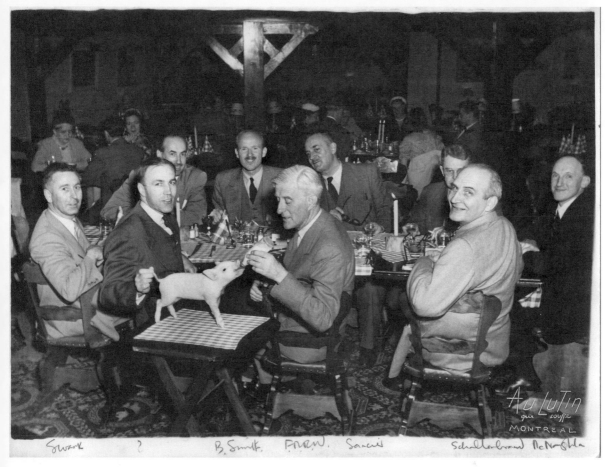

Figure 6.7 Walshe at dinner in Montréal. He seems to be feeding a piglet, 1952.

Stewart and Russell Brain also suffered at Walshe's expense. He thought Brain's textbook was 'paste and scissors'. Christopher Earl recalled that:

> Walshe once said to me, in relation to Russell Brain 'I was in court yesterday, Earl. You would think that the president of the Royal College of Physicians would know that pterygine meningioma can follow skull fracture. You would think he would know that. But he had never heard of it. You'd think the president would know that wouldn't you?[55]

Walshe had in fact published a paper on the topic of post-traumatic meningioma,[56] stimulated apparently by the behaviour of the Ministry of Pensions, which refused to entertain the relationship on the basis of the opinion of a 'psychiatrist from Blackpool' with whom Walshe was then engaged in a fight over another case.[57]

His hatred of state medicine and opposition to the introduction of the NHS in 1948 are discussed elsewhere, as are his criticisms of the university and medical school curricula. Another *bête noire* for Walshe was the 'salaried academic teacher', the professor of neurology. He told his son that anyone who aspired to be a professor of medicine was seeking 'the last refuge of the destitute', and he obstructed the creation of a professorship of neurology at Queen Square.[58] Much of his later writing was on the topic of medical education and

---

[55] McDonald archive: tape recording of a conversation between Earl and Ian McDonald.
[56] F. M. R. Walshe, 'Head Injuries as a Factor in the Aetiology of Intracranial Meningioma', *Lancet* 278 (1961): 993-6.

[57] Reply to a letter from Dr Charles Wells, correspondence dated 23 and 25 March 1963.
[58] An attitude which was shared by his friends. Critchley once told told a group of senior visiting foreign neurologists

Walshe repeatedly attacked what he saw as dumbing-down by the universities and the state with interference by academics. In the opening address to the University College Hospital Medical School in 1947, Walshe vented his spleen:

For the cloistered academic teacher life is different. He gets his patients washed and tidied and laid out in rows in Hospital wards; their importunate and exacting wives and mothers-in-law do not intrude upon his profound cogitations. No unpleasant smells or noises break in on his ordered eloquence; house-physicians and nurses wait on his bidding and tremble at his voice, and all those seeming irrelevances that are so necessary to the balanced comprehension of the patient's total situation are carefully tidied away out of his sight. He does not miss them, for he has never known them. He is rather like the florist who can arrange the plucked blooms, from which the dead leaves and the dirty roots have been removed and the earwigs shaken off, into all the combinations of form and colour his fancy dictates. I feel sure our clinical professors will greet this simple and faithful picture of their austere lives with sentiments of happy recognition.[59]

In the foreword to *Critical Studies in Neurology*,[60] Walshe reflected on the 'function of criticism in medicine' and regretted the subjugation of medicine and physiology as natural philosophy to empirical fact. He argued that these essays should be read as contributing fresh generalisations and that integration and synthesis must accompany the unresting accumulation of new facts:

For too many amongst us, also, the inadequate conception that 'science is measurement' and concerns itself with nothing but the metrical has become a thought-cramping obsession, and the more nearly a scientific paper approximates itself to a long and bloodless caravan of equations plodding across the desert pages of some journal, between small and infrequent oases of words, the more quintessentially scientific it is supposed to be, though not seldom no one can tell ... whither in the kingdom of ordered knowledge is the caravan bound.

He continued that 'there was a crying need for critical thought in neurology. By no other intellectual weapon can we hope to deal effectively with what has been called "the mysterious viability of the false".'

Walshe took issue with statistics ('a sort of propaedeutic to scientific research but little more') and genetics ('too many monographs are obsessively concerned with genetic factors in aetiology as if no other order of problem existed ... to take refuge in a noise machine is an expression of defeatism').[61] Although a staunch and devout Catholic, he also attacked the miraculous cures at Lourdes and Jesuit schoolteachers. He vehemently and repeatedly vented his opposition to establishment of the NHS and zealously attacked the idea of hospitals being state-funded and consultants no longer 'honoraries' but paid officials. Still more disliked was the concept of 'merit' awards. He was deeply antagonistic to what he perceived to be the 'socialization of medicine', and to him the NHS was an anathema. When the National Hospital was incorporated, Walshe refused to accept a salary for his work, relying for his living on private practice in Harley Street, which at its peak was very large. He retired in 1955 at the age of 70 but continued to function at the hospital and in private practice for some years. His grand-daughter remembers his rooms, with old-fashioned metal syringes on the mantle-piece and Walshe brandishing his tendon hammer. It is a sad reflection that, despite his pontifications about the superior nature of clinical neurology, by all accounts Walshe was not an especially good clinical neurologist.

The rather intolerant and tetchy picture painted above is only one side of the story. Certainly, he had many friends and genuine admirers on both sides of the Atlantic. They were loyal to Walshe and remarked on his humour and kindness. Critchley, who, of course, shared Walshe's linguistic skills, provides an affectionate portrait

For sheer intellectualism he towered above his colleagues ... but he was a nullifidian; one who could detect with uncanny sagacity the flaws or weak points in a proposition or a therapy ... there was no one like Walshe when it came to distinguishing hocus from pocus ... a figure [in the 1920s] who was rather aloof

---

who kept calling him Professor Critchley, 'In this country professor is a derogatory term.'

[59] F. M. R. Walshe, 'The Teachers of Medicine', *Lancet* **250** (1947): 817–20.

[60] F. M. R. Walshe, *Critical Studies in Neurology* (Edinburgh: Churchill Livingstone Ltd, 1948).

[61] A letter from 19 August 1964 to Dr Aubrey Lewis.

and superficially cold, for he was something of a loner. However, at the lunch table, and more particularly in the privacy of my sitting room, he would frequently converse very freely and in a most interesting fashion. In later years he mellowed, and his inherent charm came to the surface and particularly impressed his colleagues abroad.[62]

Critchley wrote, in an obituary of Walshe – perhaps too fulsomely:

It is not enough to say that he was the doyen of British neurology, for he was one of the few outstanding critic–philosophers of our time. He was a natural successor to Hughlings Jackson, but his penetration of thought went deeper, and he showed a greater mistrust of untidy speculation. Unlike Jackson, however, he was felicitous in the manipulation of prose. Walshe was the outstanding intellectual of current British neurology. Those who grumbled about his alleged lack of creative thinking or of his so-called prejudices, could never deny his alarming skill as a penetrating critic of muddled ideas, of light-hearted speculation, and of the materialism that bedevils contemporary medical science.[63]

However, Walshe's regressive attitudes – for instance, on the NHS, education, medical academics, psychiatrists, neurosurgeons and physiology – were not in tune with the times. He was the most influential physician at Queen Square in his generation and, on most of these topics, his dominant personality placed the National Hospital on the wrong side of the debates and left Queen Square sidelined. For all his achievements, one can only wonder whether the National Hospital might have fared better under a more skillful, politically astute and less prickly leader.

---

[62] Walshe could be hilariously funny, and apparently everyone had his own examples of 'Walshisms'. Critchley gave two, which somehow sum up his humour as well as his arrogance. Listening to a lecture by a lady doctor named Helen, Walshe turned to Critchley and asked what was a unit of female beauty; the answer: 'one micro-Helen; that is the face that launched one ship'. When travelling to America on the *Ile de France*, Walshe and Critchley were presented at dinner with a menu 'the size of a newspaper'. At the bottom was a note stating that invalids on special diets were catered for. The head steward was summoned and told that Walshe suffered from caviar-deficiency. 'Yes', murmured Walshe, 'severe chronic asturgeonosis'. Caviar then appeared at every meal. See Critchley, *The Ventricle of Memory*.

[63] M. Critchley. 'Obituary: Sir Frances Walshe (1886–1973)', *Journal of the Neurological Sciences* **19** (1973): 255–6.

Charles Putnam Symonds

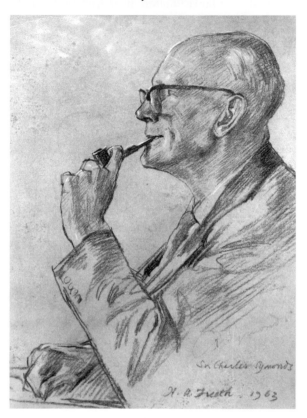

Figure 6.8 A drawing of Sir Charles Symonds by H. A. Freeth RA.

Born in his parents' house in Weymouth Street, London, on 11 April 1890, Symonds was usually known as 'Charlie' in memory of his father's favourite brother, who had drowned.[64] Symonds was educated at Rugby School, Warwickshire, supported by a scholarship. He enjoyed the rigours of enforced physical fitness and studied classics. There he met Ronald Poulton-Palmer.[65] Both went to the University of

---

[64] We are advantaged through having access in the McDonald archive papers to the typescripts of two biographical chapters that Ronald Symonds wrote on his father; these appear to be unpublished. The Wellcome Trust also has an archive, which is likely to have been provided by Ronald Symonds, contained in a box file labelled 'Papers Concerning the Life and Work of Sir Charles Symonds'. Symonds included an autobiographical introduction to *Studies in Neurology* (London: Oxford University Press, 1970), pp. 1–23.

[65] Ronald Poulton-Palmer excelled at rugby football and later captained England; he was killed in 1915. In June 1917,

Oxford, Poulton-Palmer's hometown, in 1908, where Symonds met Janet Poulton, then aged 16, whom he later married. Thwarted in his initial aim of entering the Indian Civil Service after an Oxford education in 'Greats', because he was wrongly diagnosed with a 'weak heart', Symonds defaulted to medicine, and trained at Guy's Hospital from 1912: 'At Guy's I came under the spell of Arthur Hurst who, while assistant physician, established an outpatient clinic for nervous diseases. Hurst's clinical demonstrations were superb. If there was a fault it was that they made neurology seem too easy.'

When war was declared on 4 August 1914, Symonds was three months short of qualifying in medicine but he enlisted as a motorcycle despatch rider, on 19 August, because there were no vacancies as a pilot, his preferred role. Despatch riders had to be university graduates, able to read a map, capable of some French, and the owner of a Triumph or Douglas motorcycle that the army would buy:[66] Symonds went to war sustained by a spirit of patriotism and adventure. But, like others, he was soon appalled by the terrible slaughter and suffering in the trenches.[67]

Serving with the First Division in the retreat from Mons and the Battles of the Marne and Aisne, on 7 September 1914, while delivering a message for the Second Brigade, he was challenged by a sentry.

Thinking him to be a Welshman because his diction was poor, a German bullet quickly explained where he had ended up. Surviving that encounter, Symonds was wounded in the leg two weeks later. Evacuation proved difficult and Symonds was deemed unfit to travel after developing gas gangrene.[68] On his return to England, Symonds became engaged to Janet. On 5 November 1914, he was awarded the Médaille Militaire by the president of the French Republic for gallantry during the operations in August 1914.

After his recovery, Symonds returned to Guy's Hospital, qualified in 1915, and was commissioned into the Royal Army Medical Corps and appointed as medical officer to the Royal Flying Corps squadron at Farnborough. Symonds returned to the 101 Field Ambulance in 1917 as Captain, now riding a horse over which he exerted intermittent control, rather than a motorcycle. His accounts of trench warfare are harrowing.[69] Participating in the Battle of Arras, he established a series of first-aid posts, and was twice struck on the head by bullets. On the second occasion: 'the chin strap was not fastened and the helmet went spinning away with no damage to my head. When recovered it showed a groove which I cherished as an emblem of luck.' He walked 15 miles each day on muddy ground and duckboard tracks to visit posts, and began to think that people would not believe the extent of the horror.[70]

Symonds found his grave damaged and replaced the cross with one made of oak, which was removed to Oxford after the war and set in the wall of St Cross cemetery close to that of Poulton-Palmer's sister Janet, Symonds' first wife, who died in 1919. This cross was restored by Richard Symonds in 1984.

[66] Apart from studying, while at Oxford Symonds played rugby and tennis for New College and rode a motorcycle: 'Charles had an expert knowledge of motorbikes and was seldom happier than when taking one to bits' (Symonds, *Studies in Neurology*).

[67] He wrote to Janet on 2 September 1914: 'War is a bad business: it is the worst sight in the world to see the country people leaving their homes and trekking off for safety with what they can carry on a cart. They are very brave about it though, and at all times most wonderfully kind ... even the refugees open up their bundles and give of what they have to our troops ... I have not seen very much actual fighting yet myself: mostly artillery fire. When one really gets into it, it must be the most exciting sensation in the world, if one is a decent shot, better even than the Cresta! I think it would be better still though if gunpowder had never been invented, and the fighting were still hand to hand ... I should think those men whose profession it is really enjoy war: I am mainly struck by the absolute badness of it all: the waste and the suffering.'

[68] 'Charles woke up in a hospital somewhere in France. The man in the bed next to him was dying of tetanus. A medical officer was going round the ward examining the patients. A probe was being used and Charles noticed that it was not being sterilized between uses. Charles feigned delirium, attacking the doctor and spilling the bowl in which the probe was being washed' (Symonds, *Studies in Neurology*).

[69] He wrote to Ronald, aged less than 1 year old on 22 April 1917: 'I am just going in to a very, very big battle and so I am sending you this letter for your mother to keep for you in case I should be killed and never be able to talk to you myself: so that you shall have a letter for yourself to remember your Daddy by. I am taking part in this war as are all the hundreds of men who are being killed every day, so that you and your mother and all the others should be free for all your lives to live up to the ideals which are best – without ever having to go through such a war as this. Your mother will tell what an ideal means. Her ideals and mine are the same.' Later Symonds discussed trench warfare with a great-uncle who had been a medical officer in Sebastopol during the Crimean War in the 1850s.

[70] He wrote to Janet late in 1917: 'As usual all my senses are affected by the battlefield: sight first the brown uniformity of colour, the endless pattern of contiguous shell holes, just here and there stumps of trees all splintered and stained the

Symonds was critical of the misplaced ideals that led to war but not of the enemy, whom he considered to have been humane in their treatment of British wounded. Soldiers on both sides were fellow sufferers. Any campaign of hate belonged to the home front whipped up by politicians. He was, however, critical of staff officers, finding them pompous and out of touch with reality. He retained phrases in later life that reflected wartime experience: inefficiency was 'bad staff-work', and, for more obscure reasons, a good

---

same universal brown with splashed mud, and the more particular sights, dead men and horses, and pieces of dead men and horses – shell holes full of blood: splashes of fresh blood on the duckboard tracks. Hearing comes next – the continuous crash of our guns and the strain and tension of listening all the time for the direction of the enemy shells. Last but not least comes smell – it's hardest to describe, mainly the lack of freshness in the air that comes with the absolute dearth of vegetation, and added to this the poisonous reek of rotting food and bodies mixed with whiffs of burnt cordite, and traces of shell gas. Is this too horrible for you? I don't want it to be so. But I read an article in the *Times Literary Supplement* last week, foretelling the reflections of posterity upon this war: they would forget the unpleasantness, the writer said, the filth, the agony, and the bereavements, and remember only the glorious acts of individual heroism and adventure, just as they did after the Napoleonic wars. I believe the substance of the article to be true, and so I want to leave some record of my own impressions'; and later that year: 'I saw one or two bad cases at night. Of course war could not go on at all unless there were men at the back sufficiently protected against intimate knowledge of its realities to be detached, and to drive the fighting men on from behind. It is curious to note how the spirit of the troops has changed even from two years ago. If anything it is more admirable: there is more patience and self-sacrifice: but it is infinitely more pathetic to witness. No keen curiosity now, no careless enthusiasm, not even that to carry them on: but instead a sense of duty, and a bowing down to the inevitable – the inevitable power which drives them on from behind. The troops have settled down to war as slaves to their task: if they fall short of what is expected they risk discomfort, punishment, even death: whereas if they please their masters there are certain rewards to be won in the form of holiday and rest from the line. It is a sad spectacle to see free citizens of a civilised empire thus degraded: one must admit that such a process of slavery is degrading: and looking at it from a still broader point of view – what an appalling thought it is that this is going on now in all the civilised nations of the world. It means absolute moral and intellectual retrogression. And yet – let's hope that the author of "Sonia" is right and that in the breasts of those of our generation who have survived the ordeal, there shall have been kindled desires and ambitions that will have made the war worth it: nothing else can.'

meal always elicited the remark 'tell the cook to put on his jacket ... and report to me'. Symonds' war ended in the relative safety of a casualty clearing station behind the lines.

It was while working at the Connaught Hospital in Aldershot that Symonds had met E. D. Adrian and decided on a career in clinical neurology, having, like Walshe, already been attracted to the subject through reading Sherrington's *Integrative Action of the Nervous System* while at Oxford. On demobilisation, he was appointed resident medical officer at the National Hospital. Janet and two children (Ronald and Richard) lived in Redhill, close to Symonds' parents, and it was there, on 23 July 1919, that Janet died after falling off her bicycle. Hurst had convinced his colleagues that Guy's needed a department for nervous diseases and, devoting himself to work in his grief, in 1920 (and aged only 30 years), Symonds was appointed assistant physician, although Hurst remained in charge until 1927 when Symonds was promoted to physician. At the same time, he applied successfully to Oxford for a Radcliffe Travelling Fellowship. His intention was to study neuropathology in Paris but Hurst suggested that he become interested in psychiatry and neurosurgery. This led to Symonds working with Harvey Cushing in Boston, and Adolf Meyer in Baltimore. Symonds was much in awe of Cushing.[71] Conversely, he admired and felt comfortable in Meyer's presence, with his striking physical appearance and personal manner and the ability to observe and interpret human behaviour. Whilst in Baltimore, Symonds met a young English secretary, Edythe Eva ('Peggy') Dorton, whom he married in September 1920, creating a rift with his late wife Janet's family that never healed. Symonds was reunited with his two children, living initially at 58 Portland Place and then, with two sons born to Peggy, at 74 Wimpole Street, London, where the family remained until 1939.

Symonds had obtained the MRCP by examination in 1916, making him unusually well qualified for a medical officer, and was elected FRCP in 1924. Two years later, after two unsuccessful applications, he was appointed to the consultant staff at Queen Square.

---

[71] Finding an omission in the history of a particular case written by Symonds, Cushing addressed only the resident: '[Simeon] Locke don't you know that the case history is the most important part of the case record? ... it's bad enough when I have to leave history taking to you, but when you leave it to the man who wrote this it's just terrible.'

This he relished for the companionship and spirit of competitiveness that he missed at Guy's. Symonds enjoyed meeting neurologists and trainees from the Commonwealth countries and the USA who visited the National Hospital, and, although not a person for formal entertainment, he hosted social gatherings with many of these professional acquaintances on their subsequent visits to the UK. He delivered two weekly outpatient clinics, seeing 100 patients on each occasion and, subsequently, became responsible for inpatients. Symonds rarely took a weekend away from work, and remained on-call for more senior colleagues. He retained an interest in teaching and research and was nearly always working on a manuscript.

In order to support his family, Symonds supplemented his £50 per annum honorarium from Guy's Hospital with private practice, coaching candidates for exams, working at pensions clinics and acting as an expert witness in court.[72] Most of Symonds' private

work was carried out in two nursing homes close to where he lived, each run by an ex-Guy's nursing sister as matron, and he saw cases in the 'provinces' at the request of ex-Guy's general practitioners or consultant colleagues.[73] Sometimes he was summoned at night. At first, he drove himself on a BSA motorcycle with a sidecar, next an open-top Hillman red two-seater sports car, then a series of Sunbeam motor cars, and eventually, from 1931, a chauffeur-driven Rolls Royce, driven by Smith who lived in a nearby mews house. The Rolls had a blind separating the driver from the back seats where Symonds read journals, wrote notes for lectures and ate his sandwiches.[74]

---

[72] In *Studies in Neurology* (1970), Symonds recalls two cases from this period. On these, Ronald Symonds writes: 'He gave evidence that a girl had suffered permanent injury in an accident, although there were no outward signs. Charles stated the grounds for his opinion and was subjected to a merciless attack by the opposing counsel who eventually said: "So, it amounts to this doctor, you listened to the story of the girl and her mother and accepted all they said", "not without careful cross-examination", Charles replied. To this the barrister remarked: "Your cross-examination seems to have been pretty successful, was it not doctor?" Charles was silent, whereupon the judge, Mr Justice Amory, addressing counsel said: "You see the doctor does not understand you. He means cross-examination in search of the truth." There was another case that took a more dramatic turn. A firm of solicitors tried to subpoena Charles to get him to give evidence (without a fee) in connection with a claim for damages by a former patient of his. This man had suffered a head injury in a road accident and, six months previously, Charles had said he could not exclude some permanent disability. Charles did not wish to be subpoenaed, but a lawyer's clerk hung around the entrance to 74 Wimpole Street trying to intercept him as he came out. In order to avoid the clerk, Charles made use of a fire escape which led from the roof of No. 74 to the house next door, from which he emerged into the street unnoticed. After employing this uncomfortable stratagem for several days Charles got in touch with the solicitors and suggested a meeting to settle the matter amicably. They agreed but instead immediately served a subpoena on him. Charles had to go to York where the case was being heard. Shortly before the hearing a lawyer's clerk came to his hotel and said an up-to-date medical report was needed. Charles replied that his fee would be 100 guineas. The clerk became agitated and said there was no time to lose. Charles was adamant that

he must have a cheque first. This was produced and Charles went to examine his former patient. He now found there was no indication of brain damage, only hysteria. When asked in Court if his recent examination had confirmed his earlier report he replied: "No." Counsel for the claimant tried to brush this aside, but the judge would have none of it and Charles's new evidence was accepted.'

[73] In a conversation with Ian McDonald, for which a typescript survives, Christopher Earl recalled: 'Charlie was called to Newcastle to see a young woman. He came on the sleeper. Henry [Miller] met him at the station and over his kipper, Charlie made the diagnosis and caught the 9.30 back to London.' John Walton confirms this anecdote and adds that the diagnosis was ependymoma of the fourth ventricle which was successfully operated on by John Hankinson. On another occasion, Earl was asked to see a patient whom he knew to be acquainted with Symonds: 'So I took the precaution of saying to Charlie "Would you mind, Sir, if I could go with you to see this poor man?"; "How are you going?" says Charlie; "On the train" says Christopher. "I'll tell you what I used to do before the War" says Symonds, "I would send my chauffeur off in the afternoon before the clinic and after I had finished seeing patients at 6 o'clock, I got the train from Paddington, had my dinner, got off at Swindon and there was the car to take me to the house and drive me home" ... "It was a very efficient way of doing it", which of course it was ... but times have changed', says Earl, with more than a hint of nostalgia.

[74] Earl recalled: 'Symonds had a famous dispute with a colleague at Guy's, the psychiatrist Robert Gillespie, during which, rather than the chauffeur driving up, opening the door and removing the rug from Symonds's legs, as usual, the chauffeur would get out, open the boot, undo a thermos of warm milk and give this to Symonds to provide comfort and courage for him to enter the hospital.' Symonds refers obliquely to the dispute with Gillespie (see Symonds, *Studies in Neurology*, p. 16), which arose from the latter's insistence that neurology had no place in the assessment or management of psychiatric disease. After Gillespie's death, Symonds took charge of the privately endowed York Clinic for functional nervous disorders at Guy's. In 1950, this accommodated the department of neurosurgery, to

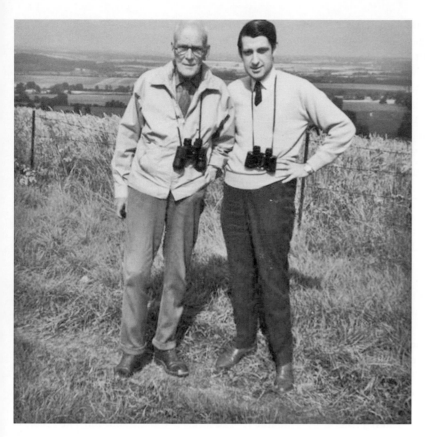

Figure 6.9 Charles Symonds and Ian McDonald. It is said that Symonds' binoculars are the pair belonging to a German officer from the First World War (collection of Alastair Compston).

His relaxations were occasional visits to the theatre, dancing and physical exercise – walking and jogging with a backpack in order to get fit for skiing. Since the First World War, he had enjoyed bird-watching, using a pair of binoculars that had belonged to a German officer, as an accompaniment to walking.

At his father's suggestion, Symonds took up fly-fishing (which he continued until age 86, when he suffered a stroke) on the rivers Test in Hampshire and Kennet in Berkshire, in Scotland and in the west of Ireland.[75] At home he read widely, including poetry. Symonds disliked London, which he designated 'The Great Wen'. In 1931, he and Peggy bought the lease of a house in Aston Ferry near Henley-on-Thames. It lacked electricity, gas or mains water but

had a boathouse on the river. The children now found their father less remote, and at the weekends he played tennis, swam in the river, invented games on the lawn and kept fit.[76] On Monday, he drove the Rolls to Slough where Smith met him at the station and returned them to London.

But this idyllic life was set to change from 1938, when war with Germany again seemed likely. Symonds was invited by Cairns to join him at the Military Hospital for Head Injuries at St Hugh's College in Oxford,[77] representing the Royal Air Force to which

which was appointed Murray Falconer, before the unit relocated to the Maudsley Hospital in 1952.

[75] On his first fishing expedition, he caught several fish and was reprimanded by a gillie for taking one underweight. Replying in his defence that no one had told him about this restriction, the gillie replied: 'I did not think you would catch any, Sir.'

[76] The Aston marathon involved running to the river, swimming across fully clothed, racing up a hill on the far side, and back – the winner receiving a small monetary reward. In the winter, the routine was a wet 14-mile walk supported by biscuits and chocolate before recovering in front of the fire.

[77] McDonald recalled the opinion of Symonds that Charles Phillips, later Dr Lee's Professor of Anatomy in the University of Oxford, was the outstanding member of the clinical neurological staff at St Hugh's during the Second World War.

Symonds had been civilian consultant in neurology since 1934. At the outbreak of the Second World War, Symonds, now a group captain, closed down the house in Wimpole Street, stored his furniture and moved to Oxford. At first, most of his time was spent at RAF Halton serving on medical boards. No doubt conditioned by experiences as a battalion medical officer in the First World War, from 1942 he became involved with 'flying stress', the equivalent of 'shell-shock', taking the view that aircrew were being misunderstood – sometimes too harshly, sometimes with excessive leniency. Symonds had a busy war and his contributions were fully recognised. He served on the Flying Personnel Research Committee from 1942 to 1963; was promoted to air commodore in 1942 and air vice-marshal in 1945; made a Companion of the Bath in 1944; and knighted in 1946. He received the Raymond Longacre Award for Scientific Contribution to Aviation Medicine from the Aero-Medical Association of the USA in 1949.

In the First World War, it had been assumed that flying stress was physiological and due to anoxia. As a member of the Brain Injuries Committee of the Medical Research Council which, in 1941, produced War Memorandum No. 4, Symonds had defined hysteria as 'a condition in which mental and physical symptoms, not of organic origin, are produced and maintained by motives never fully conscious directed at some real or fancied gain to be derived from such symptoms'. He suggested that the phenotype of hysteria is conditioned by the style of influential neurologists: Charcot expected grotesque convulsive spasms and that is what he got; Babinski was more interested in paralysis, which 'thus became more prevalent'. Symonds submitted a memorandum to the director general of RAF Medical Services,[78] which reached the Flying Personnel Research Committee, as a result of which he was charged with investigating the psychology of serving as aircrew. In this, Symonds was assisted by Wing Commander Denis Williams.[79] Their report, which was not published until after the

war, involved extensive overseas visits that were not without danger. In Bathurst, West Africa, a flying-boat needed 11 attempts to get airborne. Over New Mexico, Symonds was piloting a USAF aircraft when the engine failed and the plane started to dive. He looked for help from the crew but found them asleep, until one woke, noticed that the main fuel supply had failed and quickly made a connection to the reserve tank. Symonds and Williams argued that the load imposed by flying duties should be formulated in conventional psychiatric terms, such as anxiety or hysteria. Those unable to continue flying duties but without medical disability were designated as having low moral fibre (LMF), losing their rank and being relegated to ground duties or other services. Although considering that 'a fit man should not be able to escape the hazards of operational flying through a medical backdoor', Symonds wrote with sympathy and concern for the accuracy of diagnosis in the 2,919 cases of psychological disorder seen in the year ending 9 February 1943, of whom 419 were deemed to have 'lack of confidence'. Although it was clear that operational flying imposed strains that no one could be expected to sustain indefinitely, the need for sufficient men with operational experience to remain available to lead aircrew was paramount. The greatest strain was on members of the home-based Bomber Command, for whom the expectation of surviving a standard first tour of 30 sorties was less than 30 per cent. After a period of ground-based instruction, the routine was for a further 25 operational flights. Symonds was consulted by Group Captain (Geoffrey) Leonard Cheshire (Baron Cheshire, VC, OM, DSO, DFC), who developed 'nervous tension'. But, in Cheshire's case, this was the result of being prevented from returning to operational duties, such that Symonds was asked to record Cheshire as 'unfit for non-operational, though fit for flying duties', which he did.

Symonds' views on the psychology of flying stress formed the basis for his Croonian lectures delivered to the Royal College of Physicians in May 1943 on 'The Human Response to Flying Stress'.[80] This got him into some trouble because propaganda was immediately broadcast from Germany claiming that morale was low in the Royal Air Force. Despite the title, his position was that plain words and conventional classification of disease should be used. Those who suffered through the danger of operational flying should

---

[78] C. P. Symonds and D. J. Williams, *Air Publication (AP) 3139: A Clinical and Statistical Study of Neurosis Precipitated by Flying Duties* (London: HMSO, 1947), pp. 140–72.

[79] McDonald considered Denis Williams to be 'clever, articulate and amusing, nimble of mind and elegant in dress; much loved as a physician and admired as a teacher … he had a special capacity for helping patients to come to terms with their afflictions … [he was] interested in mechanisms even if his interpretations went beyond the facts'.

[80] See *British Medical Journal* 2 (1943): 703–6, 740–4.

not be camouflaged by spurious diagnoses such as 'flying stress', 'aeroneurosis', 'aviator's neurasthenia' – terms that were reminiscent of 'shell-shock'. Symptoms were most prevalent in those predisposed to psychological illness or with stressful domestic situations, and directly related to the intensity and duration of activity and exposure to danger, being most likely in the rear-gunners of heavy bombers on night flights. Of those affected, 79 per cent were anxious, 9 per cent depressed and 13 per cent hysterical. Symonds considered the nature of fear as a behavioural and physiological response to real, remembered or anticipated danger, conditioned by prior experience or triggers and not constrained by other emotions such as anger and loyalty. Next, he dealt with fearlessness. This sometimes arose from stupidity or lack of imagination and experience, a high threshold for acknowledging threat or blunted affective apparatus. It was not necessarily a virtue. Influenced as he was by Sherrington, Symonds explained fearlessness in terms of reciprocal facilitation and inhibition of physiological activities, and the many experimental manipulations that extinguish or modulate Pavlovian conditioned behavioural responses. The ideal was that fearlessness born of courage and nurtured by confidence would wax and wane, especially with time and unpleasant experiences, preventing the soldier being distracted from performance through the anguish of fear. This required conscious control and was likely to result in fatigue and eventual loss of efficiency.

Much later, on 27 February 1970, Symonds, then aged 80, lectured at Queen Square on 'hysteria'. In a letter to the dean, Reginald Kelly, thanking him for various practical arrangements, Symonds commented that Sir Kenneth Robson had suggested that the annotated typescript not be lost to posterity (which it has not). Two opinion leaders were quoted – Slater: 'the diagnosis of hysteria is a disguise for ignorance and a fertile source of clinical error'; and Walshe: 'the essential difference of hysteria from somatic disease is that it constitutes a behaviour disorder, a human act on the psychological level'. Symonds annotated the typescript of his lecture: 'I agree [entirely] with Sir Francis ... in this and all else that he wrote in his masterly summary. Hysteria is not a myth but a reality.' He told his audience:

> Under the conditions of the Somme, and of Pa[s] chenda[e]le, the gain to be derived from disability could be overwhelming for any normal person. The sufferer was by no means always of a hysterical personality. As a battalion medical officer I had first-hand experience of this, and successfully treated cases of hysteria without sending them into hospital. The earlier the diagnosis was made the more easily it was treated.

Symonds was scathing of the attempt to dignify these cases as due to physical disease, as proposed by Froment and Babinski, who claimed that the vascular changes of reflex paralysis proved its organicity, a view that appeared to be endorsed by Farquhar Buzzard: 'This manual translated into English under the aegis of a physician to this hospital misinterpreted the effects of prolonged disuse.' Symonds, however, did respect Farquhar Buzzard, acknowledging that his clinical judgement and advice to a young neurologist were sound:

> after the epidemic of encephalitis lethargica in 1919 ... out-patient physicians diagnosed them as hysterical because nothing like them had been seen before ... Buzzard recognised them as organic. His advice to me ... was that I should spend time in the study of the pathology of diseases with which I had become acquainted.[81]

But for Symonds, the forces driving hysteria did not end at Versailles. In his lecture at Queen Square, he continued: 'Motivation for hysteria was still prevalent in the post-war years. There was wide-scale unemployment and much hardship, and the war pension clinics yielded a considerable harvest of hysterics ... In private practice I saw as many patients with functional as organic nervous disease and found them equally interesting.'

Symonds' approach to curing hysterical illness used methods, including hypnosis, taught by Hurst, who had himself been trained by Babinski. If compensation failed to cure the complaint, recovery might require escaping from the situation with dignity, even if this involved resorting in one case to a faked religious service of thanksgiving for miraculous recovery, thereby avoiding the assumption that the illness was due to malingering. Symonds' tactic was to strike a deal with the hysteric: 'I know that your pretended loss of memory is the result of some intolerable emotional situation. Tell me your story. I promise absolutely to respect your confidence, will give you all the help I can and will say to your doctor and relatives that I have cured you by hypnotism.'

---

[81] Symonds, *Studies in Neurology*, (1970) p. 6.

After the war Symonds returned to hospital posts but had to re-establish his private practice.[82] The family moved to Harley Street and Aston was relinquished, as were Smith and the Rolls. Symonds drove himself in a Ford 8. Weekends were spent in Berkshire fishing on the Kennet, or staying at a public house as a base for walking in the Chilterns. Now famous as a neurologist, Symonds was Sims Travelling Professor to Canada, Australia and New Zealand, and visiting professor in San Francisco and Montréal.

Symonds was largely responsible for the rehabilitation of Thomas Willis' reputation as the founder of clinical neurology. Symonds started his Harveian Oration (1954) on 'The Circle of Willis' with a defence of the clinical scientist, caught between research ambition and the pressures of clinical duties, with no time to reflect and a lack of training in laboratory methods. He argued for the appointment of clinicians to senior research posts: 'every case he sees of motor neurone disease or disseminated sclerosis must become for the moment a personal issue wherein he has to acknowledge defeat. He is very often made to feel uncomfortable.' With William Feindel, Symonds arranged for the worn stone of black Belgian marble in Westminster Abbey, commemorating Willis' life and work but cracked when the great central lantern fell in 1941, to be replaced using funds (200 guineas) donated by the Royal College of Physicians of London and the Canadian Neurological Society. This was unveiled at a service conducted by Canon Adam Fox.

Symonds had served as a Guarantor of *Brain* since 1923, and a subcommittee comprising Anthony Feiling, Godwin Greenfield, Walshe, Denis Williams and Samuel Nevin met on 29 July 1952 at the Royal

Society of Medicine and decided to invite Symonds to become the next editor but, if he could not see his way to do so (as proved to be the case for reasons that are not known), then to ask Sir Russell Brain.

In retirement, Symonds produced a collection of his earlier papers.[83] The three articles on cerebrovascular disease include Symonds' account based on work with Harvey Cushing in the early 1920s on the diagnosis of intracranial aneurysm in life, before the introduction of angiography.[84] In his 1970 annotation, Symonds considers that case 5 was an example of cerebral angioma, misdiagnosed at the time. This work arose from a case in which Symonds suggested cerebral aneurysm in advance of Cushing's exploration for a presumed tumour. The patient had uncontrollable haemorrhage and died peri-operatively. At post-mortem examination, Symonds was proved correct and Cushing declared: 'Symonds, you made the correct diagnosis: either this was fluke or there was a reason in it. If so you will prove it. You will cease your ward duties as from now, and spend all your time in the library.'

Symonds' paper on cerebral infarction with contralateral hemiplegia in association with cervical rib substantiated his hypothesis, formulated as a house physician at Queen Square, of embolus as a mechanism of cerebral infarction: 'I was however unable to persuade any of my fellow residents or the staff that this could be true.'[85] Later in the book, Symonds gathers his papers on cerebral venous thrombosis,

[82] Christopher Earl recalled: 'The person [Derek] Denny [Brown] respected most was Charlie ... they had a rank at Guys: Mac [Michael 'Sean' McArdle] was the HP, Denny the chief assistant, and Charlie the boss ... Denny shared consulting rooms with Charlie. But Denny was always late and since the patients had to wait in the Symonds's dining room, they never had any dinner on the nights Denny was consulting'; 'When Sean McArdle presented a paper to the ABN on carpal tunnel syndrome, Francis Walshe, who believed the condition was due to sagging of the shoulders, commented that he did not come to the ABN to be given a lecture on anatomy by a registrar and, anyway, what would McArdle know about heavy fur coats?' Earl continues: 'Mac had reached his conclusions at Guys and nobody believed him. Charlie didn't either. I was on Charlie's firm as a student and he went to see a case while Mac was away on holiday and he said: "Oh well, if McArdle says so ... however it can't be true" ... but it was.'

[83] Symonds, *Studies in Neurology* (1970), p. 344. The collection of 21 papers and two memorial addresses, originally written between 1923 and 1967, prefaced by an informative autobiographical essay, was chosen with advice from William Ritchie Russell and Ian McDonald. Each paper has a short annotation by Symonds.

[84] C. P. Symonds, 'Contributions to the Clinical Study of Intracranial Aneurysms', *Guy's Hospital Reports* 73 (1923): 139–58. In his postscript, Cushing agonises on the many cases he must have erroneously diagnosed as cerebral tumour and concludes: 'the diagnosis of these cases during life must depend upon that form of clinical acumen, based on as thorough knowledge of normal and pathological anatomy, which has distinguished so many English clinicians, both physicians and surgeons – men of the type of the Cooper, Bright, Addison, Hodgkin and Gull, whose names have made Guy's famous'. Cushing was slow to write his addendum to the paper and, meanwhile, the subject was described by James Collier, in his presidential address to the section of neurology of the Royal Society of Medicine.

[85] C. P. Symonds, 'Cervical Rib: Thrombosis of Subclavian Artery: Contralateral Hemiplegia of Sudden Onset,

drawing attention to focal cerebral symptoms that follow dural occlusion and the late consequence of hydrocephalus. Acknowledging that, mistakenly, he had attributed the increased intracranial pressure to a change in volume of the cerebrospinal fluid, Symonds nevertheless defended the clinical observations and, with the work of Purdon Martin on puerperal conditions, the paper drew attention to the clinical importance of intracranial thrombophlebitis.[86] By 1956, Symonds had accepted that his designation of otitic hydrocephalus, later replaced by Kalbag and Woolf as cerebral venous thrombosis, was inappropriate.[87] Symonds included his paper on cataplexy as an example of a seizure disorder: 'Hughlings Jackson insisted that the characteristic feature of an epileptic seizure was its "paroxysmalness". There is something to be said in favour of the view here expressed, a view that was shared by Kinnier Wilson, who probably suggested it to the present writer.'[88]

Symonds delivered the Hughlings Jackson lecture on the physiological and chemical basis of epilepsy: 'inevitably it is now [1970] out of date but many of the questions remain unanswered'.[89] In his writings on head injury, Symonds expressed debt to the work of Ritchie Russell and Goldstein on the interpretation of organic psychological disorder – work that sits at the edge of Symonds' deep involvement with war neuroses. His views contradicted those of Wilfrid Trotter, who attributed the immediate consequences of head injury to compression and cerebral ischaemia. Symonds was eventually summoned by Trotter who declared: 'Well, I am afraid the theoretical fat is in the fire!'

Symonds wrote much on migrainous hemiplegia, but acknowledged that Wilfrid Harris had already recognised the condition:

That this is a malady *sui generis* no one would deny. Its essential features were briefly described by Harris in 1926, under the heading 'periodic migrainous neuralgia'. Harris had an immense store of knowledge of pain in the head and face, and this syndrome might well have been called after him 'Harris's neuralgia'. The American caption 'cluster headaches' has however gained wide acceptance and has some descriptive value. The paper reprinted here gave what I think was the most complete account of the condition up to that date, with details of a new and effective method of treatment.[90]

Although arguing that the entity of cough headache does exist, Symonds remained unclear as to its mechanism and, despite describing cases with structural lesions in the posterior fossa, failed to mention cerebellar ectopia as a cause.[91] We have already analysed Symonds' position on hysteria and psychological disorder, but it is revealing to see those papers that he regarded as most significant in this category. His presidential address to the section of psychiatry of the Royal Society of Medicine expressed the opinion that neurosis is best managed by a well-educated general practitioner, rather than by a specialist in psychotherapy. This analysis 'brought down on my head the wrath of a number of psychotherapists of the analytical persuasion'. Reflecting in 1970 on this paper from 1941, in which Symonds argued for a closer liaison between students of brain and mind, he claimed (perhaps with the benefit of hindsight) 'my conviction that there should be a chair of neurology at the Maudsley Hospital and a chair of psychiatry at the National Hospital, Queen Square, remains unshaken'.[92] Symonds dealt at greater length with the relationship between neurology and psychiatry in his Cairns memorial lecture.[93] The problem arose from the dominance of psychology and psychotherapy in the USA and psychopathology in the UK. The rift between psychiatry and neurology had been resisted by Symonds' mentor

---

Probably Embolic', *Proceedings of the Royal Society of Medicine* 20 (1927): 1244–5.

[86] C. P. Symonds, 'Hydrocephalic and Focal Cerebral Symptoms in Relation to Thrombophlebitis of the Dural Sinuses and Cerebral Veins', *Brain* 60 (1937): 531–50.

[87] This term evolved from the experience of cases seen after Symonds' appointment in the late 1920s to the consultant staff of the Throat, Nose and Ear Hospital in Gray's Inn Road, London.

[88] C. P. Symonds, 'Cataplexy and Other Related Forms of Seizure', *Canadian Medical Association Journal* 70 (1954): 621–5.

[89] C. P. Symonds, 'Excitation and Inhibition in Epilepsy', *Brain* 82 (1959): 133–46.

[90] C. P. Symonds, 'Migrainous Variants', *Transactions of the Medical Society of London* 67 (1951): 237–51; and see W. Harris, *Neuritis and Neuralgia* (London: Oxford University Press, 1926), pp. 301–5.

[91] C. P. Symonds, 'Cough Headache', *Brain* 79 (1956): 557–68.

[92] David Marsden was appointed professor of neurology at the Institute of Psychiatry in 1972. The events that led to failure to appoint Eliot Slater to a professorship of psychiatry at Queen Square are described in Chapter 10.

[93] The sixth Sir Hugh Cairns memorial lecture, *Tria juncta in uno*, delivered to the Society of British Neurological Surgeons, 25 September 1970 (Oxford: Seacourt Press, 1970).

Adolf Meyer, in the USA, and by Edward Mapother in the UK. Symonds, supported by George Riddoch, advocated a reconciliation in their (unpublished) memorandum to the Committee on Psychological Medicine of the Royal College of Physicians (1944). But the tone of the report was not conducive to change, arguing that psychiatry hardly deserved to be considered as a discipline alongside medicine and surgery, or a specialty, being light on understanding of aetiology and mechanisms and poor on diagnosis. Symonds blamed Gowers for neuropsychiatric dualism in dictating that 'with the much disputed relationship of mind to brain, the physician has nothing to do'.[94] In discussions at the Association of British Neurologists, the argument went that neurology would be swamped by numbers and psychiatrists spoke a language that neurologists did not understand.

The selection of miscellaneous papers in *Studies in Neurology* includes the classic account of compressive lesions at the foramen magnum, which trap the unwary into assuming a widely distributed disease process because there are symptoms referable to both the brain and spinal cord, and the false downward localisation of the spinal level through venous engorgement of the cervico-thoracic junction: on reflection, Symonds considered that his paper 'makes hard reading but is full of hard facts'.[95]

Symonds retired from his hospital posts in 1955, aged 65, but continued to see patients in private practice until his early seventies. The staff of Guy's and the National Hospital commissioned a series of three portrait drawings by Andrew Freeth RA – one for each hospital and one for the family.[96] Symonds was elected president of the Association of British Neurologists in 1956.[97] These years were marred by

the premature deaths of the two sons by his second wife Peggy – Charters and William. In retirement, Symonds bought a field outside the village of Ham, near Hungerford, close to the river Kennet, where he fished and built a house and developed the garden. He lived surrounded by books and kept in touch with developments in neurology. In 1966 he was invited to teach on two or three days each month at Queen Square, relishing the opportunity to illustrate what could be achieved through clinical analysis, rather than the use of investigations that were beginning to influence the practice of neurology. Eventually, increasing deafness,[98] Peggy's illness (haemorrhage from a cerebral aneurysm) and isolation led Symonds, with much regret, to return to London, living in a flat close to Baker Street. He walked in Regents Park and made an inventory of the bird-life and flowers. Symonds no longer saw patients, but younger colleagues came to discuss cases and he attended dinners of the (Royal College of Physicians) College Club taking the trouble to learn lip-reading in order to follow the conversation. In 1976, aged 86, Symonds developed chronic lymphatic leukaemia and suffered a stroke that reduced his mobility. He and Peggy moved to a nursing home in Totteridge, Hertfordshire, where he died after a fall on 7 December 1978. His ashes were spread over Ham Hill in Berkshire.

Ronald Symonds understood that his father's apparent aloofness reflected the many deep sorrows he had encountered during life, and his fortitude. These concealed a man of warmth and friendship. His obituary in the *Lancet*, written by Christopher Earl, made the point:

> It is probably for his skill in clinical diagnosis and his abilities as a teacher that he will be best remembered … His superb diagnostic powers rested on the foundations of high intellectual capability, profound learning, and a rigorously logical appraisal of the

[94] In his Gowers' memorial lecture 'Disease of Mind and Disorder of Brain' (*British Medical Journal* **2** (1960): 1–5) delivered on 23 June 1960 at BMA House, London, Symonds expanded on his lack of sympathy for Gowers' position on organic and functional disease, and argued for the more sympathetic attitude of Hughlings Jackson. Symonds argued that schizophrenia and affective conditions are disorders of brain function, the difference being where, in Jacksonian terms, the dissolution arose.

[95] C. P. Symonds and S. P. Meadows, 'Compression of the Spinal Cord in the Neighbourhood of the Foramen Magnum, with a Note on the Surgical Approach by Julian Taylor', *Brain* **60** (1937): 52–84.

[96] Symonds was pleased when, in 1978, a ward at Guy's was named after him. An event to mark his retirement held at the Royal College of Physicians was attended by leading doctors, including many from Queen Square.

[97] John Walton recalled that, at the 1959 meeting held jointly with the Society of British Neurological Surgeons, Symonds drew attention at dinner to the difficulty of finding a time when enough neurologists were on speaking terms with each other to schedule a meeting.

[98] Ronald Symonds wrote that, eventually, Symonds was persuaded to apply for a pension on the basis that his deafness was due to acoustic trauma during the Second World War. He arrived at the citizens' advice bureau wearing a shabby RAF coat only to be told: 'you have left it a bit late: what was your rank?' 'Air Vice Marshall' he replied, and the pension was forthcoming.

clinical evidence ... As a teacher he excelled by his example, and it was by example that perhaps he had the most influence ... He was rarely mistaken in his opinions, but when events proved him wrong there was never any 'cover-up'. No-one was more determined than he was to go over the evidence again, to pinpoint where the error lay, and to ensure that the lessons to be learned had not been lost. In this his teaching reached near perfection; here was a teacher who made it quite clear that he himself was the perpetual student. Well into his eighties he would surprise his younger colleagues by his up-to-date knowledge of the literature and his extraordinary capacity for relating the latest observations of others to his own clinical experience. His mind was always open and receptive; and his concepts of neurology and medicine in the wider sphere never assumed that fixity which often comes with advancing years.[99]

Earl wrote to Derek Denny-Brown to inform him of Symonds' death on 7 December 1978 and Denny-Brown replied:

I had a letter from [Symonds] only a few days before his death ... it was always a pleasure to write to him, and if it reported on some recent interest he would always give a reasoned criticism and review of his own ideas ... Even in 1925 when I first attended Q. Sq. as a clinical clerk, he was head and shoulders above the rest of the staff ... he had a most remarkable way of sorting and assessing historical and clinical evidence. And without any experience of experimental work he also had uncanny judgment as to the relative worth of experimental papers.[100]

Macdonald Critchley

Tall, slim and always impeccably dressed, Macdonald Critchley cast an imposing and handsome figure. His background was humble – his father had worked as a rent collector for the Bristol Gas Company but had a prodigious memory and intelligence that he passed to his son. Born on 2 February 1900, Macdonald was named after Hector MacDonald, a Boer war hero who rose from private to the rank of general.[101] This was apt given Macdonald Critchley's rise to prominence in the field of medicine. In his youth, Critchley played several

small roles at the Bristol Vic theatre. Thespian skills

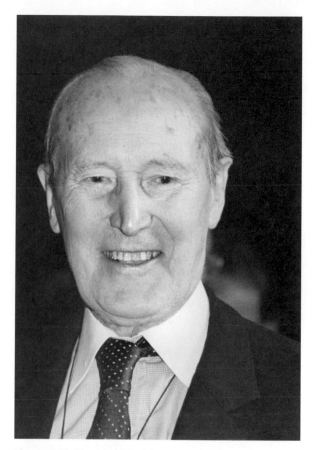

Figure 6.10 Macdonald Critchley.

proved useful and were often on display throughout his neurological career. Critchley matriculated from the Christian Brothers College, Bristol, where his talents and intelligence were recognised. Aged just 15, he was offered a place to read medicine at the University of Bristol but, deemed too young to go to university and already fluent in French and Latin, Critchley stayed on at school and taught himself ancient Greek and a smattering of Russian. Shortly after embarking on his medical training, in 1917 Critchley volunteered for the Wiltshire Medical Regiment. Reprimanded for being late on parade he found himself ordered to decapitate and fillet fish, a punishment that he later claimed turned him away from a career in surgery. A second charge of going missing without leave led to a sentence of intensive gardening. He never gardened again. His adolescent dreams of joining the Imperial Russian Army were thwarted by the Bolshevik Revolution and

---

[99] C. J. Earl 'Charles Putnam Symonds,' *Lancet* **312** (1978): 1389–90.
[100] McDonald archive: letter dated 20 December 1978.
[101] Major General Sir Hector Archibald MacDonald (spelled thus), KCB, DSO (1853–1903), also known as Fighting Mac.

Critchley completed his military service in the Royal Air Force.

Despite these delays in completing his medical training, Critchley graduated from Bristol Medical School with first-class honours at the age of 21 years. Soon after, he entered the then rather closed world of London neurology. Critchley applied successfully for a house job at Great Ormond Street and later succeeded Russell Brain as resident medical officer at the Hospital for Nervous Diseases, Maida Vale. In 1923, Critchley moved to the National Hospital where he became Risien Russell's last house physician.[102] After only three years' training in neurology, Critchley was appointed to the staff at Queen Square and then also at King's College Hospital, where he worked with Kinnier Wilson. He married twice. His first wife, Edna Morris, was a physiotherapist who suffered from hypochondriasis, with whom he had two sons.[103] Subsequently, he married his former secretary at Queen Square, Eileen Hargreaves.

Critchley was a prolific writer, publishing many books and more than 300 single-author journal articles over a period of six decades – starting in his early twenties, when he was a resident, through to his nineties. In retirement, he was seen browsing through the three box files containing his papers in the medical library at Queen Square, and with a puzzled look asking the librarian 'Did I really write that?' His interests in neurology and related subjects were many and varied, the only areas he left relatively untouched being diseases of peripheral nerve and muscle – the latter he considered to be good only to eat and unsuitable for neurological study.

As a junior doctor, Critchley published on neurological complications of disordered calcium metabolism and movement disorders. He reinforced

Marie's concepts of arteriosclerotic Parkinson's syndrome, and wrote important papers – which are still read – on essential tremors and occupational cramps. He was also one of the first neurologists to investigate the neglected field of the neurological consequences of ageing, including 'soft extrapyramidal signs', and he described the 'striatal variety' of the punch-drunk syndrome in which Parkinsonism is a striking feature. In 1980, he spoke at a symposium about his 60-page paper on arteriosclerotic Parkinson's syndrome:

> In 1929 my paper on arteriosclerotic parkinsonism … attracted no little attention and this expression passed smoothly into the currency of neurology. However, since the significance of dopamine began to unfold … some went so far as to express the view that it was an imaginary disorder … I am well aware that there are mythical maladies of the nervous system … but arteriosclerotic Parkinsonism, I strongly submit, does not belong to that category … in self-defence I will concede that it would have been appropriate to speak of arteriosclerotic pseudo-Parkinsonian but no other disclaimer will I make.[104]

During the Second World War, Critchley was asked by the Admiralty to organise neurological and psychiatric services and he became surgeon captain in the Royal Naval Volunteer Reserve. A series of interviews led to *Shipwreck Survivors* (1943), in which he recognised the frequency of certain forms of visual hallucination among survivors cast adrift in the ocean; and an article on visual and auditory hallucinations.[105] A recurring topic of interest was speech, with books on *The Language of Gesture* (1939), *Aphasiology and Other Aspects of Language* (1970) and *Silent Language* (1975) in which Critchley discusses the neurology of gesture, 'hearing eyes', the sign language of primitive communities and deaf mute signing.[106] A related interest was dyslexia. Critchley's first article on reading and writing difficulties in children appeared in 1927,[107] in which he discusses mirror-writing, a topic on which he had

---

[102] Edmund Critchley tells the story of his uncle's interviews for a post at Queen Square. In his first unsuccessful interview, he did well until the end when he was asked where his hat was. He replied that he did not possess one. By the next interview, he had a hat but did not collect it at the end, and again no luck. In the third, he held on to his hat, and got the job.

[103] One son, Julian, became a celebrated and outspoken Conservative party Member of Parliament, and his other son, Nicholas, a well-known actor. His nephew Edmund Critchley became a respected professor of neurology in Preston; one grand-nephew, Hugo, is a professor of psychiatry, with a special interest in the autonomic nervous system; and another grand-nephew, Giles, is a consultant neurosurgeon.

[104] M. Critchley, 'Arteriosclerotic Parkinsonism', *Brain* **52** (1929): 23–83.

[105] M. Critchley, 'Neurological Aspect of Visual and Auditory Hallucinations', *British Medical Journal* **2** (1939): 634–9.

[106] In his writings on neurological curiosities, he anticipated in many ways the later writings of Oliver Sacks and others, many from the United States.

[107] M. Critchley, 'Some Defects of Reading and Writing in Children; Their Association with Word-blindness and Mirror-writing', *Journal of State Medicine* **35** (1927): 217–23.

already published a small monograph.[108] Critchley returned to the topic of reading in *Developmental Dyslexia* (1964), reissued with revisions as *The Dyslexic Child* (1970). With Ronald Henson, Critchley edited a volume of essays on *Music and the Brain* (1977),[109] with a foreword by Sir Michael Tippett. This contains the definitive description of musicogenic epilepsy. Critchley edited the accounts, in *Notable British Trials*, of the Wigwam murder (1942) and the murderers Neville Heath (1951) and August Sangret (1959). On one visit to Australia, he included the subject of serial killers in his lecture programme and showed a particular interest in the 'Shark arm case' which hinged on the ownership of a tattooed arm disgorged by a shark. His many essays on medicine, literature, life and people were collected first as *The Black Hole and Other Essays* (1964).[110] In *The Divine Banquet of the Brain* (1979 – also the title of his Harveian Oration, 1966),[111] Critchley refers to T. S. Eliot's 'Who is the *third* who *walks* always *beside* you?' from *The Wasteland*, as an example of extra-campine hallucinations based on Shackleton's polar experiences.[112] Other essays were gathered later in *The Citadel of the Senses* (1986)[113] and *The Ventricle of Memory* (1990).[114] Critchley's fascination for the unusual and the bizarre led him to stray outside the conservative and formal boundaries of neurology in these essays and lectures. He touched on topics such as 'Tattooed Ladies, Tattooed Men', 'Oscar Wilde's Death', 'Man's Attachment to his Nose', 'The Idea of a Presence', self-portraiture (he himself painted), sign-language, gesture, Indian mythology and dance, and 'musical timing'.[115]

Critchley was the founding chairman of the British Migraine Trust and set up a headache clinic at King's College Hospital. At the first headache symposium in London (1966), he spoke on 'Migraine: from Cappadocia to Queen Square'. His interest in kinesics led to a close friendship with Marcel Marceau, the French mime artist. Another friend was Alexandr Luria, the distinguished Russian psychologist who visited Queen Square with an interpreter and an entourage of granite-faced, thick-set minders in black suits. Critchley wrote a monograph on Gowers[116] and with W. H. McMenemy edited a book commemorating the life and work of James Parkinson, in which Critchley contributed a scholarly chapter on the shaking palsy.[117] His last book, written with Eileen, his second wife, was a biography of *John Hughlings Jackson, Father of English Neurology*.[118]

Against this background of prolific and eclectic writing, Critchley's most important monograph was on *The Parietal Lobes* (1953).[119] This classic monograph remains an important analysis and source of reference. At Queen Square, he was considered the great authority on higher cerebral function and a worthy successor to Hughlings Jackson and Bastian. When he became senior physician in the 1960s, Critchley remained actively interested in disorders of the cortex, instructing his juniors to keep an eye out for new admissions that would interest him. After seeing an interesting patient, he would think about and memorise the findings, writing them down later in his various casebooks.[120] In later years, his secretary would sit behind him and record verbatim

---

[108] M. Critchley, *Mirror-writing* (London: Kegan Paul, 1928).

[109] M. E. Critchley and R. A. E. Henson, *Music and the Brain: Studies in the Neurology of Music* (London: William Heinemann Medical Books, 1976).

[110] M. Critchley, *The Black Hole and Other Essays* (London: Pitman Medical, 1964).

[111] M. Critchley, *The Divine Banquet of the Brain and Other Essays* (New York: Raven Press, 1979).

[112] His interest in illusions was evident from an article in the *British Journal of Inebriety* (**26** (1929): 218–22) in which Critchley described the psychedelic effects of the South American hallucinogenic vine jagé, and his own self-experimentation with mescaline.

[113] M. Critchley, *The Citadel of the Senses and Other Essays* (New York: Raven Press, 1986).

[114] M. Critchley, *The Ventricle of Memory* (New York: Raven Press, 1990).

[115] He told Lee Illis, his last houseman, that he used to go down to the south coast and stay in a hotel and write his

next paper in the tea lounge, listening to the palm court orchestra – possibly not entirely accurate, but certainly plausible to those who knew Critchley.

[116] M. Critchley, *Sir William Gowers 1845–1915: A Biographical Appreciation* (London: William Heinemann, 1949).

[117] M. Critchley and W. H. McMenemey, *James Parkinson (1755–1824): A Bicentenary Volume of Papers Dealing with Parkinson's Disease, Incorporating the Original 'Essay on the Shaking Palsy'* (London: Macmillan, 1955), p. xvi.

[118] M. Critchley and E. A. Critchley, *John Hughlings Jackson, Father of English Neurology* (Oxford University Press, 1998). The typescript, annotated mainly by Eileen Critchley, was sold at the auction of Critchley's books in 2016. Here, the book is entitled *The Sage of Manchester Square. The Life and Work of Dr. John Hughlings Jackson*.

[119] M. Critchley, *The Parietal Lobes* (London: Edward Arnold, 1953).

[120] Several, listing a variety of cases seen at the National Hospital and in private practice, together with notes made

everything that was said by the patient and Critchley and, by a process of telepathic communication, even that which had been left unsaid. In the introduction to *The Parietal Lobes*, Critchley refers to the wealth of features associated with parietal lobe dysfunction. The first two chapters review the comparative anatomy and physiology of the parietal lobes, and the remaining 12 are a remarkable summary of symptomatology and the features found on examination. Critchley, referring to an American visitor designating the pre-war psychiatric clinic of Vienna as 'the posterior parietal lobe Institute of Europe', hastened to point out that – in recognition of his own work – a similar claim had been made on behalf of Queen Square. The monograph is the first devoted exclusively to the subject of parietal symptomatology, but also probably the last, since the parietal lobes are an empirical concept and future works have focused on individual faculties associated with parietal lobe function, such as calculation, rather than being based on an anatomical structure. In his summing up, Critchley echoes Hughlings Jackson in emphasising the fallacy of conflating localisation of lesions with function. After the Second World War, the study of higher cerebral function came to be considered by many as more philosophical than medical and not amenable to scientific inquiry. In that sense, Critchley's work may have become unfashionable in the broader world of scientific medicine, although it was vindicated and massively resurrected with the advent, after his time, of structural and functional brain imaging. Some of his outstanding neurological achievements continue to resurface, including a well-documented case of a patient with clinical features that would have fulfilled all the consensus criteria for semantic dementia, not widely recognised until the 1980s but fully described in his case notes of 1938.

Critchley is remembered for his silvery tongue, élan and awe-inspiring erudition. His turn of phrase was both punctilious and arresting, and his prose polished. His Goulstonian, Harveian, Sherrington, Croonian, Gowers and Hughlings Jackson lectures were meticulously prepared and delivered. Critchley had the great gift of being able to distil ideas and make these accessible to other people. He was a brilliant teacher, who attracted students from around the world, and his controlled showmanship guaranteed a packed house at the Wednesday afternoon and Saturday morning clinical demonstrations at Queen Square. His delivery was unhurried, given without notes, and his interaction with the patient showed great tact and ingenuity. His style was to place diseases of the nervous system in their historical context and, although competent at eliciting physical signs, this was not his forte. He used various ingenious instruments: a black-and-white tie, which he sometimes removed to demonstrate optokinetic nystagmus; a tendon hammer inscribed 'with admiration ... from the Mayo clinic'; a large coloured hatpin; an alarm on his watch that he used to startle students; and, for eliciting the plantar response, a carved ivory hand given to him by Babinski, a gold cornuto purchased in Italy by his second wife Eileen, and a feather, discarded by a pigeon in Queen Square and provided to him by Sister Magnusson, or one from a flamingo picked up in San Diego zoo. Critchley carried a special bag filled with unusual objects which he would ask the patient to handle or answer questions about when examining the higher centres. He opened his letters with a silver paper knife given to him by Francis Walshe, passed down to others, and engraved with the name of each owner. Displayed on the desk in his *pied à terre* in Queen's Court was a human skull given to him on a visit to the Brain Institute in Vienna and on which Dr Franz Gall had placed and painted various phrenological centres.

When a particular finding interested him, Critchley would often digress for long periods, but the enthralled students were carried with him, and his ability to communicate meant that he was remembered much more than other more didactic teachers. When demonstrating a case of Huntington's disease, Critchley always began by describing the history of how the disease reached the east coast of the USA with the Winthrop fleet of the Pilgrim Fathers. His presentations on multiple sclerosis might include readings from W. N. P. Barbellion's moving pathography *The Journal of a Disappointed Man* (1919).[121] After the demonstration, he would be seen driving away from the hospital in a fine black vintage Rolls Royce heading for King's College Hospital, or the Garrick Club for dinner with overseas colleagues. Critchley was an excellent clinical neurologist. Always singular in his approach, he was remembered by Michael O'Brien, one of his junior

during his time as a medical student in Bristol, survive and were sold at the auction of Critchley's library in 2016.

---

[121] W. N. P. Barbellion, *The Journal of a Disappointed Man* (London: Chatto and Windus, 1919). Wilhelm Nero Pilate Barbellion was the *nom de plume* of the diarist Bruce Frederick Cummings.

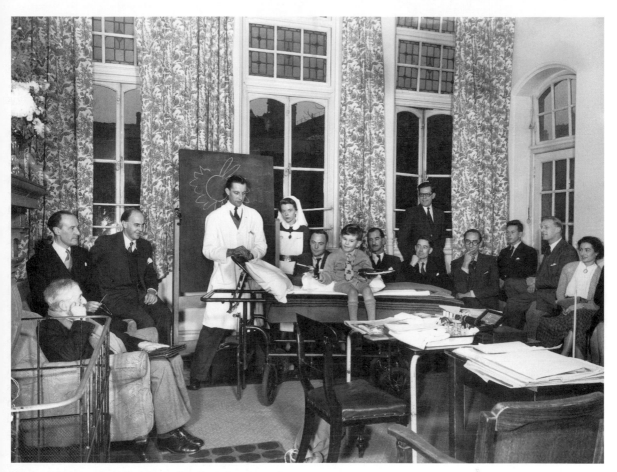

Figure 6.11 Macdonald Critchley (far left) teaching on a ward.

staff, as habitually scribbling notes on the back of referral letters, which were then typed for the case notes by his secretary. He also frequently counselled patients that exercise could seriously damage their health. On one ward round, he flexed the terminal phalanx of his little finger and remarked that 'even this slight movement will shorten your lifespan'.

Domestic recognition came with his appointment as dean to the Institute of Neurology and clinical vice-president of the Royal College of Physicians, and he was particularly proud of his election as master of the Worshipful Association of Apothecaries. But, as with his teacher, Kinnier Wilson, Critchley was a neurologist appreciated far more in continental Europe and the Americas than at home. In fulfilling his responsibilities as president of both the World Federation of Neurology and the International League Against Epilepsy, he was the first Queen Square physician to travel extensively and lecture all over the world.

He spoke French and German and had many international friends. In private, he was relaxed, generous and always helpful, and his mischievous wit enlivened many official occasions. At one meeting in Florence, his Italian colleagues repeatedly introduced him as Lord Critchley. One can understand the assumption, and why Critchley must have relished this elevation. Although he was appointed CBE, several contemporaries at Queen Square, including Walshe and Symonds, were knighted. Reasons for the lack of comparable recognition for Critchley remain matters of speculation.[122] When asked about the matter, Critchley stated that it was

---

[122] It has been said by some that this was because his son, the MP Julian Critchley, was a thorn in the side of the then Prime Minister, Margaret Thatcher, but this is denied by the family. It seems more likely that this was because of his contretemps with Russell Brain (personal communication, Edmund Critchley).

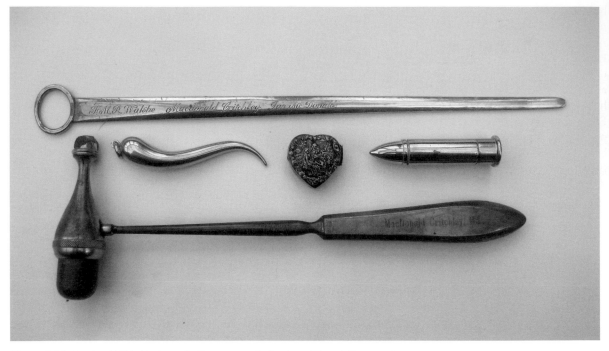

Figure 6.12 Macdonald Critchley's medical instruments (collection of Alastair Compston).

because he had once driven the wrong way up a one-way street in Portugal.

Ian McDonald recalls that Critchley was always calm, unhurried and civil. His reputation amongst some of his colleagues for being vain and aloof nevertheless concealed a sympathetic concern for others.[123] He was aware of appearing distant and impenetrable, and explained this as due to a developmental difficulty in recognising faces (he had quite severe prosopagnosia). He was a shy man, and the prosopagnosia exacerbated this tendency making social interactions sometimes difficult. At times he failed to recognise and therefore ignored his colleagues, magnifying an air of apparent aloofness. When introduced to an overseas colleague on a ward round, he would bow his head, offer his hand as he looked to the ground, and utter a curt 'Good morning'. Unlike many at Queen Square, he was an intellectual, who briefly considered leaving neurology to try his luck on the stage. Jealous of his brio, sharp cutting wit and charisma, some detractors considered him to be a facile dilettante who bent the truth.

Sharing several characteristics, Francis Walshe remained a great friend, and they enjoyed each other's intelligence and humour. Critchley held strong opinions about some of his colleagues but remained outwardly loyal and respectful. Any antipathy he might have held towards particular individuals never stood in the way of his tireless support and belief in the importance of the National Hospital. His lucid biographies and colourful essays on Jackson and Gowers, and his teachers Holmes, Ferrier, Wilson and Collier, enriched for many years the hagiography and folklore of Queen Square for its many alumni and visitors from around the world.

A Festschrift was held at the Medical Society of London in 1980 to celebrate Critchley's eightieth birthday, under the aegis of the World Federation of Neurology.[124] It was a fitting tribute to one of the 'grand seigneurs' of British neurology, who represented a living link by oral history to Jackson, Gowers and Ferrier, and who was by then acclaimed as a founding father of modern cognitive and

[123] Ian McDonald, 'Macdonald Critchley', in *Lives of the Fellows (Munk's Roll)* (London: Royal College of Physicians), Vol. **X** (1994–1997), pp. 83–5.

[124] M. Critchley *et al.*, *Historical Aspects of the Neurosciences: A Festschrift for Macdonald Critchley* (New York: Raven Press, 1982).

behavioural neurology. He was still seeing a few patients and occasionally lecturing at Queen Square.

The final years were spent at his home – Hughlings House at Nether Stowey in his beloved West country of the UK. He continued correspondence with friends and students using a felt pen and magnifying glass to help his failing sight. He had a particular interest in French Second Empire style and was a collector of this period. He remained slim and upright and, with his broad-brimmed black hat and cane, still resembled the epitome of a Parisian *flâneur*. His enthusiasm for writing was intact, and, in completing the biography on John Hughlings Jackson, he contested vehemently the heretical grammatical and spelling changes enforced by his publishers with their commercial eye on the American market. His characteristically indefatigable iron will and infinite capacity for hard work had a dictionary planned as the next project. Despite the arrival of molecular biology and functional imaging in neurology, Critchley's watchful gaze from his portrait in the Wolfson lecture theatre at Queen Square has ensured that the relevance and importance of classic clinical investigation are preserved by his successors on the staff of the National Hospital.

The NHS Arrives and the Hospital Celebrates its Centenary 1946–1962

Chapter 7

The end of the Second World War was followed by a prolonged period of austerity in Britain. National finances were in ruins and the country reflected on its fading role as the world order began to change. Abroad, its position as headmaster of a worldwide empire was rapidly evaporating and the domestic imperative, however, was for social change. 'Modernity', the new catchphrase of the 1950s, became an obsession. Nostalgia for the pre-war decades vied with a desire to move on from the recent past.

A new liberalism had grown up, and, after the Second World War, the academic discipline of Social Policy took centre-stage in Britain. After the election of the first majority Labour government in 1945, a whole raft of new legislation on social reform was enacted (including the 1946 National Insurance Act, the 1946 National Health Service Act, the 1948 National Assistance Act and the 1948 Children Act), accompanied by widespread nationalisations including the industries of coal and steel, railways, electricity and gas, and the Bank of England. There was a major transformation of society and social values, and at its centre, and most significant of all social reforms, was the creation of the National Health Service (NHS) on the 'appointed day', 5 July 1948. There were critics from the right and the left, but the NHS itself was welcomed by most of the population – to the extent that it was not reversed with the replacement of the Labour by a Conservative government in 1951. Indeed, it was an aspect of welfare reform which enjoyed the support of many Tories, socialists and liberals, although controversy on its detail continued (in fact, it was the Labour government in 1951 which introduced prescription charges, prompting Bevan's resignation as Minister of Health).

The medical profession was in large part opposed to the formation of the NHS, and this was on the grounds that turning doctors into government employees was an assault on their freedom and their professional status, as well as the fear amongst hospital doctors that their right to private practice would be abolished, with a substantial loss of earnings. Between 1946 and 1948, the BMA conducted a vigorous campaign against the legislation. It published the results of a poll of doctors in 1948, and claimed that only 4,734 out of the 45,148 surveyed were in favour of a National Health Service. In the teeth of this controversy, Aneurin Bevan managed to negotiate his way through the minefield, splitting the doctors' lobby and bringing down their united opposition. He promised the consultants that they could keep their private beds and retain their private practice – stuffing their mouths with gold, as he put it – and promised to pay GPs by the number of NHS patients on their lists. Although, when the final bill came to Parliament, the Tory amendment stated that it was 'a Bill which discourages voluntary effort and association; mutilates the structure of local government; dangerously increases ministerial power and patronage; appropriates trust funds and benefactions in contempt of the wishes of donors and subscribers; and undermines the freedom and independence of the medical profession to the detriment of the nation', it was passed with a large majority (261 votes for, and 113 against) and enacted into law. Although the views expressed in the amendment were shared by many at the National Hospital, the introduction of the NHS also promised the end of decades of recurring financial crisis, and so, when the hospital was taken over by the government, there was a sense of relief amongst the members of the Board of Management.

With the passage of the 1948 Act, all voluntary, teaching and municipal hospitals were subsumed into state ownership, and this included the National Hospital. At the time a whole series of weighty issues challenged the existing order: take-over of management and functions by the NHS; merger with Maida Vale Hospital; incorporation of the medical school into the British Postgraduate Medical School (BPMS) and the London University; investment in academic positions and their acceptance by a reluctant body of consultants; the severe financial situation; and the ambitious but repeatedly frustrated plans for rebuilding. Queen Square had survived the war largely unscathed but the recurring issue of specialist versus general medicine and what constituted 'neurology' again bubbled to the surface, threatening the authority of the National Hospital. The impact of increasing intervention by the state and marginalisation of the voluntary hospital ethos, which had sustained Queen Square since 1860, could not be ignored. By the time of its centenary, the National Hospital had become a very different place from that which it had been in the pre-war days, elite and confident as the undisputed leader of neurology nationally and internationally, and had begun its transition into a more forward-looking institution.

The National Hospital 1946–1962

This transformation evolved over several decades and affected many aspects of the hospital. One important thread running through the history of Queen Square in the immediate postwar years was the estranged attitude of the senior staff to the rapid evolution of academic medicine. The position taken by the physicians, led by Francis Walshe whose influence was all-pervasive in the decade after the Second World War, was out of step and backward-looking. Queen Square became isolated on major issues, with the senior staff continually backing the wrong horse, with the result that they were repeatedly sidelined.[1] Not all his colleagues shared Walshe's opinions but long experience, power of invective, strong personality and chairmanship of the Medical Committee ensured a level of influence that made him the key figure at Queen Square after the war. For a while, his ivory tower attitude opposing change prevailed. As time passed, more forward-looking opinions were voiced, and a watershed event was the vote of the Medical Committee in favour of establishing a readership in neurology, which set the Institute of Neurology on a new course and resulted in the rise in academic medicine. During the 1950s, attention began to be paid to the positive changes brought by the National Health

Service, expansion in subspecialties, merger with Maida Vale and integration into London University. By the time these changes were worked through during the 1960s and 1970s, the National Hospital had developed into an altogether more modern establishment.

The medical staff changed in the ten years after the war, with many of the older consultants retiring, and with the appointment of several gifted young neurologists. Throughout the period, however, the image of neurology as an elite pursuit, at an intellectual level above that of other medical specialties, and of the neurologist as polished, cultured, urbane and confident in his own superiority, still characterised the style of the physicians, with – in their different ways – Walshe, Critchley, Hallpike, Symonds, Kremer and Williams each exemplifying these traits. But some at least of the new appointees also exhibited more empathy and emotional intelligence than was shown in previous years, and this slowly altered the perception that the staff were aloof and distant from the needs of patients and their relatives.

Despite all, the name 'Queen Square' retained its cachet. The brand was assiduously protected, and much of the political and professional manoeuvring in British neurology continued to revolve around the National Hospital. In 1954, Holmes described the achievements of the hospital in a way that would have resonated with many around the world:

> [the National Hospital] has grown from eight beds in an old and ill-adapted house to a modern institution, with accommodation for two hundred patients, and in its later years over fifty thousand visits made annually to its out-patient departments. It had treated or offered advice to more than a quarter of a million persons, and its medical school, unrecognised and unsupported by the state or by any academic body, had attracted medical practitioners and students from almost every country in the world.

Postwar Financial Crisis

During the war, financial solvency had been achieved only through government subsidy for treating service personnel – a 'windfall', as Ewart Mitchell observed. This explained the slight surplus of funds in 1945, but when, in 1946, this resource was removed, expenditure (£101,121) rapidly exceeded income (£73,159). As the reader will have seen, financial crisis was a recurring theme, and rapidly the National Hospital again careered towards insolvency. A large overdraft developed and the hospital fell into arrears at a rate of

---

[1] There is a curious parallel here with Burford Rawlings' traditionalist position at the end of the nineteenth century. Queen Square, it seems, has always maintained a strong conservative streak and resistance to change.

over £1,000 per week. The situation was so bad that the longstanding bankers, Coutts, threatened on 4 September 1946 not to honour cheques, and the National Hospital was, as had been the case at the end of the First World War, effectively bankrupt, with closure looming again.

Many of the cost increases could not be avoided. The reopening of wards required more nursing staff for whom accommodation in Guilford Street had to be rented at over £2,000 p.a. The cost of maintaining each inpatient increased to £20 per week, and 13s a week for each outpatient. Voluntary donations had been an important source of income before the war but, with the new austerity and wealth redistribution, charitable income did not keep up with hospital needs. Urgent representations were made to government, indicating that £80,000 was needed immediately. A one-off grant of £50,000 was made, with the hospital required to realise the remaining £30,000 from investments. Coutts agreed initially to an overdraft, but as the financial situation worsened they reneged on 8 October 1946. The government was asked to confirm that it would provide further sums, and only with this assurance was the hospital able to continue trading. The overdraft was agreed, with quarterly payments, albeit with arguments about the interest rate, which Coutts agreed to reduce.[2]

From the financial point of view, the Board was hardly in a position therefore to oppose incorporation of the National Hospital into the NHS. Indeed, the transfer of their liabilities to government was a source of much relief, and it is absolutely clear that the hospital could not have continued as an independent voluntary hospital for very much longer. Costs increased further after July 1948, as the medical staff became salaried, and the number of house physicians and surgeons rapidly increased. Appointments in the immediate postwar period were reduced from three years to six months so that the many returning military doctors could gain experience and employment, but there was a cost in making so many short-term appointments.[3] Salaries for nurses also rose.[4]

The first financial strains in the new NHS did not take long to surface, and the financial issues at the National Hospital were shared by many other hospitals around the country. These have recurred regularly ever since. In 1950, the Board of Governors was told that capital expenditure had to be reduced and spending caps must be introduced. The annual estimates of income and expenditure, submitted to the Ministry of Health, had escalated progressively during the early years of the NHS. In 1948, expenditure at Queen Square was £321,725 (and for Maida Vale, £2,420), £382,930 in 1950, and £996,100 by 1961.[5] Another phenomenon that appeared for the first time was litigation against the hospital by a patient complaining of medical negligence. This was a harbinger of things to come, with complaints later becoming a regular feature.[6]

Incorporation of the National Hospital into the NHS

The first mention of the NHS in the hospital minutes is a report by the new secretary, Ewart Mitchell,[7] to

---

Hurwitz (1957), Peter Ebeling and Richard Hornabrook (1958) and Frank C. Rose (1959).

[4] Nursing salaries at that time were very low. The Medical Committee minutes in 1948 (27/48) mention that nurses, after one year of postgraduate training at the hospital, were paid £40 per annum (in the same year, Slater's salary was raised to £1,250 per annum).

[5] The annual 'estimates of expenditure' were published each year by the Finance Committee for the Board of Governors and after negotiation, were approved by the Department of Health. The figures were: 1951, £490,230; 1952, £605,030; 1953, £625,755; 1954, £624,280; 1955, £709,000; 1956, £760,200; 1957, £849,312; 1958, £868,080; 1959, £880,200; 1960, £929,172; and 1961, £996,100.

[6] In those days, the hospital had to bear the cost of any legal settlement, since there was no crown indemnity as is now the case.

[7] Ewart Mitchell was secretary between 1945 and 1958. He took over from Lionel Thomas, who had resigned due to ill health and contributed little. Although a Lancastrian by birth and upbringing, Ewart Mitchell had previously worked as an administrator at the Royal South Hampshire Hospital, Winchester, and brought with him to Queen Square a number of former colleagues from Winchester, notably the new hospital steward, William A. Graham. Shortly afterwards, the future secretary Geoffrey Robinson also arrived, initially as accountant, becoming Ewart Mitchell's deputy in 1948, and eventually succeeding him in 1959 when Mitchell retired early through ill health. According to Robinson, Ewart Mitchell 'had great

---

[2] Letters in the Board of Management minutes, from Coutts 19 July 1946, 4 September 1946, and letter to Coutts 4 October 1946, and minute 110/47.
[3] The list of postwar resident medical officers includes some names later highly distinguished in their branches of neurology: E. C. O. Jewesbury (1946), C. Harold Edwards (1947), William Gooddy (1948), Reginald Kelly (1948), Raymond Hierons (1953), Roger Gilliatt (1954), Chris Earl and M. T. F. Yealland (1956), Fritz Dreifuss (1956), Louis

the chairman of the Board of Governors in January 1946, summarising activities during his first year in office. He reported, with remarkable prescience:

> It is known that the Minister of Health [Aneurin Bevan] has seen the representatives of the local Authorities, the representatives of the medical profession and the representatives of the BMA and he has in fact not discussed with them, but told them, what he proposes to do to form a National Health Service for the future ... There are many rumours circulating in the hospital world and I wonder if it might be as well if I told the Board what the rumour is which I personally feel is the true one ... Ownership of all the public, municipal and voluntary hospitals will be taken over by the Minister subject to special arrangements in the case of the teaching hospitals; provision for the protection of existing officers and servants; buildings, equipment and other assets will vest in the Minister and existing liabilities will be taken over; the setting up of a Central National Health Service Council to advise the Minister on technical aspects; the country will be divided into about 20 areas or regions for health organization; in each there will be a regional Health Board appointed by the Minister.[8]

Mitchell noted that the teaching hospitals would probably be granted special status, and a degree of independence from the Ministry, but with close association to the university. He predicted that teaching institutions would have their own independent Boards of Governors – unlike the non-teaching hospitals – separate financial arrangements allowing 'fullest possible discretion in expenditure', 'arrangements to retain their various endowments in their possession', and the ability to attract funds from other sources for 'experimental work and innovations in organisation'. He expected that government would give the teaching hospitals 'full freedom to appoint their own staff advised in making appointments by a special selection committee'. For Mitchell, therefore, the imperative for the National Hospital was to gain designation as a teaching hospital and thus still retain administrative control, with freedom to make progress and set standards that others might choose to follow. To achieve teaching hospital status was going to be a high hurdle, and by no means certain. He continued:

> It seems to me if a scheme of this kind came into operation there is just a terrific responsibility on you, Sir, and on your colleagues on the Board, to see that this Hospital stands for something just a little more than a National Health Service, and I think your responsibility, Sir, is to get every international contact you can to establish this Hospital as an international hospital which can stand just a little apart.

In order to secure these aims, Mitchell urged the Board to enter into 'a close association with, and be organised to meet the requirements of, the University'. This was to prove difficult, but his advice and predictions on all these matters proved wholly correct. In turn, the Board recognised that it was powerless to obstruct the larger political movements in the country that resulted in the formation of a National Health Service. It recognised that state take-over was the best and only way to ensure a secure financial future since, by 1947, the hospital was again in deep financial crisis and already completely reliant on government subsidy. In that rather important sense, the NHS seemed to offer a route to salvation. The violent opposition to state control, with loss of voluntary status, an anathema to the pre-war Board, was dissolved away.

Mitchell's report was very influential, and the main focus of concern for the Board of Management in 1946–8 was not loss of its independence as a voluntary hospital, as had been the case in the past, but, rather, now to ensure that teaching hospital status was granted within the new NHS. Therefore, it was with

---

imagination, energy and drive', insisting on 'everything being done yesterday'. He 'did not spare himself in the pursuit of his objectives', expecting his close colleagues 'to work all the necessary hours and at any jobs which needed doing – including, if need be, scrubbing the floors'. He was an exacting taskmaster and subjected the employees to frequent and sometimes prolonged 'progress-chasing' meetings. In the immediate postwar period, Ewart Mitchell's skills as an emergency fund-raiser and his talent for crisis management were also important assets. Ewart Mitchell's official responsibilities and titles underwent similarly rapid change and growth. From being secretary of the National Hospital and secretary to the Board of Management in 1945, he became secretary to the National Hospitals and the newly enlarged joint Board of Governors in July 1948, as well as serving as one of two representatives on the newly created Association of Postgraduate Teaching Hospitals. Given the variety of tasks, skills and challenges which these various roles involved, it is perhaps not surprising that Ewart Mitchell seems to have had little by way of a social life outside the world of hospital administration, or that he should have been forced to retire early due to ill health, dying in March 1960.

[8] Board of Management minutes, January 1946. His information came, he said, from reports in the *Yorkshire Post*.

much relief that, in 1948, Queen Square received this status, granted to only a handful of the small voluntary hospitals in London. The Board and staff had reason to be proud of their success.

Also, as urged by Mitchell, in those years the Board did what it could to ensure that the National Hospital was seen not only to be the leader of neurology in Britain but also to play an international role. This ambition permeated thinking on the Medical Committee and Board of Governors, but failure on the part of Aneurin Bevan to appreciate their position proved a source of frustration. Understandably, whatever else was on the Minister's mind at the time, the position of the National Hospital in world neurology was hardly a priority.

In 1947, Mitchell presented his next annual report, writing rather grandly, in a section headed 'International Asset':

> My impression of this hospital is that it is not a London hospital, it is a National Hospital situated in London. It is not truly a National Hospital, it is an international asset situated in England ... You will remember that when we approached the Minister of Health for financial aid, he promised full financial support on the condition that we went ahead with the policy of re-establishing this hospital as an international centre of learning and I believe that we have just over a year of freedom in which to set a standard which will enable us to offer a really first class service to the nation, but at the same time place us in the unique position of being rather bigger in conception than the National Health Service itself ... We are now taking patients from all over the world and doctors from far and wide are coming here to study our specialty, and, while we shall probably have a very close relationship with the London University, I feel that we have a very great interest in our associations with every other university in the world.[9]

The sense of being bigger in concept than the NHS itself was reminiscent of the attitude of previous generations at Queen Square, and the notion of the National Hospital as an international asset underpinned much of the Board's planning. Now the perceived role of the hospital began to alter. In earlier years, the clinical work was centre-stage, with teaching also important but research a poor third. However, as new regional centres opened throughout the United Kingdom, the clinical service available at Queen Square was no longer unique. One senses that

the hospital was being forced to fall back on its role in training, and to re-emphasise research, in order to maintain its status as an elite institution. The provision of a superlative clinical service, the hallmark of the hospital over the previous 90 years, was no longer considered sufficient justification for the National Hospital's special position.

The doctors at Queen Square were more discomforted by the establishment of a National Health Service than was the Board. With misplaced conceit, the physicians assumed that their conservative views would be heard. Bevan despised this attitude, which he saw as indicative of arrogance and self-interest. Walshe, who initially was chairman of the Medical Committee, was an implacable opponent of the NHS and one of its leading public adversaries. His excoriating and verbose articles in the medical and national press must have been a serious irritant to the Labour government. One presumes he carried with him the Medical Committee, but the collective displeasure at the proposed NHS was out of tune with the public mood and weakened the negotiating position of the hospital. A flavour of Walshe's position, his elite view of medicine and doctors coupled with distaste for the common man, can be gained from a letter published in 1948:

> Sir – Any one of us who seeks to grasp first things first amidst the clamour of voices contending on the merits of the National Health Act, and to preserve his equanimity under the buzz of certain lectures, prosy and splenetic, which *The Times* newspaper presumes to give us, may well feel that we are in danger of concentrating unduly upon details and of omitting a general diagnosis of the situation which confronts our profession. Details our negotiators had perforce to attend to, but those of us who have not been thus thanklessly engaged are at leisure to take a more general view and to look beyond the apparently hostile figure of the Minister of Health, who is after all an ephemeral phenomenon, to the state of affairs of which he is symptomatic. What does this import in our disturbed society? I think the Spanish writer Ortega y Gasset sums up the situation in his well-known book *The Revolt of the Masses* with a harsh candour we shall do well to ponder.
>
> The characteristic of the hour is that the commonplace mind, knowing itself to be commonplace, has the assurance to proclaim the rights of the commonplace and to impose them wherever it will. The mass crushes beneath it everything that is different, everything that is excellent, qualified and select. Anybody who is not like everybody, who does not think like

9 Board of Management minutes, January 1947.

everybody, runs the risk of being eliminated. And it is clear, of course, that this 'everybody' is not 'everybody.' 'Everybody' was normally the complex unity of the mass and the divergent specialized minorities. Nowadays, 'everybody' is the mass alone. Here we have the formidable fact of our times, described without any concealment of the brutality of its features … Where, indeed, could we look for a more manifest expression of the coarse ferocity of the power of mere numbers when challenged than in the speech of the Minister of Health in last week's Commons debate, or in the proposal to abolish the university representation in Parliament? What good, in the Greek sense of that word, can the community hope for from government carried on in such a spirit? Do men gather figs of thistles?

There are, I believe, qualities of rare excellence in our profession, though like every human institution it has its imperfections. I submit that this excellence and an unworthy envy of it are the basis of much of the odium to which we are now being subjected in the hope of bending us and our profession to the ends of a retrograde political ideology. We should be too guileless to deserve to survive as a free profession serving the State through the community if we supposed that the nationalization of medicine is the pure expression of a burning and altruistic desire to see a wider measure of social justice, or that the forces now mustered against us are anything but levelling and intellectually and morally destructive in their essence under whatever sophistries and platitudes they hide themselves.

It is, I believe, now given to our profession to have the place of honour and to stand in the gate against ruthless and levelling forces that will, if not resisted in time, crush yet other excellences than ours and make the word 'democracy' as nauseating and as compact of cynical falsehood in Western as it is in Eastern Europe. This is the real issue before us. – I am, etc., FMR Walshe, London W1.[10]

Notwithstanding the heat generated in the Medical Committee, as the appointed day of inauguration (5 July 1948) came closer, the Board of Governors paid less and less attention to the NHS, presumably partly because of public enthusiasm for the project and recognition that the time for protest had passed. Furthermore, the proposals on control and lack of independence, as they evolved, seemed less threatening than initially had been feared, and

there was the great comfort of financial protection. As it turned out, when the day came and the NHS was inaugurated, this fact was hardly noted in the minutes of either the Board or the Medical Committee.

In 1948, the hospital did achieve teaching hospital status, and this ensured that it retained its own Board of Governors responsible directly to the Minister of Health and with no statutory connection with the Regional Health Board. The justification for this arrangement, as expressed at the time, was that it would ensure that the advancement of medicine was not subordinated to the provision of routine hospital services, teaching hospitals would not be starved of resources by cash-strapped general hospitals, and that the high standard of teaching hospital staff would not be diluted by the inferior abilities of those working in general hospitals. Also influential was the view that the London teaching hospitals served national not local needs, and their medical schools and institutes should retain a strong influence on policies of the associated hospitals, which might not be possible if answerable to Regional Health Boards. Teaching hospitals in London also considered that they should have special access to the Minister in setting policy, and, in some instances, were keen to retain control of their considerable endowments. For all these reasons, the National Hospital clung to the coat-tails of the larger and more powerful London hospitals with which it was grouped at the birth of the NHS.

Despite this relative independence, the minutes of the Board after 1948 do in fact show the increasing hand of government in all major policy decisions. The Board was obliged to consult the Department of Health on a range of matters that previously would have been decisions for the hospital: property purchase, nursing and medical salaries, medical staffing complements, medical appointments and rebuilding. Furthermore, under NHS provisions, the Minister was responsible for appointing a new Board of Governors. Sir Ernest Gowers was approached to be chairman. Initially, he was reluctant, in view of the hostility of the Medical Committee to the various government proposals, but acquiesced on condition that he could influence the exact composition of the new Board.[11] As it turned out, Sir Ernest was a popular choice with the doctors as he sided with them

---

[10] F. M. R. Walshe, 'The Commonplace Mind', *British Medical Journal* **1** (28 February 1948): 407. A typical example of Walshe's prose style, elegant and scholarly, and laced with venom.

[11] In the event, all the lay members of the previous committee were reappointed, namely the Countess of Rothes, the Hon. Mrs Richard Lyttleton, Miss Kathleen Cooper

subsequently on many occasions. And he was, after all, a 'Gowers'.

Merger with Maida Vale Hospital

One item that greatly occupied the Board of Management and Medical Committee in these years, and to which they strongly objected, was the proposed merger of the National Hospital with Maida Vale Hospital. The grounds for opposition were embedded in the view that the National Hospital had an elite position relating to postgraduate teaching and an international role, each of which would be damaged by the merger. This was not a strong case, but the Board was again very much advised by the Medical Committee, led by Walshe, which was utterly opposed to any form of amalgamation.[12]

Merger had been discussed intermittently for half a century, and had come close to happening in 1940, when it had been strongly backed by the King's Fund on financial grounds. Indeed, the closing down or merger of smaller hospitals was a recurring feature of British health policy, and an issue which applied especially in London, where many such hospitals

existed. In subsequent years, whenever the topic arose, the Medical Committee fielded a flurry of documents opposing merger and waved these at the King's Fund, the University of London and the Post Graduate Medical Foundation. However, Aneurin Bevan (Walshe's 'ephemeral phenomenon') took the opportunity of postwar reorganisation of health services to bulldoze this through. The logic for merger was obvious, but the opposition from the physicians at the National Hospital was surprisingly intense. It was an interesting episode, which also exposed the perfidy of the university and reinforced the fact that, buffeted by the seismic changes occurring in this postwar period, the power and influence of the National Hospital was now far less than perceived by its Blimpist medical staff.

The merger again showed up the extent to which central government was taking charge. On 16 February 1948, the Minister wrote to the chairman of the Board informing him of the intention to designate the National Hospital as a teaching hospital merged with Maida Vale.[13] This came as a shock. The letter was referred to the Medical Committee which held an emergency meeting on 26 February 1948 to consider the proposal. Walshe wrote back to the Board pointing out that the medical school at Queen Square had carried out organised teaching for over 50 years and had 'an international prestige for its methods and principles of teaching, and that the present staff have inherited the accumulated experience of this half century of highly specialised work'. He railed at the fact that the Medical Committee had not been consulted and that the university seemed covertly to have supported the merger. Walshe explained that, over the past decade, the university had on a number of occasions been appraised of the hospital's opposition to merger. He wrote:

> After full discussion, the Committee decided unanimously that such an amalgamation would not be in the best interests of neurological teaching or research but, on the contrary, would inevitably be detrimental to both …
>
> (a) The hospital is the only one in the British Commonwealth in which organised and systematic postgraduate teaching of the highest order has been carried on hitherto. This state of affairs has been made possible because the hospital has consistently recruited its medical staff from the best men available at any time, not infrequently admitting amongst its

---

Abbs, Mr Donald Black, Mr Piers Danvers Power and the Rt Hon. the Lord Rayleigh. Other external members were Mr Barker (Maida Vale) and Russell Brain (university representative). It is noticeable too that 6 of the 21 members of the Board were doctors at the National Hospital (Purdon Martin, Julian Taylor, Russell Brain, Arnold Carmichael, Denis Brinton and Francis Walshe). Other new members were P. McHugh, William Taylor, the Hon. Mrs Waley Cohen, Sir Archibald Gray, Austin Longland, Professor Hughes-Parry and John Vaughan-Morgan. Sir Ernest Gowers was a distinguished civil servant who sat on a range of committees and commissions, and was the author of *Plain Words* and other books, and the editor of *Fowler's Modern English Usage*. His contributions to British life were enormous. As far as the National Hospital was concerned, however, being the son of Sir William Gowers was sufficient eminence.

[12] At the end of the war, Maida Vale Hospital was in a very difficult position. It had suffered bomb damage, had severely reduced services and was in danger of closure. According to Robinson, the hospital at this stage considered the options of amalgamation with St Mary's Hospital and also of moving to a site south of the river. Later, under pressure from the University of London, the option of merging with the National Hospital at Queen Square was favoured. In 1946, Maida Vale had been granted training status by the British Postgraduate Medical Federation, under a scheme to train doctors released from the armed services, and this no doubt contributed to the government decision to force a merger with Queen Square.

[13] Board of Management minutes 51/48.

number young men who had served their apprentice-ship at the Maida Vale Hospital. Election to the honorary staff at the National Hospital has always been, and continues so far to be, the highest distinc-tion to a neurologist in the United Kingdom, and such election carries with it unique prestige in the world of neurology both here and abroad.

(b) The National Hospital Medical School, thus steadily built up over the years, has attracted post-graduate students from the entire English-speaking world and from the countries of Europe, and there are now few neurologists of international repute abroad who have not at some stage in their careers worked in the National Hospital as postgraduate students or as research workers.

The preservation of this tradition and this activity, so laboriously built up and maintained throughout the disturbances of two wars and attached to the name of the National Hospital, is in the judgement of the Medical Committee a matter of the highest importance to British medicine, and no considera-tion of administrative convenience should be allowed to threaten or to impair the tradition of the asset.

(c) The diluting of the staff of the hospital and of its medical school which this amalgamation would involve would impair both the value of the tradition and the quality of the present intellectual asset. It would do so by adding to the present staff a number of men who have not reached the standard hitherto regarded as essential. Furthermore, the total number of beds available on amalgamation is insufficient for the increased medical staff, the resulting redundancy of staff would restrict the clinical opportunities of each member, and would postpone for a period of between 10 and 16 years in all probability, the entry of young and promising recruits to the staff.

Such a block must induce a stagnation in which the activities of the hospital would progressively dwindle and its prestige perish, for it is only by the steady recruitment from below that research and teaching activities of a hospital can be maintained.

That there is a real disparity between the academic quality of the two hospitals is made clear by the absence of any systematic postgraduate teaching, or of any steady stream of research work, from Maida Vale Hospital throughout its history.

(d) Since the end of the war, the National Hospital has worked steadily and not without success, to revive its teaching activities and to render those more comprehensive and effective, and the returning stream of postgraduates from the Dominions and foreign countries indicates that the hospital's tradi-tion under an active and enthusiastic Board of Management and with a medical staff eager to coop-erate is so far secure.

The Medical Committee believe that the dilution proposed would weaken this tradition and lessen the facilities now available for high grade postgraduate teaching and for research. In this last regard, it may be pointed out that the Medical School houses the research units under the aegis of the Medical Research Council and directed by members of the National Hospital medical staff.

(e) Finally, the Medical Committee believe that such facilities as Maida Vale Hospital offers for teach-ing can best be utilised by leaving it as a separate entity, to which could be assigned teaching functions of the order in which it has hitherto been engaged, e.g. refresher courses for general practitioners, and courses for candidates of the MRCP and the DPM diploma. Such a function would not require amalga-mation and would not be facilitated by it, while an assignment of this order, administratively simple, would leave the National Hospital unhampered to pursue its normal activities undisturbed by an undue burden of elementary postgraduate teaching, not weighed down by an excessive staff, and not faced by a long prospect of a complete block in the addition of new blood to the school.

The Medical Committee therefore expresses its strong conviction that such an amalgamation as is proposed would gravely threaten an asset of incalcul-able value to British medicine, and views such a prospect with profound disquiet.[14]

This was an extraordinarily arrogant view, and the arguments were not strong. Mention that a merger would be 'adding to the present staff a number of men who have not reached the standard hitherto regarded as essential' was gratuitously and grossly insulting.[15] Russell Brain was the leading physician at Maida Vale and he and Walshe were not close. Walshe considered Brain not only 'not up to standard neurologically, but also insufferably boring'. In turn, when Brain was invited to join the Queen Square staff in January 1948, the suggestion was met with the frosty reply that Dr Brain was 'gratified to receive, but was not free to accept, a proposed invitation to join the staff of the National Hospital'.[16] He must have been

---

14 Minutes of the Board of Governors, 24 March 1948.
15 The approach to the National Hospital to discuss merger was led by Brain, with his colleagues Ironside, Feiling and McAlpine. The National Hospital representatives at the discussions were Walshe and Purdon Martin.
16 Russell Brain then became highly influential in British medicine. He served on many government bodies and com-mittees and, between 1950 and 1957, was president of the Royal College of Physicians. His disdainful treatment by the

thoroughly annoyed by the attitude towards his own institution, which Walshe seemed to think was staffed by a second-eleven fit only to teach refresher courses for general practitioners.

The Board approved the stance adopted by the Medical Committee, and wrote to the Minister reminding Bevan that, in 1946, he had urged the National Hospital to strengthen its role as an international centre of learning. This they had done and the proposed merger would seriously impede the role of the hospital in its future service to the international community. A meeting was requested to discuss the proposal prior to a final decision. The Ministry replied on 18 March 1948 saying that a meeting was unnecessary since the views of the hospital were clearly known and 'will be given full weight in arriving at a decision'. The secretary continued to press for the meeting but, appearing to realise that too much pressure might prove counter-productive, retracted the request at the instigation of Sir Ernest Gowers. In fact, as chairman, he was granted a meeting with Sir Wilson Jamieson, the principal medical officer to the Ministry of Health. Gowers pressed his case and Jamieson seems to have listened but, on 23 April 1948, a note was duly received informing the National Hospital that it was designated as a teaching hospital (1 of 26 in London) amalgamated with Maida Vale. On 30 April, Gowers again wrote to the Minister asking for a meeting before the 'decision becomes irrevocable'. On 10 May, Bevan replied:

> It is because I appreciated the feelings of the National Hospital regarding the amalgamation with Maida Vale Hospital that I asked you to come to see Sir Wilson Jamieson in April. It was only after this meeting that I came to the conclusion that joint designation was the only proper course. In a question of this kind, I must be largely guided by the views of the University, and those are, as you know, strongly in favour of joint designation. In my view there is no reason why this course should be detrimental to neurological teaching, and I feel that the decision must stand. I do not therefore feel it would be valuable to take up your time in covering ground which has already been covered in discussions with Sir Wilson Jamieson.

Gowers replied on 11 May 1948, expressing disappointment and surprise that the university had expressed strong support for the amalgamation. He arranged to see the vice-chancellor and asked for the decision again to be postponed. A special joint meeting of the Medical Committee and medical school had been held on 7 May, and Walshe wrote to the Board reporting its conclusions. He noted that, in the absence of formal recognition by the university, the medical school was 'in no way under its authority', and yet the university had, without consultation, influenced the future status and activities of the school. Walshe surmised that the decision reflected the initiative of the director of the Postgraduate Medical Federation (Francis Fraser), who was also then acting vice-chancellor of the university. He explained that the Medical Committee had lost confidence in the university's conduct and had a 'strong sense of lack of candour and courtesy in which the hospital's Medical School had been treated'. Gowers then wrote to the vice-chancellor supporting the conclusions of the Medical Committee and reiterating the arguments against merger and how this had been handled. But this was to no avail for, on 12 May 1948, a letter was received from the Minister enclosing a Statutory Instrument concerning the designation of teaching hospitals, in which the amalgamation was confirmed.[17] The National Hospital and Maida Vale were now to be considered united, under a single Board of Governors, as one teaching hospital, to be known as the National Hospitals for Nervous Diseases.

Thus ended a sorry saga, but one which was, it seems to us in retrospect, a storm in a teacup. The episode also shows how strong the influence of the Medical Committee was on the Board of Management over this period. One might have expected Sir Ernest Gowers to have shown better judgement in his dealings with government, and the fact that he did not was surely a reflection of how he was constrained by the doctors. The stated objections of the National Hospital seem rather weak. The issue of teaching served as a smokescreen for a more arrogant and unworthy set of arguments. Others would have seen opportunities where the Medical Committee saw only problems. Perhaps the only objection that held sway

---

National Hospital cannot have helped the hospital negotiate the very tricky environment of the years 1945–60, and he was a formidable foe. Queen Square must have rued their disparagement and caustic attitude.

[17] The National Health Service (Designation of Teaching Hospitals no. 2) Order 1948. Statutory Instrument 1948 no. 979. National Hospital Board of Governors' minutes 1, 1948–1996 (NHNN/A/5).

was that the amalgamation of staff might act as a block on new appointments, but even this did not happen. More generally, the events revealed the impotence of the hospital in the larger politics of London. The Medical Committee's longstanding disparagement of the university also came home to roost. In the end, the doctors' retrograde attitudes were ignored. Not only did the National Hospital authorities, and particularly its Medical Committee, manage to insult Maida Vale and the university, but Bevan also must have been irritated by what he saw as the hospital's obstructionism and resistance to change. As the NHS gained in momentum, Queen Square was back on the wrong foot and facing a difficult period in its relationships with the university, just as academic medicine was starting to blossom elsewhere.

Despite the fierce opposition of the physicians at Queen Square, and the unkind comments made about their staff, the merger was welcomed by those at Maida Vale, not only because it prevented closure of the hospital but also because teaching hospital status was conferred. By 1949, all the Maida Vale consultant staff were joined administratively with those at Queen Square, and, in 1950, the physicians at the National Hospital hosted a dinner for their new allied colleagues to discuss future relationships in an informal way, but it is not recorded whether this dinner was convivial or helped to thaw relations. In March 1951, the Medical Committee at Queen Square held an extraordinary meeting to discuss the question of a joint committee with Maida Vale, and this idea was rejected.[18] In time, a more cooperative approach developed and the icy atmosphere of the enforced merger slowly began to thaw. The logic of a single joint Medical Committee seemed increasingly evident and, in September 1962, this was finally agreed. On 10 December 1962, ten years after the possibility was first suggested, the consultants from both hospitals held a meeting of their combined committees: Jack Elkington was chairman, Redvers Ironside his deputy,

and Christopher Earl[19] the secretary. Perhaps the main catalyst behind this more forgiving arrangement was the prospect of rebuilding both hospitals as a single 300-bedded hospital on the Queen Square site.

Maida Vale Hospital After the Merger

The merger brought some benefits to Maida Vale. Michael Kremer, universally respected as dean of the medical school at Maida Vale, resigned in 1948 and was appointed to the staff of the National Hospital,[20] but he remained favourably disposed to Maida Vale. He was

---

[18] The Queen Square Medical Committee was still a selective group, and in 1948 comprised: Walshe, Purdon Martin, Symonds, Critchley, Carmichael, Brinton, Elkington, Meadows, Williams, McArdle, Kremer, Taylor, Harvey Jackson, McKissock, Slater, Harding, Williamson-Noble, Lyle, Cawthorne, Hallpike, Davies, Bull, Greenfield and Cumings. The Maida Vale Committee was more democratic: all physicians, assistant physicians, surgeons, assistant surgeons, the ophthalmic surgeon, surgeon to ENT, physicians in psychological medicine, gynaecologist, radiologist and pathologist were members.

[19] Christopher Joseph Earl was born at Ashbourne, Derbyshire, where his father worked as a manager for Nestlé. From a staunch Roman Catholic family, he was sent to Cotton College boarding school in Staffordshire, from where he won a scholarship to study medicine at Guy's Medical School in London. Earl did his National Service with the RAF at Biggin Hill before returning to Guy's to continue his training. In 1952, he spent a research year at Harvard with Derek Denny-Brown, who had a particular interest in Wilson's disease at the time. Earl also honed his clinical skills during his time in Boston and returned to England to complete his clinical training in neurology. In 1961, he replaced Lord Brain as consultant physician in neurology at the London Hospital, Whitechapel. From then on, Earl resolved to focus his career on the diagnosis and treatment of people with neurological disease, and teaching. In 1970, he moved to the Middlesex Hospital, where he continued to pass on his expertise to generations of juniors and medical students. As for research, the bedside became his laboratory, in the tradition of the great neurologists. Earl maintained a particular interest in neuro-ophthalmology and disorders of the central visual pathways, holding an honorary appointment at Moorfields Eye Hospital. For the last 20 years of his career, he was regarded – almost universally by his colleagues – as the best diagnostician in London, and was frequently called on to see difficult cases all over the United Kingdom. His many patients included neurologists who had confidence in his wise counsel. He was much involved in medical jurisprudence and served for many years as an adviser to the Medical Defence Union, advising his juniors to make sure they wrote detailed case notes and follow-up records (which he never did himself). He served as president of the Association of British Neurologists (ABN) and of the section of neurology of the Royal Society of Medicine, and also as a consultant adviser to the Chief Medical Officer. In 1996, he was awarded the ABN Medal.

[20] Michael Kremer trained in medicine at the Middlesex Hospital and in neurology at the National Hospital. Working in the RAMC during the war, he was neurologist to a neurosurgical unit in the Middle East, and then at St Hugh's in Oxford. After the war, he was retained as civil consultant in neurology in the Army. He was appointed to

replaced by Redvers Ironside who also nurtured that medical school. By 1950, 89 students from all parts of the world were attending Maida Vale, of whom 28 were full-time employees of the hospital. The bomb-damaged wards were enlarged and the outpatient department refurbished. New hospital buildings were erected, and property acquired. A museum and research space were provided. Laboratories for pathology were opened, and William McMenemey appointed as pathologist. Facilities for radiology were expanded. In 1949, EEG equipment was installed and Sam Nevin[21] appointed to supervise the newly formed department of electroencephalography. A second

machine was bought in 1951 for electrocorticography in the operating theatre. The department of psychological medicine expanded. Alexander Kennedy left to become professor of psychiatry in Glasgow and was succeeded by P. H. Tooley. He resigned in 1952 and was replaced by the greatly admired Richard (Dick) Pratt. Valentine Logue was appointed as neurosurgeon in 1948, Ronald Henson[22] and William Gooddy in 1951 and Reginald Kelly in 1955 as physicians.[23] Each

---

the consultant staff of the Middlesex Hospital as a neurologist, and to the Maida Vale Hospital as a physician in 1945, but resigned that appointment to take up the post of assistant physician at Queen Square in 1948. He remained in these posts until retirement in 1973, and served as dean of the Institute of Neurology between 1954 and 1962. Kremer was renowned as an accomplished and compassionate clinician, to whom his patients and colleagues were devoted. His clinics were enormous and he made a point also of following up his patients and compassionately guiding their long-term management, a skill not many of the physicians at Queen Square had. Gautier-Smith recalls that his many patients literally mourned his retirement. He completed some clinical research but his main contributions were as a clinician and inspirational teacher. His life was not easy, caring for his wife who became paraplegic as the result of a road traffic accident that occurred as they left for their honeymoon, but she managed to give birth to three children. Kremer remained, despite the difficulties, always cheerful, urbane and conscientious. Elkinton said of him that he was the 'most Christian man in the hospital', which was an interesting remark as he was Jewish (Gautier-Smith unpublished papers). Sadly, though, early in retirement, Kremer had a major brain stem stroke and spent 18 months as a patient on his own neurology ward at the Middlesex Hospital.

[21] Samuel Nevin was an Ulsterman, graduating in medicine from Queen's University, Belfast, in 1927. After house appointments in Belfast, he moved to London, and after other posts worked in the clinical research unit at Queen Square. He was appointed assistant physician and neuropathologist at Maida Vale Hospital and, on the death of Kinnier Wilson, in 1937 became assistant neurologist at King's College Hospital. In addition to running the EEG department at Maida Vale, he was director of the research laboratory of the Institute of Psychiatry and professor of mental pathology in the University of London. With D. P. Jones, Nevin was the first to describe subacute spongiform encephalopathy in 1954, and was interested particularly in muscle and nerve disorders, having an eponymous peripheral nerve disorder named after him. He was a retiring and devout person, remembered with great affection by those who knew him.

[22] Ronald Alfred Henson trained in medicine at the London Hospital. He worked at the London and at St Hugh's during the war and was appointed consultant at the London after the death of George Riddoch in 1947, having been turned down in the previous week for a post on the house at Queen Square. He was a man of culture who edited *Music and the Brain* with Macdonald Critchley (1977), and wrote a definitive monograph with Henry Urich on *Cancer and the Nervous System* (1982). Henson served as deputy editor of *Brain*, and president of the Association of British Neurologists and the neurological section of the Royal Society of Medicine. Henson had acute bulbar and limb poliomyelitis in 1953 and left a sensitive and informative account, in which the altered mental state left him feeling as if he was sitting in his own medulla oblongata watching the fallout of cells from the nucleus ambiguus. He wrote that 'it is difficult to imagine a more terrifying predicament than that of the patient with bulbar poliomyelitis who lies in the care of the ignorant'. And, as any physician who has been unwell recognises, the illness provided 'an opportunity to show the way in which the sick should be treated ... doctoring will never be quite the same again': see Anon. (R. Henson), 'Poliomyelitis', *Lancet* **261** (1953): 1196–7.

[23] Reginald Edward Kelly was born in London, where his father was in the Diplomatic Corps, and educated at St Ignatius College. On qualification, he joined the Royal Naval Volunteer Reserve (RNVR) and served in Home Fleet destroyers, and later with the Royal Marine assault group attached to the Eighth Army and as a surgical specialist during the Normandy invasion. He graduated in 1945, and was resident medical officer at Queen Square in 1948–9, and then senior registrar. He spent six months at the Salpêtrière, and was appointed in 1950 as consultant neurologist to Queen Mary's Hospital (Sidcup), then the Prince of Wales Hospital, Mount Vernon Hospital and St Thomas' Hospital, and Maida Vale in 1955. He was a gifted clinician and his teaching was legendary because of his deep voice, clear diction and sense of the theatrical. He had a compassionate nature and sound judgement and attracted a large National Health Service and private practice. He was appointed to Queen Square and then dean of the Institute of Neurology from 1968 to 1975, and steered the Institute through a period of great expansion in basic science in the early 1970s. He served as chairman of the medical research advisory committee of the Multiple

proved effective and significant figures in postwar neurology. In September 1958, the Medical Committees of Maida Vale and the National Hospital took an important step towards integration when they agreed that future junior and senior staff appointments should, where possible, be linked to both hospitals.[24]

Other physicians who were on the Maida Vale staff at the time it merged with Queen Square were Brain,[25] McAlpine,[26] Nevin, Ironside,[27] Feiling,[28] Dimsdale,[29]

Sclerosis Society and was instrumental in the award of grants to Queen Square for research on magnetic resonance imaging. A larger-than-life figure with tremendous energy and humour, Kelly was a born leader and strode the international stage as an ambassador for British neurology.

[24] The members of this committee reflect the changing power structure of these days: from Queen Square, Gilliatt, Critchley and Paterson; and from Maida Vale, Brain, Henson and Kelly. The first two joint consultant appointments were of Roman Kocen and Bruce MacGillivray. A later appointment was that of Joseph Norman Blau. 'Nat' Blau was born in Berlin to Polish parents and, aged 10 years, on 29 August 1939 fled Poland on one of the last boats to England. His parents and sister were shot by the Nazis, and he was evacuated to live with his cousins in Cambridgeshire. He was educated at the Jews' Free School and Owens School, and entered St Bartholomew's Hospital Medical School from 1947. He served at the RAMC hospital in Wheatley and, in 1962, won a Nuffield medical scholarship to the Massachusetts General Hospital. He trained at Maida Vale under Lord Brain and in 1962 was appointed as a consultant neurologist at the National Hospitals, the Royal National Throat, Nose and Ear Hospital, and Northwick Park Hospital. In 1980, Blau joined Marcia Wilkinson in opening the City of London Migraine Clinic, a medical charity, and worked there for one day a week as an honorary consultant neurologist for the next 30 years. At the National Hospital, he specialised in migraine (the first physician at the hospital to be appointed with this interest). Unkindly, his appointment to the National Hospital was designated 'Brain's revenge'. He died in 2010 of prostate cancer.

[25] Walter Russell Brain was born in Reading and educated at Mill Hill and Oxford, and the London Hospital. He was appointed to Maida Vale in 1925 and then to the London and Moorfields, and continued to work at Maida Vale until his retirement in 1960. No short biography can do justice to his achievements. He wrote the standard British textbook of neurology, and was editor of *Brain*. He was president of the Royal College of Physicians from 1950 to 1957, and also of the Association of Physicians, Association of British Neurologists, neurological section of the Royal Society of Medicine, and the International Society of Internal Medicine. He was elected FRS in 1964, knighted in 1952, created baronet in 1954 and made an hereditary peer in 1962. He became a Quaker in 1931, and was a pacifist. He wrote poetry and essays, and lectured on philosophy, as well as being the most well-known physician of his generation.

[26] Douglas McAlpine, son of Sir Robert McAlpine, was educated in Edinburgh and qualified in medicine in Glasgow. He was in active service on the front in France and in a hospital ship in the First World War, and in 1920 worked with Greenfield at the National Hospital on post-encephalitic Parkinsonism. In 1924, he was appointed physician in charge of nervous diseases at the Middlesex Hospital, and assistant physician and pathologist at the Maida Vale Hospital. In the Second World War, he was appointed adviser in neurology for the Middle East, in 1941, initially as part of the India Command and finally for South East Asia. He was a celebrated physician and a renowned expert on multiple sclerosis, and, in 1955, published the first edition of *Multiple Sclerosis*, now in its fourth edition and entitled *McAlpine's Multiple Sclerosis*.

[27] Redvers Noel Ironside was born and educated in Aberdeen and graduated from Aberdeen University. He held a registrar appointment at Queen Square and served in the Royal Air Force Volunteer Reserve (RAFVR) in the Second World War, reaching the rank of air commodore in 1944, and completing his book *Aviation Neuropsychiatry* in 1945. He was appointed assistant physician to Maida Vale Hospital and was dean from 1948 to 1951 when the school at Maida Vale merged with that at Queen Square. In 1956, he served as president of the neurological section of the Royal Society of Medicine, and in 1963 as master of the Society of Apothecaries. He had a well-displayed collection of Leeds cream-ware in his third-floor flat at 22 Wimpole Street, and enjoyed his membership of the English Ceramic Circle. According to McMenemey, he showed 'the courtesy and elegance of a more gracious age'.

[28] Anthony Feiling was born at Epsom, educated at Marlborough, and graduated in medicine from Cambridge and St Bartholomew's Hospital. He was appointed physician to the Maida Vale Hospital in 1914, served in the RAMC, and in 1923 was appointed assistant physician to St George's Hospital and then dean of the medical school from 1926 to 1936, and later senior physician. He was a founder member and, later, president of the Association of British Neurologists, and president of the neurology section of the Royal Society of Medicine. He was Lettsomian Lecturer of the Medical Society of London in 1942, speaking on the topic of epilepsy, and president of the Society in 1944. He retired in 1951 and later wrote *A History of the Maida Vale Hospital for Nervous Diseases* (Butterworth, 1958).

[29] Helen Easdate Dimsdale was born at Stretford, educated at Culcheth Hall and Hayes Court, and graduated from Cambridge University. Her house appointments were in Windsor, University College London Hospital and the Elizabeth Garrett Anderson Hospital, London. In 1941, she began her training in neurology at Maida Vale, and was appointed physician there in 1947, and at the Royal Free Hospital in 1950. She retired due to ill health in 1967. The first woman to hold the position of consultant

Sandifer[30] and Pritchard.[31] Many were major figures in British postwar neurology, and all had spent some time in their training at Queen Square, but none were granted beds at the Queen Sqaure site despite being listed as members of the consultant staff.

Thus, within ten years of the amalgamation with Queen Square, Maida Vale was flourishing in many ways, but its triumph was to prove short-lived for, with the disastrous failure of united redevelopment of the two hospitals in the 1960s and 1970s (see Chapter 2), Maida Vale Hospital withered through lack of investment and low NHS priority, and finally closed in January 1994. Ironically, there was great sadness expressed by the Queen Square staff who by then respected the hospital in which many of its staff had worked as trainees, and who valued the quality of its services and the intimate atmosphere. That it did close was due essentially to financial pressures in the

straitened circumstances of the NHS, and not, as argued by Walshe and his colleagues, through inferiority or inadequate teaching and research.

A Link with the Chalfont Colony for Epileptics

In the postwar period, there was renewed interest in the social aspects of epilepsy. Writing from Harley Street in 1947, Denis Williams approached Swithin Meadows,[32] chairman of the Medical Committee, proposing a 'separate branch of the Almoners department to be responsible for the home care as well as help in finding employment, and maintaining the cooperation of employers of epileptics'. One social worker and one clerk would be employed.

> The National Hospital has made itself responsible for the medical treatment of a large body of socially well-adjusted and employable epileptics, but a great gap

---

neurologist, she also served as treasurer of the ABN from 1961 to 1966.

[30] Paul Harmer Sandifer was educated at Mill Hill School and graduated from the Middlesex Hospital. He was house physician to Dr Douglas McAlpine, and held various junior appointments, including at the Maudsley Hospital. He was then appointed first as house physician and, in 1937, resident medical officer at Queen Square. In the war, he served as neurologist to the EMS Sector 5 hospitals, and then as a neuropsychiatrist in the RAF, rising to the rank of wing commander. In 1946, he was appointed assistant physician to the Maida Vale Hospital and the Royal National Orthopaedic Hospital, and later to Mount Vernon Hospital, the Radium Institute and to the Oxford hospitals. He took a special interest in the neurology of childhood and was one of the first British paediatric neurologists. In 1953, a department of neurology was created at the Hospital for Sick Children, Great Ormond Street, and Sandifer was appointed as consultant in charge. He was renowned as a brilliant and enthusiastic physician and teacher. He specialised in the 'floppy infant' and in infantile and early childhood illnesses, and has an eponymous syndrome named after him.

[31] E. A. Blake Pritchard was educated at Whitgift School, where his father was headmaster, and then at King's College Cambridge. He served in the Friends' Ambulance Unit in the Second World War and contracted poliomyelitis. He completed his clinical training at University College, qualifying in 1924. He was appointed physician to University College and to Maida Vale in 1932. He was a founder member of the ABN. He wrote on the treatment of myasthenia and was a conscientious clinician with an eye for detail. He was said to be a quiet and gentle person and well liked. He suffered increasing respiratory problems in his later life, perhaps as a late deterioration of his polio, and died after a protracted illness.

[32] Swithin Pinder Meadows was born in Wigan, where his father was editor of the *Wigan Observer*. He was educated at Wigan Grammar School, from where he won a scholarship to Liverpool University for his pre-clinical studies and St Thomas' Hospital, where he qualified in 1927. He was resident medical officer at the National Hospital in 1932 and appointed to the staff of Westminster Hospital, then Maida Vale and Moorfields Eye Hospital, and to the consultant staff at Queen Square in 1946. He specialised in neuro-ophthalmology. He had an extensive NHS practice from which he retired at the age of 65, and also a large private practice which he continued for a further ten years. He was appointed Hunterian Professor at the Royal College of Surgeons in 1951–2, visiting professor at the University of San Francisco in 1954, and president of the neurological section of the Royal Society of Medicine in 1964. Meadows did not publish a great deal, but was considered to be one of the outstanding clinical neurologists of his generation. He was, according to Gautier-Smith, 'a burly, ruddy-complexioned man, who always looked slightly rumpled, he had the appearance of a jovial farmer, and also spoke with a slight regional accent' (unpublished papers). He was modest, courteous, approachable and free of the pomposity and arrogance which was, sometimes fairly, attributed to the neurologists of his generation, and there is a story of how he shocked a distinguished Eastern European professor when he said that he had not made a correct diagnosis for weeks. Ralph Ross Russell, in his generous obituary published in the 1992/3 annual report of the Institute, tells of how he asked Joe Pennybacker's advice about taking a house position at Queen Square. About the medical staff, Pennybacker said: 'There are some who sound good, there are some who really are good, but the one worth all the rest is Meadows.'

exists between this treatment and the meagre social services which at present cater for them. It is perfectly clear that the medical treatment of the epileptics should include advice as to methods of living and of gaining a livelihood, as well as education of the people with whom they live … In this time of transition, there is a tendency for many of the more liberal charitable undertakings to be supplanted by more rigidly organised state-controlled schemes. Because of this it seems that the National Hospital should take the lead by providing an extension of its services to the epileptic – an extension which will put life into otherwise sterile legal provisions.[33]

Ewart Mitchell proposed in January 1947 that negotiations be re-established with the Chalfont Colony for Epileptics as one way of providing social care facilities, and also of extending the range of medical facilities for patients with epilepsy.[34] As a consequence of the 1910 schism, the colony had evolved into what was essentially a residential nursing home and was totally isolated from the mainstream of medicine or neurology. After the Second World War, it housed 520 people with epilepsy in a farm setting, with medical input provided by a visiting general practitioner and with up to 100 new cases admitted each year. Contacts between the National Hospital and Chalfont then resumed, with proposals for closer collaboration made by the chairman of the colony, Sir John Stewart Wallace, and, in 1953, Sir Ernest Gowers accepted an invitation to become vice-president of the National Society for Epilepsy.[35] Williams, Carmichael and Dimsdale were asked to develop a plan for closer links and to bring the colony back into the medical fold. They visited Chalfont in 1953 and reported back that there was a need for greater medicalisation, proposing the creation of a small unit of six beds, under the control of the NHS and staffed with a registrar, EEG technician, social worker and nurses. This would

provide a significant medical service and valuable material for the National Hospitals, at a modest capital outlay, estimated to be £5,000, and an annual cost of £5,000 a year. The Medical Committee at Queen Square was enthusiastic, but Maida Vale baulked at the cost. The Ministry of Health then reported that the plans were impractical, because staff employed by the NHS could not work on the premises. It was then agreed by the Medical Committee that a Medical Board be established to advise on the 'general treatment of the colonists and other relevant matters' and that all patients scheduled for admission to the Centre should be admitted for a prior neurological assessment at Queen Square, a procedure that lasted for a few years and then petered out.

Not much further contact occurred until 1956 when consideration was again given to the establishment of a unit at Chalfont for the long-term study of epileptic patients, no doubt partly in response to the publication of the Cohen report,[36] which had recommended specialised clinics and facilities for the investigation and treatment of epilepsy. The Board of Governors agreed to rent a house in the colony (to be called the National Hospitals unit), and to request funds for refurbishment from the Chartered Society of Queen Square, establish daily transport between the Colony (with 'such as a Volkswagen bus') and the National Hospital, and staff the unit as originally proposed but with all medical investigation and treatment carried out at the National Hospital.

'The first purpose will be to convert the patient's stay at the colony into a therapeutic period directed wholly to his return to a normal constructive life.' All treatment was to be applied through the NHS, despite the fact that the colony was statutorily independent. But, in the event, progress again faltered due to failure of agreement over details by the National Hospital and the colony, and the lack of financial approval from the Ministry. At this stage, all communication broke down, and the colony looked to the Oxford region for neurological support, which was supplied by a monthly visit from the Oxford neurologist Dr John Spalding.

Many changes occurred at the Chalfont Colony in the subsequent decade, reflecting alteration in the

---

[33] Denis Williams, 8 November 1947 (NHNN/A/10/6/35).

[34] The colony had been established in 1893 with intimate connections to the National Hospital, but these links were severed in 1910 due to a schism between the Queen Square physicians and the colony's lay management. See J. W. Sander, J. Barclay and S. Shorvon, 'The Neurological Founding Fathers of the National Society for Epilepsy and the Chalfont Centre for Epilepsy', *Journal of Neurology, Neurosurgery, and Psychiatry* **56** (1993): 599–604.

[35] Distinguished vice-presidents were appointed with Gowers, raising the profile of the Society, and including Lord Inman, Lord Terrington, Sir Henry Aubrey-Fletcher (Lord Lieutenant of Buckinghamshire) and Dr H. J. Carpenter (Bishop of Oxford).

[36] Central Health Services Council, *Ministry of Health Medical Care of Epileptics: Report of the Sub-committee of the Central Health Services Council* (London: HMSO, 1956) (Chairman: Lord Henry Cohen).

social attitudes to epilepsy and growing public pressure, campaigning by the British Epilepsy Association, and lobbying by its president, Lord Hastings, in the House of Lords. In 1968, the Seebohm Report recommended that responsibility for support of residents at facilities such as the Chalfont Colony should be transferred from the local authority to the Department of Social Services.[37] This led to renewed effort in housing handicapped persons in small community homes rather than large asylums or colonies, and as a result the number of cases referred for long-term residential care began to fall. Dr John Laidlaw was appointed senior physician, and he began admitting, for the first time, 'transit patients' for relatively short-term assessments (6–24 months). At his instigation, there were moves to modernise the ethos and role of the institution. The term 'colonists' was changed to 'residents' or 'patients'; 'epileptic' became 'the person with epilepsy'; and the name 'Chalfont Colony' was altered to 'Chalfont Centre'. Then, in 1969, the Reid Report was published and this proved a watershed in the history of epilepsy in Britain, and of the Chalfont Centre.[38]

The Reid Committee was a subcommittee of the Cohen Committee, which had been reconvened by the government in view of lack of progress on the recommendations made in the 1956 report. Sir John Reid already had connections with the Chalfont Centre in his capacity as chief medical officer for Buckinghamshire, as did several other of the 11 members of the Committee. Denis Williams was the key connection with the National Hospital. In relation to 'colonies', the Reid Committee agreed with the stance of John Laidlaw and found this nomenclature old-fashioned and inappropriate. The Committee noted that there were then 2,129 residents in UK institutions for people with epilepsy, and advised that no one should be admitted without a full medical and social assessment. The report also recommended the establishment in Britain of multidisciplinary specialised epilepsy clinics and, for the first time, sanctioned the

clear subspecialisation of epilepsy within neurology. The aim was to establish around six 'special centres', modelled on the Comprehensive Epilepsy Program established by the National Instituts of Health in the United States. These centres would have a hospital and residential component and, in addition to caring for the residents of the colonies, would serve as a short-to-medium-term facility for the comprehensive medical and social assessment of non-residential patients. Together, the National Hospital and National Society for Epilepsy proposed that the Chalfont Centre be designated in this way, and, in October 1971, Ministry approval was granted, as one of three special centres in Britain, the others being at Bootham Park in York and the Park Hospital in Oxford (for children). The Special Centre at Chalfont was to be managed jointly by the National Society for Epilepsy and, through the National Hospital, by the NHS. A ward staffed by Queen Square medical and nursing employees was to be established, effectively constituting an off-site part of the National Hospital. The plan was for 180 patients a year to have detailed assessments at the Centre. Dr Roman Kocen was the physician from the National Hospital given responsibility for the Centre,[39] and he worked with Laidlaw, who remained senior physician at Chalfont, now with an honorary appointment at Queen Square. The Special Centre opened in 1972, and over the next eight years admitted around 1,000 patients. The Ministry commissioned a review of all the special centres, published in 1980, which demonstrated moderate but sufficient utility and advised that the arrangement be continued.[40] Thus, through a

---

[37] F. Seebohm et al., Report of the Committee on Local Authority and Allied Personal Social Services, Cmnd 3703 (London: HMSO, 1968).
[38] People with Epilepsy: Report of a Joint Sub-Committee of the Standing Medical Advisory Committee and the Advisory Committee on the Health and Welfare of Handicapped Persons (Chairman J. J. A. Reid) (London: Department of Health and Social Security, 1969).

---

[39] Roman Stefan Kocen was born in Lodz, Poland, the son of a clinical pathologist. He was rounded up into the Warsaw ghetto but escaped in 1943, at the age of 11, and, travelling alone across Europe, reached England in 1946. He learned the language and, seven years later, was awarded a state scholarship to study medicine in Leeds, qualifying in 1956. He served in Malaysia and then, on demobilisation, trained in neurology at the Middlesex Hospital and Queen Square, and was appointed consultant at the Brook Hospital in 1968, and then Queen Square, Maida Vale and Edgware General Hospital in 1970. He was an original thinker, totally dedicated to the National Hospital and served its many committees, including as chairman of the Medical Committee. He had a large private practice and was considered an excellent neurological opinion. Kocen served also as civilian consultant adviser to the Royal Air Force. His last years were marred by severe Parkinson's disease.
[40] J. D. Morgan and A. E. Bennett, The Development of Services for Epilepsy in the 1970s (London: DHSS, 1980).

curious twist of fate, a relationship was forged which had many echoes of the pre-1900 link between the Chalfont Colony and the National Hospital. It also provided the opportunity for the renaissance of epilepsy work at Queen Square, with subsequent expansion of both clinical work and research from the late 1970s.[41]

The Consultant Staff and Medical Committee

Given the attrition of staff during the Second World War and the rapid rise in activity of the hospital in the pre-war period, there was an obvious need to expand medical staffing. Despite the foreboding of some senior staff that appointments to the National Hospital might be based on clinical imperative rather than quality (see later), several new consultant neurologist appointments were rapidly made between 1946 and 1948: Meadows, Williams, McArdle and Kremer. The seniors should not have worried for the new appointees were excellent choices and each became an important figure in their respective fields.[42]

Other new consultant appointments at Queen Square and Maida Vale in the period before and around the founding of the NHS were: McKissock in neurosurgery (and Logue at Maida Vale); Slater and Shorvon in psychiatry (and Tooley at Maida Vale); Hill and Cobb in neurophysiology;

Blackwood, Cumings and McMenemy in pathology; Bull in radiology; Harding in orthopaedics; and Aserman in anaesthetics. Thus, the hospitals had greatly expanded their consultant staff with a young and talented group by the end of 1948.

The National Hospital at Queen Square had 14 physicians classified into four categories: three consulting physicians (retired physicians who retained admitting rights – Holmes, Hinds Howell and Stewart); four physicians (Walshe, Martin, Symonds and Critchley); four physicians to outpatients (Brinton, Carmichael, Meadows and Elkington); and three assistant physicians (Williams, McArdle[43] and Kremer). At Maida Vale, there were eight physicians at the time of merger: Brain, McAlpine,

---

[41] It was noted by some at the time that Queen Square was again proving loyal to its origins as 'The National Hospital for the Epileptic', at least in part – a designation not justified since the schism from Chalfont in 1909. There was a large increase in the facilities devoted to epilepsy, which was made possible by bringing together the resources for epilepsy of the NHS hospital, the university and the national charity. By 1996, there were 11 consultants, including professorial posts in neurology, neurosurgery and behavioural psychiatry, and five senior non-clinical scientists in the epilepsy group. Over the seven calendar years of 1990-6, 72 postgraduate research workers had passed through the group, most obtaining higher degrees, and 37 books, 137 chapters and 378 articles in scientific journals were published by the group (details listed in *Epilepsy: A Seven Year Report of the Clinical and Research Work of the Epilepsy Group* (London: Institute of Neurology, 1997).

[42] The physicians were appointed initially as associate physicians, and then, on the death of Riddoch in 1947, Kremer was appointed, Critchley promoted to physician, and Meadows took Critchley's place as a physician to the outpatients.

[43] Michael John Francis McArdle, always known as Sean, was of Irish extraction but educated at Wimbledon College and at Guy's Hospital Medical School. He was resident medical officer at the National Hospital in 1935, and then won a Rockefeller travelling scholarship, spending a year in France studying neuropathology with Bertrand. He served with the RAMC as neurologist in Edinburgh, St Hugh's and in Europe. In 1946, he was appointed to Guy's and Queen Square, and subsequently to Kingston Hospital, where he held outpatient clinics and conducted ward rounds each Saturday. He had no sense of time: his clinics and ward rounds began at odd hours and proceeded at a leisurely pace, but no one minded as he was one of the greatest clinicians of his age, with a brilliant grasp of clinical neurology and tremendous compassion. He was eccentric but devoted to neurology and to his patients, spending hours eliciting the smallest clinical signs. His special interest was peripheral nerve and muscle disease. He described many features of the carpal tunnel syndrome, incurring the waspish tongue of Walshe, amongst others. He was a main contributor to several editions of *Aids to the Investigation of Peripheral Nerve Injuries* (first published in 1942) where his hands are much in evidence demonstrating the position of muscles. Towards the end of his career, McArdle developed essential tremor but persisted in carrying out alcohol injections of the trigeminal ganglion under local anaesthetic, a technique learned from Wilfrid Harris and performed after his ward round at Queen Square on Friday evenings, much to the discomfiture of his young assistants and some of the patients, one of whom leapt from the table and threw off his surgical gown leaving the hospital somewhat *deshabillé*, never to be seen again in the vicinity of Queen Square. As McArdle was short in stature, equally unnerving was the ride home for a house physician in McArdle's car, the latter's head barely raised above the dashboard, regaling his junior with details of his culinary prowess and anticipating the delights of the fish that he would be cooking for his wife on arrival home.

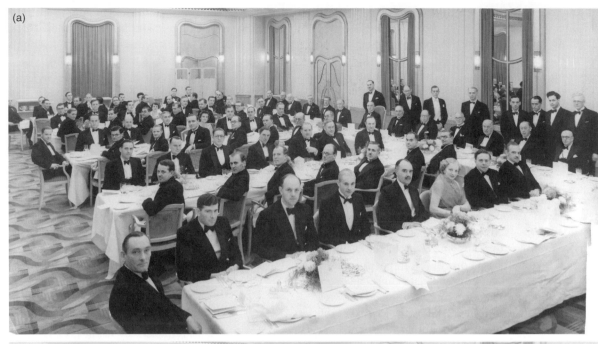

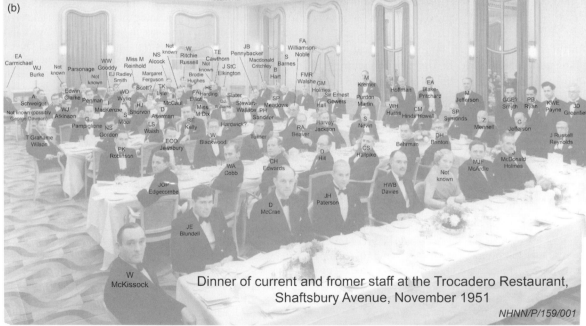

Dinner of current and fromer staff at the Trocadero Restaurant, Shaftsbury Avenue, November 1951

NHNN/P/159/001

Figure 7.1 Staff dinner in 1951 (a. original photograph; b. overlaid with staff names).

Ironside, Nevin, Feiling, Dimsdale, Sandifer and the newly appointed Pritchard.

In addition, the following staff were listed in the hospital's 1947 annual report (the last of its type, and with the staff lists dated '1948'): Greenfield (pathologist);

Carmichael (as director of the neurological research unit); Hallpike (as director of aural research and aural physician); and Purdon Martin (as dean of the medical school). Williams, Hill and Cobb were listed as physicians to the electroencephalographic department, and

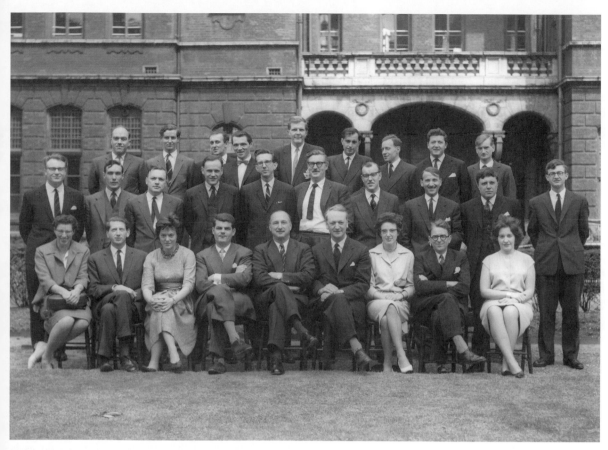

Figure 7.2 The registrars and houseman, 1962.

Zangwill as an honorary psychologist. Russell Reynolds was consulting radiologist, Davies radiologist, and Bull and Sutton assistant radiologists. The junior medical staff included the registrar, resident medical officer, three house physicians, a resident surgical officer and two house surgeons. Sir Stanford Cade retained the grand title of honorary radium registrar, but the post of electro-therapeutics officer had disappeared.

The other staff listed in the annual report were: Hart (consulting psychiatrist), Cawthorne (aural surgeon; and McKenzie at Maida Vale), Williamson-Noble (ophthalmic surgeon of) and Lyle (assistant ophthalmic surgeon), Harding (orthopaedic surgeon) and Hardwick (dental surgeon). The Queen Square anaesthetists were also acknowledged for the first time. Zebulon Mennell was listed as consulting anaesthetist, and Hall, Edith Taylor (the only woman in the hospital staff), Beaver,[44]

Aserman and Cobb as anaesthetists. There were two consulting gynaecologists, Hedley and Lockyer; a consulting dental surgeon, Smale; and a consulting ENT surgeon, Scott.

The 14 Queen Square neurologists continued to regard themselves as firsts amongst equals. Up until 1948, a smaller establishment had been considered sufficient by the Medical Committee to meet the demands of the hospital and, following the victory over Burford Rawlings at the start of the century, its position had been consolidated as the arbiter of medical matters

---

[44] Beaver was a charming and multi-talented larger-than-life figure at Queen Square. He ran the Batten Unit with

John Marshall and invented a celebrated mechanical ventilator, the Beaver breathing machine. He had also been a racing driver. At the end of Powis Place, as space was so tight, there was a turntable to allow cars and ambulances to be turned around manually, but Beaver would race up to the space, slam on the brakes and skid around before accelerating off in the opposite direction – a movement he perfected. His mechanical ventilator used an automotive wiper motor to drive the bellows used to inflate the lungs.

with the Board of Governors largely rubber-stamping decisions. Over time, the Committee had strengthened its grip on strategy, dictated the number and appointment of medical staff at all grades and their terms of service and salary scales, controlled the distribution of beds to the various consultants, and vetted publications by staff, study leave allocations and research projects. After 1948, this dominant role was eroded not so much by the Board of Governors, which continued largely to approve its recommendations, as by the increasing imposition of directives from the Ministry of Health on matters over which previously the hospital had absolute authority. In the early years after the Second World War, membership of the Committee was still self-appointed and restricted largely to physicians,[45] leaving the surgeons, in particular, heavily outnumbered.[46] By 1960, however, although membership had broadened, this remained selective. The loss of influence inside the NHS was partly mitigated by Sir Ernest Gowers as chairman of the newly constituted Board of Governors, who was sympathetic to their concerns and aspirations and on very good terms with the physicians. He appointed four of the medical staff to the Board, thereby ensuring that their voices were heard. But this respite was temporary and, as central government control tightened, tensions arose and the Medical Committee had a number of skirmishes reflecting its loss of influence. Particularly sensitive was the Ministry's circular in 1950 concerning the constitution of 'appointment committees' for senior staff, stipulating the involvement of four members of the university, and four others, only one of whom might be a member of the consultant staff, drawn from the Board of Governors, the regional authorities and the Royal College of Physicians. Despite protestations, this structure was endorsed, but the hospital finessed the situation to some extent by appointing members of the consultant staff as the university representatives. A further tension arose from the new contractual requirement that all doctors should retire at the age of 65 years, with the possibility of annual extensions up to the age of 70. The Medical

Committee produced a paper showing that, in 1894, when the retirement age was raised from 60 to 65 years, four doctors then aged over 60 but still employed (Ramskill, Jackson, Buzzard and Bastian) were reclassified as 'consulting physicians', with each allocated ten beds up to the age of 75. Similar arrangements had later been made for Hinds Howell, Holmes and Grainger Stewart. This matter was of much concern to Walshe who was himself now past retirement age.[47] Eventually, it was agreed to consider extensions on a case-by-case basis, and the Board of Governors conceded to a request from the Medical Committee that it should be the body advising on any modified contract or extension of employment.

A most profound change from the perspective of the doctors, however, was that, as NHS employees, the consultant medical staff were salaried by the state and no longer 'honoraries' giving their services unpaid to the hospital whilst earning their living in private practice. Temporary contracts were initially offered to the medical staff, and accepted, other than by Walshe who was bitterly opposed to socialised medicine and who continued to work at the hospital until his retirement without remuneration (and the ophthalmic surgeon Williamson-Noble who similarly refused to accept payment). There was little complaint among the other Queen Square consultants about the financial aspects of the contract, at least as far as is recorded. One striking feature of the contracts was the small number of sessions the consultant neurologist staff were required to commit to the hospital – in 1949, this was fixed at three sessions[48] for the senior physicians, and four for the assistant physicians and physicians for outpatients. The three surgeons together had 13 sessions, but others in the hospital were committed more heavily.[49] Central control was exercised in other ways, including emphasis on economies of scale and record-keeping in X-ray departments, reflecting the general desire of the Ministry to lessen the power of the consultant body

---

[45] Attendance in the immediate postwar years was restricted to Walshe, Elkington, Hallpike, Harvey Jackson, Purdon Martin, Riddoch, Carmichael, Symonds, Cawthorne and Williamson-Noble.

[46] In 1948, the consultant anaesthetists also applied to join the Medical Committee, but were refused.

[47] The Maida Vale Medical Committee objected to allowing Walshe to continue after the age of 65 years, no doubt contributing to bad feeling between the two committees.

[48] A 'session' was half a day's work. The distribution and allocation of 'sessions' remain a continual matter of concern up to this day.

[49] All the physicians also had duties at other hospitals, and, of course, their private practices, without exception carried out in Harley Street and its surrounds.

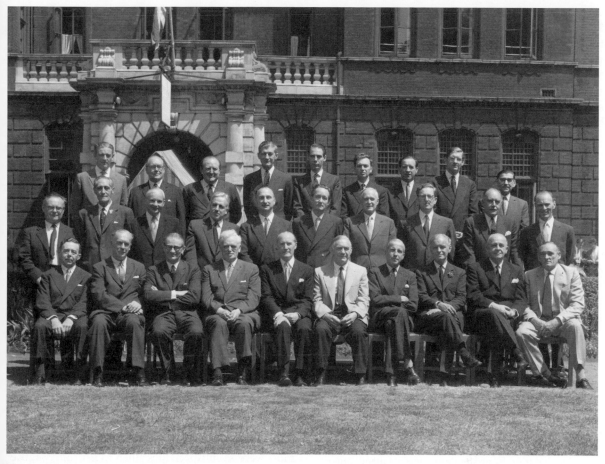

Figure 7.3 The consultant staff, 1960 (left to right: back row – unknown, unknown, Beaver, Bull, Gilliatt, Marshall, Mair, Farl, Shorvon; middle row – Dawson, unknown, Marrack, Hallpike, Kremer, Gooddy, Cumings, Blackwood, Davies, Cobb; front row – McArdle, Meadows, Brinton, Carmichael, Critchley, Jackson, Elkington, Williams, Cawthorne, McKissock).

in management matters – attempts that were frustrated whenever an opportunity arose.

The expansion in the number of consultants working in the NHS could not continue indefinitely and, in the 1950s, the Ministry of Health started to introduce 'manpower planning'.[50] At Queen Square, after much wrangling, an establishment of 63 medical staff was agreed in 1956. The division of the consultant neurologists into three categories was also seen as old-fashioned,

and William Gooddy,[51] by then secretary to the Medical

---

[50] The first attempt at centralised manpower planning at Queen Square seems to have been in March 1951 (Board of Governors' minutes); subsequently, various letters were sent by the Ministry instructing the Board that it had to approve consultant and junior staff posts. Over the years, this process proved very difficult, and predictions of the required number of doctors were notoriously inaccurate.

[51] William Walton Gooddy was educated at Winchester College, where many of his lifelong passions were kindled. He went on to read medicine at University College London. He intended to become a surgeon but, while working as a junior doctor on the medical unit at University College Hospital (UCH), came under the influence of Sir Francis Walshe. After completing his training at the Military Hospital for Head Injuries at Oxford and then at the National Hospital, Queen Square, Gooddy eventually succeeded Walshe in 1951 as consulting physician to UCH and the National Hospital. His annual leave was occasionally spent as visiting neurologist to Mauritius. His main academic contributions were in the field of higher cerebral function, and particularly on time and the nervous system, on which he published papers in the *Lancet* and *Brain*. His ideas were summarised in *Time and the Nervous System* (New York: Praeger Publishing, 1988). He was

275

Committee, informed the Board of Governors that, although 'traditional, internally useful, and acceptable to all of us, the divisions are now indistinct and at variance with the terminology of the National Health Service'. Each neurologist was now designated as 'physician to the National Hospital, Queen Square'. An accompanying 'report on medical establishment' sent by Gooddy, on behalf of the Medical Committee, to the Board of Governors in May 1955 described the role that neurologists envisaged for themselves and the criteria for their appointment:

> As a general policy the number of consultant neurologists on the staff of the hospital should remain small, while the number in other centres, particularly outside London, should be increased. The consultant staff should be selected entirely for the needs of the hospital and for the advancement and teaching of neurology. Expansion of neurological services to meet the needs of the population should take place elsewhere, and the staff of the hospital should contribute to that expansion by leading in the field of neurology, and providing suitably trained candidates for consultant posts. This staff need not be increased beyond the present number of twelve physicians, unless the hospital takes on further commitments ... in general appointments to the staff should, as in the past, be determined by the potential contribution of a physician to the hospital, not upon expediency. Provided the clinical needs are supplied it might be better to refrain from appointment if a suitable candidate is not available, or to create such an appointment for an exceptional man.[52]

an intensely private man who reluctantly took on responsibility for hospital committees and served as president of the Association of British Neurologists. Later in his career, he became interested in the importance of trace elements in neurological disease, combining adolescent interest in the periodic table with his clinical work. Gooddy was one of the first physicians to become interested in cognitive impairment in private and public life, concluding that the arrival of non-invasive neuroimaging should lead to routine neurological and psychological assessment of world leaders. Unlike many neurologists of his generation, he was amusing and charming, lacking the austere asceticism and obsessional approach of some of his Queen Square colleagues. He hated to give bad news, leaving much of this to his juniors. He was an idiosyncratic teacher who sometimes took students round the Circle Line on the London Underground looking for signs, or spending an entire session talking about Proust. In his ninth decade he completed a second book, *Neurological Cosmology: The World, the Brain and I* (London: Minerva Press, 2000) which encapsulates much of his view of life.

This stance perpetuated the vision of Queen Square consultants as the elite of the medical establishment,[53] and they indeed were prominent in national positions and committees in this period, serving the Royal College of Physicians and Ministry neurology committees. They also exerted influence though external appointments. Holmes, Walshe, Brain and Williams were at various times editors of *Brain*; Kinnier Wilson and Carmichael, editors of the *Journal of Neurology and Psychopathology* (then known as the *Journal of Neurology and Psychiatry* and now the *Journal of Neurology, Neurosurgery, and Psychiatry*); and Purdon Martin, editor of the *Journal of Neurology*. Macdonald Critchley was president of the World Federation of Neurology (1965–73) and the International League Against Epilepsy (1949–53), and vice-president of the Royal College of Physicians of London (1964). As a mark of Queen Square's influence on British neurology, it is instructive also to look at the officer positions of the Association of British Neurologists. Of the first ten honorary secretaries (in post between 1933 and 1984), nine were Queen Square consultants, and, of its first 13 presidents (in post from 1933 to 1964), eight were consultants and four of the remaining five had been resident medical officers at the National Hospital. Three-quarters of its first 100 members had at least part of their training at the National Hospital (and, of the few who did not, most were in subspecialties allied to neurology rather than the mainstream subject).

An Impression of the Neurologists and their Practices

Although in somewhat short supply, contemporary memoirs give an indication of how the National Hospital was viewed during this period. The 1960 centenary was an occasion for self-congratulation which those involved did not resist, the various

---

[52] Elkington, in particular, expressed this view, but also emphasised the importance of attracting those capable of original research. At the time it was also recommended that all patients should be available for research and teaching by any member of staff with permission of the treating physician: see G. Robinson, *The National Hospital for Nervous Diseases 1948–1982* (London: National Hospital for Nervous Diseases, 1982).

[53] See S. T. Casper, 'One Hundred Members of the Association of British Neurologists: A Collective Biography for 1933–1960', *Journal of the History of the Neurosciences* 20 (2011): 338–56.

commentators basking especially in the glories of the nineteenth century.[54] Those outside took a more measured stance. One perceptive observer was Lord Walton. His description of Queen Square in 1951, not altogether flattering, is worth quoting at length. Walton described how, as a clerk arriving at Queen Square, he was free to attend outpatient teaching sessions and ward rounds 'in order to sit at the feet of some of the great men of twentieth-century British neurology'.

Critchley was invariably entertaining, suave, elegant, accurate and lively, even if he gave, perhaps through a degree of innate shyness, more than a hint of aloofness ... Elkington, too, was clinically efficient but rather cold and distant, and I cannot readily recall anything of note which he taught me. Carmichael was calm, pragmatic, physiological in his approach, and thoughtful, if rather deliberate. Most deliberate of all, however, was Purdon Martin, whose ward rounds were punctuated with long periods of painful silence, justifying fully the epithet which has been applied to many other similarly uninspiring teachers of 'shifting dullness' as one moved from bed to bed. Nevertheless his knowledge of extrapyramidal disease was original and encyclopedic. Denis Brinton struck me as being an exceptionally nice man to whom one could always talk on equal terms, but his teaching was not particularly inspiring ... Michael Kremer, almost as suave, elegant and polished in his approach as Critchley, was an outstandingly sharp clinician with that kind of insight into the nature and significance of clinical phenomena which identifies the great diagnostician. Sadly, in out-patients especially, his apparent lack of compassion and somewhat cavalier management of patients were occasionally distressing ... Denis Williams, the flamboyant, oozed Welsh charm ... I came to respect him greatly as a most able consultant. Larger than life, at least in terms of personality and flow of language, was Sir Francis Walshe ... who could never resist the sharp incisive and at times wounding comment, which, however clever, witty, and memorable, must nevertheless have regularly left emotional scars upon those with whom he came into conflict. ... But the sheer brilliance of his discourse and even of his repartee left an indelible impression. Paradoxically, he was not a good clinical neurologist and all too often, perhaps through carelessness, perhaps through lack of clinical skill, he was

led into error ...[55] Swithin Meadows was an exceptionally competent clinical neurologist, who was often taken around the ward by the houseman after the great man, Walshe, had passed by in order to correct his all-too-frequent diagnostic errors ... MJ (Sean) McArdle was perhaps the most obsessional of all the Queen Square physicians to whom time seemed irrelevant and who often spent interminable hours studying and examining a single patient. Technically he was brilliant ... but by the time the diagnostic denouement was reached, clerks and house officers alike had often lost interest, not through boredom, as his demonstration of clinical skills was invariably arresting, but simply through exhaustion ... Towering above them all, however was the great Sir Charles Symonds ... never before or since have I come across a physician with such a remarkable ability to dissect and analyse the details of the clinical history in a way which, in over 90% of cases, led him to draw the correct conclusions about the nature of the patient's illness. Invariably, however, the final brick in the diagnostic edifice was drawn from a prodigious clinical memory and an unrivalled experience of clinical neurology. 'Charlie' ... was an incomparable clinician, but despite the enormous respect and admiration in which he was held, there was perhaps here, too, a hint of shyness, even aloofness, which meant that few younger colleagues, however well they came to know him, seemed to achieve closeness to him as a person ... If Carmichael had a fault, it was that he found writing extremely painful (every word a drop of blood, as he said). He therefore published far less than he could and indeed should have done, so that some of his most important original observations never saw the light of day in print ... Martin Halliday was an able clinical neurophysiologist, and Alex Elithorn was doing some important research on the physiological effects of anxiety. There was a strong culture of elegance and panache, mixed with a sense of the superiority of the hospital in neurology and of its staff amongst their peers. There was also an interest in good living and in style personified by Critchley and Williams perhaps more than any other. Many a good evening was had by the physicians at the Athenaeum.[56]

[54] See, for instance, M. Critchley, *Developmental Medicine and Child Neurology* **2** (1960): 5–6. This was Critchley's oration at a hospital reception held on 22 November 1959.

[55] It has been said of Walshe that if he held an opinion forcefully, then you could be sure it was wrong.

[56] J. N. Walton (Lord Walton of Detchant), *The Spice of Life. From: Northumbria to World Neurology* (London: William Heinemann, 1993).

John Pearce, another contemporary observer, also felt that Sir Charles Symonds was 'without doubt the most distinguished neurologist in Britain in his day', who immeasurably advanced the bedside and clinic disciplines, and rational thinking, in clinical neurology. His prodigious memory for previous cases and approach and techniques were, according to Pearce, unrivalled, and he was 'the neurologists' prime choice for the ultimate second opinion'.[57]

Purdon Martin also published his reminiscences and noted that the outpatient department of the hospital had changed greatly during his years, but not as much as the patients:

There is, of course, a great change in their social state – they are better off, better dressed, better

forms of neurosyphilis, no post-encephalitics, almost no cases of cerebral abscess or of meningitis, no Pott's disease, no subacute combined degeneration of the cord, no poliomyelitis, no Sydenham's chorea, no diphtheritic palsies.[58]

The Balance of Clinical Work, Teaching and Research, and the Crisis in Academic Neurology

Despite the earlier manoeuvring of the hospital to ensure designation as a teaching hospital, the fact is that the focus of the physicians in this period was, almost without exception, on clinical practice. Most pursued large private practices, the journey to and

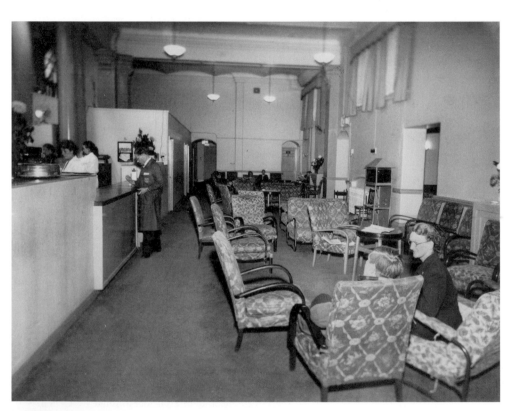

Figure 7.4 Outpatients hall in the Powis wing, 1954.

educated – but what I have in mind is the medical change; there are no cases of tabes, general paralysis of the insane (GPI), syphilitic ocular palsies or other

---

[57] John M. S. Pearce, *Fragments of Neurological History* (London: Imperial College Press, 2003).

[58] J. P. Martin, 'British Neurology in the Last Fifty Years: Some Personal Experiences', *Proceedings of the Royal Society of Medicine* **64** (1971): 1055–9. He notes that the number of outpatients at Queen Square in 1969 was only five-eighths of that seen in 1920, although numbers of inpatient admissions were two and a half times greater.

from Harley Street and its environs being negotiated by the most successful in a chauffeur-driven Rolls Royce. Success and the maintenance of a thriving practice depended on polish and good connections. The consultant staff were members of the better London clubs and societies, and occupied positions in professional life that would ensure good networks for referral of private patients. Justifiably, the reputation for being superb and skilful diagnostic clinicians, of the old school, had grown in the 1920s and 1930s, and was milked repeatedly, even though the suffering of the patients was not always relieved.

The academic focus in these years was on teaching, much more highly rated than on research, and for which the physicians were also held in high regard. A period at Queen Square was almost mandatory for anyone wanting to pursue a career in neurology, especially in the south of England, and through its central training role, the National Hospital retained an iron-like grip on appointments in British neurology. In the early postwar period, experimental research had almost completely vanished from the National Hospital. Any investigative work carried out was clinically based, and usually descriptive. In terms of research or original discovery, the hospital was standing still, and had clearly been overtaken, especially by American institutions, which thrived vicariously during the war at the expense of their European counterparts. The tendency to place a premium on clinical rather than laboratory research was noted by William Lennox, from Harvard, who observed: 'The influential men of the staff have gained their reputation and knowledge by the use of pin, cotton wool, and reflex hammer and are scornful (and fearful) of the new paraphernalia of the laboratory.'[59]

Walton reminds us of Henry Miller's description of Queen Square at this time as 'one of the great silent areas of neurology', and his own conclusion was that 'As a cradle, therefore, of world-wide teaching and practice in clinical neurology, Queen Square was outstanding and had a well-deserved international reputation, but as a fountain-head of neurological research in the UK, it lagged progressively behind.'[60]

In 1958, Elkington visited hospitals in the University of California and reported on neurological practice and conditions that were markedly different from those at Queen Square. The typical Californian hospital was built 'without regard of cost', with paying and non-paying patients sharing many facilities 'without embarrassment to either party' and with 'differences in sex appearing to be of no significance'. He found the teaching of junior staff in the USA much more organised, and benefitting from a large number of departmental and inter-departmental conferences. He was surprised about how high the charges were for patients and how much debt was incurred.[61] He concluded that the most interesting aspect was comparative life-style in the two countries:

> No-one worked on Saturday or Sunday, and during the remainder of the week at least half of each day was at their disposal for reading and writing or pursuing any other interest which might suggest themselves ... The most important difference was in the relative priority given to the activities of a consultant in the university teaching hospital in the two countries. In London, one's primary function is the care of patients and, next in importance, the teaching of one's subject whether this be to undergraduates or post-graduates. Advancement of knowledge and academic activities for their own sake are very much third. If a member of the hospital staff, during a busy life, is successful in advancing his subject, this is to be regarded as a bonus rather than as an obligation for which proper facilities should be provided. In America the position is reversed ... I prefer the English system. But the Americans are at least logical in that, since they expect their staff to do original work and to keep abreast of the academic advances of the times, they provide leisure and physical facilities which make it possible for them to do so. It would be inconceivable in any American hospital that I saw for a senior member of the staff not to have an office of his own with adequate secretarial assistance, as well as the leisure and medical assistance to make it possible for him to use it.

The link between Queen Square and American neurology remained strong during this period, and both Gordon Holmes and Francis Walshe were approached and asked whether they wished to take up directorships of newly developing neurology units. British neurology still regarded itself as superior to that in the United States but, as could be inferred from Elkington's analysis, this reputation was based on past

---

[59] Cited by S. T. Casper, 'The Idioms of Practice: British Neurology 1860–1960' (PhD thesis, University College London, 2007), p. 317.
[60] Walton, *The Spice of Life* (1993).

[61] He mused: 'I found the American public surprisingly docile but I should be surprised if, in the next twenty years, some form of national health service is not forced on an at present unwilling medical profession.'

glory rather than the declining credentials of postwar hospitals in the United Kingdom.[62] Even Carmichael, who was salaried entirely by the MRC, published very little. The crisis in academic matters came to a head with the debate over whether to establish professorships in clinical neurology and other disciplines. In 1959, Walshe gave an address at a meeting of the Neurological Institute of New York, to celebrate its 59th anniversary, entitled 'The Present and Future of Neurology'. This was a trenchant analysis in which he proclaimed that physiology, the predominant research focus in the previous 50 years, had contributed little to an understanding of human disease (and he included his own research in this pessimistic analysis).

> Supposing, and it is perhaps an idle thought, that half the human energy and money that in the past twenty years have gone into electroencephalography had been given to the study of disseminated sclerosis, or the myopathies, or the metabolic and inborn disorders of the nervous system, or even to any single one of these problems, what achievements in the relief of human suffering we might by now have been able to acclaim.[63]

Walshe maintained the importance of the traditional clinical examination, but went on to press for more neurochemistry and neuropathology. It is therefore not surprising that the first two professorial positions at Queen Square were in those specialties. He could not resist a further withering attack on psychiatry, and he reaffirmed that neurology should not be separated from general internal medicine. On 3 December 1959, in support of the rebuilding programme, the Board of Governors submitted a memorandum to the Ministry of Health listing what it perceived to be the most important achievements of Queen Square in neurology. Compared with the academic prowess of earlier generations, the catalogue is underwhelming, and interesting not least for the large contribution of physiology, despite Walshe's dismissive analysis:

> The anatomy of the spinal cord and cerebellum have been largely rewritten as a result of the clinico-anatomical studies made at the hospital. The EEG pattern of subacute inclusion body encephalitis was first described in the EEG department, and the introduction of the measurement of conduction velocity in peripheral nerves as a diagnostic tool was the work of the electromyographic unit. The Batten Unit played a valuable part in the treatment of poliomyelitis. The Beaver respirator invented here is now used around the world. The operation of hemispherectomy for one particular type of 'spastic child' was developed in the hospitals. The cause of minor, but ubiquitous and troublesome, acroparaesthesiae was first recognized by members of the staff, and relief by decompression of the median nerve in the carpal tunnel.[64]

The Clinical Service in the Postwar Years

Ewart Mitchell and Matron Ling both left descriptions of the state of the hospital at the end of the war.[65] The buildings were coated in bomb-dust and appeared rather derelict. Large sections of the hospital were damaged and the roof required extensive work before wards could again become habitable. There were problems with heating, the interiors needed cleaning and re-plastering, old windows and sashes had to be replaced, and the wards required refurbishment and decoration. New stocks of linen, crockery, instruments and all manner of equipment had to be purchased. However, the hospital was coming to life. Matron Ling paid tribute to the small, but valiant and enthusiastic, body of staff who had kept the

---

[62] Of the 28 consultants, two were knighted and two elected FRS, compared with five knights and seven Fellows of the Royal Society among the first 20 appointees (1859–86). In terms of publications, 436 papers appeared between 1950 and 1960; only Walshe, Symonds, Critchley, Williams, Hallpike and Cawthorne published more than 20 papers in this period. Many of the papers were opinion pieces, political or administrative pieces (especially those of Walshe) or reviews. Even allowing case reports, updates on therapy, and descriptions of techniques, only 247 could be classified as research publications. Only Hallpike (27 research papers), Cawthorne (25 papers) and McKissock (20 papers) published consistently. Given that a cursory search of PubMed for 1950–60 using the keyword 'neurology' picks up over 2,200 papers, the relative decline of Queen Square as a central institution in the academic development of the discipline is all too apparent.

[63] F. M. R. Walshe, 'The Present and Future of Neurology', *Archives of Neurology* 2 (1960): 83–8.

[64] Board of Governors minutes, 3 December 1959.

[65] Ewart Mitchell wrote in the annual reports for 1946 and 1947 as secretary to the Board of Management; Matron Ling gave a lecture at the 1960 centenary celebrations (NNHN/EN/9/11).

National Hospital functioning during the war. Mitchell describes the spirit of the staff and especially the leadership of Carmichael and Elkington:

> who had done a very big job, without any troubles of any kind. All have been very willing. Some of them have been here very late at night and for some holidays have been almost unknown ... [progress was due] to what I may call 'The National Team' because the whole of the staff in this hospital during this last year has been pulling as a team.

The medical staff began to resume civilian work after demobilisation from their military service. The neurosurgical unit returned from Haywards Heath, and the theatres were reopened (aural, orthopaedic and ophthalmic surgery also returned) with 16 beds allocated. Julian Taylor, who had spent harrowing years as a prisoner of war, was now the senior surgeon. 'A temporary surgeon', Mr Wylie McKissock, was appointed to assist him. Many wards, closed during the war, were still out of commission and being used as storage areas. Albany, Annie Zunz and Chandler wards reopened in 1946, and Gibbens and John Back in early 1947. The last to reopen was Bentinck ward in 1952. But, even in 1960, the old fabric was still evident, with chairs in the wards dating from 1887, and a much-used wheelchair boasting a plate 'presented by the Ladies Committee 1865'. Doctors were summoned to the wards by bells, the forerunner of the bleep.

The postwar outpatient department was also modernised. Before the war, the hall had been described by Geoffrey Robinson as:

> Typically institutional. The wooden floor was highly polished, the benches, which offered a maximum of discomfort to the occupants, had been shined by the sliding bottoms of the patients as they edged their way along them towards the consulting room door. This was to change – the benches were removed and armchairs of various types were introduced; patients were called by name to see the doctor – although there was as yet no appointments system. The sad green paint on the walls was replaced by a grey, white and blue decor that enhanced the intrinsic beauty of the architecture of the out-patients hall itself, the floor was carpeted as, surprisingly, the cost of carpeting was only £595 whereas the estimates for linoleum or rubber flooring were £1085 and £1992 respectively. An additional feature was a large tank of goldfish and other exotic piscatorial creatures which attracted much attention. Mr Dickson Wright was known to comment on one

occasion that the goldfish at the National Hospitals were better fed than the patients.[66]

The Member of Parliament for Willesden West, Mr Laurence Pavitt, recorded his view on the importance of creative planning in a debate on the topic of hospitals:

> Without a great deal of extra expenditure, tremendous advantage could be secured to the hospital services ... [such as] the National Hospital Queen's Square (*sic*) and Maida Vale Hospital where there was a marvellous arrangement and fine organisation and administration. There were comfortable chairs, little tables and a small cafeteria in a corner of the room. Patients are made to feel that they were not a lot of sheep being pushed past hurdles but human beings suffering from illness and being treated with sympathy and understanding. If this can be done in two hospitals why can it not be done elsewhere? ... Out-patient departments are now the only survival from pre-war days when employment exchanges treated the unemployed man as if he were a criminal. We still have not got out of that attitude of mind in the matter of treating people in the out-patient departments of some of our hospitals.[67]

The X-ray department was initially split on two sites, in the outpatients and adjoining the theatres. It was re equipped partly with gifts from Sweden by Erik Lysholm and, in 1947, moved to a new site on the third floor of the old hospital. Massage and electrical treatment were on the wane, and each was absorbed into the physiotherapy unit when this was formed a few years after the end of the war. In 1946, an approach was made to provide radiotherapy for cancer at the National Hospital as an 'outlying centre' of the main centre at University College Hospital. This followed the government directives in 1946 to concentrate the treatment of tumours in certain centres.

There was a slow but steady rise in hospital activity. The number of beds increased gradually, with only 80 available in 1946, increasing to 142 by the end of January 1947, and 194 distributed across 14 wards by 1957.[68]

---

[66] Geoffrey Robinson, *The National Hospitals for Nervous Diseases 1948–1982* (London: The Board of Governors of the National Hospitals for Nervous Diseases, 1982).

[67] Hansard, 21 July 1960, vol. 627, col. 825.

[68] These beds were assigned as follows: 60 to the four physicians, 40 to the four physicians to outpatients, 15 to the three assistant physicians, 18 to the three surgeons, five to the psychiatrist and four to the otologists. Ward 14 was for post-operative patients under joint care of a surgeon and physician.

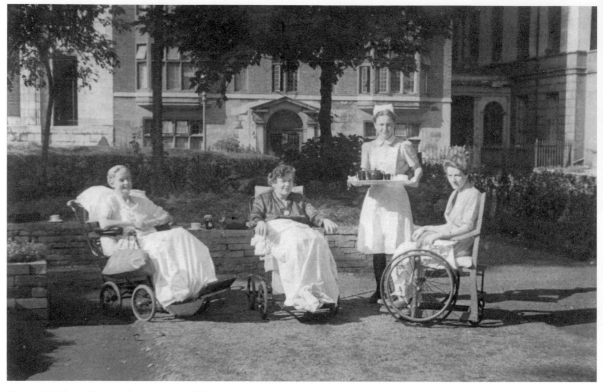

Figure 7.5 Nurse Bird and three patients, 1947.

The inpatient admission numbers for the three years 1956–8, respectively, were: 2,226, including 410 emergencies; 2,651 including 513 emergencies; and 2,893 including 631 emergencies. These numbers were substantially higher than in any pre-war period and possibly due to much shorter lengths of stay. New outpatient rooms were opened and the consultants were encouraged to do their private practice in the hospital so as to be on-site. A deafness clinic was opened. The Parkinson's Disease Society initiated a specialist clinic.

By 1954, the Medical Committee could state that the number of beds for general neurology 'is at present adequate'. Any increase should be made for special needs, such as viral diseases (presumably referring to poliomyelitis), acute neurosurgery, and research or academic units. However, by 1954, the Medical Committee had noticed a reduction from the pre-war number of outpatients reflecting the mix of new and old cases, the complexity of referrals, the fact that 'patients do not now return simply for repeat prescriptions' (as these were now provided by general practitioners, which was not often the case in pre-NHS days), and the policy of acting mainly as a tertiary centre.

The Batten Unit and the Birth of Intensive Care

A wave of poliomyelitis epidemics in Britain was the trigger for another important development in the hospital – the opening, in 1953, of a respiratory ward. The unit was named after Frederick Batten, in recognition of his work at Queen Square on poliomyelitis. After studying cases from an epidemic in London during 1902, Batten wrote definitive papers on polio and later gave the Lumleian lectures on 'acute infective poliomyelitis'.[69] The major outbreaks in Britain occurred, however, some decades later, with

---

[69] F. E. Batten, 'The Epidemiology of Poliomyelitis', *Proceedings of the Royal Society of Medicine* (section on epidemiology) **4** (1910–1): 198–221; and F. E. Batten, 'Acute Poliomyelitis', *Brain* **39** (1916): 115–211. Poliomyelitis had aroused the interest of other Queen Square physicians. The first was James Collier, whose theories on transmission were savaged by Francis Walshe in the 1930s. Walshe's own theories were in turn later criticised by Purdon Martin but, in contrast to the enmity induced in other opponents of Walshe, no lasting damage to their relationship seems to have occurred.

over 8,000 notifications in some years and many hundreds of deaths. The 1945 epidemic exposed the woeful lack of respirators, and it required gifts by Lord Nuffield to supply large numbers of 'iron lungs' to hospitals around the country. This form of tank respirator was first used for polio in the Children's Hospital in Boston in the 1920s, powered by an electric motor attached to two vacuum cleaners. As technology improved, assisted respiration became widely used. However, the machines had many drawbacks, not least the strong negative inspiratory pressure which tended to suck secretions into the lungs in patients with bulbar paralysis.

During the severe 1962 polio epidemic in Copenhagen, a patient was treated as an emergency with tracheostomy and manual 'bagging'.[70] This proved so successful that, within weeks, 40–70 patients were managed in this way, with 200 medical students working day and night to perform manual bagging. In the summer of 1953, when further polio epidemics spread through London, the Board of Governors, noting that 'reports on the treatment of poliomyelitis from Denmark and from the Royal College of Physicians had been received', established a subcommittee to consider equipment and details of treatment at Queen Square. This resulted in the establishment of an isolation unit for the treatment of polio under the supervision of Michael Kremer. Once in place, in October 1953 the Medical Committee recommended that, when no cases of polio were present, the 'poliomyelitis Batten Unit' might be used for other neurological diseases also requiring respiration. In the following year, Kremer reported on the first 16 cases admitted to the Batten Unit: four with polio and two suspected cases, eight with polyneuritis, one case of myasthenia gravis, and one patient with myelitis. Four had died: three with polyneuritis and the patient with myasthenia gravis. The Medical Committee agreed to appoint to the unit a medical officer who had no other responsibilities in the hospital, and that the main function of the unit now 'should be for neurological diseases with respiratory or circulatory

embarrassment, and that straightforward cases of polio might have to be turned away'.[71]

Thus, although the Batten Unit was conceived as an emergency response to potential polio epidemics, it was very soon transformed into what was, it seems, the first respiratory unit in the world devoted to neurological cases.[72] Poliomyelitis was now rapidly diminishing in importance as an epidemic disease, with introduction of the Salk vaccine in 1956 and, then, the Sabin vaccine. By 1963, the number of deaths in the country had fallen to single figures. The National Hospital showed great vision in establishing the unit, which maintained the hospital at the forefront of neurological intensive care for many years.

In 1961, John Marshall, who succeeded Kremer as physician-in-charge, summarised the work of the Batten Unit over its first six years.[73] A total of 229 patients had been treated, of whom 48 had polio (mortality rate 6 per cent), 49 stroke (53 per cent mortality rate), 39 polyneuritis (26 per cent mortality rate), 16 myasthenia gravis (44 per cent mortality rate), 15 spinal cord lesions (17 per cent mortality rate) and 13 cerebral tumours (85 per cent mortality rate). Other cases treated in smaller numbers included polymyositis, motor neurone disease, encephalitis, meningitis, multiple sclerosis, head injury, barbiturate poisoning, tetanus (only a single case in five years), status epilepticus and miscellaneous chest conditions. Of these cases, 61 were treated with intermittent positive pressure respiration, 13 with tank respirators (in the earlier years, until these were discontinued in 1959), 22 with tracheostomy, two with endotracheal intubation, and 134 only needing expert nursing and supportive care. The paper summarised the methods and principles of therapy, and showed how quickly medicine had advanced in this area. Marshall emphasised the importance of early ventilation as an elective procedure and methods for eventual weaning, recognition of the clinical signs of

---

[70] Blegdam Hospital, the only institution in Copenhagen for communicable diseases, admitted 2,722 cases over a five-month period, of whom 319 had respiratory symptoms. Lassen was the director of the hospital and Ibsen his anaesthetist: see H. C. A. Lassen, 'A Preliminary Report on the 1952 Epidemic of Poliomyelitis in Copenhagen with Special Reference to the Treatment of Acute Respiratory Insufficiency', *Lancet* **261** (1953): 37–41.

[71] It was suggested that the Western Fever Hospital might be an appropriate unit, and also used for cases with chronic respiratory problems.

[72] According to Wijdicks, Walter Dandy opened the first neurosciences intensive care unit at Johns Hopkins in 1932; this was not specifically a respiratory unit, but rather to care for sick neurosurgical patients: see E. F. M. Wijdicks *et al.*, 'The Early Days of the Neurosciences Intensive Care Unit', *Mayo Clinic Proceedings* **86** (2011): 903–5.

[73] J. Marshall. 'The Work of a Respiratory Unit in a Neurological Hospital', *Postgraduate Medical Journal* **37** (1961): 26–30.

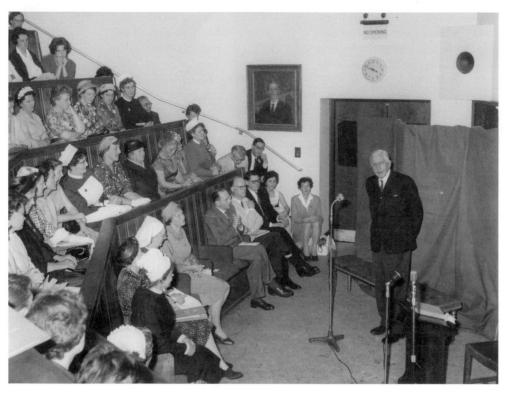

Figure 7.6 Sir Ernest Gowers addressing guests at the centenary celebrations in the Queen Mary wing lecture theatre, 1960.

respiratory embarrassment ahead of changes in blood gases, general and nursing management, and the appropriate use of antibiotics. All these principles still apply today.

The Centenary Celebrations in 1960

The National Hospital celebrated its centenary in June 1960 with a week-long programme that offered 100 demonstrations, including films and static images, scientific and clinical presentations, a service of thanksgiving and dedication, an opening ceremony by the Minister of Health (Derek Walker-Smith), a visit and tour by the Duke of Edinburgh, a keynote lecture relayed to the outpatient hall, a lecture series at BMA House, cocktail parties at the Royal College of Physicians and Royal College of Surgeons, a sherry party for the 'Alpha guests', a wine and cheese party for women, and a centenary luncheon for the staff. Attendance at these various events was by invitation, and 780 home and 180 overseas visitors were expected. The centrepiece was a banquet at the Mansion House for over 280 people, including 50 of the more favoured guests, almost all of the present and past hospital consultant staff, and leading figures of the

medical establishment outside Queen Square and in international neurology.[74]

A temporary exhibition of paintings by John Piper, Jacob Epstein and Carel Weight, among others, was hung in the corridors of the hospital. An interesting historical exhibition of 55 items was mounted by Hunter, Gooddy and Hamilton-Paterson.[75] A

---

[74] The rather conventional menu for the banquet on 24 June is to be found in the Board of Governors' minutes: paté; lobster Newburg; Tournedos chasseur with croquette potatoes and French beans; peaches au kirsch and tuiles; fromage frappé; and coffee. The wines were not exceptional, Pouilly Fuissé 1953, Chateauneuf du Pape 1955 and Quinta Port. The table plan is in the archive, showing Sir Ernest Gowers at the head. Penfield and Walshe are both present, but at different ends of the top table. Others present included Lord Adrian, Alajouanine, Monrad-Kohn, Percival Bailey, Russell Brain, Lord Cohen of Birkenhead and Harry Platt.

[75] John Hamilton-Paterson was born in Jiangxi Province in China, the son of two medical missionaries. He was educated at University College Hospital and worked at Leavesden with Wyllie McKissock and then at St Hugh's, serving later with the Army in France, Belgium and finally in Delhi. In 1946, he was registrar at University College Hospital to Walshe and, in

rather fetching red-and-blue ashtray, valued at 4s, was given to all patients and 950 members of staff, in a gesture not conducive to public health. A new book – anonymous, although everyone knew the author was Critchley – entitled *The National Hospital Queen Square*, with a foreword by Sir Ernest Gowers, was published at 30s per copy.

Critchley gave the Centenary Oration on 'Jacksonian Ideas and the Future with Special Reference to Aphasia'. Sir Charles Symonds delivered the second Gowers memorial lecture on 'Disease of Mind and Disorder of Brain'. Norman Dott delivered the Victor Horsley lecture on 'Brain, Movement and Time'.[76] Pierce Bailey, from Bethesda, spoke on 'The National Hospital and the Growth of Neurology'. Other addresses were given by Théophile Alajouanine ('Recollections of Queen Square'), Henri Gastaut ('Present State of the Post-hemiplegic Epilepsies, Described by Gowers')[77] and Jerzy Chorobski from Warsaw ('Hughlings Jackson and Focal Epilepsy'). Members of the staff were also involved: Michael Kremer spoke on 'C. H. Beevor – the First Dean of the Medical School', Meadows on 'C. B. Radcliffe and his Contribution to Neurology', Gooddy on 'Brown-Séquard and his Associations with the Beginnings of the National Hospital', Marshall on 'Batten and the Developments and Future of Research into Poliomyelitis', Davies on 'The Growth of Neuro-radiology', Cawthorne on 'Sir Charles Ballance and his Work', Hamilton-Paterson on 'Dr Charlton Bastian and his Contribution to Neurology', Blackwood on 'The National Hospital and the Development of Neuro-pathology', Cumings on 'The National Hospital and the Growth of Neuro-chemistry', Lyle on 'The Early Neuro-ophthalmologists at Queen Square', Hunter and Hurwitz on 'The Case Notes of the National

Hospital for the Paralysed and Epileptic before 1900', Harvey Jackson on 'Changes in Neurosurgery' and J. Purdon Martin on 'Observations on the Function of the Basal Ganglia'. Professor Grashchenkov from Russia, scheduled to lecture on 'The Role of the National Hospital in Russian Neuropathology', and John Fulton from America, speaking on 'Elihu Yale', failed to attend.

The Duke of Edinburgh's tour involved much shaking of hands with the physicians (but not all, and for some reason not the neuropsychiatrists) and a series of visits to different departments: Marshall demonstrated a tremor machine, Carmichael explained the principles of stereotaxis, Cumings showed a stage-by-stage procedure for examining cerebrospinal fluid, Beaver demonstrated his breathing machine and heart pump, Blackwood prepared material for microscopy, Hunter and Etlinger showed a tachistoscope and apparatus for the determination of depth perception, Williams demonstrated the electroencephalograph, Gilliatt stimulated peripheral nerve at the wrist and recorded ascending action potentials, and Hallpike demonstrated the revolving chair – a dizzying and possibly rather dull tour, although Walshe later remarked that the Duke 'claimed to have enjoyed himself'. Nursing was celebrated: Miss Ling, the Nightingale-like matron of Queen Square, wrote in the *Nursing Times*:

> The main event was a pageant ... [It was] a verbal panorama of the history of neurological nursing. Reciting singly, in pairs, or in chorus, the six girls told the story of nursing in their hospital, from the early days, when patients came from the streets around the square, and a lady caused a great stir by coming all the way from Brighton to be a patient, to the present when the hospital draws its patients and its staff from the four corners of the earth ... It is impossible to convey in print how moving this all was, and the whole audience felt humble and immensely grateful for the enthusiasm of Miss G Rubin, the sister tutor, who had planned the pageant.[78]

The rather limited interest of the national newspapers was in marked contrast to the extensive comment that had attended the opening of the hospital 100 years earlier, but the *Manchester*

1951, appointed assistant physician at Queen Square and St George's Hospital. He acted as sub-dean to the Institute of Neurology, and held various international administrative positions. His main contribution to academic medicine was a paper on the symptomatology of auditory nerve tumours published in 1951 in *Brain*, described as a minor classic by his obituarist in the *British Medical Journal*. He was a kind, gentle and scholarly person much loved by his colleagues, but the last two years of his life were complicated by illness and he died aged only 46.

[76] These three lectures were published back-to-back in the *British Medical Journal* 2 (1960): 1–15.

[77] Although Alajouanine was well known to Queen Square, Gastaut was a surprising choice having had little to do with the hospital, and having fallen out badly with Walshe during Walshe's editorship of *Epilepsia*.

[78] *Nursing Times*, 16 December 1960.

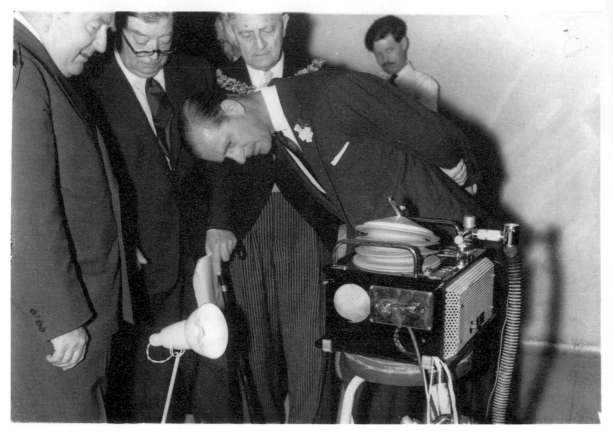

Figure 7.7 Prince Philip examining Beaver's breathing apparatus during his tour for the centenary celebrations, with Dr Beaver looking on, 1960.

Guardian for 18 June 1960 told its readers that 'nerve specialists from 37 countries attended the celebrations and that invitations were sent to 2500 specialists who were trained at "Queen Square"'.

All were agreed that the celebrations were a success and, as for the practice of neurology, Queen Square could still claim, in 1960, to be the National Hospital.

Beyond the Walls: British Neurology Outside Queen Square

The gradual separation of neurology from internal medicine began in the mid nineteenth century but took many decades to gain full acceptance. The declaration by the Chandlers that they were founding a National Hospital for Paralysis and Epilepsy provided some impetus but, although the establishment of a neurological hospital was universally welcomed, the trend towards specialisation more generally in medicine caused considerable controversy. The senior physicians in the larger teaching hospitals were largely opposed to change and for various reasons. They saw specialist hospitals and experts in defined areas as threats to their lucrative private practices. They argued that the establishment of specialties in subjects such as ophthalmology, ear nose and throat disease, orthopaedics and urology had been tainted by association with quacks and charlatans. They considered isolation damaging to medicine. Many generalists remained openly hostile to specialism, doubting that the work of neurologists was worthwhile because the subject was descriptive and lacked any therapy or practical applications. As a result, departments of neurology, as such, were not formed in any general hospital until the turn of the twentieth century.[1] But specialisation was inescapable as the science of neurology advanced, knowledge increased, and the diagnosis and management of neurological diseases grew more sophisticated. Slowly, momentum gathered pace, and the number of doctors who considered themselves to be 'neurologists' increased in London, and then, more generally, throughout the United Kingdom.

Neurology as a Specialty, and Its Relation to General Medicine, Psychiatry and Neurosurgery

Although some degree of specialisation was inevitable, the extent to which neurology should separate entirely from general medicine was a contentious issue (and so it remains today). In the nineteenth century, there was no consensus, even amongst those who took an interest in diseases of the nervous system, in seceding from general medicine. Much more agreement on specialisation was apparent in the United States and in Europe. Even at Queen Square, the physicians supported a strong attachment to internal medicine and, well into the twentieth century, almost all continued to practise general medicine in their teaching hospital positions, as well as neurology. As a result, until around 1970, consultants were appointed to Queen Square as 'physicians' not 'neurologists',[2] and styled themselves thus in letters and documents.[3] Reconciling these views was not helped by those who practised neurology barely concealing the fact that they regarded themselves as elite among physicians, preferring the title 'consultant' to 'specialist', an attitude that did not fade and which was nicely encapsulated in an editorial (anonymous, but

---

[1] The first department of neurology was established at St Mary's Hospital in 1907, with Wilfred Harris – who had been the resident medical officer at the National Hospital in 1895 – as director, having succeeded Armand de Watteville in 1899 as electrotherapeutics officer at St Mary's.

[2] Nonetheless, many designated themselves as 'neurologist' in their writings. The origin of the term is discussed in Chapter 1. By the early 1900s, 'neurologist' was being widely used in its modern sense to describe a doctor who specialised in the treatment of organic diseases of the nervous system.

[3] At the time of writing, government – faced with a crisis of recruitment into internal medicine – is again proposing that doctors who wish to be neurologists must also be trained and practise as general physicians. This politically driven stance based on short-termism goes against the drift of the last 150 years and cannot be seen as in the interests of people with neurological disease, who, self-evidently, want to be managed by doctors committed full-time to the study of their illnesses.

in the style of Walshe) reflecting views expressed in the 1945 report of the Neurology subcommittee of the Royal College of Physicians:

> Clinical neurology has for a century been one of the cynosures of British medicine ... The function of the neurologist in one way differs from that of the practitioners of some other aspects of medicine – e.g., psychiatry, tuberculosis – for the neurologist is a consultant rather than a specialist; he is a judge who sums up and advises as to the nature, origins, outcome of an illness, and the disposal of a sick person, and he is not the purveyor of a particular line of treatment. Hence neurologists have been comparatively few in number, self-selected, highly trained and experienced. If schedules of training should become necessary – and such may of course be deplored – then they must be exacting, eclectic, and extensive.[4]

The role of the National Hospital within the specialty of neurology in Britain was another controversial issue and the topic of several prestigious lectures. Henry Miller spoke at Queen Square in 1957 defining the role of the hospital in ways that still very much apply: 'The provision of second opinions as a court of appeal ... [the hospital is] an inestimable boon to every neurologist working outside London, and to his patients ... teaching and the development and application of new knowledge and new methods'.[5]

Miller pointed out that neurology as practised in district hospitals differed in a number of important ways from that taught at Queen Square. The district neurologist was able to take a much broader overview of neurological disease in the community; he (*sic*) dealt with acutely ill emergency cases rarely seen at Queen Square; and he encountered neurological aspects of general medical conditions, especially in haematology, cardiology and rheumatology. Miller was critical of specialist hospital neurologists, including those at Queen Square, for not being interested in treatment.

> The rather unkind observation of a medical colleague that only three out of the last hundred papers published in *Brain* held out any hope for the patient is perhaps not entirely without significance. In fact, there have been two and a half papers in that journal devoted to treatment during the past three years, and two of these dealt with the not exactly day-to-day problem of the control of myotonia. It is difficult to

rebut in its entirety the imputation that neurologists are not very interested in treatment.

Russell Brain, in his Frederick Price lecture to the Royal College of Physicians of Edinburgh in 1957, was more generous on the role of the National Hospital, although recognising that the type of neurology seen there (both Queen Square and Maida Vale) was not representative of practice elsewhere.

> Nothing can take the place of the special neurological hospital. It has an essential part to play in the training of neurologists and provides a unique forum for the interchange of ideas and a continuing stimulus to the thought of the neurologist already in practice. Moreover, it is also the most suitable place for the expansion of neurology into some of the new fields which recent scientific developments, especially in biochemistry and electronics, are opening.[6]

Both he and Henry Miller considered the issue of whether neurologists should be specialists in their own right or whether neurology could once again be the responsibility of 'general physicians with an interest'. Both recognised the advantages and disadvantages of each view, and both stressed the importance of embedding neurology in general medicine. Brain, though, considered 'it to be a mistake to suppose that his [the neurologist's] place there [in the general hospital] can be supplied by the general physician'. Miller took the opposing view and believed that a general physician with an interest in neurology was both the only practical solution to the manpower problem and also better equipped to deal with the type of neurology that occurs in the context of general medicine, and which rarely graced the corridors of Queen Square. Each recognised that, as Brain put it, the 'growing relationship between neurology and general medicine might well now be more widely recognized in the training of the neurologist'.

The debate has continued to this day, with opinion veering towards and away from the extremes of 'specialization' versus 'the integration of neurology into general medicine'; and the 'decentralization of neurology to district level', with physicians practising general medicine as well as neurology, versus the 'maintenance of national centres' having a concentration of neurologists, many of whom subspecialise

---

[4] Anon., 'The Training of Neurologists', *British Medical Journal* **2** (1 September 1945): 292–3.

[5] H. Miller, *British Medical Journal* **1** (1958): 477–80.

[6] R. Brain, 'Neurology: Past, Present and Future', *British Medical Journal* **1** (1958): 355–60.

within neurology.[7] This debate has rarely been based on the the advancement of knowledge and best practice but, rather – in a National Health Service driven by the expediencies of providing a workforce capable of dealing with the volume and case-mix of medicine in its entirety – on manpower.

It was not only in its relationship to general medicine that the question of specialism was constantly debated, but also in the differentiation of neurology from psychiatry. Again, opinion has fluctuated. In Britain, neurology and psychiatry have traditionally remained almost entirely distinct. This is partly because the practice of psychiatry had, since the eighteenth century, been based in asylums and mental hospitals, and therefore outside the orbit of general medicine.[8] Furthermore, with registration by examination, psychiatrists qualified through the Diploma in Psychological Medicine and Membership of the Royal College of Psychiatrists,[9] rather than through recognition by the Royal College of Physicians. However, many argued for closer integration of the two disciplines, not least because there are very many psychiatric features in neurological conditions which affect the brain (for instance, in epilepsy or movement disorders), and because many psychiatric conditions have a biological and 'neurological' basis.[10]

Only now, riding the crest of the wave of biological rather than analytical psychiatry, is there revival of the wish to bring these two medical specialties closer under the rubric of 'brain and mind sciences'.

Another factor in determining the pace of specialisation was the relationship of neurology to neurosurgery. Queen Square was a hospital founded on neurology and, after the death of Horsley, investment in and the nurture of neurosurgery were not prioritised. Sir Charles Symonds argued forcibly for closer union, citing the example of ophthalmology, but the attitude of the neurologists for whom any form of surgery was a craft carried out by barbers proved a barrier to fusion. Not surprisingly, neurosurgeons were keen, early in the twentieth century, for emancipation, having their own beds and units.[11] Attitudes outside Queen Square were more progressive and in tune with the times. The Second World War stimulated the rapid development of neurosurgery regionally, and, from this point onwards, surgery led and neurology trailed in its wake, as units were established throughout the British Isles. Indeed, it was in part the ostrich-like attitude at Queen Square to neurosurgery that led the development of regional centres which, paradoxically, then undermined the national role of Queen Square in clinical neurology.

The Emergence of Specialist Societies

The rise of the medical society in the second half of the nineteenth century was a striking phenomenon, and in these societies specialisation was much debated. Several sought to engage with professional affairs in the wider arena of national medical politics, and others adopted an educational position. Some faded, were amalgamated into bigger groupings, or reappeared phoenix-like, and as a result and over time, neurology as a speciality grew in stature within the societies if not on the wards of the great teaching hospitals. The staff of the National Hospital were prominent in the activities related to neurology in these forums and in the eventual separation of neurology from the general medical societies.

---

[7] Reviewed by R. Langton Hewer and V. A. Wood, 'Neurology in the United Kingdom. I: Historical Development', *Journal of Neurology, Neurosurgery, and Psychiatry* **55** (supp.) (1992): 2–7.

[8] Even in 1938, there were only nine psychiatric beds out of 6,700 in the London teaching hospitals.

[9] And its predecessors: the Association of Medical Officers of Asylums and Hospitals for the Insane founded in 1841 which in 1865 changed its name to the Medico-Psychological Association, which was awarded a Royal Charter in 1926 and became the Royal Medico-Psychological Association. In 1971, the latter was converted, by a supplementary royal charter, into the Royal College of Psychiatrists.

[10] The view of Sir Charles Symonds, expressed as late as 1970 in his lecture *Tria juncta in uno*, shows the strength of feeling on this topic, but at that time this view was largely rejected. Henry Miller agreed with Symonds that the neurological trainee should spend at least six months in a busy acute psychiatric unit, 'where he will learn an enormous amount of neurology', and recalls that Charles Symonds viewed 'a neurologist as a neuropsychiatrist specialising in the management of nervous disease that is already known to have a structural basis, and a psychiatrist a neuropsychiatrist concentrating on syndromes (mostly of unknown causation) that present with predominantly psychological symptoms': H. Miller, *Proceedings of the Royal Society of Medicine* **61** (1968): 18–24.

[11] This was pithily put by Professor George Gask, in his inaugural address as president of the Medical Society of London, *British Medical Journal* **2** (26 October 1935): 816 – 'In neuro-surgery there was a strong and growing tendency for the surgeon undertaking operations on the brain and spinal cord to carry out his own examination of the patient and make his own diagnosis. He was no longer content to act the plumber for the physician.'

The Medical Society of London and the Medical and Chirurgical Society (Later the Royal Medical and Chirurgical Society)

>Before Hughlings Jackson and colleagues founded the Neurological Society of London in 1887, physicians interested in the nervous system participated in meetings of one or other of two London societies. From 1773, they could attend the Medical Society of London, founded – 36 years after the Medical Society of Edinburgh (1737) – by John Coakley Lettsom and a small number of London physicians. Lettsom had been brought up by the Brotherhood of the Society of Friends (the 'Quakers'). His concept was to bring together the disparate but independently influential communities of physicians, apothecaries and surgeons.[12] The society sought to extend its influence beyond the constraints imposed by the religious affiliation required in order to study medicine in the Universities of Oxford and Cambridge, and extended membership to the graduates of Scottish, Irish and foreign universities, in contrast to the rules of the fellowship of the Royal College of Physicians. Neurologists participated in its activities from the outset. Members of the staff at Queen Square who served as presidents of the Medical Society of London included Hughlings Jackson, Brudenell Carter, Ballance, Ferrier, Symonds and Armour, along with Crichton-Browne who served on the Board of Governors at Queen Square, and Feiling from Maida Vale. Gowers and Horsley were recipients of the society's Fothergill gold medal.

In the early nineteenth century, the 'age of reform', new clubs and groupings were being created in many areas of public and professional life. In 1805, the Medical and Chirurgical Society was formed by 'seceders' from the Medical Society of London seeking a more inclusive and academic body. The society flourished and, in 1834, became the Royal Medical and Chirurgical Society. In the 1860s, it had over 600 fellows and retained its academic focus by holding meetings and publishing a journal. But, at the same time, 21 specialist medical societies had been established in

London alone, and this profusion led to repeated proposals for merger. With the usual mix of entrenched isolationism and more liberal attitudes, these overtures came to nothing until 1907 when the Royal Medical and Chirurgical Society and 14 specialist organisations amalgamated to form the Royal Society of Medicine (RSM). Two of these specialist societies were of especial relevance to physicians and surgeons who studied diseases of the nervous system.

The Ophthalmological Society of the United Kingdom

The Ophthalmological Society of the United Kingdom was founded in 1880. This society strove to identify ophthalmology as a specialty separate from medicine and surgery, based on expertise and an interest in practice as 'oculists'. In 1880, 'a few gentlemen in London … sent to ophthalmic surgeons and others … in the three kingdoms … likely to be interested … a circular suggesting the formation of an Ophthalmological Society'. By 23 June, 50 acceptances had been received and 28 (of whom four were based out of London) attended a first meeting. From the outset, the society nurtured a close relationship with neurology. The founding president, Sir William Bowman, had worked with Robert Bentley Todd at King's College Hospital, and Hughlings Jackson was appointed as one of the six vice-presidents at the inaugural general meeting held on 6 July 1881.[13] Several of the 140 foundation members were well-known neurologists: Thomas Barlow and Sir William Broadbent, and, from Queen Square, Buzzard, Gowers, Jackson, Beevor and Ormerod. Bowman wrote: 'I advert with special pleasure to the fact that a large and important part of the total communications received by the Society has come, as was hoped and anticipated, from … physicians largely concerned with disease of the nervous system.'[14]

---

[12] There were 30 members in each category, with some corresponding members. The purpose was 'to establish a society to give practitioners in medicine frequent opportunities of meeting together and conferring with each other concerning any difficult or uncommon cases which may have occurred, or communicating any new discoveries in medicine which have been made either at home or abroad'.

[13] In addition to bimonthly meetings, attended on average by 32 members, two extraordinary ones were arranged in the first year: one was a discussion led by Hughlings Jackson 'On the Relation of Optic Neuritis [papilloedema] to Intracranial Disease'. The communications brought before the society in its first year were grouped by anatomical structure: on the optic nerve – Gowers describing cases of optic neuritis with nerve VI palsy due to meningitis and optic neuritis with loss of upgaze – and paralytic affections; and Hughlings Jackson writing on eye symptoms in locomotor ataxy.

[14] W. Bowman, 'Inaugural Address at the First Meeting of the Society on June 23, 1880', *Transactions of the Ophthalmological Society of the United Kingdom* 1 (1881): 1–5.

The theme of specialism was taken up by Hughlings Jackson in his 1885 Bowman lecture to the Ophthalmological Society in which, speaking on 'Ophthalmology and Diseases of the Nervous System', he expounded the doctrine of using clinical phenomena as the basis for developing ideas on cerebral physiology; from these analyses emerged new ideas on the organisation of the central nervous system that resonated with the emerging concepts of evolution and the structure of social systems.[15]

The Neurological Society of London (Later the Neurological Society of the United Kingdom)

Crichton-Browne's successor as director of the West Riding Lunatic Asylum in Wakefield, Herbert Coddington Major, indicated that he was not willing to continue publication of the *West Riding Lunatic Asylum Medical Reports*, which ran to six annual volumes between 1871 and 1876. Consequently, Crichton-Browne, Bucknill, Ferrier and Hughlings Jackson, closely associated with Wakefield but all now in London, decided to start a new journal, and the first issue of *Brain* was published in July 1878. Armand de Watteville joined as a fifth co-editor, in 1882. He was appointed acting editor from 1884 and sole editor from 1887 to 1900, with an editorial committee made up of Bucknill, Buzzard, Crichton-Browne, Ferrier, Jackson and James Ross. Three months after Jackson's Bowman lecture was published, de Watteville hosted a meeting in his house at 30 Welbeck Street (London W1) on 14 November 1885 at which Broadbent proposed, and Jackson seconded, that 'it was desirable to form a Neurological Society'.[16] Events moved forward at further meetings on 14 January 1886 (also at 30 Welbeck Street), and at the home of Jackson (3 Manchester Square) on 23 January 1886 and 13 January 1887, resulting in an initial announcement that the Society had been formed. A

subcommittee comprising Drs Broadbent, Bristowe, Ferrier, Jackson and Crichton-Browne, and Messrs Hutchinson and Schäfer, with Dr de Watteville as secretary, drew up the constitution and rules of the Society and elected council and office bearers for the year 1887.[17] It has been said that the stimulus for establishment of the Neurological Society was a meeting of the Royal Medical and Chirurgical Society in May 1885, at which Rickman Godlee described his removal of a cerebral tumour. Neurology and neurosurgery were entering a feverish period of growth, and Jackson and Broadbent decided that the formation of a society dedicated to the new specialism of neurology was opportune. In the event, there was considerable overlap between the membership of the Ophthalmological Society of the United Kingdom and the Neurological Society of London. Buzzard is recorded as saying that, at its foundation, the Neurological Society was established 'on no narrow basis', and its presidents and officers rotated in a reasonably egalitarian manner. But not everyone was pleased: Gowers refused to join because of the involvement of de Watteville, and is reported to have said 'that the society was founded by a charlatan [de Watteville] to keep out a quack [Julius Althaus]'.[18]

During its first year, the Neurological Society met on eight occasions. Jackson delivered an inaugural presidential address at the National Hospital on 'The Scope and Aims of Neurology' (24 March 1886). Horsley and Schäfer introduced a discussion on sensory and motor localisations at the physiological laboratory of University College (26 May 1886). A clinical meeting was held, at which, among others, James Anderson presented a case

---

[15] J. H. Jackson, 'Ophthalmology and Disease of the Nervous System', *Transactions of the Ophthalmological Society of the United Kingdom* **6** (1886): 1–22.

[16] This meeting was chaired by Samuel Wilks and attended by Anderson, Barlow, James Bristowe, Buzzard, Crichton-Browne, Sir Horatio Donkin, Ferrier, Samuel Gee, Walter Baugh Hadden, David Bridge Lees, Sir Stephen Mackenzie, Angel Money, William Miller Ord, William Pasteur, Sidney Philip Phillips, Sir George Savage, Semon, Octavius Sturges, Tooth and de Watteville, and Messrs Horsley, Herbert Page and Sir Edward Sharpey Schäfer.

[17] The foundation officers were: *President*: John Hughlings Jackson; *Vice-presidents*: Samuel Wilks and James Crichton-Browne; *Council members*: Charlton Bastian, William Broadbent, John Bucknill, Thomas Buzzard, David Ferrier, Francis Galton, Jonathan Hutchinson, George Romanes and Edward Schäfer; *Treasurer*: John Bristowe; *Secretaries*: Hughes Bennett and Armand de Watteville. *Other founder members*: Charles Beevor, Frederick Gowland Hopkins, Robert Maguire, Charles Mercier, Joseph Ormerod, George Poore, Seymour Sharkey, William Hale White, Isaac Yeo and Messrs George Gould, Marcus Gunn, John Lunn, Edward Nettleship, John Tweedy and Professor William Stirling.

[18] 1907 minutes of the Committee of Management of the neurological section of the Royal Society of Medicine, cited by P. Hunting, *History of the Royal Society of Medicine* (London: Royal Society of Medicine Press, 2002).

of 'basal tumour affecting the left temporo-sphenoidal lobe' (24 June 1886). Savage hosted a discussion at the Bethlehem (*sic*) Hospital (17 November 1886); and Bastian spoke 'on the muscular sense' (16 December 1886) which, with the ensuing discussion, occupied the whole of the April 1887 issue of *Brain*. At the second annual general meeting for election of office bearers, councillors and new members (27 January 1887), Buzzard presented a case of Thomsen's disease. Clinical cases and pathological specimens were presented at a 'subsequent' clinical meeting (23 February 1887). Finally, in its first year, the Society met again at the physiological laboratory of University College, where Semon discussed the topic of the 'laryngeal cortical centre', and Horsley and Schäfer stimulated a discussion that led to the creation of a subcommittee to consider facts bearing on the localisation of the visual and auditory centres (26 March 1887). It soon became clear that the Neurological Society of London needed a means of publishing its activities and leaving a permanent record of the lectures given at its meetings. In 1887, the Society adopted *Brain* (in which many of the presentations had already been published) as its official journal. In marking this affiliation and rehearsing the history of the Society, de Watteville wrote 'From this sketch of the activity of the Society, during the first period of its existence, the reader will readily perceive how advantageous for *Brain* its more intimate connection with such a Body is sure to prove.'[19]

The rules and list of office bearers and members of the Neurological Society of London, and the annual reports listing growth in membership, communications and meetings held, and the financial balance sheets, were published in *Brain* in 1891, 1894, and annually from 1896 to 1906. In 1897, a 'Hughlings Jackson Lectureship' was established in recognition of 'the discoverer of cortical epilepsy', the first lecture being given by Jackson himself on 8 December 1897.[20] When de Watteville resigned in 1900, Council

recorded its thanks for his stewardship over a 20-year period:

> Parting with Dr de Watteville is an event of great moment to the Society, for he has not only brought *Brain* to a high standard of perfection and secured for it a great European reputation, but even the existence of the Journal at the present time is due to his energetic action at a critical juncture in 1880. Moreover the Council is mindful that the Society itself took origin on Dr de Watteville's initiative, at a meeting held at his house 30 Welbeck Street on 14 November 1885.[21]

Between 1886 and 1900, the Society held only two provincial meetings (both in the physiological laboratory in Cambridge). But, by 1903, of 230 members, 107 were living outside London (England, 73; Scotland, 10; Wales, 5; Ireland, 3; and foreign, 16). As a result, the name was amended to the Neurological Society of the United Kingdom from 4 February 1904. To celebrate this change, the Society agreed to meet in Edinburgh, but only 34 members attended. In a further attempt to encourage more distributed engagement, a meeting accompanied by an 11-course dinner was hosted in 1905 by 37 London members for 47 of their provincial colleagues. Notable was the election to membership of two women in 1905: Helen Stewart and Mary Sturge. The membership had reached 253 by the time the Society was disbanded in 1907 and its activities incorporated into the newly formed Royal Society of Medicine.

The Neurological Section of the Royal Society of Medicine

With the Royal Medical and Chirurgical Society leading the initiative, 14 specialist societies amalgamated to form the Royal Society of Medicine (RSM) in 1907.[22] A special meeting on 6 December 1906

---

[19] See (A. de Watteville) 'Editorial Note', *Brain* **10** (1887–8): 1–4, following p. 576.
[20] Jackson's lecture was entitled 'Remarks on the Relations of Different Divisions of the Central Nervous System to One Another and to Parts of the Body'. On 29 November 1901, the lecture was delivered by Professor Hitzig (Halle) on 'Hughlings Jackson and the Cortical Motor Centres in the Light of Physiological Research'. In 1904, Sir William Broadbent gave the third Hughlings Jackson lecture on 'Hughlings Jackson as Pioneer in Nervous Physiology and Pathology'; and in 1907, Sir Victor Horsley spoke 'On the

Illustration by Recent Research of Dr Hughlings Jackson's Views on the Functions of the Cerebellum'.
[21] See *Rules and List of Office Bearers and Members of the Neurological Society of London 1901* (London: John Bale, sons and Danielsson Ltd, 1901), 20 pages bound in at the end of *Brain* **24** (1901): 672.
[22] The Medical Society of London and the Ophthalmological Society of the United Kingdom chose not to be involved: the former remains an independent and successful society; although an ophthalmological section was formed at the Royal Society of Medicine in 1912, and a Faculty of Ophthalmologists was founded as a professional body in 1946 by Sir Stewart Duke-Elder as an offshoot of the Royal College of Surgeons, these merged in 1988 to

recommended that 'the Neurological Society of the United Kingdom join in the scheme for the amalgamation of Medical Societies', and Henry Head[23] was appointed as delegate to the new committee. There was no opposition from the 256 members, who voted unanimously to disband the Neurological Society of the United Kingdom and join the Royal Society of Medicine. Merger of the specialist societies was strongly supported by influential figures in the medical establishment, such as Sir William Osler, Sir Frederick Treves, Dr Archibald Garrod, Sir William Broadbent and Sir Henry Morris. The *Lancet* welcomed the decision, emphasising the advantages of amalgamating the libraries and the high quality of the proceedings. The *British Medical Journal* noted that 'men are tired of subscribing to so many societies, tired of listless, ill-attended meetings, tired of the old customs, formalities and conventions'.[24] By 1908, there were 2,025 fellows of the new society, including 290 who had not previously belonged to any other organisation. The finances were sound, and a new journal (*Proceedings of the Royal Society of Medicine*) had been formed. In 1912, new premises were acquired at number 1 Wimpole Street and the building completed.

The first meeting of the section of neurology was held in July 1907, with Beevor as president. Subsequent meetings included visits to Queen Square, alternating with Maida Vale Hospital. Charles Sherrington was elected president in 1909. Early lecturers included Gordon Holmes and Robert Foster Kennedy. Important addresses were given by Head, Holmes, Collier, Sargent, Cairns, Golla, Mapother and Jefferson, amongst others. Cushing was an honorary member. For the next 16 years, the Royal Society of Medicine was the only forum for neurological debate in Britain. Many Queen Square physicians have been appointed as president of the section, including in recent years. Although its influence waned after the formation of the Association of British Neurologists (ABN) in 1933, that organisation did not become dominant until the 1960s, when Russell Brain took over the presidency at a time of

crisis for British neurology in relation to manpower and organisation of services. In 1997, the section was renamed 'clinical neurosciences' in order to incorporate all the relevant disciplines, but it has never regained the political role that was assumed in the early years and functions mainly as a club hosting educational meetings.

The Association of British Neurologists (ABN)

On 28 July 1932, Holmes held a meeting at 9 Wimpole St, London W1, to discuss the formation of another society dedicated to neurology.[25] As a result, many individuals defected from the section of neurology at the Royal Society of Medicine in 1933 and joined the newly formed Association of British Neurologists.[26] There were several reasons for this fracture. It promised resolution of the debate over specialism in neurology, which had struggled to gain acceptance for many years and was, for a while, suppressed by establishment of the Royal Society of Medicine. It recognised the need to emancipate neurology outside London. It expressed frustration over lack of ambition in activities of the Royal Society of Medicine, and loss of patience with the social and professional atmosphere of the neurological section. And it made clear that meetings dominated by clinical case presentations did not satisfy the appetite of the scientifically minded neurologist at a time when other disciplines were starting to inform the study of mechanisms in neurological disease. Nevertheless, initially, most physicians with an interest in neurology were members of both societies, and for several decades the RSM section did retain a dominant influence – for instance hosting, in 1935, both the Hughlings Jackson centenary and the International Neurological Congress.

---

form the College of Ophthalmologists, which received its Royal Charter in 1993.

[23] Head had been elected to membership of the Neurological Society of the United Kingdom in 1891, served on Council in 1900, and was secretary from 1901 to 1904.

[24] See Anon., 'Union of Medical Societies in London', *British Medical Journal* **1** (4 March 1905): 490–1.

[25] This was attended by William Adie, Edwin Bramwell, Henry Cohen, James Collier, Donald Core, Anthony Feiling, Ronald Gordon, Godwin Greenfield, George Hall, Wilfrid Harris, William Johnson, Frederick Nattrass, Kinnier Wilson and Cecil Worster-Drought.

[26] For a brief history of the Association of British Neurologists, see P. K. Robinson, *The Association of British Neurologists: 1933–1983* (Privately printed, 1985). A fuller account is provided by S. T. Casper, *The Neurologists: A History of a Medical Specialty in Modern Britain c. 1789–2000* (Manchester University Press, 2014). This is based in part on his PhD thesis, 'The Idioms of Practice: British Neurology, 1880–1960' (2006).

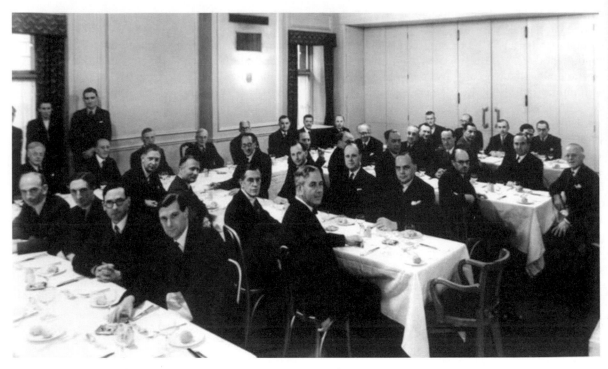

Figure 8.1 Association of British Neurologists at dinner in 1948 (courtesy of ABN).

The founding officers of the Association of British Neurologists were Harris (president), Kinnier Wilson (treasurer) and Holmes (secretary). When the council met in December 1932, there were 51 founding members comprising 'those actively engaged in any branch of neurology', and not necessarily involved in clinical practice. Macdonald Critchley described it as 'a select neurological club ... restricted to full-blown consultants', and, in the event, almost all of the early members were physicians with an interest in neurology. At first, the meetings were held annually. In the early years, the proceedings were not published but, in time, the *Journal of Neurology, Neurosurgery, and Psychiatry* printed the abstracts and, *de facto*, represented the Association. As intended, the meetings were more scientific and research-oriented than those of the section at the Royal Society of Medicine.[27] From 1937, joint meetings with foreign societies were held, and overseas members admitted. There were only three female members of the

Association, often in attendance in the 1930s: Dorothy Russell, Helen Dimsdale and Miss G. Griffiths. Towards the end of the Second World War, the Association aspired to a more political role and recognition as the voice of neurology, although even by the mid-1960s there were still only 125 'ordinary' members. The Association became increasingly interested in training and manpower and took over those dialogues with government from the Neurology Committee of the Royal College of Physicians. Biannual scientific meetings were introduced in 1950, usually with one held in London and the other elsewhere. The atmosphere was not always relaxed, performance being valued as much as the content of presentations. Many who attended meetings as late as the 1970s recall the authoritarian style maintained by senior members of the ABN, and some of the caustic comments made in discussion of papers directed at colleagues or trainees.

Thus, not for the first time, the more enlightened staff of the National Hospital had exercised their leadership role by correctly sensing that neurology must offer more than clinical description, and that the subject had to develop a scientific basis

---

[27] Papers attracting most interest were on physiology from E. D. Adrian and Thomas Graham Brown; those who spoke most often as presenters or in discussion were Holmes, Symonds, Kinnier Wilson, Ritchie Russell, Cloake, Riddoch, Adrian, Greenfield and Carmichael.

building upon the physiological doctrines of the past and engaging with emerging disciplines. However, there was something of an impasse. Although the staff at Queen Square were not the ones to deliver the scientific transition, there was almost no infrastructure elsewhere ready to take on the mantle. Therefore, the situation arose in which the National Hospital dominated leadership of the ABN in the first two decades of its existence, but, paradoxically, held back full realisation of the ethos that it had spawned by breaking away from the Royal Society of Medicine. This combination of vision inhibited by resistance to change resulted in stagnation of neurology as a recognised specialty and, crucially, in early application of postwar scientific medicine. So entrenched were the attitudes that, by the early 1960s, the universities and British neurology were losing patience with Queen Square and making their own plans for modernisation. Whilst this analysis may seem harsh and lacking generosity with respect to excellent doctors and basic scientists, many relegated to basement premises and corridors at the National Hospital, it is undoubtedly the case that a number of figures who might have provided Queen Square with a new and national role in the science of neurology during the period before 1960, chose to function elsewhere. Several people from whom Queen Square might have benefitted in the first half of the twentieth century included Sherrington and Adrian in neurophysiology, and Head, Brain, Miller, Ritchie Russell and Walton in clinical neurology. Denny-Brown, Cairns and Jefferson had a look but were lured away elsewhere. That said, much talent was available at Queen Square, and yet, in the case of Carmichael, Greenfield and others, it remained held in check by the dominance of the clinical neurologists with Walshe as their spokesman, for whom maintaining the reputation of the National Hospital as the only place where diseases of the nervous system were properly understood and could be managed was the mantra. But, in this, they were doomed to fail as the steady take-over by the National Health Service, the emergence of the ABN and regional centres for the clinical neurosciences, and the final emergence of neurology as a specialty were crowned by forces greater than the Canute-like stance of some physicians at Queen Square.

The Neurology Committee of the Royal College of Physicians and the ABN: Medical Manpower and Training

After the Second World War, doctors showed a new willingness to engage in national planning, a change of mind which was influenced by the establishment of state-run medicine in the form of the NHS, but also by Riddoch's success in setting up the special neurosurgical centres and Emergency Medical Services in London. This had shown, at least for one specialty, what could be achieved by central planning and engagement with the Ministry.

It was partly in this spirit that a Committee on Neurology was established by the Royal College of Physicians. This proved a watershed for British neurology, and the committee published a series of reports over the next 30 years that were to prove especially influential.[28] In the later years, particularly after 1980, its lobbying role in this regard was superseded by the work of the services subcommittee of the Association of British Neurologists (ABN). The second half of the twentieth century proved to be a time when central 'manpower planning', directed by the state, became an important issue for many medical specialities in Britain and much time and effort was devoted by the ABN and College committees to this topic. The role of the National Hospital within the developing framework of British neurology was a recurring topic for discussion during these meetings.

The 1945 College Committee was constituted to consider the training of specialists in neurology, the 'conditions of recognition as a consultant or specialist in neurology', and the relationships of neurology to general medicine and psychological medicine. It was one of 15 such committees (five representing specialties) at the College. The staff of Queen Square dominated the membership, ensuring that the hospital could protect its own interests at a time when the political imperative was to increase the provision of neurological services in the regions and redress the imbalance of metropolitan and regional services. Of the 14 members in 1945, ten were consultants at the National Hospital or Maida Vale, and others had former connections with Queen Square.[29]

---

[28] See Royal College of Physicians, 'Report of the Committee on Neurology', July 1945, April 1954 and January 1970; 'The Neurology Services in Great Britain', 1965; 'The Neurology Facilities in the United Kingdom', November 1986.

[29] Queen Square and Maida Vale members were: Elkington (secretary), Critchley, Symonds, Riddoch, Greenfield,

The recommendations of the 1945 report show how much more systematised neurological training had now become, and they also reflected the elevated status of the specialty. The situation was summarised by the editor of the *British Medical Journal*:

> 18 months' whole-time study of general medicine after registration; the MRCP Lond., or its accepted equivalent; six months in the whole-time study of pathology, physiology, and anatomy of the nervous system, together with normal psychology; a year's devotion to psychiatry (including six months' hospital residence); and 18 months' study of clinical neurology (including a year's hospital residence). This means that the neurologist will be around 27 or 28 years of age before he leaves the embryo stage. At the end of that time he is advised to embark upon a period of foreign travel or of research. A hard apprenticeship indeed, but one that is necessary if the prestige of consulting neurology is to be maintained in international medicine. No discipline has yet suffered from the austerities of its regime, and the best types of anchorite will not be deterred by exacting conditions of entry or pupillage.[30]

In fact, the report recommended not just 'a year's hospital residence' as part of the neurology training, but one year spent as a resident medical officer in a 'neurological hospital'. This stipulation ensured the central positions in training, as the only specialist neurological hospitals at the time, of the National Hospital and Maida Vale.[31] The 1945 report did not

support the creation of a special diploma nor the idea of a 'statutory register' of neurologists. The committee also failed to address the relationship of neurology to neurosurgery, an omission which led to the spat between Walshe and Jefferson.

Although the main function of the 1945 committee had been to make recommendations on training, what again dominated discussion was the extent to which neurology should be a 'specialism' and the position of neurology *vis-à-vis* general medicine and psychiatry. Although neurology had been one of the first of the medical specialties to claim status of its own, the committee articulated the arguments for and against concisely and elegantly, and the debate provided a snapshot of Queen Square thinking at the time on this important issue. As the report stated:

> The consideration of the future of neurology quickly brings the enquirer face to face with a problem which is common to all specialists and which is one of the most important and debatable matters that confront the profession at the present time. This is the question of how far specialisation can proceed without detriment to the specialty itself and to the larger subject of which it is a part.

It noted that specialisation is the 'natural and inevitable result of growth of knowledge' because no one can keep pace with the literature and progress of all branches of medicine, but also acknowledged that intensive study leads to important advances. Nevertheless:

> An exclusive preoccupation with one branch of medicine, especially if this is undertaken too early in a practitioner's career, inevitably leads to deficient knowledge of the subject [medicine] as a whole. This in turn promotes an unbalanced outlook and tends to lead to an artificial division of the subject into a number of watertight compartments, a separation, which though convenient from the administrative point of view, is not in the best interests of the patient ... It is also true that many advances are brought about by the application of knowledge from one branch of medicine transferred to another ... too rigid a restriction of a worker's activities to a limited field endangers the growth of individual

---

Brinton, Feiling, Meadows, Nevin and Brain. The chairman was Stanley Barnes, a retired dean of the medical school in Birmingham and president of the ABN, and a neurologist who had trained at Queen Square. Other members were Aubrey Lewis, a psychiatrist, council member and president of the ABN; Professor Philip Coake, a neurologist and professor of medicine in Birmingham, who had trained for a period at Maida Vale; and Professor R. V. Christie, who was not a neurologist but an academic involved with the MRC, and also College lead on postgraduate education. Riddoch, Symonds and Brain were also members of the Specialty Committee in Psychiatry.

[30] Anon., 'Neurological Training', *British Medical Journal* 2 (1945): 292. This editorial puts the Queen Square view of neurology perfectly, and one presumes that it was written by a Queen Square neurologist, probably Walshe or Critchley.

[31] The committee felt that a period of 18 months in the neurological hospital was ideal, but recognised this was not practical given the small number of posts, and so extended the training to teaching hospitals, specifying that 'it may even be found necessary during an interim period to reduce the

period of residence in a neurological hospital to six months, but we hold strongly the view that a year of such residence is the minimum period upon which a satisfactory neurological training can be based, and that this should be insisted upon as soon as the necessary facilities can be made available'.

initiative which is such an important quality in any-one who hopes to advance knowledge in his subject.

The problem of how far to go down the road of specialisation formed 'a constant background to the Committee's discussions', as did the amount of general medical training needed before specialisation. It was felt that the recommendations made by the committee should do nothing that might isolate neurology from general medicine, should take account of widely differing degrees to which medicine had evolved in different parts of the country, and give full scope to the varying interests and potential of individual workers. Neurology, it was argued, should not be separated, and it was essential 'that the neurologist should base his specialised knowledge on a foundation of sound training and experience in general medicine'. In relation to psychiatry – remarkably, when one recalls Walshe's near-contemporaneous vitriolic attack – the committee considered the relationship with neurology to be so intimate that drawing a line between the two was not possible. Thus, both psychiatry and general medicine featured prominently in the proposed training of neurologists. However, exposure to neurosurgery, a topic that was to induce much subsequent debate, was ignored.

The 1945 report was also the first of a series that addressed the issue of 'manpower planning' and how many experts in neurology were needed in the country as a whole. At the time, there were only 60 practising neurologists, all based in large centres of population and dominated by London, compared with a total of 25 (19 in London) in 1939. The report commented that 'it is certain that there will need to be a considerable increase in the total number of neurologists and a more even distribution of them throughout the country'. It was recommended, as a first aim, that all medical teaching centres should establish a department of neurology, with a minimum of two neurologists supported by junior staff, and adopting the hub-and-spoke structure of servicing clinics in district hospitals. Rather quaintly to the modern reader, the committee concluded, in relation to neurological posts, that all neurologists 'need a degree of leisure which is an indispensable requirement of any one who is to lead satisfactorily the life of a consultant and teach in any branch of medicine'.

The insufficient number of fully trained staff able to deal with diseases of the nervous system in all hospitals, especially in thinly populated areas, was also acknowledged. In these settings, the committee

recognised that a physician with an interest in neurology, whose practice combined neurology and general medicine, but who was not a fully fledged neurologist, was a viable alternative. This issue was another that was to resurface repeatedly in future years.

It was the example of the Emergency Medical Service (EMS), deemed to have worked well, that inspired the hub-and-spoke model recommended by the committee. The central hub would be the regional neurological centre based in a teaching or large urban hospital, from which consultant staff would visit district general hospitals and repatriate cases to the centre for specialist investigation and further care. Russell Brain argued that the example of the EMS had shown how neurology could be organised on a regional basis despite responsibility devolving to more than one municipal authority:

> A specialist service has become available to many patients who would otherwise have been admitted to hospitals where they would not normally be seen by a neurologist. Such a system as this could readily form the basis of a post-war organisation ... with perhaps ten or twelve sectors of the emergency medical services type [being] needed for a neurological medical service ... it would probably be impossible to have as many neurosurgical units and arrangements would have to be made whereby two or more sectors would be served by a single neurosurgical unit.[32]

The contemporary views of the Queen Square physicians concerning the qualities of a neurologist, and on 'manpower planning' at the National Hospital, were well illustrated by the memorandum sent from Gooddy to the Board of Management, and the letter from Walshe and Symonds. But, despite the over-representation from Queen Square, the tone of elitism and London-centricity was partly suppressed in the College Committee's 1945 report.

The next document was published in 1954, now with Russell Brain, who was by then also president of the College, as chairman of the committee. Opinion on specialism and 'neurology with an interest' had changed. The report made a much more definitive statement about what constitutes a neurologist and who should oversee neurological care. After almost 100 years, specialism in neurology had finally arrived: 'A neurologist is a trained physician ... who has received the necessary special training and experience in neurology, and proposes thereafter to devote himself to

32 Cited by S. Casper, *The Neurologists* (2014), pp. 136–7.

297

that specialty. This definition does not include those general physicians … who include an interest in neurology as part of their practice.'[33]

The problem was that, despite the general expansion in consultant numbers that followed the introduction of the National Health Service, the manpower situation in neurology was no better than in 1945. At the time, there were around 50 to 60 neurologists working in England, providing 1 neurologist for every 400,000 persons in metropolitan areas, and 1 per 1.2 million elsewhere, and with large areas lacking any specialist cover. The 1954 report condemned this failure of expansion, and again recommended a significant increase and more even distribution around the country. Its refusal to solve the problem by acceding to the further appointment of 'physicians with an interest' was a departure from existing dogma. The College Committee emphatically stated that the time when a general physician with an interest in neurology could provide a neurological service was past. The failure to develop the specialty was put down to low priority afforded by administrators for increasing manpower at times of financial stringency, and the dogged stance of some senior physicians who remained of the view that neurology could be performed adequately by general physicians. The committee decried this attitude and pointed out that trainees took up neurology on the very reasonable assumption that more consultant posts in neurology were needed and would become available.[34] The committee explained that it

> desires to draw attention to the serious long-term effects of the policy at present adopted in the Health Service in relation to neurology. After the war, relying on the promised expansion of the consultant services and being aware of the need for more consultant neurologists, a considerable number of ex-service graduates undertook and completed their

training as neurologists. Of these, only 15 per cent have been able to find reasonable employment … in this country. At least five have emigrated. Promising graduates now regard the prospects as so discouraging that they are becoming increasingly reluctant to enter a branch of medicine in which this country is pre-eminent.

The prejudice against neurology, not least based on its reputation for arrogance and elitism, and the resistance to its specialisation, was still strong amongst many other physicians, and the College Comitia (remarkably, since it was chaired by Lord Brain) distanced itself from the conclusions of the College Committee, which it considered 'exaggerated'. A member of Council commented:

> If they looked at the work done by the present neurologist, they would find that his time was completely taken up with a very long waiting list in outpatients, with chronic epileptics and similar cases, most of whom he cannot help at all … many physicians would not welcome neurologists. They would rather have another general physician with a special interest in neurology.[35]

A similar view was also expressed by some influential neurologists, and Henry Miller, for instance, strongly believed that the general physician with an interest was the only reasonable solution to the undersupply. Not surprisingly, the ABN strongly supported the conclusions of the 1954 report and formed a subcommittee to consider the status of neurology in the National Health Service, and to advise on action to be taken. Notwithstanding the Comitia's lack of support, by 1955 the Joint Consultants Committee sided with the ABN and the Neurology Committee and recommended to the Minister of Health that he should have a consultant adviser in neurology to assist with the expansion of the specialty. This was accepted and Russell Brain was appointed in 1958. He was followed by a succession of neurologists working with the Chief Medical Officers of the Department of Health until 2001, when the posts were abolished by Sir Liam Donaldson, who felt that he could always ask for advice should that be necessary.[36]

Denis Brinton, in his 1959 president's address to the section of neurology of the Royal Society of

---

[33] See Royal College of Physicians, Committee on Neurology, 'Interim Report', 1954; Committee on Neurology, 'Document 11. Discussion of the interim report of the Committee on Neurology by the Council', April 1954, 1–7, 13C; and minutes of the Committee of Neurology, Vol. I (1944–66).

[34] There were 41 neurologists in London, covering a population of 15,732,700, and 18 neurologists in the rest of the country, covering a population of 29,357,300. This compared with the number of consultant general physicians (668), psychiatrists (515) and total number of consultants in England (6,384). Furthermore, there were only 14 senior registrar posts in neurology, out of a total of 1,068.

[35] Cited in S. Casper, *The Neurologists* (2014), p. 145.

[36] Subsequently, but in different guises and reporting to different individuals or bodies, specialist advice to government has been reinstated.

Medicine, recorded that, although the number of neurologists in the United Kingdom had increased by more than 250 per cent between 1939 and 1959, the establishment was still too small, and the inadequate provision of neurological services in the country remained a vexed subject. Outside London, many neurologists were single-handed and responsible for clinics that were widely separated geographically, some with no connection to a teaching centre, without access to neurosurgery and inadequately supplied with junior medical assistants. Most consultants were appointed on a maximum part-time contract and worked at capacity. Brinton was particularly critical of the care of the 'epileptic' and the 'neurological chronic sick', whom he said were 'left to rot, physically and spiritually'. However, despite this depressing picture nationally, as one of its senior physicians, Brinton defended the National Hospital:

> Current criticism [is] that British neurology in general and the National Hospital (Institute of Neurology) in particular are tending to drift away from general medicine. Some physicians have even given their opinion that the day of the special hospital is ended ... As a place of reference for the difficult clinical problem, as a school for part of the training of doctors who have an interest in neurology, as an institute of research, and as a national or even an international headquarters for all neurologists, there cannot be any substitute for the special hospital ... With the increasing complexity of the medical sciences, it is inconceivable that any of these functions could be efficiently discharged by general physicians or by scattered neurologists, each with his own small department in a general teaching hospital. Nearly all the part-time consultants at the National Hospital also work in the general hospitals of the undergraduate medical schools of the University of London. Not one of the staff of the Institute need be out of touch with general medicine.[37]

Brinton also concluded that physicians with a special interest in neurology 'are unquestionably useful in a few parts of the periphery of England and Wales in covering the present serious shortage of neurologists'.

The next important contribution to this debate was the report of a Joint Working Party of the Department of Health on the topic of medical staffing structures in hospital, chaired by Sir Robert Platt, president of the Royal College of Physicians, and published in 1961. It was written partly in response to the problem of the 'time-expired' senior registrar, whose plight the 1954 College report had raised.[38] The report recommended that there should be 2.2 consultant neurologist sessions per 100,000 of the population, and expansion by four posts per annum, in addition to replacements arising from retirement and death. The role of specialisation was also the subject of an excellent editorial by the chief medical officer at the Department of Health, Sir George Godber, in 1961:

> It is not uncommon to hear comment upon the increasingly rapid scientific developments in medicine during the last two decades. This is often accompanied by reference to the increasing extent of specialisation within medicine, sometimes with laments about the slow progress in some special fields. But often one hears criticism of the narrowness of specialisation which leads to the patient being regarded less as a person than as a vehicle for a disease.[39]

Godber pointed to the very large increase in consultant numbers since the inception of the National Health Service and mentioned that the Royal College of Physicians' recommendations on regional centres for neurology and cardiology had met with considerable resistance 'in many places' concerned about 'surrender of some or even part of this work to a special department'. He also noted that there were new specialisms and techniques, singling out electroencephalography:

> which began to be used generally in neurology, neurosurgery, and psychiatry only after the war, and its

---

[37] D. H. Brinton, 'President's Address: The Development of Neurological Services under the NHS', *Proceedings of the Royal Society of Medicine* **53** (1960): 261–3.

[38] Ministry of Health, Department of Health for Scotland, *Medical Staffing Structure in the Hospital Service: Report of the Joint Working Party* (London: Her Majesty's Stationery Office, 1961). There were more senior registrars than consultant posts becoming available, and the career prospects for outstanding young neurologists in Britain were bleak. Then, and over the next 20 years, trainees had little choice but to take a consultant post as it arose, wherever situated and whatever the facilities. Queen Square lost the opportunity of recruiting a number of talented young doctors in this period, amongst whom were Louis Hurwitz (who went to Belfast), Michael Espir (to Leicester) and Fritz Dreifuss and Oliver Sacks (who both emigrated to North America).

[39] G. Godber, 'Trends in Specialisation and their Effect on the Practice of Medicine', *British Medical Journal* **2** (1961): 5256–8.

future has not yet become firmly established. Yet there is a clear trend toward concentration of this work in a few hands, and a breed of neuro-electro-physiologist (if that is an admissible term) is emerging in main centres and the need to provide a regional consultative service rather than more machines is now recognized.

More generally, he debated the thorny issue of specialism, arguing that separation from general medicine was in the interests of people with disease of the brain and spinal cord.

In some regions, even their exclusion from particular major hospitals, prevents the development of the attainable level of clinical service. I do not suggest that we are likely to see such elaborate specialization as the emergence of a specialty I have seen identified in New York as 'vestibulotomist' – the man who does fenestration for otosclerosis – but rather that the increases in specialists should be proportionately greater in them than in the main older specialties … If, then, we are facing a progressive increase in specialization, how are we to avoid the division of the care of the patient and the failure of communication of knowledge between the specialists and the rest of medicine? How are we to balance the need to include the stimulus of new specialties in the work of teaching hospitals and at the same time preserve sufficient work on the medical problems of every day to give all-round experience to the student? These are the great dilemmas of medicine as I see them.

As chief medical officer having the ear of the Minister, Godber's view was important and, in the decades that followed, there was a steady increase in specialist numbers. The Neurology Committee of the Royal College reported again in 1965. It recommended, as had the previous reports, that neurologists should be based in regional centres as part of large district general or teaching hospitals and linked in a hub-and-spoke pattern to other local hospitals. It also recommended that neurologists should not work in isolation, the neurological unit having full facilities for neurosurgery, neuroradiology, neuropathology and all ancillary services. The report also noted that there were still only 90 neurologists employed in the National Health Service, with wide regional variations. Again, the view was expressed that the concept of the 'physician with an interest' was 'outmoded', and the 'demands of the subject precluded such a spurious solution to the problems of neurological staffing'. For the first time, this report also emphasised the importance of research, noting

that there were by then three professorial departments of neurology (Queen Square, Glasgow and Newcastle) and making the case for appointing more neurologists to academic posts.

Contrast between neurology and neurosurgery was also made. In 1965, 0.8 per cent of all consultants were neurosurgeons, compared to 1.1 per cent who were neurologists, and there had been a 100 per cent increase in the number of consultant neurosurgeons appointed over the previous 15-year period.[40]

These reports moved along the debates on manpower and the organisation of neurology in the country. Once again, the number of neurologists needed to provide an adequate service became a pressing issue. In its next report, in 1965, the College Committee on Neurology reiterated that the general physician with an interest was now 'an outmoded concept' (Henry Miller disagreeing).[41] But even when doctors were appointed as specialists in neurology without commitment to general medicine, their numbers remained small until the 1990s, resistance to change perpetuated to some extent by the rigid hegemony of Queen Square on training and being granted the perceived 'licence' to be regarded as competent. One factor was the perception that more and larger regional centres posed a potential threat to the privileged position of the National Hospital. Questions about the role and position of a mono-specialty hospital were repeated. It was an uncomfortable period in which the National Hospital again had to justify its existence, and counter feelings of resentment.

A number of leading neurologists weighed in on the argument. Miller,[42] for instance, felt that in the smaller district hospitals, the general physician with a neurological interest could provide an adequate

[40] P. Harris, *Proceedings of the Royal Society of Medicine* **61** (1968): 1001–4.

[41] Royal College of Physicians, Committee on Neurology, *The Neurology Services in Great Britain* (London: RCP, 1965); Royal College of Physicians of London, *Report on Neurological Manpower* (London: RCP, 1970). Its subsequent report in 1986 also considered that the only solution to the lack of neurological services was the expansion in the neurological consultant establishment, backing the ABN's work on this topic: see Royal College of Physicians, 'Neurological Facilities in the United Kingdom'. Prepared by the College Committee on Neurology, London, November 1986.

[42] H. Miller, 'The Organisation of Neurological Services and Neurological Training', *Proceedings of the Royal Society of Medicine* **61** (1968): 1004–10.

neurological service, and indeed one that might be better than deploying a fully trained neurologist because of the wider perspective and experience, given that the main function of the visiting neurologist was merely to select patients for transfer to the regional centre. As for the 'special hospitals' (his target was Queen Square), Miller noted that the ABN's plea to the Todd Committee to retain this facility was not surprising given the Association's 'composition and history' and that

> in fact of course, the special hospitals are an expensive anachronism, exemplifying a familiar and deplorable national reluctance to adapt its institutions to changing conditions ... no hospital of 200 beds can be economic ... we are the only country in the world that clings to the concept of the special hospital ... the modest claim that the special hospital is essential as a centre of excellence is entirely affirmative and inherently improbable.

Luckily for Queen Square, the onslaught from figures such as Henry Miller failed to make much impression in the London corridors of power.

Denis Williams had been appointed as consultant adviser in neurology to the Department of Health and, in 1968, published a further report entitled 'A Survey of the Neurological Needs of the United Kingdom', in which he pointed out that neurology was lagging behind 'because neurological physicians tend to have less political drive and administrative zeal than those in more obviously utilitarian vocations, so that their voice is not heard ... many of them would say that they are so overworked that they have little chance of making it heard'.

Williams had arranged a meeting at the National Hospital in February 1968, to which all consultants in neurology were invited. 'Over 90% accepted' and the outcome was the decision to conduct in-depth interviews in each of 11 random sectors within the United Kingdom. These inquiries formed the basis for a further report submitted to the Minister and published on behalf of the Neurology Committee of the College of Physicians in January 1970.[43] That report painted a devastating picture of inadequate neurology services. Expansion since 1961 had occurred at a rate of only 4.4 per annum (almost all arising from retirements at a rate of 4 per annum) not the proposed 8 each year recommended by Platt. There were by then

112 neurologists in Great Britain, providing 1.7 clinical sessions per 100,000 of the population but with grossly uneven distribution, leaving wide areas of the country with no provision of neurological services. Reaching the requisite 2.2 consultant sessions per 100,000 would require the appointment of 33 new full-time-equivalent posts. The position on the old question of the 'physician with an interest' was now unambiguous: 'We advise most strongly that the appointment to these centres of physicians with an interest is a relic of 19th-century medicine and is in all respects retrogressive. Neurology is far too difficult a subject to be practised by any other than highly trained and carefully selected specialists.'

Williams' recommendations and the College's efforts in support, together with increasing prominence given to documents produced by the ABN, were gaining traction. By the mid-1980s, the number of consultant neurologists had increased to 190, with an overall ratio of 1 full-time-equivalent per 373,000 of the population. However, 55 per cent worked in the Thames Region (representing 1 full-time-equivalent neurologist per 250,000). Still, the issue of the 'physician with an interest' would not go away until, at the June 1982 meeting, the Neurology Committee of the College 'agreed to reject the concept absolutely'. Supporting the case with such issues as safety for driving, services for stroke, number of beds and junior staff conditions, the 1986 College report, now with Christopher Earl as chairman, again pressed for an urgent expansion in the consultant establishment and reiterated that chronic under-staffing could not be solved by appointing general physicians.

The College Committee had proved very influential in consolidating the concept of the consultant neurologist distinct from general medicine and in lobbying for expansion of manpower. The National Hospital was well represented on the membership of the Committee from its inception, and the chairman was more often than not based at Queen Square. In this way, its influence was protected despite the rapid expansion of neurology elsewhere in the United Kingdom. In the 1970s, the ABN began to lobby in an active and politically effective manner and became the main advocate for neurology. The Association established a services subcommittee in 1984 to advise on all matters relating to standards, staffing, organisation and distribution of neurological services in Britain, and manpower became a predominant issue. Surveys were carried out and, in 1990, the ABN

---

[43] The 1970 Committee was chaired by Denis Williams and, of its 13 professional members, five were from Queen Square or Maida Vale: Williams, Earl, Kelly, Bull and Marshall.

published an influential report pointing out severe deficits in neurological services and issuing a policy statement recommending 1 full-time neurologist for every 200,000 people.[44] Two independent papers were published by Richard Langton Hewer and Victorine Wood, from Bristol, summarising the findings on which the ABN survey was based.[45] They noted that there were 152 whole-time-equivalent neurologists practising in the United Kingdom, whereas 284 posts would be needed to meet the 1 in 200,000 target. Significantly, in not one of these various reports was there any extended mention of Queen Square or the role of the special hospitals. Whether this was because the place of Queen Square was considered secure, or its interests were being suppressed by the emerging voice of provincial neurology, is not clear, but it was obvious to all that the National Hospital was, once again, in an anomalous position and on the back-foot. Langton Hewer and Wood paid lip-service to

> The role of the National Hospitals for Nervous Diseases (in Maida Vale and Queen Square) [which] has changed over the last 40 years as a result of the establishment of regional centres and district services. However, the hospitals have continued to provide a valuable secondary and tertiary referral service for much of the United Kingdom. The National Hospitals also provide a unique teaching service for neurologists who will in the future work elsewhere in the United Kingdom and abroad. In addition, the National Hospitals, together with the Institute of Neurology, are a major focus for neurological research.

It seems that, even in an age of numbers and statistics, the basic message was that Queen Square still had a national role for quality: and the staff must have breathed a heavy sigh of relief that the new brooms were not seeking to sweep them totally aside.

In 1995, there were 250 consultant neurologists in the United Kingdom, a population ratio of 1 per 233,600, still many fewer than in most other countries. At this stage, the ABN upped its ideal target to 1 per 100,000, justifying this change with a number of revised assumptions. The number of junior staff committed to neurology had increased to 158 and the ABN concluded that two extra trainees should be appointed each year in order to reach the desired number of consultants by 2008.

Given the national shortage, Queen Square had conspicuously more neurologists than elsewhere, leaving the National Hospital again vulnerable to threats of redistribution. In the event, further specialisation within neurology was to some extent its salvation, as it was through its subspecialty clinics that the National Hospital differentiated itself and offered a unique service. This further partitioning of neurology did not feature in any of the College reports and took much longer to develop than in Europe or the USA. Apart from epilepsy, for which special clinics had been established by the end of the nineteenth century, key opinion leaders remained opposed to such fragmentation of neurology. In the 1960s, Roger Gilliatt had refused to allow the establishment of special clinics at Queen Square and these only flourished with the appointment of David Marsden in 1987.[46] In the event, the rise of subspecialisation within neurology, promoted by a marked shift in public perception that patients with less common conditions deserved the best possible care, came to the rescue, and allowed the National Hospital to finesse the situation and remain ahead of the game.

The Growth of Neurology Outside Queen Square

In the years between 1945 and 1995, one can see that the National Hospital faced threats to its very existence as external forces started to loosen its stranglehold on the practice and organisation of neurology, and this topic is taken further in Chapter 13. What was surely crucial was that the hospital maintained flexibility and responded to changing currents of opinion, as exemplified by the

---

[44] Association of British Neurologists, *A Policy Statement on the Number and Distribution of Consultants in Adult Neurology* (1990).

[45] See R. Langton Hewer and V. A. Wood, 'Neurology in the United Kingdom. I: Historical Development; II: A Study of Current Neurological Services for Adults', *Journal of Neurology, Neurosurgery, and Psychiatry* 55 (supp.) (1992): 2–7, 8–14. Langton Hewer had served as a house physician at Queen Square from 1958 to 1960 but had no other connection with the hospital, and was not widely perceived as a supporter.

[46] Opinion has oscillated between and away from the extremes of complete specialisation in centres versus decentralisation of neurology to district level. However, specialisation, supported by extravagant claims for the number of neurologists needed to serve a population, has proved inflationary; and general medicine is now chronically under-staffed.

move to subspecialisation. Nevertheless, its perceived role throughout this period, and today, remains essentially unchallenged – to provide a tertiary service for other neurologists (a court of last appeal), to deliver postgraduate teaching, and to remain at the cutting edge of research and development. The hospital's performance was judged on these criteria. How much of a local service the hospital should provide, and how differentiated it should be from regional neurological centres, seemed of less importance, at least until the 1990s when these issues became much more explicit, and again making the provision of subspecialist clinics a priority.

Elsewhere, neurology was on the move. Both World Wars had underlined the role of neurosurgery, and the inception of the National Health Service had revealed the need for regional centres where neurosurgery was supported by clinical neurology and related disciplines. The period after 1948 saw the development of regional centres that took trade away from Queen Square. Many were associated with universities and, in time, they also had aspirations to develop academic departments. In turn, trainees felt comfortable and adequately educated without necessarily enduring the rite of passage through Queen Square, previously essential for any aspiring neurologist. What follows is a brief survey of how neurology existed and eventually flourished outside Queen Square over the 100 years after the founding of the National Hospital in 1859.[47] This reveals a story of painfully slow and uneven growth. This pattern remained essentially unchanged, with increases in workforce kept under tight central control until the 1990s, when a more rapid expansion of consultant appointments was seen throughout the United Kingdom, which could not be met by maturation of a cohort of trainees nicely polished at Queen Square.

Neurology in Britain Prior to the First World War

Before the First World War, there were a few London physicians not working at Queen Square who nevertheless considered themselves to be experts in diseases of the nervous system. Most, but not all, had passed through the National Hospital. These Victorian and Edwardian neurologists included Julius Althaus at King's College Hospital; Wilfrid Harris, who started the first neurology department at a London teaching hospital, St Mary's; Herbert Campbell Thompson at the Middlesex Hospital; Sir Frederick Mott and Robert Smith at Charing Cross Hospital; Cecil Worster-Drought at the West End Hospital; Sir Arthur Hurst and Sir Maurice Craig at Guy's Hospital; Leonard Guthrie at the Great Northern Central Hospital and Paddington Green Children's Hospital; John Bristowe, Sir Seymour Sharkey, Sir Thomas Barlow and Horace Turney at St Thomas' Hospital; Frederick Golla at the Maudsley Hospital (and later the Burden Institute in Bristol); and Sir James Purves-Stewart at the Westminster Hospital.

Outside London, there was activity that could be described as neurology, although this was firmly embedded in general medicine. Three cities were dominant: Edinburgh, Manchester and Newcastle. As one of the leading medical schools in Europe, it was inevitable that Edinburgh should have been home to distinguished physicians who were interested in the nervous system. Those active before the National Hospital was founded included Alexander Monros (Primus, Secundus and Tertius), Robert Whytt, Sir Charles Bell and Douglas Argyll Robertson. Between 1861 and 1876, Thomas Grainger Stewart (father of the Queen Square physician of the same name) progressed steadily from lecturer and consultant in pathology and medicine to professor of physic at the Royal Infirmary of Edinburgh. He introduced the examination of tendon reflexes into routine medical practice in the United Kingdom, and used electrical excitability to study function in the limbs. Described as one of the most brilliant lecturers in the University of Edinburgh, *A Practical Treatise on Bright's Disease of the Kidneys* (1868) was well received, but Grainger Stewart's most influential books were *The Teaching of Medicine in Edinburgh* (1877) and *An Introduction to Disease of the Nervous System* (1884).[48]

Another figure of significance was Thomas Laycock, professor of medicine at Edinburgh after

[47] The account is based on our own knowledge and scrutiny of various sources, conversations with others active in neurology over the last 50 years, and information available to the Royal College of Physicians; we recognise that it is certainly incomplete, but does at least provide a framework for understanding the story of British neurology in this period.

[48] Attendance grew steadily at his lectures in the Extra-Academical School in Edinburgh. The two manuscript notebooks in which Grainger Stewart drafted these 141 lectures cover 594 pages. Lecture 98 includes a section on 'Paralysis and other conditions due to disease of nerve endings or

working at the York Infirmary, where he wrote *A Treatise on Nervous Diseases of Women* (1840). Laycock had studied with Charles Bell and Marshall Hall. Sir Byrom Bramwell spoke in 1922 to the Royal Medical Society on his own education in Edinburgh. He had special praise for Laycock as an original thinker and intellect, whose theory of the division of the brain into the basilar corresponding to animal life, the middle to sensorial life, and the higher to the intellectual and inhibitory functions anticipated the work of Hughlings Jackson, who was also much influenced by Laycock.[49] David Ferrier, an Edinburgh graduate, was Laycock's assistant and he lectured each Friday 'summarising for the students Laycock's lectures for the previous week … [his] practical teaching was a valuable adjunct to Laycock's theoretical discourses'. But because it is argued that neurology was fully integrated with general medicine prior to the 1860s, Bramwell himself might be dubbed the first Edinburgh neurologist. He worked in Newcastle upon Tyne between 1874 and 1879, where he was closely associated with Drummond.[50] Bramwell moved to coincide with the opening of the Edinburgh Royal Infirmary at Lauriston Place in 1879. He was an influential teacher and can claim to have advantaged the work of the National Hospital through Edinburgh alumni whom he nurtured and who were subsequently appointed to its consultant staff: Marcus Gunn, Risien Russell, James Taylor, Thomas Grainger Stewart, Kinnier Wilson,

William Adie and Joseph Greenfield. Bramwell was disappointed at not being appointed to the chair of medicine in Edinburgh on the occasion when John Wyllie was elected in 1899. Bramwell wrote monographs on *Diseases of the Spinal Cord* (1882) and *Intracranial Tumours* (1888), based on lectures delivered in Newcastle and Edinburgh, in which there is a description of pituitary disease and acromegaly. His *Studies in Clinical Medicine* (1889–90) contains many neurological cases, as does the three-volume *Atlas of Clinical Medicine* (1892–6) and the eight volumes of *Clinical Studies: A Quarterly Journal of Clinical Medicine* (1903–10).

Byrom's son Edwin Bramwell knew he would be in the shadow of his illustrious father but learned neurology during visits to Germany and thereafter moved to the National Hospital in 1888. Edwin returned to Edinburgh in 1901 and was appointed to the Royal Infirmary and, in 1919, as lecturer in neurology.[51] In 1934, his lecture on aneurysm and third nerve palsy was the first paper delivered to the newly formed Association of British Neurologists.[52] James Graham Brown was an Edinburgh medical graduate, later a lecturer in neurology, elected as president of the Royal College of Physicians of Edinburgh in 1912, and a lifelong friend of Sherrington. William Barnett Warrington studied with Sherrington in Liverpool where, later, he practised as a neurologist.

Sir David Drummond studied neurology in his early years and worked in Newcastle and Durham.[53] As was often the fashion, Drummond was initially a pathologist before appointment as consultant physician. He was subsequently vice-chancellor of the University of Durham and president of the British Medical Association (1921–2). He wrote *Diseases of the Brain and Spinal Cord* (1883). George Hall was a physician who practised neurology in Newcastle and other hospitals in the north-east before 1914.

nerves [neuritis, peripheral neuritis, multiple neuritis, alcoholic paralysis]'.

[49] See B. Bramwell, 'The Edinburgh Medical School and its Professors in My Student Days, 1865–69', *Edinburgh Medical Journal* **30** (1923): 133–56. Bramwell describes Laycock as a poor teacher, 'too pernickety and apt to dwell on small points, too keen to make hasty, physiognomic diagnoses. One day in going round the ward, he came to a new patient, a woman with well-preserved strong teeth. "Gentlemen, observe the teeth of this patient; they are highly characteristic of the sanguine arthritic diathesis." The patient, seeing that he was interested in her teeth, took them out and asked if he would like to see them closer.'

[50] Drummond described Bramwell as combining the thoroughness of the German with the courtesy, qualities of heart and scientific enthusiasm of the best type of British physician. Bramwell was taught by John Hughes Bennett, who died after surgery for a stone but had a large extradural tumour at post-mortem examination, and whose son Alexander diagnosed the tumour that Sir Rickman Godlee first removed on 25 November 1884 – for details, see B. Ashworth, *The Bramwells of Edinburgh: A Medical Dynasty* (Royal College of Physicians of Edinburgh, 1986).

[51] Dr Christopher Clayson recalls that Edwin Bramwell 'looked like an agnostic and taught like a Jesuit; that is with admirable logical simplicity': see Ashworth, *The Bramwells of Edinburgh*.

[52] Cleverly, Bramwell drew together strengths of Edinburgh neurology down the ages in his last paper on pupil reactions: Robert Whytt who described the light reflex; Argyll Robertson and the light accommodation-dissociated pupillary response in tabes dorsalis; Kinnier Wilson and the same features in mesencephalic disease; and William Adie and the Holmes–Adie pupil disease.

[53] A useful cricketer, Drummond could still turn over his arm and strike the ball forcibly in the nets after the age of 60.

Neurology continued at the West Riding Lunatic Asylum after the departure of Ferrier and Hughlings Jackson, especially under the direction of Joseph Shaw Bolton, later professor of mental diseases in Leeds. James Ross and Richard Williamson functioned as neurologists in Manchester. Jefferson considers that, with this pair and William Thorburn, Manchester in the nineteenth century rivalled Queen Square and Edinburgh as a centre for diseases of the brain and spinal cord.[54] Working as a general practitioner and doctor on a Greenland whaler until his early forties, Ross wrote on *Diseases of the Nervous System* (1881) and important papers on referred pain. Williamson studied as resident at Queen Square with Hughlings Jackson, Ferrier and Gowers. But on leaving London he had to work as a registrar for 14 years before eventually obtaining a post as physician at the Manchester Royal Infirmary in 1903. He was lecturer in neurology, and wrote *Diseases of the Spinal Cord* (1908), but resigned after developing a depressive illness. His immediate successors in Manchester were Judson Bury and Ernest Septimus Reynolds.

The first physician in Belfast with specific neurological training was John McGee McCormac, who had attended the National Hospital as a postgraduate student and was a member of the Neurological Society of London. His house became 'The Belfast Institution for nervous diseases, paralysis and epilepsy' and he helped to establish the 'Victoria Hospital for diseases of the nervous system, paralysis and epilepsy', later the Claremont Street Hospital. John Michell Clarke worked as a neurologist in Bristol. Sir Thomas Clifford Allbutt was a physician in Cambridge, from where he published his *System of Medicine* in eight volumes between the years 1896 and 1899. He had previously invented the short-stemmed clinical thermometer and was a renowned ophthalmoscopist.[55] But, whilst previous history and geographical distance acted to maintain the independence of cities in the northern United Kingdom in terms of expertise in diseases of the nervous system, elsewhere Queen Square had no rivals.

The Second Wave of Neurologists After 1914

One consequence of the First World War was a modest expansion in the number of neurologists working outside London. Most were required to retain activities in general medicine, and in the early years neurological practice was a relatively minor part of their work – for instance, in the case of Francis Purser in Dublin, Henry Cohen in Liverpool and Donald Core in Manchester. For others, neurology became the major interest: Richard Allison and Hilton Stewart in Belfast, William Johnson in Liverpool, Fergus Fergusson in Manchester, Ronald Gordon in Bath and Hugh Garland in Leeds. Frederick Nattrass was professor of medicine in Newcastle, but functioned as a neurologist, having served in the First World War and written his MD thesis on nerve injuries. Stanley Barnes worked as a neurologist in Birmingham, with Philip Cloake, the first person to be styled as a professor of neurology, from 1947,[56] and then Gilbert Hall.

The Second World War provided another set of lessons on the need for specialists in diseases of the nervous system. The emphasis was on neurosurgery, with Cairns, Jefferson and Dott leading developments and working in Oxford, Manchester and Edinburgh, respectively. Their war work proved influential when the National Health Service was founded. But it was clear that neurosurgery could not be managed by general surgeons, or by individuals working in isolation without access to facilities that supported surgical practice. Furthermore, it made no sense to create neurosurgical posts without there also being local provision for consultants in neurology. Now

---

[54] Sir Geoffrey Jefferson, *Selected Papers* (London: Pitman, 1960): see 'James Ross, Sir William Thorburn, R. T. Williamson – Pioneers in Neurology', pp. 195–209, reprinted from the *Manchester University Medical School Gazette* (June 1948).

[55] See *On the Use of the Ophthalmoscope in Diseases of the Nervous System and of the Kidneys* (London: Macmillan and Co., 1871), p. 405.

[56] Cloake was an advocate of treating disseminated sclerosis with arsenic, which he gave four times annually for the first five years and three times thereafter. This work was described in his (the first) Humphry Davy Rolleston lecture to the Royal College of Physicians in 1947, on 'The Treatment of Disseminated Sclerosis by Artificial Pyrexia and the Prolonged Administration of Arsenic'. The lecture remained unpublished and the then Harveian Librarian, Sir Charles Dodds, and his successor, wrote serially to Professor Cloake between 1953 and 1966 trying to extract a manuscript, but (despite promises of imminent dispatch) with no success. This correspondence closes with an unanswered note of condolences to Philip Cloake's widow, dated April 1969, adding that the College still hoped to acquire the 1947 manuscript should this be found among Cloake's papers. It never arrived.

neurology followed neurosurgery into the English countryside. This emphasis on neurosurgery was one significant reason for development of regional services away from Queen Square, such as at Atkinson Morley Hospital (Wimbledon) and the Maudsley Hospital in London, and in Oxford, Cambridge and Southampton. At the same time, the older established provincial centres, such as those in Edinburgh and Glasgow, Newcastle and Manchester, gained in numbers as their neurosurgical departments strengthened or were newly formed.

Modest expansion did also occur in London. Some physicians held joint appointments with a teaching hospital and Queen Square or Maida Vale. But a new breed emerged, working in other London hospitals, and deprecated by Walshe even more than the 'amateurs at Maida Vale'. Some of these specialists in neurology had trained during the war in military settings, without necessarily ever having worked at the National Hospital(s). Amongst these in the immediate postwar period were Michael Ashby (Whittington), Peter Croft (Whittington), Simon Behrman (Brook and Bromley Hospitals), Harold Edwards (St Mary's), Kenneth Heathfield (Oldchurch), Norman Hulbert (West End Hospital), Eric Jewesbury (Royal Northern Hospital), J. N. Milnes (West End Hospital), John Phemister (Central Middlesex Hospital), Robert Porter (Central Middlesex), Finlay Graham Campbell (Croydon), Eric Arnold Nieman (West End Hospital and Charing Cross), John Aldren Turner (St Bartholomew's), Basil Parsons-Smith (West End Hospital and Charing Cross), Frank Clifford Rose (Charing Cross), J. Small (Croydon) and Marcia Wilkinson (Elizabeth Garrett Anderson Hospital, South London Hospital and Hackney Hospital).

The impetus for developing regional centres coincided with the debate on neurology as a specialty. Taken with the sustained pressure to increase manpower, the number of doctors practising neurology outside London increased, gradually redressing the imbalance in metropolitan versus provincial provision and reducing the number of people for whom each specialist had responsibility. John Gaylor, Gervais Joly Dixon, Stewart Renfrew and Ian Simpson were appointed in Glasgow. Andrew Lenman and Alan Downie worked in Aberdeen. Appointees in Edinburgh included Walter Sneddon Watson,[57] Kate Herman, John Marshall before moving to London, John Stanton, Clifford Mawdsley,

Bryan Ashworth and J. K. Slater. In Newcastle, neurology flourished with the appointment of the charismatic Henry Miller, who followed Nattrass and was then joined by John Walton, John ('Jack') Foster, David Shaw and Peter Hudgson.

The tradition of neurology in Northern Ireland was maintained by Louis Hurwitz and Harold Millar. John Millar, Eddy Martin and Hugh Staunton were appointed in Dublin. Neurologists in Manchester included Fergus Ferguson, George Smyth, Laurie Liversedge, Bryan Matthews (before his move to Derby and then Oxford as William Ritchie Russell's successor) and Neil Gordon, who was the first paediatric neurologist in the north of England. J. P. P. Bradshaw and Maurice Parsonage set up the neurological service in Leeds. Clifford Astley was the lone neurologist in Teesdale, John Cook maintained the tradition in Wakefield, and James Carson worked in Sheffield, where Sir Arthur Hall had maintained an interest in neurology whilst professor of medicine after the First World War. Philip Buckley was based in Chesterfield.[58] Charles Hutchinson and James Heron were in Stoke-on-Trent. In Birmingham, Edwin Bickerstaff, Michael Jefferson (son of Sir Geoffrey Jefferson), John Holmes and Isadore Guest established a department of neurology at the Midland Centre for Neurosurgery at Smethwick.

Arthur Stewart-Wallace and John Penman provided services in East Sussex, based at Haywards Heath after the neurosurgeons returned to Queen Square, and John Foley worked in Worthing and Chichester. In Bristol, Golla and Grey Walter ran the Burden Neurological Institute, and neurology was managed by (Archibald) Malcolm Campbell, Francis Page and Richard Langton Hewer, with Graham Wakefield based in Bath after the retirement of Henry Lovell Hoffman. Ritchie Russell left

---

[57] It is significant that, after gaining experience in psychiatry serving with the Royal Army Medical Corps in the Middle East from 1940 to 1946, Watson returned to Edinburgh as physician in the department of surgical neurology, where he remained as medical neurology developed in Edinburgh at the Northern General Hospital.

[58] According to Stephen Casper, Buckley 'reflected that morbidity was so high through neglect that each case took time to evaluate; and there was no cover for holidays or sickness. Difficult cases always had to be referred elsewhere. Consultants need to be educated at regional centres and manage their complex cases. This is turn would allow centre neurologists to learn things of interest that they might never encounter.'

Edinburgh and moved to Oxford with Honor Smith, John Spalding, Charles Whitty and Bryan Matthews. Michael Espir provided services in Leicester with Paul Millac. In East Anglia, Michael Yealland, based in Cambridge, worked alone until joined by Colin Brown in Norwich. Frederick Lees was the neurologist in Essex, Alan Barham Carter in Ashford (and also at St George's and Atkinson Morley Hospital, working with McKissock) and Raymond Hierons at the Brook Hospital looked after Kent, with Surrey covered by David Kendall at Guildford and Kingston. Ian Mackenzie was appointed to Maidstone and Bedford. Southampton appointed Stanley Graveson, who attracted Jason Brice and John Garfield to develop the Wessex Neurological Centre, where Peter Robinson, Lee Illis and Jeremy Hallpike were also neurologists. John (Jerry) Spillane, Charles Wells and then John Graham were appointed in Cardiff, and Esmond Rees in Swansea. North Wales was served by Geoffrey Lloyd and also the neurologists from Liverpool, who included Robert Hughes and Kenneth Slatter. T. G. Wilson and Nathaniel ('Barney') Alcock were responsible for Devon and Cornwall.

It is fitting to end this catalogue (dutiful, but certain to be incomplete) of regional expansion in the provision of neurological services outside Queen Square in the 1950s and 1960s with the recollections of Barney Alcock, one of the last surviving neurologists who knew the National Hospital before the Second World War. He had worked at the Royal Postgraduate Medical School, Hammersmith Hospital, and planned to emigrate to Australia, but moved to Cornwall on demobilisation. He 'saw the need to serve the community by travelling to patients and having busy outpatient clinics in several locations and to form links with general practitioners'. Interviewed by Ian McDonald, in the Royal Clarence Hotel, Exeter, Alcock (then aged 92) recalled his training at Queen Square, and early years in the west of England.

> I qualified in 1931 and was house physician to Edwin Bramwell in Edinburgh also being taught by Ritchie Russell before arriving at Queen Square to work with Greenfield on Huntington's disease ... relationships between consultants were guarded ... Purdon Martin was someone from whom you needed to know what he thought but as soon as he started lecturing, it was v. dull ... he had a facility for making it duller than anyone else ... Adie was quite the nicest person I met amongst the consultants ... SAK Wilson had a magnificent command of English (and of himself) ... Symonds was aloof and very well dressed ... I was rather embarrassed one day when Collier asked what I thought of Critchley ... Holmes was in full swing ... he always read notes taken by clerks ... his crossness always took place with clerks, and he was perfectly nice to most HPs ... When George Vth died Holmes said 'we'll walk over to Southampton Row to see the coffin on its way up from Euston' ... with the PoW [Prince of Wales] walking behind, the crown fell off the coffin ... There was practically no neurology outside London ... Manchester was just beginning and Newcastle starting ... In Bristol, Golla was a thoroughly tiresome man ... Malcolm Campbell came back from the war and there was Grey Walter. I was appointed in January 1948 and started as assistant to a general physician in Truro ... I took the post because the physician said there would be an opening for a neurologist and was then appointed in Exeter, Plymouth and Truro ... found suitable GPs to be assistants in each place.[59]

---

[59] See McDonald archive: manuscript, 20 July 2001.

Neurosurgery and War Neurology at Queen Square

Neurosurgery

In the first years of the hospital, three surgeons[1] were appointed, all renowned figures in London surgical circles, but none carried out neurosurgery. This discipline became part of the fabric of the National Hospital only from the time of Sir Victor Horsley's appointment in 1886. Horsley, in effect, invented modern neurosurgery and, for many years, dominated the world of neurosurgery in Britain and abroad, and Queen Square became renowned as *the* neurosurgical centre. Horsley died during the First World War, and it was that conflict and the Second World War which drove the subject forward outside Queen Square, and although, with Horsley's work still recent, the First World War might have been an opportunity for the National Hospital to exploit its dominant position, in the event, neurosurgery at Queen Square simply trod water between 1918 and 1945, and the opportunities for innovation and leadership were missed.

War was an important stimulus. Before the First World War, Horsley's researches into gunshot injury and the practical management of head wounds on the battlefield had been a significant influence on the practice of military neurosurgery. Whilst working in France during the war, Percy Sargent and his colleague Gordon Holmes made further theoretical and practical contributions to the topic. In the First World War, key staff were deployed to the front, and surgical activity largely ceased at the National Hospital. It did not regain its previous emphasis, and, in the inter-war years, the focus on neurosurgery was lost. Again in the Second World War, no operating took place at Queen Square. Elsewhere though, the recognition of neurosurgery as a specialty in its own right, and the need for expertise to be available across the country, stimulated the development of regional centres that, after 1948, rivalled the National Hospital. It was only

after 1960 that there began a renaissance in neurosurgical studies at Queen Square, not least due to the establishment of an academic unit. In recent years, inpatient work at the hospital has increasingly been dominated by neurosurgery, which, with the National Health Service managed as an internal market from the 1990s, remains crucial to its financial security.

Neurosurgery at the National Hospital before 1918

Horsley, whose work is described in earlier chapters, was the only consultant dedicated to neurosurgery based at the National Hospital until 1891, when Charles Ballance was appointed, no doubt at Horsley's instigation since they were close friends and had worked together at the Brown Institution. Although Ballance resigned his appointment in 1908, he remained close to the National Hospital and on cordial terms with its staff. In 1906, two more surgeons were appointed, Percy Sargent[2] and Donald

---

[1] Sir John Fergusson, J. Zachariah Laurence and William Adams.

[2] Sir Percy William Graham Sargent was trained at St Thomas', and his greatest contributions occurred whilst working with Holmes in the First World War. Together, they formed a small neurological unit in 1914, and later he took charge of a department established for the treatment of those still suffering from remote injuries of the nervous system. For his military services, he was awarded the DSO in 1917 and the CMG in 1919, and he was created a Knight Bachelor in 1928. He was a charming man and a renowned and entertaining teacher. His obituarist in *Plarr's Lives* comments that 'as a surgeon he was also famous for his dexterity, rapidity, and gentleness. His operations were models of skill and almost perfect restraint.' He appeared in many surgical meetings in London, but, it has to be said, published relatively little, although he did write substantial papers on glioma, posterior fossa surgery and pituitary surgery. His obituary in the *British Journal of Surgery* mentions that 'he was never a robust man, and a physical disability told heavily on him at times, though it was hidden from view', but what this was is not clear. He was said to be a benevolent man interested in charity, and was an active Mason, being appointed a senior

Armour,[3] with the express purpose of supporting

Horsley.[4] Their duties were to receive referrals from the outpatient and assistant physicians[5] on two afternoons, and to operate on two mornings each week.

The surgical facilities at Queen Square were thoroughly inadequate. At first, Horsley operated in a side-room on Margaret Gibbens ward. The first operating theatre was constructed in the Westminster wing in 1891. This also proved unsatisfactory and was replaced in 1905 by a new, but not much improved, theatre. Thus, by 1910, there were three neurological surgeons at Queen Square working in poor facilities. By then, Horsley had become heavily involved in campaigning on social matters and political affairs, and these interests kept him away

---

grand deacon in the United Grand Lodge of England in 1915. His friend at medical school, William Eardley, published a eulogy about Sargent on his death, in the *British Medical Journal*, which, even allowing for exaggeration, paints an attractive picture, revealing: 'the nobility of his character, the strength and splendour of his manhood, his high principles and sense of honour, the strength and loyalty and faithfulness of his friendship, his unbounded sympathy and consideration for others, his constant devotion to duty, his dauntless courage, his brilliant intellect, his wit and humour, his beautiful gentleness and kindness, courtesy and tact, his innate modesty (Sargent never boasted), not to mention his erect and handsome figure, his radiant countenance and cheerful disposition, which spread happiness among all around him'. Clearly, Sargent was a cultured, urbane figure and an excellent surgeon and teacher, but not a pioneer or with the innovative or experimental flair of Horsley or Cushing. He died suddenly in 1933.

[3] Donald Armour was a Canadian who trained in Toronto and then came to England, where he was appointed demonstrator in anatomy at University College. There he met Horsley and they became great friends. Armour often remarked that he was guided by Horsley, and certainly Horsley did everything he could to get the young surgeon elected to the staff at the National Hospital, as he was in 1913 at the same time as Percy Sargent. Armour was a man of great energy, and with a large private practice. He was president of the neurological section of the Royal Society of Medicine, the West London Medico-Chirurgical Society, the Medical Society of London and the Society of British Neurological Surgeons. He gave the Lettsonian lectures before the Medical Society of London, which were widely recognised as an accurate description of modern surgery of the spinal cord and membranes, becoming the standard work on the subject. He wrote extensively, including papers on the surgery of the posterior fossa and of the spinal cord. According to his obituarist, the influence of Horsley was obvious in his approach, but Armour did not have the skill of his master. He did, however, invent new machinery and instruments, and 'as an admirer of de Martel of Paris, he had introduced that surgeon's electric motors, saws, trephines, and pumps into the theatre at the National Hospital'. This analysis adds details that still chime with the experience of some surgical practice today: 'It would not be correct to say he was easy to work with, but his criticisms were always made in such a way that it was impossible to take offence at his apparent impatience, and he always managed to get the best of service from his assistants.' The obituary in *Plarr's Lives* also recounts: 'Not an easy man with whom to work, he retained many of the characteristics of individuality and resourcefulness which must have led his ancestors to leave their native country and act as pioneers (!).' Geoffrey Jefferson provided a more tender account: 'He was deeply interested in the welfare of the National Hospital, and most anxious to help everybody who came within his sphere of

influence ... He was President of the Society of British Neurourgeons for two years (1929–30, 1930–1) and was able to present to the society the old wooden mallet that Horsley had used, suitably embellished with a silver plate to bring it into currency again as a gavel for the president's use at meetings ... No one who has had the privilege of his hospitality will be likely to forget the perfection of the settings in his print-lined rooms ... Armour had his disappointments, and to those who knew him he was not shy of revealing them, but he did this without weakness, and above all without malice. It was the entire absence of rancour that made Armour so pleasing a personality; his tongue knew no bitterness, so that disagreements remained just that and never grew into quarrels that left scars. We who knew him well will miss that deep voice, that tall figure, and that genial smile.' He retired in 1933 and died relatively suddenly, shortly afterwards.

[4] The recommendation that an assistant surgeon be appointed is recorded in the Medical Committee minutes of 2 February 1906, with Horsley acting as secretary. Applications were received from Armour and Sargent, and also from four others. These were: (Sir) Thomas Crisp English, who became a famous general surgeon in London; James Sherren, who wrote a book on injuries to peripheral nerves and sectioned Henry Head's radial nerve in the famous experiments on nerve regeneration; and L. B. Rawlins and Mr Buckrall, about whom less is known. A ballot was held by the Medical Committee on 11 May 1906. Armour received seven and Sargent five votes, Rawlins two, and Sherren and English one each. A second ballot was held and Armour and Sargent each received eight votes and both were appointed. They attended the Medical Committee meeting on 1 June 1906, showing how rapidly appointments were then taken up.

[5] See Medical Committee minutes for 1906. Presumably Horsley received his referrals from the senior physicians, but this was not stated. Other regulations included the requirement that one of the surgeons always had to be in London, and operations were to be performed on Tuesday and Friday morning starting at 9 a.m.

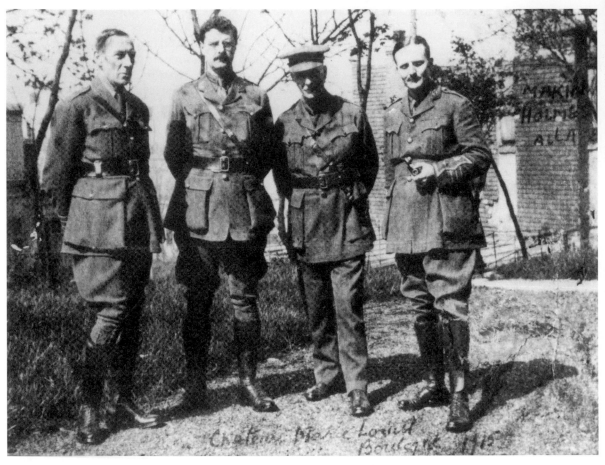

Figure 9.1 Geo Makins, Gordon Holmes, Cuthbert Wallace and Percy Sargent in Boulogne in 1915.

from the hospital, and Sargent took on an increasingly important surgical role.

With the outbreak of war in 1914, the surgical team at Queen Square was dispersed. Horsley and Sargent were both posted abroad on military service for long periods, and then, in 1915, the hospital was deeply affected by Horsley's death in Mesopotamia. Meanwhile, Sargent had become extremely active as a surgeon in France. He and Gordon Holmes worked together in Boulogne at Hospital No. 13. Cushing provides a vivid picture of conditions there in a visit he made in 1916:

> After tea, Holmes and Sargent took me back to No. 13, where I saw an amazing number of head and spinal wounds, for they often received daily convoys of 300 recently wounded. With the proper backing these two men have an unparalleled opportunity, not only to be of service to the individual wounded,

but, when this is all over, to make a contribution to physiology, neurology and surgery which will be epochal ... On the whole, I take No. 13 to be a good example of the large overseas hospitals of the RAMC. The comforts are slight, the attendance insufficient, the work, though it naturally varies, is simply overwhelming – perhaps as many admissions in a day as the American Ambulance might get in a month ... This is truly a man-sized job, in the midst of which the Britisher stops for tea, and everyone – even down to the Tommie – has time to shave; and its taking-it-quietly that possibly enables them to see things through with some measure of composure ... After a pick-up supper, learning that Sargent was winding up a busy operative day at No.13, Holmes guides me down there – literally so, for it is black as tar and he has to count the steps as we descend the twisting path down the hillside. And we are in time to see his final case, a bad shell wound of the right parietal region with a big piece of *obus* and countless fragments of bone, and a definite though well-localised infection. It was a very careful, neat and expeditious performance.[6]

It is said Sargent was the only person who could discuss the nervous system with Gordon Holmes on equal terms, and even survive teasing him.[7] Donald Armour was often the only Queen Square surgeon who remained working in London. He was commissioned in the Royal Army Medical Corps (RAMC), as lieutenant-colonel, and nominally attached to numerous metropolitan hospitals for officers. Not shy of increasing his private work from 1914, in the absence of the only other two London neurosurgeons, most of his civilian work took place in the Canadian hospitals in general surgery and neurosurgery.[8]

Neurosurgery at the National Hospital 1919–1930

The First World War proved a watershed in the neurosurgical fortunes of the National Hospital. During the war, when the surgical staff were deployed in the services abroad, almost no surgery was carried out and, even after the war, interest in the topic had waned. The specialty made little progress over the next 15 years in Britain, where it was perceived to be merely a branch of general surgery. Apart from Sargent and Armour, only a very small number of surgeons were performing brain or spinal operations, no one of whom had a practice confined to neurosurgical cases. Neither Sargent nor Armour dissented from the view that neurosurgery was subsidiary to general surgery, and each retained general surgical practices at other London teaching hospitals (Sargent at St Thomas', where he was nicknamed 'Pretty Percy'; and Armour at University College Hospital). Although neurosurgical activity at the National Hospital had stagnated, with only 98 major operations carried out in 1923 and 110 in the first ten months of 1924 – fewer than in Horsley's day – Sargent was nevertheless frequently referred to in medical circles as 'the leading neurosurgeon in Britain and abroad'.

Neurosurgical procedures were largely confined to dealing with tumours, trigeminal neuralgia, obstructive hydrocephalus, head injury and brain abscess. Surgical mortality was high, the outcomes were often disappointing, and neurosurgery had a low priority and poor reputation amongst the grandees of general surgery. This situation was in marked contrast to advancement of the specialty in the United States. With the National Hospital hesitating to maintain the leadership that Horsley had established, Harvey Cushing, at Peter Bent Brigham Hospital in Boston, increasingly dominated the subject by nature of his style, personality and manifold achievements. He challenged the general surgical approach practised at Queen Square and introduced novel surgical techniques, with an emphasis on the avoidance of collateral injury to the brain, delicate handling of tissue, meticulous haemostasis, and closure of the wound. His surgery was thorough and extremely slow. Sargent typified what became the Queen Square approach, based on more traditional general surgical principles, and was 'vocally critical of [Cushing's] slow and painstaking methods'. Harvey Jackson describes Sargent removing a meningioma with his finger and dealing with haemorrhage merely by packing the cavity with gauze. Nevertheless, Sargent was renowned as a fast and skilled surgeon, and indeed was acknowledged to be so by Cushing himself.[9]

One consequence of the attitude to neurosurgery in London was that plans for a new operating theatre

---

[6] From H. Cushing, *A Surgeon's Journal 1915–1918* (Boston: Little, Brown and Company, 1936), ch. 2, Wednesday 5 May 1915. Cushing also emphasised the research potential of the war, highlighting Holmes and Sargent's work on traumatic brain injury, including 'gutter wounds' caused by ill-advised exposure of the head in the trenches, and complete transection of the cord, neither of which conditions Cushing had previously encountered.

[7] M. Critchley, *The Black Hole and Other Essays* (London: Pitman Medical, 1964).

[8] There were two Canadian military hospitals for officers in London: the hospital at No. 1 Hyde Park Place in Bayswater had 25 beds and was known for its comfort and elegant surroundings, but with cramped operating facilities. It was founded by the Imperial Order of Daughters of the Empire, and functioned between 1916 and 1919. The other was the larger Canadian Red Cross Hospital, known as the Petrograd Red Cross Hospital for Officers, in North Audley Street. This had excellent operating facilities and was considered to be the best-equipped military hospital in London during the war. There were also five Canadian auxiliary hospitals for convalescence which formed part of the network of over 300 small military and auxiliary hospitals (and many more outside London), based in residential houses but with facilities for surgery, required to deal with the massive flow of casualties returning from the front.

[9] See T. T. King, *Origins of the Society of British Neurological Surgeons 1926–1939* (2006), www.sbns.org.uk/index.php/about-us/history.

at the National Hospital, first discussed in the early 1920s, and then repeatedly mooted in the hospital committees, moved slowly. Throughout the 1920s and 1930s, there were only seven surgical beds at the hospital, and this had increased merely to 24 by 1938, when new theatres and dedicated surgical wards were completed in the Queen Mary wing. This development, funded by the grant from the Rockefeller Foundation, was, as mentioned earlier, partly motivated by the wish of the Foundation (and championed by Gregg and O'Brien) to proselytise Cushing's approach to neurosurgery and to disseminate the use of his techniques in Europe.

Representing the old school of Queen Square neurologists, Walshe was highly contemptuous of the Cushing method, condemning it 'as the triumph of technique over reason'. Indeed, some blame for the neglect of neurosurgery at the National Hospital in these years is due to this attitude shared amongst the senior physicians. They resented Cushing's influence and retained the view that neurosurgery was a 'craft' specialty lacking the intellectual rigour of neurology. Post-Horsley, the surgeons at Queen Square were treated as technicians, physicians sometimes insisting on being present during operations. It is said that Sargent would rarely operate without Holmes standing over him and indicating with his finger-tip on the skull the site of the underlying tumour.

In what was to prove a particular flashpoint at Queen Square, the longstanding policy that surgeons were not allowed to admit patients directly to the hospital was maintained in the inter-war years.[10] All patients were admitted into a physician's bed, where management was decided, and then transferred for surgery, returning to the safety of medical care once the technical procedure was completed. Conversely, Cushing ruled over his neurological colleagues and took charge of his patients. He made it his business to train neurosurgeons, and a 'Cushing school' grew up, with surgeons from around the world spending part of their training in Boston. This was to have repercussions for Queen Square.

Amongst the most renowned of the Cushing school were his 'British disciples' Sir Hugh Cairns, Sir Geoffrey Jefferson and Norman Dott.[11] All three trained in Boston and then returned to Britain, where they invigorated British neurosurgery in units at the London Hospital and Oxford (Cairns), Edinburgh (Dott) and Manchester (Jefferson). Regarding them as close friends, Cushing visited England several times to promote their cause and make neurosurgery a specialty led by the surgeon, not the physician. However, despite Cushing's efforts, prior to 1948 neurosurgery did not separate from general surgery, just as the same conservatism retained clinical neurology as part of general medicine.

In 1929, Hugh Cairns reported to the MRC on his stay in Boston working under Cushing in 1926–7, giving a flavour of what constituted the practice of neurosurgery at the time.[12] In the 12-month period, Cushing admitted 463 cases, of whom 369 had intracranial tumour, 37 trigeminal neuralgia, 23 head injury, 20 lesions of the spinal cord and 14 other miscellaneous conditions. Surgery for epilepsy, which had inspired Horsley in the nineteenth century, had now ceased. Diagnosis was made by history, examination, plain X-ray, ventriculogram and exploratory craniotomy. Surgical mortality was low at 10 per cent. Cairns also emphasised in the report that Cushing believed the surgeon should be 'shouldered with the responsibility of acting largely on his

---

[10] Only Horsley in his later years had been exempt from this ruling.

[11] Norman Dott was born in Edinburgh, the son of an art dealer. Initially training as an engineer, he sustained a leg injury in a motorcycle accident in 1913 and was admitted to

the Royal Infirmary of Edinburgh. The injury affected him physically for the rest of his life. Amputation was considered by Sir Henry Wade, but Sir Harry Platt later fused his hip; Sir Walter Mercer shortened the leg; Sir Geoffrey Jefferson carried out cordotomy for chronic pain; and Tom McNair performed a colostomy. Despite the severity of his injury, admission to hospital in 1913 led to Dott studying medicine at Edinburgh University where he graduated in 1919. He was awarded a Rockefeller Travelling Fellowship in 1923, and spent a year with Cushing. Thereafter, he worked as a neurosurgeon, founding Scotland's first dedicated neurosurgical ward in 1938 and, in 1960, the department of surgical neurology at the Royal Infirmary of Edinburgh. During the Second World War, Dott set up the Brain Injuries Unit in Bangour General Emergency Service Hospital in Broxburn, West Lothian, and was appointed CBE for this work in 1948. He retired in 1963. His archive documents the many cases treated in Ward 20 of the Royal Infirmary of Edinburgh.

[12] H. Cairns, *A Study of Intracranial Surgery 1929*, MRC Special Report 125 (London: HMSO, 1929). Joe Pennybacker, Cairns' successor in Oxford, considered that Dott was probably the best technical surgeon; Jefferson had the most genial personality and philosophical turn of mind; and Cairns was the great teacher. See J. B. Pennybacker, 'Sir Hugh William Bell Cairns', *Surgical Neurology* 4 (1975): 347–50.

own diagnosis'. The *Lancet* published an effusive editorial about Cairns' report, emphasising Cushing's genius and technique, and drawing unfavourable comparisons with British neurosurgery and neurology. The main strength of the British system was considered to be physiological enquiry. The editorial concluded that 'it is clearly in the patient's interest that Cushing's methods should be practised as widely as possible'.[13] Cairns sent the report to Richard Pearce at the Rockefeller Foundation, who was impressed. On 9 April 1929, Cairns wrote: 'Today I had a letter from Gregg saying that the Rockefeller people wish to finance the distribution of my MRC report on a large scale to all the important people between the Caspian sea and the English Channel.'[14]

Cairns considered the report to be the single most important factor in establishing his reputation in neurosurgery and it re-stimulated interest in neurosurgery at Queen Square, including efforts to induce Cairns to join the consultant staff.

One development of great importance to the future of British neurosurgery was the establishment in 1926 of the Society of British Neurological Surgeons (known by some as 'the Nutcrackers Union'). Jefferson was a prime mover, urged by Louis Bathe Rawling 'for God's sake to keep it to surgeons, we don't want anyone impractical', an obvious reference to excluding neurologists.[15] Jefferson's initiative was endorsed and encouraged by Ballance and Cushing, who had 'inherited Osler's belief in the virtues of medical societies as centres for the exchange of knowledge and the encouragement of warm and friendly relations'. The Society was formed at the Athenaeum Club on 2 December 1926 during a dinner hosted by Ballance. There were 17 people present, including (from Queen Square and University College Hospital) Armour, Sargent, Ferrier, Trotter and Scharpey-Schäfer. Ballance was elected as the first president and Jefferson as secretary (a post he held until 1952). In

his presidential address, Ballance said 'I look forward for a future when a window in the skull will be made by the surgeon with the like gentleness, precision and ease that a pane of glass is fashioned by the glazier by means of a diamond.' The following day the first scientific meeting was held at the National Hospital, with four operations demonstrated in the morning. Partial removal of a suprapituitary tumour and a craniotomy for a suspected parietal endothelioma were carried out by Sargent on two of Holmes' patients, and cordotomy for tabetic gastric crises and exploratory surgery for a possible acoustic neurofibroma performed by Armour for Grainger Stewart and Adie.[16] The delegates then departed for lunch at the Holborn Restaurant. Jefferson recalls the day in his eulogium for Ballance:

> It was Ballance who invited us to the remarkable dinner at the Athenaeum on the occasion of the foundation of the society, when he induced Sir

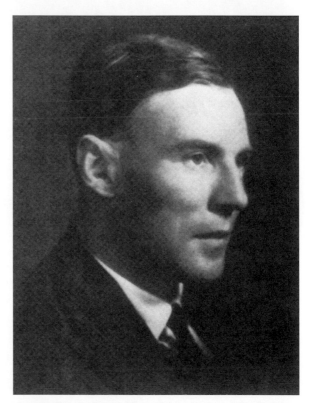

Figure 9.2 Sir Hugh Cairns.

---

[13] The editorial continued in rather strange vein: 'though it must not be that British neurology has nothing to contribute to neurological surgery … [this], in fact, offers a great opportunity for the union of different but complementary mental qualities of the American and British peoples'.

[14] See G. J. Fraenkel, *Hugh Cairns* (Oxford University Press, 1991).

[15] Louis Bathe Rawling was a general surgeon at St Bartholomew's Hospital and, after the war, at the West End Hospital for Nervous Diseases. See also King, *The Origins of the Society of British Neurological Surgeons*.

[16] The case records provide details of these four patients and it has been said that, in at least two, surgery proved unnecessary, and three of the four had a fatal outcome.

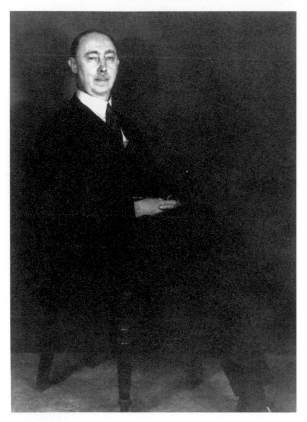

Figure 9.3 Sir Geoffrey Jefferson.

David Ferrier to come out of his retirement to allow a younger generation to hear him speak. With him were Sir E. Sharpey-Schafer, Sir Grafton Elliot Smith, and Sir Arthur Keith. Had it not been for Ballance the society might have had more difficulty than it had in getting itself born. He was its first president, and characteristically refused to hold office for more than one year, insisting on relinquishing office for Wilfred Trotter to carry on. The society replied by making him honorary president.[17]

The Society of British Neurological Surgeons proved enormously influential in promoting specialisation and gaining recognition for neurosurgery in Britain, acting as its unofficial governing body.[18]

---

[17] See *British Medical Journal* **1** (1936): 340.

[18] There was only one other specialist society in Britain at the time, of orthopaedic surgeons, set up by Sir Harry Platt, and only in the USA was there another neurosurgical association. There was no such society in Europe, and many European neurosurgeons became foreign members of the British Society.

Cairns and Jefferson at the National Hospital 1929–1939

With this move towards better recognition of neurosurgery as a specialty, in the late 1920s the younger consultants at Queen Square became concerned about its future in the hospital. Armour and Sargent were nearing the end of their careers, and Cairns[19] and Jefferson[20]

---

[19] Sir Hugh William Bell Cairns was born and educated in Adelaide, Australia, where he entered medical school. He interrupted his studies to enlist with the Australian Army Medical Corps, being based on the Aegean island of Lemnos, supporting the Gallipoli campaign. He won a Rhodes Scholarship to work in Oxford and arrived at Balliol College in 1919 after war service in France. In Oxford, he was taught by Sherrington, earned a rowing blue and married the daughter of the Master of Balliol College, where he had matriculated. Because there was no academic interest in surgery in Oxford, he moved to the London Hospital to work with Sir Henry Souttar, and was appointed honorary assistant surgeon in 1926. He was interested initially in genitourinary surgery but turned to neurosurgery after being awarded a Rockefeller Fellowship in 1925 and going to work with Harvey Cushing, whom he had first met at tea with Lady Osler in 1922. On his return to London, Cairns was keen to extend Cushing's methods to British neurosurgery but was considered an irritable and difficult person, nicknamed 'pepper-pot' by his students, and had little support from London neurologists.

[20] Sir Geoffrey Jefferson was born in County Durham, and trained in medicine in Manchester. He emigrated to Vancouver in 1914 aiming to develop a surgical career in Canada, but returned when war was declared and joined the staff of the Anglo-Russian Hospital in Petrograd. Later, he went to Volhynia attached to General Kaledin's corps, which was besieging Warsaw, and operated in a field station during 1916. There were horrifying conditions, but Jefferson kept a Fabergé cigarette case given by Alexei, grandson of the writer Aleksay Khomiakov, 'en souvenir de Lutsk et de tout de que c'est passé de gai, de triste et de macabre'. After witnessing the Russian revolution, Jefferson went to France with the 14th General Hospital, and, despite skills in managing head injury, realised the consequences of uncontrolled infection. In 1918, he spent a year in Boston, training with Cushing, and on his return was appointed consultant surgeon in Manchester. He was considered a subtle and original thinker, a very scholarly person and also a brilliant surgeon, unlike Cairns. He wrote on many neurosurgical topics and made several technical and surgical contributions. He also played a vital role in the EMS and the organisation of neurosurgical services during and after the war, and it is no exaggeration to say that the postwar direction of British neurosurgery was forged to a large extent by the work of Jefferson and Cairns. He was knighted in 1943 and elected FRS in 1947, and the last decade of his

potentially represented a strategic investment. Cairns was informally approached in 1929 about a post at Queen Square and expressed interest. In 1930, a new consultant post was duly advertised. Cairns, Jefferson and Dott each applied. They were the three most promising neurosurgeons in the country and their surgery was very much in the mode of Cushing, their teacher. Cairns described doing the rounds of the senior physicians in their Harley Street lairs to discuss his application, and gleefully reported that the forthcoming election was 'the talk of Harley Street'. He quickly realised, though, that Holmes was opposed to his appointment, mainly due to Cushing's insistence that the surgeon should take charge of cases, including 'making the diagnosis and determining management'. Symonds was more sympathetic to Cairns' position. He also had worked as an intern with Cushing and had come to the conclusion that the prospect of successful brain surgery by Cushing's methods was 'a great deal better than it was in London, and that neurosurgery should be practised as a specialty'.[21] In fact, he usually referred his patients to Cairns at the London Hospital, rather than to the Queen Square surgeons.[22] Sargent argued that Dott was ineligible

because he had only the Edinburgh, not the London, fellowship, and so the post was contested by Cairns and Jefferson. An acrimonious debate ensued. According to Cairns, the senior physicians, with the gynaecologists and orthopaedic and aural surgeons recruited to their side, remained firmly 'anti-Cushing'.[23] The Medical Committee voted and Cairns lost by seven votes to Jefferson's nine, but the Board refused to accept this decision. The two consultant neurosurgeons were also split: Armour voting for Cairns but Sargent threatening to resign if he was appointed. As Symonds recalled in his Hugh Cairns lecture: 'Cairns had the support at the London of Riddoch and Russell Brain, but at Queen Square the senior members of the staff clung to the idea that a general surgeon with an interest in the nervous system was the right choice. Holmes, who carried great weight, was of this opinion.'

This was a defining moment in the history of the hospital. Cairns now devoted his energies to establishing a department of neurosurgery at the London Hospital, supported by Riddoch and Brain. In 1931, Julian

---

life was spent serving the Medical Research Council and other committees. Jefferson was a bibliophile who collected widely and was the subject of a scholarly biography by one of his previous trainees: see P. Schurr, *So That Was Life: Biography of Sir Geoffrey Jefferson* (London: Royal Society of Medicine Press, 1997).

[21] See C. P. Symonds, *Tria juncta in uno* (Oxford: Seacourt Press, 1970). This was the sixth Sir Hugh Cairns lecture, addressed to the Society of British Neurological Surgeons on 23 September 1970. 'Tria juncta in uno' is the motto of the Order of the Bath and derived from the lustral ceremony before knighthood; Symonds ends with a quote from John Milton: 'Fame he sought and won in his day, till there came the blind Fury with th'abhorréd shears, and slit the thin spun life. But not the praise.'

[22] Christopher Earl later did the same for his patients with acoustic tumours, whom he referred to Tom King at the London Hospital. One such patient was his redoubtable and loyal secretary Enid Halsey. The London Hospital had a distinguished neurological unit at the time. One interesting footnote in the history of neurology of that period, emanating from both the London and Queen Square, was the Hexagon Club. Symonds, Brain, Riddoch and Cairns were, with Critchley and Denny-Brown, members. In *The Citadel of the Senses* (Oxford: Raven Press, 1986), pp. 109–20, Critchley describes the club: 'The idea was to dine in private somewhere neutral and where the cuisine was above criticism. Rules? We had none. We took turns in alphabetical

order to ventilate some neurological topic of the speaker's choice for 20–30 mins, after which a frank, fierce, but friendly discussion went on well into the night ... Many a paper which eventually found its way into *Brain* had been tried out as an immature unpolished, and tentative contribution to the Hexagon, where it was debated censured and modified ... sometimes the gestation period was so stormy that the foetal version never went to term.' From 1930 to 1939, 30 meetings were held, and minutes were kept. Guests were invited if they were visiting London; and these included Foerster, Lhermitte and Brouwer of Amsterdam. The club met first in the Grand Central Hotel, and then in the fashionable Pagani's restaurant in Great Portland Street. The meetings were stopped by the Second World War when the restaurant was destroyed by aerial bombing. Macdonald Critchley acted as secretary of the club and he arranged preparation of the minutes, and typescripts of lectures, annotated and signed by the presenters, all of which were preserved. These were eventually handsomely bound in half-vellum and blue cloth by the firm of Bumpus, with various letters from guests in manuscript retained. When Critchley's library was dispersed at auction in 2016, following the death of Eileen Critchley, this volume was purchased and the single copy documenting activities of the Hexagon Club is now safe in private ownership. The Hexagon was one of the several clubs which occupied the spare time of some of the Queen Square physicians, including the 'Pants down' club and the 'Ratio' club.

[23] In 1929 the gynaecologist on the staff was Cuthbert Lockyer, the orthopaedic surgeon George Perkins, and the aural surgeons Sydney Scott and Theodore Just.

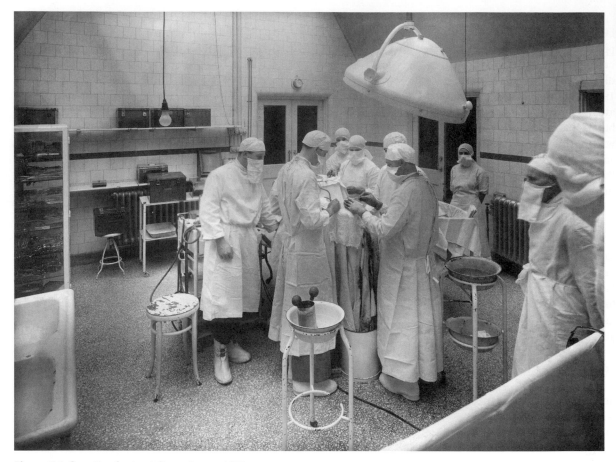

Figure 9.4 Operating theatre at Queen Square, 1935.

Taylor,[24] whom the physicians held in great estseem, was

appointed at Queen Square. Cairns disregarded Taylor on the basis that he was not a specialist.

[24] Julian Taylor was born in London, educated at University College School and trained in medicine at UCH. He was appointed chief assistant to the UCH surgical unit, then gazetted into the RAMC and awarded an OBE for his war services. Having completed his training he was appointed to the consultant staff at UCH and the National Hospital in 1931. He was essentially a general surgeon with an interest in neurosurgery. Trained by Wilfred Trotter, he 'imitated that great man in manner, in outlook, and even in walk. Like Trotter, he took all surgery within his ambit, and has been known to do a brain tumour, a gastrectomy, and a tonsillectomy in the same list'. At the onset of the Second World War he again volunteered for the RAMC, although by then over the age of 50, and was posted to Malaya as Colonel. Like James Bull, he was captured by the Japanese at the fall of Singapore, and was interned in Changi prison for three and a half years where he suffered terrible ordeals. In the camp, he carried out operations with remarkable ingenuity and was said to be an inspiration to the younger men maintaining morale: 'with his wide range of knowledge and

experience he could lecture on English history, French history, the City of London, the tides round the English Coasts and the sailing of small boats, thus relieving the tedium and hopelessness of the situation'. On his return after the war Taylor was so malnourished that he broke both arms. His account is published as chapter 24 in the volume on surgery in the *History of the Second World War, United Kingdom Medical Services* (HMSO 1953) and shows his courage. He was appointed CBE in 1946. He retired from his hospital practice at UCH and the National Hospital in 1954, became vice-president of the Royal College of Surgeons and in 1956 accepted the Chair in surgery in the University of Khartoum, and became a key figure in the development of surgery in the Sudan, a country and whose people he loved. He was a man of outstanding character, and his obituaries celebrate his altruism, bravery and exceptionally high standard of conduct and action. (Details from *Plarr's lives; The Times* 18 and 20 April 1961; *Lancet* (1961) **1**: 952; *Brit med J* 1961, **1**: 1255; *Ann Roy Coll Surg Engl* (1961) **28**: 389).

The failed attempt to appoint Cairns had a chastening effect at Queen Square, and amongst the younger physicians there was increasing discontent over the lack of neurosurgical leadership. Matters came to a head with the intervention of the Rockefeller Foundation, which, in 1933, opened discussions with the National Hospital on awarding a large grant. Alan Gregg and Daniel O'Brien, both strong supporters who had already provided Cairns with significant financial support, indicated that they wished to create a centre for neurosurgery in London that would apply the Cushing method to surgery in Britain, the Empire and Europe, and, through research and practice, develop the subject using his approach. Cushing recommended to the Foundation that they should invest in Cairns, who lobbied hard for the grant to be diverted to the London Hospital. When it was decided that this centre should be at the National Hospital, Gregg envisaged Cairns and Jefferson moving to Queen Square and working with the more forward-looking neurologists – Critchley, Carmichael, Riddoch and Symonds – in creating a world-class neurosurgical centre. This vision was a primary motivation for the Foundation's donation.

Armour retired from Queen Square in 1933, and died unexpectedly the same year, as did Sargent. Now faced with having almost no presence in neurosurgery despite the prospect of the Rockefeller award, the physicians changed tack and agreed that neurosurgery should be revitalised along the Cushing lines.[25] In January 1933, Collier, as chairman of the Medical Committee, again asked Cairns if he would consider moving and taking over Sargent's position; and, in May 1933, the Board of Governors sent formal invitations to Cairns and Jefferson to join the staff. Cairns accepted but stipulated that he would transfer all his cases to the London until suitable facilities were provided at the National Hospital. In the event, he operated on only one patient at Queen Square during his whole appointment. Almost immediately, the London Hospital offered Cairns the post of full honorary surgeon and director of a new department of neurosurgery without any general surgical duties, which Cairns accepted,[26] thereby becoming the first

neurosurgeon in Britain free from any general surgical duties. Jefferson had also just been appointed to the Royal Infirmary in Manchester and was then offered the chair of neurosurgery in 1934. He also decided to use Manchester as his main base, although he did visit Queen Square and operated on two days each month. But neither surgeon was prepared to commit full-time to Queen Square because of the dismissive attitudes of the senior physicians. This spilled out in its most forcible manner in 1945 with a row between Jefferson and Walshe in the pages of the *British Medical Journal*. The Queen Mary wing, including its two new theatre suites and modern neurosurgical facilities, was completed in 1938, and it still seemed possible that Cairns and Jefferson could be persuaded to remain at the National Hospital and develop the subject in line with the expectations of the Rockefeller Foundation, but the coming of the Second World War put paid to these plans and both Cairns and Jefferson resigned their Queen Square practices.

The failure of Queen Square to retain Cairns and Jefferson was a lost opportunity. Each had the potential to transform the hospital into an internationally recognised neurosurgical centre. The vision of the Rockefeller Foundation was not realised, and the course of neurosurgery at the National Hospital took at least two decades to reassert its nineteenth-century prominence. It must represent one of the worst botches in the whole history of the National Hospital. In the event, Harvey Jackson was appointed on Cairns' resignation and served at Queen Square for more than 30 years.[27] A

---

[25] This 'conversion' is evidenced by the note in the Medical Committee for March 1933: 'the medical committee have received with pleasure the Chairman's letter in which he recognises the immense importance of proceeding with the rebuilding of the surgical wing and they desire to impress upon the Board their view that this work should be put in hand with the least possible delay'.

[26] The London Hospital department was the first dedicated neurosurgical department in Britain, and became a well-

known centre, with famous surgical figures working there over the years, including Northfield, Pennybacker, Krayenbühl and Watkins.

[27] Harvey Jackson was educated at the Royal Grammar School in Newcastle upon Tyne, and studied medicine at the Middlesex Hospital Medical School, qualifying in 1923. He was appointed consultant surgeon at Acton Hospital (1930) and West London Hospital (1935), and then spent time in America. On his return, Jackson trained with Percy Sargent and was then appointed as consultant neurosurgeon at the National Hospital, St Thomas' and the Westminster Hospital. He was said to be a technically skilful and conservative surgeon, and was involved with work on orbital tumours, psychosurgery and stereotactic surgery for Parkinson's disease. During the war, he served as director of the Emergency Medical Service Head Injury Unit at Hurstwood Park, Sussex. He was Hunterian Professor at the Royal College of Surgeons in 1947 and 1951, a founding member and later president of the Society of British Neurological Surgeons, and also president of the neurological section of the Royal Society of Medicine. Jackson and McKissock did not get on and

rather unkind, and undeserved, anecdote survives that, although he shared his name with a distinguished neurosurgeon and a neurologist (Harvey Cushing and Hughlings Jackson), he had no characteristics in common with either. In the event, only with the appointment of Wylie McKissock in 1946 did neurosurgery again start to prosper at Queen Square.

Queen Square and Neurosurgery 1939–1945

Once again, all neurosurgery ceased at Queen Square between 1939 and 1946. The main reason was the fact that hospitals in central London were vulnerable to air raids, although, as described in Chapter 5, the obstructive attitude of the physicians in the pre-war period may have played a part, and when, later in the war, the hospital again offered the services of its mothballed theatres, the offer was turned down. Harvey Jackson, his surgical team and its equipment were transferred to Hurstwood Park hospital in Haywards Heath, where the majority of operations were carried out on civilians, mostly dealing with brain and spinal tumours, and the staff played little part in the management of neurosurgical military casualties.[28]

Many members of the medical staff at Queen Square enrolled into either the military or the Emergency Military Services, which took over control of several large mental hospitals of the Metropolitan Asylum Board located in the London suburbs. A head injury neurosurgical unit was established at Leavesden Hospital under the leadership of Wylie McKissock and soon gained an excellent reputation for its work. As a result of the relocation of its staff and surgical facilities, and although its individual surgeons and physicians held prominent roles in the services, as an institution the National Hospital itself played no significant part in the developments in neurology and neurosurgery that occurred during the Second World War.

When the war was over, the tensions of the 1930s relating to the relative prestige of neurology and neurosurgery at the National Hospital still had not gone away.[29] In 1945, a further spat developed involving

Walshe, Symonds, Cairns and Jefferson. A rather benign editorial had been published in the *British Medical Journal* about the 1945 Royal College of Physicians' report on neurology, in which mention was made that the relationship between neurologist and surgeon had not been addressed in the report. Walshe and Symonds responded:

The problem that confronts us is that of harmonizing the roles of physician and surgeon in the field of neurology, and a clue to its rational solution is given in your remark that the neurologist is 'a judge who sums up and advises as to the nature, origins, outcome of an illness, and the disposal of a sick person, and *he is not the purveyor of a particular line of treatment*' (italics ours) ... If we are to take this view of the neurologist's functions and it is impossible to suppose that any less comprehensive view is practicable – certain consequences follow of necessity. The neurologist must be so trained that he is competent to act over the whole field of neurological illness, and, what is not less essential, over the entire range of clinical material that may be referred to him – even though erroneously – as neurological. For no neurologist of experience will dispute that an appreciable proportion of the cases that come under his observation are not neurological in nature, but include many and diverse illnesses, somatic and psychological. He has therefore to be vigilant and reasonably competent over the whole field of medicine if he is to be expert within his own. He has diagnostically to handle neurology and whatever his colleagues may believe to be neurological, whether in fact it is so or not.

If this be a fair and reasonable statement of his position, it is clear that to exclude from his purview all clinical neurological material which investigation may ultimately show to call for surgical intervention is arbitrarily to mutilate his proper field of experience, and to do so upon no scientific basis nor in accord with any nosological categories. Such a mutilation must cripple his competence both as diagnostician and as teacher, and have unfavourable consequences for those who seek his advice as patients. Therefore the preservation of a coherent and complete field of experience is essential, and a condition of his competence within any

---

refused to speak to each other or cooperate in any way. Jackson was popular amongst the neurologists at Queen Square, but disliked by those at St Thomas', who would not refer cases to him, for reasons which are not clear.

[28] John Rees, privately published history of neurosurgery at Hurstwood Park. After the war, Harvey Jackson continued to operate at the Hurstwood Park.

[29] An interesting example of how raw these tensions were is evident in the Medical Committee at the end of 1945, for

which the minutes report that a paper was adopted which formally restated that surgical patients were to be admitted under physicians initially (although it was also accepted that patients could stay under the care of surgeons in the whole post-operative period until discharge, and that surgeons could receive outpatient referrals directly). There was only one surgeon present at the meeting, Harvey Jackson, who was said to have agreed. However, he objected to the minutes, saying they did not reflect the discussion, but his objection was over-ruled.

part of that field. How does the position of the neuro-surgeon compare with that of the neurologist in these respects? Of its nature his is primarily and predominantly a therapeutic specialty, and that this is so is implicit in his training, for he passes directly from the general surgical to the neurosurgical clinic in all but the rarest instances – instances too few to invalidate the statement. He does not undertake a general neurological training, and whatever he may chance to see of what we may call nonsurgical clinical neurology comprises no more than those cases that come into a neurosurgical clinic because someone outside it – in error or in doubt – happens to think them in need of surgical intervention.

The dominance of therapeutic thinking is also reflected in the routine to which these cases are commonly subjected once they enter the neurosurgical clinic. The bulk of the neurosurgeon's non-traumatic cases is made up of space-occupying lesions of one kind or another, and the great ingenuity and skill of the modern neurosurgeon have provided him with a range of diagnostic methods peculiarly his own for the recognition or exclusion of such lesions. These are ventriculography, encephalography, and arteriography, which are indeed amongst the major achievements of modern neurological diagnosis within their proper field. It is therefore not surprising that they should come to constitute the neurosurgeon's diagnostic weapons of choice.

The neurologist, faced by a new case, instinctively asks himself, 'What is the matter with this patient?' and he is prepared to find the answer anywhere within the field of medicine. Whereas the neurosurgeon instinctively asks, 'Has this patient a space-occupying lesion, and where is it?' It can scarcely be maintained that this is an ideal approach, for it carries a tacit assumption which it is neither safe nor reasonable to make as a routine. That upon occasion it has its striking triumphs few would deny, but it remains a method in which far too wide a margin of diagnostic error or failure is implicit – a margin far wider than that of the individual variations in diagnostic acumen possessed by different individuals, be they physicians or surgeons. It leads also, no less inevitably, to the undue use of the particular surgical techniques enumerated and, when these fail to yield relevant information, too often to a negative diagnosis, and to the ultimate handing over of the patient to the neurologist, to whom in such cases – if we are to be perfectly frank – it would have been better to refer him in the first instance.

All this is not to depreciate the importance of the neurosurgeon in the field of neurology. It is simply to indicate that his role is different from that of the physician ... Thus it would appear that, for the present, physician and surgeon have each a proper role, and each a different role, in neurology, and it would be as unreasonable for the physician to claim to be

able to employ surgical techniques without due training and practice as for the surgeon to ask to be accepted as completely equipped to meet the wider range of diagnostic requirements it is the physician's prime duty to acquire.[30]

This was certainly an extraordinarily arrogant letter, but entirely consistent with the general attitude of Queen Square. Walshe, who concurrently was also vehemently attacking the idea of state-run medicine and the dumbing-down of the medical curriculum, and disparaging psychiatrists, was exceeding even his own standards of acerbic rhetoric. To throw into the mix the word 'mutilate' was surely too much. Cairns wrote to Jefferson saying that he had decided not to reply since 'Queen Square has decided to revert to the old practice of admitting all cases under the physicians.'[31] Jefferson, however, with barely suppressed rage, wrote to the *British Medical Journal*, hitting back at the old-fashioned Queen Square attitude that had proved so influential in the decision not to move his practice from Manchester to London.

I must take the letter by Dr FMR Walshe and Dr CP Symonds (Sept. 15, p. 364), who will always be heard with respect, as an invitation to express my own views, even though time proves that they do not coincide with the consensus of my brethren.

Your correspondents are concerned about an ideological concept of the neurologist, but since this does not admit of realistic treatment they resolve the problem into a statement of the relative function and required training of the medical neurologist and the neurosurgeon. They regret that the medical neurologist has lost too much valuable clinical material to the latter, and believe that this stunts the growth of the physician.

It is a fact that the neurological physician no longer sees each and every case of suspected brain tumour before it goes to the surgeon, as was the custom in former days. It needs little imagination to comprehend that this is disappointing to the physician, but it has happened in many branches of medicine and is a sign of (at least) commencing maturity.

What Dr Walshe and Dr Symonds do not say is that the state of affairs which causes them anxiety has not been brought about as the result of a deliberate policy of exclusion laid down, or likely to be laid

---

[30] F. M. R. Walshe and C. P. Symonds, 'Neurologist and Neurosurgeon', *British Medical Journal* 2 (1945): 364. It has been said that the instigator of this letter was Walshe and that Symonds later regretted being a signatory.

[31] P. Schurr 'So That Was Life: A Biography of Sir Geoffrey Jefferson, Master of the Neurosciences and Man of Letters'. London: RSM Press, 1997.

down, by neurosurgeons, but has occurred as a natural process which needs a new adjustment – that of partnership.

I am well aware that the emancipation which the neurosurgeon now enjoys carries with it heavy responsibilities. He is called upon to make the greatest contribution that he can to our knowledge of the nervous system (for which he has exceptional opportunities), and, more important from the humanitarian point of view, to avoid the infliction of unnecessary trauma … The lodestone that draws the surgeon into neurosurgery is not surgical technique but neurology. We must do our utmost to see that the younger generation has a balanced training and adequate remuneration to enable a man to obtain it, a vital condition on which many planners are silent. I know from a long personal experience that a happy relationship, mutually educative, to say nothing of friendship, between the medical and surgical subdivisions of neurology is possible, and is, moreover, already exemplified in many neurological centres in this country – and elsewhere. Any further schism, if such it be, will be prevented by the development of Regional Neurological Institutes with common laboratories and services, such as is planned for

Manchester. No good will come of repressive action in which one branch seeks to dominate the other.[32]

Politically, the letter from Walshe and Symonds was badly timed because Cairns, then president of the Society of British Neurosurgeons, was at that moment in discussion with the Department of Health about the training of neurosurgeons. Details of the programme eventually accepted were drafted by Cairns and Jefferson, and it was clear that the surgeons were no longer prepared to function as hand-maidens of the neurologists, whatever Walshe might think. Furthermore, neurosurgical leadership in the country, which had once emanated from Queen Square, had moved to provincial centres during the Second World War and, as far as Cairns was concerned, there it was going to remain. The argument over admission rights lingered on for years, although belatedly the surgeons at Queen Square were granted independence from physicians. Ironically, in 1990, when the name of the hospital changed to the 'National Hospital for Neurology and Neurosurgery', one senses that the old argument was one factor in the insistence by Lindsay Symon upon having neurosurgery inserted into the title.

Sir Wylie McKissock and the Renewal of Neurosurgery at the National Hospital: 1946–1965

The return of neurosurgery to the National Hospital in 1946 was of great significance, not least since the experience of war had convinced the hospital that the surgical facilities must be improved. The two neurosurgeons, Julian Taylor who had returned from active service, and Harvey Jackson who had moved back from Haywards Heath,[33] resumed operating at Queen Square, and they were joined by Wylie McKissock in 1946.[34] They had a re-equipped theatre and a ward of

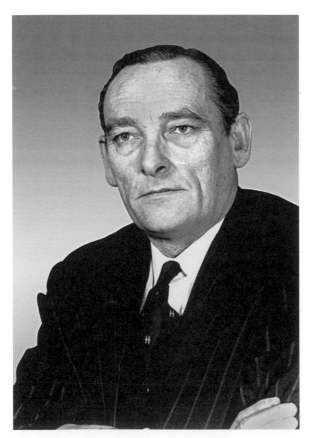

Figure 9.5 Wylie McKissock.

[32] Jefferson, 'Neurologist and Neurosurgeon', *British Medical Journal* 2 (1945): 473.

[33] Although he continued also to operate there during the rest of his career.

[34] Sir Wylie McKissock was born in Staines, educated at the City of London School, and studied medicine at King's College and St George's Hospital Medical School, from where he qualified in 1931. He began his career in neurosurgery in 1934 as a registrar at Maida Vale Hospital and, in 1936, spent a formative period visiting the unit of Herbert Olivecrona in Sweden. Later that year, McKissock was appointed to the staff of Maida Vale Hospital, and in 1937 he won a Rockefeller Foundation Fellowship to visit units in the USA. In 1939, he was appointed as the first paediatric neurosurgeon at the Hospital for Sick Children, Great

15 or 16 beds in the Queen Mary wing, as well as use of Ward 15 jointly with the physicians. Several junior surgical staff were resident within the hospital,[35] and a new anaesthetist, Dr Aserman, was appointed to join R. A. Beaver. The equipment loaned to the Ministry was also returned. Surgical activity increased rapidly, so that, in 1950–1, 858 operations were carried out, of which 423 were 'of a major cranial or spinal nature'. Most procedures dealt with tumours, but there were also an increasing number of operations on cerebral aneurysms and an interest in psychosurgery that achieved some notoriety. Of these three surgeons, it was undoubtedly Wylie McKissock who was the driving force behind the postwar renewal of interest in neurosurgery at the National Hospital.

McKissock was a man with manic energy and a prodigious work output, whose interest moved from wartime practice in head trauma to psychosurgery, epilepsy surgery, focal radiosurgery for tumours and cerebrovascular surgery. He performed large numbers of operations for each condition, all carried out extremely quickly. His focus on any one branch of surgery was sometimes short-lived once another attracted his attention. Happiest in the operating theatre, McKissock spent rather little time talking to patients (in contrast to his successor Valentine Logue), considering himself to be 'a man of action not words'. Although entitled to admit cases to Queen Square, he preferred to use

Atkinson Morley Hospital, soon the largest neurosurgical unit in Britain at that time, and which McKissock always regarded as his natural base, no doubt finding the freedom of the smaller hospital and the unopposed clinical command more to his taste. Anthony Bell, a trainee under McKissock, described a typical day:

> The ventriculograms and the previous day's angiograms were taken to McKissock's office where they would be examined through a cloud of cigar smoke which every now and again would be wafted away with a vigorous gesture when visibility was threatened. By 10.00 am the order of the operating list was determined, McKissock would have had coffee in the surgeons' room, exchanged greetings and news with his colleagues, and be ready to start the list. Away from the rest of the staff he changed alone in the sister's office, and emerged in white trousers and a Harvey Cushing-style wrap around white shirt which bore no visible means of fastening so that strips of white elastoplast were used for this purpose … He refined his neurosurgical technique until his operating time for a major craniotomy was under 2h, achieving this by economy both of movement and of the number of instruments used. He frequently enjoyed the sense of disbelief of visiting neurosurgeons who saw four craniotomies completed by 5 pm, when in their own units one craniotomy would have taken all day. Watching him operate gave no impression of haste, onlookers were caught up in the action and swept along at almost mesmeric pace, and it was only when the clock was checked that the speed of his surgery was realized … His theatre was a haven of silence and order no matter what was happening in the rest of the hospital and this contributed to his trainees' sense of awe. He demanded meticulous postoperative care and each patient undergoing major surgery had constant nursing care for at least 24h. McKissock was perfectly capable of carrying out four or five craniotomies in a day plus a laminectomy or two and in order to do this he would open the first case which the first assistant would close and then join him for the second case in sequence.[36]

Psychosurgery, a particular feature of his work from the 1940s, provides a good example of McKissock's surgical approach. Prefrontal leucotomy and its variants were attracting considerable interest, stimulated by Fulton's advocacy and the fashion for this operation in America. McKissock carried out his first case in 1941,

---

Ormond Street, but the Second World War then intervened. His application for active service was refused on health grounds, and McKissock was appointed surgeon-in-charge of the head injury treatment centre at Leavesden Hospital. In 1941, the unit was moved to Atkinson Morley Hospital in Wimbledon. This was intended as a temporary measure but McKissock remained as the neurosurgeon at Atkinson Morley for the rest of his career, apart from a brief period when the unit relocated to a hutted hospital in Bath because of air raids in Wimbledon. He was awarded an OBE in 1946 for his war service. In addition to Queen Square, Great Ormond Street, Atkinson Morley and St George's, McKissock was also appointed to the Metropolitan Ear Nose and Throat Hospital (London), St Andrew's Hospital (Northampton), Graylingwell Hospital (Chichester), St James' Hospital (Portsmouth), Park Prewett Hospital (Basingstoke), the Welsh Regional Hospital Board and the Royal Air Force. He was knighted for his services to neurosurgery in 1971, the year in which he retired.

[35] A minute for the Medical Committee in 1946 reports that approval was given to the surgical registrar (Dr Schwatzwald) to live outside the hospital 'due to exceptional circumstances, and on the understanding that this did not create a precedent'. (NB: the spelling of 'Dr Schwarzwald/Swarzwald' differs in the Medical Committee and Board minutes.)

[36] See B. A. Bell, 'Wylie McKissock – Reminiscences of a Commanding Figure in British Neurosurgery', *British Journal of Neurosurgery* **10** (1996): 9–18. Anthony Bell was later himself appointed the first professor of neurosurgery at St George's and the Atkinson Morley Hospital.

and became quickly convinced of its benefits. He adopted the Freeman–Watts technique and became a most prolific leucotomist, touring the country and operating in many hospitals. As he wrote: 'This is not a time-consuming operation. A competent team in a well-organised mental hospital can do four such operations in 2–2½ hours. The actual bilateral prefrontal leucotomy can be done by a properly trained neurosurgeon in six minutes and seldom takes more than ten minutes.'[37]

McKissock developed his own variant, rostral leucotomy, in 1948, because he judged that the trans-orbital approach contravened aseptic surgical principles, and also because the undercutting was less extensive, resulting in fewer adverse effects on personality. By the mid-1950s, he had personally carried out more than 3,000 operations. That he was in demand can be seen from the Board of Governors' minutes at Queen Square, which granted him study leave for one week in 1967 to perform leucotomies for the Maltese government.[38] In time, his enthusiasm for this operation waned, perhaps because of mounting public and professional criticism, and the rostral approach was then seldom practised.[39] This was a period when neurosurgery, and even psychosurgery, could be performed experimentally without much ethical oversight. An interesting example was the study of prefrontal leucotomy performed for severe tinnitus. The Institute of Neurology annual report noted: 'In a small series of patients he found the results very encouraging. He pointed out that no patient became free from tinnitus but all were able to adjust better to the noises. Though some patients were loath to admit improvement the relatives clearly noted that the patient became less concerned with the tinnitus.'

With John Bates, McKissock also explored the effects of hemispherectomy for severe epilepsy associated with infantile hemiplegia and, by 1952, more than 40 cases had been treated. They were investigated peri-

operatively by Bates, with corticography and stimulation. Bates' main interest was in the opportunity this operation offered for the study of human physiology and he published important papers on this topic.[40] In 1952, McKissock was one of the first in the world to initiate a series of temporal lobectomies,[41] and wrote rather presciently, although this seems not to have been an argument he applied to prefrontal leucotomy: 'In this type of surgery it is wise to have a reasonably large series of well documented cases backed by a follow up period of several years before making any pronouncements on the relative merits of surgical and conservative forms of treatment. Several more years of work in this field are yet required.'[42]

This influenced Murray Falconer, who developed a specialist service at the Maudsley Hospital and became Britain's leading epilepsy surgeon.[43] Then, in the late 1950s, McKissock's attention turned to neurovascular surgery. Between 1958 and 1961, his personal collection included over 780 cases of ruptured aneurysm, and over 200 of intracranial haemorrhage. McKissock was also by then looking at the stereotactic implantation of radioactive gold seeds for the treatment of glioma. With Harvey Jackson, he assessed the effects of ablation within the globus pallidus in the treatment of Parkinson's disease. By the early 1960s, there was no mention of epilepsy surgery or prefrontal leucotomy in McKissock's clinical and research portfolio, as he moved on to other fields. McKissock's drive resuscitated neurosurgery at Queen Square, and John Garfield, one of his early trainees, recalls that period:

> McKissock had a foot in the door of the establishment through working at Maida Vale, Great Ormond Street and St George's before establishing his own neurosurgical department, first at Leavesden Emergency Hospital before this was moved to the Atkinson Morley's. One must not underestimate the natural

[37] W. McKissock, 'Rostral Leucotomy', *Lancet* **258** (1951): 91–4.

[38] The operation had then become extremely popular, and, in Britain between 1948 and 1952, 7,225 leucotomies were carried out according to a note in the public record office in response to a question in Parliament: see R. Barrett, 'Manhandling the Brain', lecture at the annual meeting of the Faculty of Neuropsychiatry, Royal College of Psychiatrists, 10 September 2015.

[39] See D. Kelly *et al.*, 'Modified Leucotomy Assessed Clinically, Physiologically and Psychologically at 6 Weeks and 18 Months', *British Journal of Psychiatry* **120** (1972): 19. Desmond Kelly was a psychiatrist at St George's Hospital and an authority on psychosurgery.

[40] See, for instance, J. Bates, 'Stimulation of the Medial Surface of the Human Cerebral Hemisphere After Hemispherectomy', *Brain* **76** (1953): 405–47.

[41] McKissock's contribution to this operation has been largely overlooked in the many historical reviews of the topic, but was significant.

[42] Institute of Neurology annual report 1952–3.

[43] Murray Alexander Falconer was a New Zealander, trained in Dunedin and in Oxford (by Cairns), and promoted by Symonds for the post at Guy's, where he had a distinguished career as consultant neurosurgeon from 1949 to 1975: see P. F. Bladin, 'Murray Alexander Falconer and the Guy's-Maudsley Hospital Seizure Surgery Program', *Journal of Clinical Neuroscience* **11** (2004): 577–83.

desire to out-do the established centres, their tendency to chauvinism and self-aggrandisement, and resentment of challenge from centres outside central London. Neurosurgery could by-pass this resentment, and it had a certain freedom to develop in its own way.

In 1946 there were two neurosurgical teams at Queen Square; one led by Wylie McKissock and the other by Harvey Jackson. The relationship was such that the teams only met in the residents' mess – a hangover from the days of great competition in building up surgical practices. The notion of a cohesive joint department of neurosurgery simply did not arise. McKissock's only interest in his colleague lay in finding out from his juniors how long the other's operations were taking, compared to his own reputation for speed and less blood loss. Of the neurologists, Denis Williams and Swithin Meadows were the two with whom McKissock most often dealt. Lawrence 'Tickey' Walsh from Atkinson Morley's would also operate during McKissock's lists, especially on patients with Parkinson's disease. Most of the pre-operative contact was done by Denis Williams explaining to the patient where Mr Walsh would place the burr hole – Walsh being the technician instructed and guided by the great neurologist.[44]

McKissock rarely appeared other than for operating sessions. He very rarely entered his own, let alone the neurology wards. The neurosurgery ward was mainly filled with routine neurosurgical cases from the elective Atkinson Morley admission list, operated upon by the senior registrar. Referrals from within the National were somewhat different. The route might be through a neurologist's specific request – 'refer to Mr McKissock' – or via the junior staff. An important link was through McKissock's secretary, June Marson, who received all telephone calls and was often his eyes and ears as the neurologist knew well. Her instant

availability did much to bolster neurosurgical practice especially from within Queen Square, as did the theatre sister, Barbara Tell. The resident medical officer was an important line of communication and he certainly was entitled to an audience with McKissock. Very rarely would a neurologist appear in the office. The impression gained was that surgeons were of a lower stratum, servants of the neurologists, to be reluctantly called upon when action had to be taken and more needed than the usual brilliant diagnosis and prognostic pronouncements. The only exception to this style came from Swithin Meadows. Occasionally, the selection of a particular neurosurgeon was countermanded by the neurologist so that all major or difficult problems came to McKissock. The only exception was pituitaries which went to Harvey Jackson.[45]

When he arrived at the National Hospital, there was virtually no surgical research, but McKissock rekindled the academic tradition for neurosurgery which had largely been in abeyance after Horsley's death. He brought rigorous documentation and the routine use of investigations to research in neurosurgery. The involvement with neuroradiology dated from his time in Sweden, where he met Eric Lysholm, a 'strange little man who would be sent for by Herbert Olivecrona to come up to theatre'. This interest in the new science of neuroradiology served McKissock well. He pioneered ultrasound and isotope scanning and, with James Ambrose, was the first clinician to see the potential for computerised tomography scanning. Having met Sir Godfrey Hounsfield, plans were laid under McKissock's influence for the installation of the world's first CT scanner at Atkinson Morley Hospital (now in the Science Museum in London) but he retired just before the initial images were produced in 1971. Again, John Garfield comments:

> McKissock challenged the establishment and conducted research. This was essentially clinical and dependent upon a large intake of patients from a wide region, coupled with the existence of a single unit in which policies of management could be planned. Up to the end of the war, any meaningful research in neurology – and especially clinical neurology – had been largely confined to Queen Square where almost every neurologist had been trained. In a curious way, neurosurgeons were better able to challenge the neurological establishment than were obedient neurologists. There were no competing interests and, at least in the early years, no separation of patients under the care of different consultants. Thus protocols

---

[44] Lawrence Sutcliffe Walsh was born in East London, South Africa, educated at Selbourne College and graduated from Cape Town University. He came to England in 1947 and was house surgeon to Hamilton Bailey, and then to Wylie McKissock at the National Hospital. He spent some time in Stockholm training in stereotactic surgery. Walsh was appointed consultant neurosurgeon at Atkinson Morley Hospital in 1957, and in 1965 to the National Hospital and St Mary's Hospital. His specialist areas were in stereotactic surgery, especially for Parkinson's disease, radioactive implants for pituitary tumours and craniopharyngioma, and cerebrovascular disease. He retired early in 1981, due to respiratory problems, for which he needed supplementary oxygen, and suffered increasing disability until his death in 1986. Of diminutive stature, Walshe was also known as 'Tickey' after the small South African threepenny coin, and was a skilled neurosurgeon well liked by his colleagues. One of his sons, Richard Walsh, also became a distinguished neurosurgeon.

[45] John Garfield, personal communications.

were easily established and, once agreed, strictly followed. This principle enabled efficacy to be assessed and the emphasis was upon management rather than surgical outcome. The great multicentre subarachnoid haemorrhage (aneurysm) trials demonstrated this approach to perfection; they required considerable courage especially in the early stages when mortality following surgery could be very high. Once a trial had been approved a very careful statistical validation system was in operation; the trial was stopped as soon as the advantage of one arm of treatment was shown to be more effective and statistically verified. Virtually no patients were treated without strict randomization. There was no real opportunity for objection by referring physicians who were usually only too glad to have their patents admitted without delay. Previously, all patients with a ruptured aneurysm went straight to theatre from X-ray; sadly with very high mortality.

All this was made possible through the background and origins of the unit, and above all upon the determination of McKissock. He felt – rightly – that without such organisation and control the best course of management could never be established. Also there had to be unity of pre-operative and post-operative care, and standardized surgical methods in theatre were all part of the 'diktat'. Another essential factor which made the work possible was a superb system of clinical notes which were typed immediately by a secretary on each ward from tapes dictated by the housemen. One of the secretaries was McKissock's daughter, Araminta. The results of investigations including radiology and all correspondence were pasted into the notes chronologically with any follow-up notes. A complete copy went back to the referring hospital with the patient. McKissock felt so strongly about notes that in the very early days he typed them himself. This was another mark of his demand for highest standards.

Another feature of McKissock's success was the application of advances in neuroradiology learned in Sweden. The neuroradiologists were very much an intrinsic part of the neurosurgical team, and the relationship was very close. It was never called a 'department' of neuroradiology, it was one team. Thus, ultrasound was used to detect shift of the midline and extracranial lesions; and operations were done on this basis especially in head injury. Similarly isotope scanning was used as the safe investigation of mass lesions, such as meningioma, glioma and abscess. Operation was done without any other radiology. Although not strictly research, these attitudes certainly bolstered the standing of neurosurgery in the evolution of neuroscience and the methods could be used on large numbers of patients. With its concentration of neurosurgical material, the unit had a great opportunity for co-operation with other specialties –

especially ENT (otology). The experience of acoustic Schwannomas was considerable, and the ENT surgeons from St George's often appeared in theatre, as did the ophthalmologists. In neuropsychiatry, leucotomy 'in-house' was a considerable banner to be waved widely, and brought a certain fame to the department.

Valentine Logue and the Gough-Cooper Bequest

McKissock may have encouraged the rise of neurosurgical research at the National Hospital, but the greatest stimulus to change was the establishment of an academic unit by McKissock's trainee Valentine Darte Logue.[46] Logue had trained initially as a general surgeon but moved to McKissock's service at Atkinson Morley Hospital to learn neurosurgery, and went with McKissock when the unit was moved to Bath, where

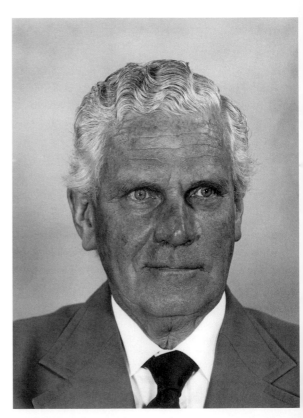

Figure 9.6 Valentine Logue.

---

[46] Valentine Darte Logue was born in Perth, Western Australia, with Scottish ancestry, and came to London in 1922, where, like McKissock, he trained in medicine at King's College and St George's Hospital, qualifying in 1936.

he remained for a while after others had returned to London. Logue then served in the Far East, and returned to Atkinson Morley Hospital to rejoin McKissock at the end of the war. In 1948, he was appointed consultant neurosurgeon at Atkinson Morley (until 1957, when he transferred to the Middlesex Hospital) and Maida Vale Hospital. At Maida Vale, he was the first surgeon to be given admitting rights, and on his arrival a new operating theatre was built to his design and a large ward provided for his patients. He operated there until 1965, despite having rights at Queen Square, largely because he liked the more relaxed and indulgent atmosphere of the smaller hospital.[47] In 1965, however, he was awarded a personal professorship, and Logue moved his work to Queen Square to found the academic unit. Despite their background and friendship, the two neurosurgical units – McKissock's department of neurosurgery and Logue's department of neurological studies – worked in almost complete isolation.

In August 1975, following a bequest from the Gough-Cooper family, the university department of neurosurgery was established with Logue appointed to the foundation professorship. Harry Gough-Cooper was a household name in the UK and South Africa after the Second World War. Starting from very modest beginnings, he built up a successful company making well-built affordable houses 'for the average man to buy'. In 1951, he developed severe pain in his back and difficulty walking. Over the next 15 years, he had fluctuating recurrences and, in 1969, consulted Allan Bird in Johannesburg, who found cord compression. Gough-Cooper was transferred to the care of Denis Williams in London. Exploratory operations were carried out but the nature of the illness escaped diagnosis until July 1972 when it was confirmed on bone marrow examination that he had a reticulum cell sarcoma. This proved untreatable and his condition slowly worsened. Denis Williams had founded the Brain Research Trust in 1971 as a charity devoted to funding research at the Institute of Neurology,[48] and he brokered the bequest of £300,000 from Gough-Cooper, who knew he was dying and

generously decided that his company would endow the professorship of neurosurgery.[49]

On taking up the professorship, Logue relinquished his private practice (a sacrifice not made by many neurosurgeons), resigned from the Middlesex Hospital, and devoted his time to academic work at Queen Square. His clinical work was meticulous and he was the 'neurologist's neurosurgeon', spending a great deal of time taking a history from his patients and performing the clinical examination. He was a fellow of both the Royal Colleges of Physicians and of Surgeons, a rare feat which emphasised his neurological as well as neurosurgical expertise. Logue had a major interest in cerebrovascular disease and spinal arterio-venous malformations. He made various significant contributions to neurosurgery. He developed the 'Logue' procedure for treating ruptured anterior communicating artery aneurysms and made various important studies of intracranial pressure. He was also renowned for work on cranio-cervical dysplasia, arterio-venous malformations of the spinal cord, Chiari malformations and syringomyelia. He collaborated with Martin Halliday on measuring evoked potentials from the thalamus in patients with Parkinson's disease undergoing stereotactic surgical therapy. Logue evaluated results of the Cloward procedure compared to posterior laminectomy for cervical spondylosis, and operation for the treatment of acoustic neuroma. He accumulated a very large series of meningiomas, most of which he operated on personally, and was scrupulous in documenting and describing the outcomes of surgery. Towards the end of his career, the operating microscope was introduced and Logue delighted in exploring its potential, despite the fact that this technical advance was going to render redundant much of the neurosurgical technique he had so painstakingly developed.

Valentine Logue was the first of McKissock's trainees to develop an international reputation and carve out an independent career, thereby helping to restore the status of Queen Square (and indeed of Britain) in the field of neurosurgery. He was also a renowned teacher and will be remembered for his advocacy of the place of research in the training of young neurosurgeons, and

---

[47] See M. Powell and N. Kitchen, 'The Development of Neurosurgery at the National Hospital for Neurology and Neurosurgery, Queen Square, London England', *Neurosurgery* **61** (2007): 1077–90.
[48] Williams was the driving force behind the charity, and spent much time and energy fund-raising on its behalf. He did so altruistically, purely for the benefit of the Institute of Neurology, and had neither personal research ambitions nor clinical interests that might benefit from the charity funds.

[49] Gough-Cooper's condition deteriorated progressively. By 1973, he had lost all feeling in the legs, his memory was affected and his speech slowed. He was treated by deep X-ray therapy but by the end of 1973 was in an akinetic mute state. Lawrence Walsh inserted a ventriculo-atrial shunt in February 1974 but without improvement, and Gough-Cooper died on 27 February 1975 (information from Harry's daughter Jennifer Gough-Cooper, who is writing a memoir about her father).

many of his trainees became major figures in the next generation of British neurosurgeons. Logue was a shy man, made president of the Society of British Neurological Surgeons in 1974, played an active role in the development of the European Association of Neurological Surgeons, and held many other honours. Although he was a workaholic who spent long hours in theatre and on the wards, Logue absented himself completely from the hospital on retirement in August 1977, and never returned. In his obituary of Logue for the World Federation of Neurology, Lindsay Symon, his successor, wrote:

> He was himself a meticulous and careful surgeon, notable not only for superb operative technique, but also for the care which he lavished on the preoperative assessment of his patients and on their postoperative care. Not for him the view from the end of the bed, he was a neurologist of magnificence, whose examination would often reveal nuances which had escaped others.

Neurosurgery at Queen Square after 1965

After seven years at Atkinson Morley Hospital as McKissock's assistant, Lawrence ('Tickey') Walsh was appointed consultant neurosurgeon at the National Hospital in 1965 on Jackson's retirement. McKissock retired in 1971 and was succeeded by Norman Grant, another of his trainees, who also worked at the Hospital for Sick Children, Great Ormond Street. Walsh and Grant were employed by the hospital and formed the NHS department of neurosurgery, which conducted its business entirely separate from the academic department headed by Valentine Logue and then Lindsay Symon. Each department had its own catchment area in London, and also nationally and internationally. Neither Walsh nor Grant contributed much to research, but each provided a good clinical service and was trusted and admired by the new generation of physicians. In 1978, Alan Crockard was appointed to join them, and, in 1980, Walsh retired and was replaced by Richard Hayward. At this stage, it was reported that about 500 patients a year were admitted into the 21 beds in the department of neurosurgery. By 1985, Crockard was specialising in skull base and spinal surgery, and the department was expanded with the appointment of Michael Powell in 1985. Although he focused initially mainly on spinal work, Powell developed a special interest in pituitary surgery. Grant retired from the hospital in 1990, and Hayward took up a larger commitment in paediatric neurosurgery at Great Ormond Street, but retained an appointment at

the National Hospital until 1994 when he stopped all adult neurosurgery. In 1991, the team was joined by Mr William Harkness, who was appointed to expand the epilepsy surgery work started by David Thomas at Queen Square and also at Great Ormond Street. In 1993, with closure of Maida Vale, Harkness, Hayward and Crockard formed a new department of surgical neurology based entirely at Queen Square.[50]

A major change in academic neurosurgery was the arrival of Lindsay Symon.[51] He had been appointed to the National Hospitals in 1965, the year in which Logue moved to an academic post at Queen Square, and based his work largely at Maida Vale before taking up the Gough-Cooper professorship on Logue's retirement in 1977. On Symon's departure from Maida Vale, his beds were used by David Thomas and Alan Crockard, but, with the closure of Maida Vale in 1993, the entire neurosurgical practice moved to Queen Square. Lindsay Symon was Logue's most brilliant trainee, and, under his direction, the department expanded its interest in cerebrovascular disease with laboratory and experimental work on cerebral ischaemia and on subarachnoid haemorrhage. The experimental work was carried out largely on baboons, and important advances made in relation to blood flow, ischaemia and cerebral oedema. David Thomas was appointed as senior lecturer and consultant neurosurgeon in 1976. His research was focused initially on neuro-oncology but then extended to stereotaxy, functional neurosurgery and (in the 1990s) epilepsy surgery. Throughout the 1980s and 1990s, with Symon and Thomas as the two senior clinicians, and the non-clinical senior lecturer Neil Branston, the department produced between 40 and 90 research publications each year. David Thomas became head of department, with Branston as reader and two new clinical senior lecturers (Neil Kitchen and James Palmer) by the time Symon retired in 1995. The work on vascular surgery and head trauma was

---

[50] Crockard was initially appointed to the academic department but in 1980 formed what was in effect a second hospital department of neurosurgery. He also set up the surgical skills teaching facility at the Royal College of Surgeons, and from 1997 to 2000 was appointed director of education at the College. He retired from Queen Square in 2006 to work as national director of Modernising Medical Careers, a move that may not have brought unbridled satisfaction to him or young trainees in medicine.

[51] In line with editorial policy in this book, biographical aspects and detailed analysis of the work of living persons are not discussed. But it should be mentioned here that both Professor Lindsay Symon and Professor David Thomas were outstanding researchers.

continued by Kitchen, Palmer and Branston. During these years, neurosurgery at Queen Square again became internationally renowned. Lindsay Symon was appointed president of the World Federation of Neurosurgical Societies, with both he and David Thomas each prominent on the international stage.

The Contribution of Queen Square Neurologists and Neurosurgeons in War

Many of the National Hospital staff and alumni served with distinction in the two World Wars, but, gazetted into the British military across the world, their clinical and research work was remote and not at the hospital. The technical surgical advances of the period were primarily in the fields of trauma to the head, spine and peripheral nerves, but the evolution of wartime neurosurgery was also of significance by stimulating the growth of neurosurgery away from the National Hospital. The wartime experience of surgical specialisation and organisation proved to be an experiment that set the pattern for the postwar development of regional centres of neurosurgery and neurology.

In the First and Second World Wars, the neurology of trauma advanced, much as it had done earlier in the American Civil War with the work of Silas Weir Mitchell.[52] However, the twentieth century saw the mechanisation of war, advances in the manufacture of armaments, and their liberal use resulting in injuries on a scale that had not previously been encountered. It has been calculated, on best estimates (although accurate figures are difficult to derive) that the First World War resulted in over 17 million deaths and 20 million wounded, including over 900,000 military deaths from the British and Empire forces. In the Second World War, the number killed is estimated to be over 60 million (more than 3 per cent of the 1939 world population) with 400,000 military deaths in the British and Empire forces.

In both World Wars, in contrast to earlier conflicts, more of the casualties were from bombs and blast injuries rather than bullets. The head and the spinal cord were particularly vulnerable. New types of injury were encountered, for instance the so-called gutter injury of trench warfare in the First World War. Many limbs were severed or required amputation, leading to a high rate of subsequent phantom limb and causalgia. In the pre-antibiotic era, infection was a major cause of death in the weeks following injury. Entirely new concepts of managing trauma were required: Henry Head considered that the First World War changed medicine by shaking the belief in reliance on diagnostic labels, 'anodynes to the conscience that explained nothing and put to sleep the need for further thought and investigation'. He derided 'penny-in-the-slot' medicine that confused diagnosis with naming. Rather, he saw war as having liberated ideas in line with the Jacksonian concept of evolutionary organisation within the nervous system.[53]

The Organisation of Neurological and Neurosurgical Care

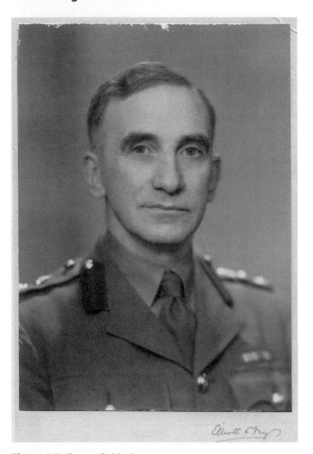

Figure 9.7 George Riddoch.

---

[52] It was at the request of William Hammond, surgeon-general of the US Army that, in 1863, Weir Mitchell and George Morehouse established a 400-bed hospital at Christian Street (moving, later, to Turner's Lane) in Philadelphia, to which was referred 'a vast collection of wounds and contusions of nerves including all the rarest forms of nerve lesion of almost every great nerve in the human body' suffered during the American Civil War.

[53] See I. S. Jacyna, *Medicine and Modernism: A Biography of Sir Henry Head* (London: Pickering and Chatto, 2008).

In the First World War, there were few advanced preparations for dealing with military casualties, and the organisation of neurological care evolved, but in a chaotic fashion. Medical responsibility for the military lay mainly with the RAMC. Soldiers injured at the front were removed by stretcher-bearers to the regimental aid post, then taken by stretcher to an advanced dressing station near the front line and, if required to be removed from the battlefield, transported by wagon, motor or horse ambulance to a casualty clearing station. These were basic hospitals, often in requisitioned houses, chateaux, barns or tents, behind the lines, where acute surgery was sometimes carried out, including amputation or wound debridement. Seriously ill individuals were moved by barge, train or motor vehicles to a 'stationary' or 'general' hospital, usually arranged according to nationality. In France, large British hospitals were situated in Wimereux, Étaples and Boulogne. Where necessary, the injured were repatriated to Britain, by hospital boat or ambulance train. These tortuous journeys added to the already considerable morbidity. Senior staff from Queen Square working in the military during the First World War were based in the stationary hospitals (Holmes and Sargent, for instance, in Hospital No. 13 in Boulogne) or, if still in Britain, in one of the large number of small military hospitals in London. Horsley did not operate but was very active in administrative roles, touring several battlefronts and inspecting the medical facilities, such as that in Mesopotamia where he died.

In the Second World War, the country was very much better prepared for neurological injuries. Neurosurgery was organised in an impressive and highly effective manner, which had profound consequences not only for injured soldiers at the time, but also for the postwar development of neurology and neurosurgery in the country. On the battlefront, an effective system of hospitals and special units was established, and a faster system of evacuation to large stationary hospitals, and then to Britain, often by air, put in place. One innovation was the establishment of mobile neurosurgical units travelling just behind the front lines. At home, the Emergency Medical Service (EMS) arranged care on a sector basis, providing a rapid triage system for serious civilian injuries. This proved highly efficient and was a much admired model of care. The neurosurgical unit set up at Haywards Heath and the head injury units at Leavesdon and Atkinson Morley Hospital were very

successful parts of this scheme. Many Queen Square medical and nursing staff were redeployed to these units during the war. The effective organisation of neurological and neurosurgical services, both in the war-zones and at home, was to a significant degree due to the work of people associated with Queen Square, in particular Riddoch, Symonds, Cairns and Jefferson.

In parallel with these arrangements, a series of 12 remarkable Special Neurosurgical Centres for the treatment of head and spinal injury was established between 1939 and 1944. These included the facilities at St Hugh's in Oxford and at Stoke Mandeville. London was avoided because of the constant risk of air raids, and so Queen Square was excluded from this arrangement. Jefferson mentions that the 'famous National Hospital, Queen Square, was closed for surgery, and was hit and burned by incendiaries … but otherwise it remains [at the time of writing] intact, and its staff unhurt'.

By 1943, 5,638 cases had been managed at these specialised centres and an analysis of 3,045 admissions to six centres showed that 50 per cent were primarily for head trauma, 7 per cent for spinal cord injury, and 3 per cent for peripheral nerve lesions. Arrangements were made for quick evacuation to the centres for the rapid treatment of open and closed injuries, and then onward rehabilitation.

The Medical Research Council formed influential committees to consider the treatment of neurological injury. The committee on head injury was established in 1940 under the chairmanship of Adrian, and with Cairns, Jefferson, Riddoch and Symonds amongst its members. It produced a glossary of terms and programmes of research, and much useful clinical guidance. The committee on spinal and nerve injury was chaired by Riddoch and produced expert guidance for urgent therapy and rehabilitation.

A word here is appropriate about George Riddoch.[54] He has been called the forgotten man of British neurology, and there is a certain truth in this, since he was profoundly influential in both World Wars and the years between. Born in Keith, Banffshire, he was educated at Gordon's College Aberdeen and then Aberdeen University, from where he qualified in 1913. He was house physician

---

[54] J. R. Silver and M.-F. Weiner, 'George Riddoch: The Man Who Found Ludwig Guttmann', *Spinal Cord* **50** (2012): 83–93; G. Storey, 'George Riddoch (1888–1947)', *Journal of Medical Biography* **18** (2010): 35-7.

at the West End Hospital and was then put in charge of injured patients in the Empire Hospital for officers, Vincent Square, during the First World War. There he carried out work which greatly advanced the understanding and clinical management of spinal injuries. After that war, he was appointed with assistance from the MRC as physician to the medical unit at the London Hospital, working with Head, and, from 1919, also as assistant physician to Maida Vale Hospital. In 1924, he was given the post of supernumerary assistant physician at the London, resigned from Maida Vale, and joined the staff of the National Hospital. In these inter-war years, he developed very large private and hospital practices and was one of the most renowned figures in neurology. In the Second World War, he was responsible for organisation of neurology for the army and the clinical services of the EMS. From the mid-1930s until his untimely death in 1947, Riddoch devoted his huge energies to assisting government and ministries, and also the MRC, in planning the organisation and implementation of neurological and neurosurgical care. Casper[55] put it well when he wrote 'from 1938–1947, Riddoch's name appears everywhere in files pertaining to neurological subjects'. Through his efforts, neurology and neurosurgery evolved in this period into a shape that is still recognisable. In the Second World War, it was Riddoch who persuaded the reluctant Ministry of Health to recognise neurology and neurosurgery as specialties distinct from orthopaedics in the emergency treatment centres, a very important step in the subsequent separate identity for these two specialties. By common consent, Riddoch was driven and energetic, but overworked to the extent that eventually his health was affected; and he died at the age of 58, after surgery for a peptic ulcer. He was a man adored and admired by all. Lord Adrian regarded Riddoch very highly and described him as a man of great ability, great personal charm and great integrity.[56] Critchley's biography paints a touching picture:[57] 'George Riddoch was a man of outstanding personality, universally beloved – by his students, colleagues, and above all by his patients. He had a disarming sense of fun. Beneath his charm was a quick intelligence, and thought, and a profound interest in the physiological attributes of neurology.'

Head Injury

Head injury was, in numerical terms, the commonest neurological condition encountered in both World Wars, in each of which significant progress was made with respect to treatment.[58] Horsley was the first surgeon in Britain systematically to study the effects of gunshot wounds to the head. On the basis of his work before the First World War, elaborated upon by Sargent and Holmes working together in Boulogne, where experience of more than 2,000 head injuries was gained,[59] and later by Cushing, the neurosurgical principles for treating head injuries were laid out and widely applied during the First World War, providing the first significant step in improving management.

At the beginning of the First World War, the mortality from open head injury was extremely high and, in the absence of antibiotics and other active interventions, most patients died of secondary infection. Where it could, the British Army segregated cases of head injury, in view of their likely demise and to avoid too much despair amongst troops. As a result, very few surgeons had any experience of operating on the brain. In the event, the dividend from this terrible conflict for neurology was the work of Holmes on injuries to the visual cortex and cerebellum – which were areas of the brain particularly vulnerable to injury due to the design of the British Army helmet which stood high on the head leaving the occiput exposed – and the practical recommendations of Sargent and Holmes for the management of head and spinal trauma. Holmes published 18 papers during the war, on the topics of spinal injury, head injury, and occipital and cerebellar function as revealed by acute traumatic injury.

Tatsuji Inouye had previously published his analyses of gunshot wounds of the head occurring in the Russian–Japanese war of 1900 and 1904–5.[60] Drawing

[55] S. T. Casper, 'The Idioms of Practice: British Neurology 1860–1960' (PhD thesis, University College London, 2007).

[56] E. Adrian, 'George Riddoch: Obituary', *The Times*, 1 November 1947.

[57] M. Critchley, *The Ventricle of Memory* (New York: Raven Press, 1990); Anon. (Macdonald Critchley), *Queen Square and the National Hospital 1860–1960* (London: Edward Arnold Ltd, 1960).

[58] Note that shell-shock, and the work on head injury by Holmes and by Horsley, are dealt with in other chapters.

[59] P. Sargent and G. Holmes, 'Preliminary Notes: The Treatment of the Cranial Injuries of Warfare', *British Medical Journal* 1 (1915): 537–41.

[60] See T. Inouye, *Die Sehstörungen bei Schussverletzungen der kortikalen Sehsphäre, nach Beobachtungen an*

on more than 400 cases of penetrating occipital injury, with post-mortem examination in 23, Holmes was able more precisely to map visual function in the occipital cortex.

These injuries made it possible to construct a map of the projections of different portions of the retina on the cortex. It was placed beyond doubt that the maculae are represented unilaterally and at the posterior extremity of the lobe, surrounded by concentric rings of retinal topography expanding out across the neighbouring cortex. He showed that the peripheral portions of the retina anteriorly, its upper and the lower portions in its lower or ventral part, and the vertical sectors of the retinae adjacent to the vertical meridians, correspond to the portions of the area striata exposed on the medial surface of the hemispheres, and the horizontal sections to the cortex lining the depth of the calcarine fissure.

Holmes noted that the macula had much more extensive cortical representation than the peripheral retina, and later added details on altitudinal paracentral and sector scotomata, congruity of field defects in the two eyes depending on the anteroposterior positioning of the lesion, and disorders of visual attention with lesions of the angular and supramarginal gyri, especially bilateral depth perception and appreciation of colour. He opposed the view that simple visual phenomena such as shape, colour and movement are differentiated from more complex visual perception. He also recognised that the anatomical basis of visuospatial perception is subserved by the association fibres projecting from the visual cortex to other parts of the brain. Detailed maps of the occipital cortex were drawn by Holmes,[61] the remarkable accuracy of which are a testament to his extraordinary analytical skills, and all the more notable for the fact that they were produced in the turmoil and chaos of the head injury wards of Hospital No. 13. Holmes

worked until 5 a.m. on his studies, dressed in his British 'warm', wrapped in a rug and with his hands in mittens, assisted by Colonel William Lister. His observations were made using a small hand-held perimeter, a McHardy perimeter and an adapted Bjerrum screen. The anatomical correlations were further constrained by primitive radiography and the conditions under which surgical exploration took place in the Red Cross Hospital. Without a secretary, Holmes wrote up all his own notes and performed all the post-mortem examinations

Holmes also made detailed studies of 70 soldiers with acute cerebellar lesions, which were rare in civilian life, defining alterations in tone, posture and reflexes; the features of asynergia, dysmetria and adiadochokinesia; observations on 'asthenia', astasia, fatigability, appreciation of weight and various sensory phenomena; and the presence of nystagmus and abnormal eye movements. He showed that the symptoms of cerebellar dysfunction are most severe for complex movements, and also that there is the possibility of some recovery. The descriptions, which formed the basis of his four Croonian lectures in 1922,[62] consolidated Holmes' already high reputation for clinical observation.

Holmes and Sargent described another condition, the so-called 'gutter injury'. By October 1915, they were in the position to write a paper based on 70 cases, of another condition seldom seen in civilian practice.[63] Typically, this occurred when a soldier, unwisely raising his head above the trenches, was hit by a bullet which traversed the skull tangentially but superficially in the midline, causing a depressed fracture with thrombosis of the superior longitudinal sinus, sometimes in the absence of direct brain injury by either the bullet or bone fragments. The clinical features depended on the site and extent of injury, but typically the soldier would instantly develop hemiplegia or tetraplegia and with marked rigidity. Each hallux was described as being often in a state of permanent extension, and there would be variable sensory loss. Holmes found these cases fascinating from the physiological point of view. Deciding whether or not to operate was difficult, not least because many cases made a remarkable spontaneous recovery, in Holmes' view 'probably owing to the free

Verwundeten der letzten japanischen Kriege (Leipzig: Engelmann, 1909); translated as M. Glickstein and M. Fahle, 'Visual Disturbances Following Gunshot Wounds of the Cortical Visual Area. Based on Observations of the Wounded in the Recent Japanese Wars: 1900, 1904–5', *Brain* **123** (supp.) (2000): 1–101.

[61] G. Holmes, 'Disturbances of Vision by Cerebral Lesions', *British Journal of Ophthalmology* **2** (1918): 353–84, 449–68, 506–16; W. T. Lister and G. Holmes, 'Disturbances of Vision from Cerebral Lesions, with Special Reference to the Cortical Representation of the Macula', *Proceedings of the Royal Society of Medicine* (section of ophthalmology) **9** (1916): 57–96.

[62] G. Holmes, 'The Symptoms of Acute Cerebellar Injuries Due to Gunshot Injuries', *Brain* **40** (1917): 461–535.

[63] G. Holmes and P. Sargent, 'Injuries of the Superior Longitudinal Sinus', *British Medical Journal* **2** (1915): 493–8.

venous anastomosis permitting a re-establishment of the circulation'.

The work of Holmes and Sargent demonstrated the potential for new research, even under the extreme and adverse conditions of war and made without access to any sophisticated equipment. Sir Wilmot Herringham, consultant physician to the Army in the First World War, could not have described Holmes' work better when he wrote:

The War has shown the immense services which original research can render to preserve the efficiency of an army ... results could be obtained by the union of clinical and pathological research, not only at home, but also in the actual area of military operations ... clinical medicine and surgery in war time is not of necessity rough in method and imperfect in attainment; but is susceptible of a high and exquisite perfection and affords scope for the finest scientific work.[64]

As early as 1915, Sargent and Holmes had also gathered considerable practical experience, and their writings on the management of head trauma due to blast and missile injuries were of great importance. They stressed the need to get the patient immediately to a base hospital.[65] They emphasised the over-riding importance of infection, and that if the dura was not breached it must not be opened (as was frequently done by general surgeons in debriding the wound). If, as often happened, the dura had been breached at the time of injury, they considered that the brain would invariably become infected. Their description of the typical subsequent clinical course of these unfortunate soldiers was vivid:

Let us briefly consider the usual course and fate of a patient in whom the brain is exposed through a relatively small opening, whether produced by a bullet or by a timid trephining operation. These patients are usually unconscious immediately after the infliction of the wound, and are drowsy and obviously suffer from the effects of shock on regaining consciousness. A gradual improvement may be observed in the general condition and in the direction of recovery of function during the next few days, but soon some protrusion of the brain is observed, together with symptoms of progressive loss of certain functions according to the site of the injury. The patient becomes duller, apathetic, and more drowsy, or may be restless and noisy, and often complains of headache [commonly recognised as an ominous sign in all those writing in the period]; optic neuritis [i.e. papilloedema] frequently develops, together with other symptoms which point to a pathological increase of intracranial pressure. This naturally leads to further protrusion of brain matter which then becomes strangulated and more and more septic. Even at this stage the septic process may come to an end and the patient survive[s]; but if so, it is often at the expense of an irremediable loss of function.

Like Horsley before them, Sargent and Holmes stressed the importance of avoiding where possible raised intracranial pressure, 'fungus cerebri',[66] brain herniation and sepsis. In terms of treatment, they followed generally the principles laid out first by Horsley, such as thorough and wide resections, the removal of all foreign particles and bone fragments, and debridement of the wound. Unlike Horsley, however, they recommended closure of the wound and also discussed the need for large craniotomies, wide excision of dura, methods of drainage, the use of dural and pericranial flaps, and the value of constant irrigation of the wound with carbolic and the brain track with peroxide during the operation. They also described the indications for second operations, and dealing with meningitis and brain fungi, including the use of clean contralateral decompressions. Sargent recommended finger palpation of the brain track to identify any deep-seated fragments, a procedure criticised by Cushing, and the use of a metal drainage tube covered in glycerin for its hypertonic action. Their 1915 paper was born of considerable practical experience, which had already been gained despite the fact that the war had been in progress for less than a year.

Jefferson, who 'cut his teeth neurosurgically on active service' in the British military during the First World War, published an interesting retrospective account of the pre-antibiotic trauma surgery.[67] He was proud of the fact that, by 1918, his mortality rate after surgery on open head injuries was only 37 per cent, and better than that of Cushing (41 per cent). Jefferson made the point that the high mortality was

---

[64] W. Herringham, *Medical Services, Diseases of the War, History of the Great War* (London: HMSO, 1922).

[65] P. Sargent and G. Holmes, 'Preliminary Notes on the Treatment of Cranial Injuries of Warfare', *British Medical Journal* **1** (1915): 537–41.

[66] The term then used to describe a hernia of infected brain tissue protruding from a scalp wound.

[67] G. Jefferson, 'Head Wounds and Infection in Two Wars', *British Journal of Surgery* **55** (supp.) (1947): 3–6.

not due to lack of ingenuity, equipment or surgical planning. Surgery had in his view by then reached a high standard, but morbidity and mortality were caused to a large extent by infection: 'Looking back, we remembered the long periods of invalidism imposed by chronic infection, the endless dressings, the wearing repetitions of the early post-war years of operations on sinuses and sequestra. It was this large residuum which told its bitter tale.'

Antiseptics were far less useful in wartime than in peacetime surgery, for the simple reason that the wounds were already infected by the time they reached the operating theatre. Once infection had invaded brain tissue, the horse had bolted and antiseptic methods, designed to prevent not to treat infection, were too late. Almoth Wright, the leading bacteriologist of the time, recommended the application of gauze with hypertonic salt solution to open wounds in order to draw out fluid. However, it was quickly realised that the best hope was very early removal of contaminated tissue. Horsley had recommended the same when he remarked that 'the fatal and detestable practice of "leaving head cases alone" … is the outcome of ignorance'. It was this recognition that drove the Army to move their surgical theatres close to the front line, and to evacuate soldiers with significant head wounds as quickly as possible.

After the First World War, W. J. Adie, who was appointed assistant physician at Queen Square in 1921, published for the Army Council and the MRC the first of a series of 'Statistical Reports'[68] analysing cases of 'gunshot wound to the head' admitted to Hospital No. 7 in Saint-Omer between May 1916 and December 1917. These cases were all well enough to be transported from a casualty clearing station, a journey of three hours by motor ambulance (a pulse rate under 100 constituting fitness to travel), or, for those previously operated upon, by barge. Of the 656 cases, 119 had dural penetration requiring operation before transfer, and were received an average of 9.2 days after injury. In 86 of these cases, further operation was performed. In 119 cases of dural penetration, there had been no previous surgery and the patients underwent surgery on arrival, as did 36 with a fractured skull and no dural penetration. Based on this

experience, a number of recommendations were made about surgical therapy. First, wherever possible, surgery should be carried out at the base hospital where appropriate facilities and expertise were available, and not the clearing station, even if this involved several hours of rough transportation. Second, transfer should be rapid and surgery carried out preferably within four hours of arrival at the base hospital, giving time simply for X-rays to be obtained and morphia and scopolamine administered. As for the surgery itself, the principles outlined by Holmes and Sargent (which were based on Horsley's work) were largely accepted. All fragments of shell should be removed, and a finger inserted to explore to a depth of 1½ inches in order to locate debris. Strict antisepsis was vital and best served by constant irrigation with warm saline. The flap should be large and all damaged bone removed to leave an intact surrounding margin, with a quarter of an inch of healthy dura left around all perforations. A drainage tube should be placed and the skin closed (here was a divergence from Horsley's approach). Initially, it was suggested that surgery should take no longer than 30 minutes from the time of first incision to removal of the patient from theatre but, with more experience, careful debridement was recommended, even if the longer procedure increased the risk of surgical shock. Good post-operative nursing care was vital and the patients were kept still, even if this required sedation with morphia. The report stated: 'In fact, we may say that the success or failure of the treatment is largely in the hands of the nursing staff … of all the surgical patients that one sees in military hospitals, head cases are, as a whole, the hardest and most exacting to nurse.'

In this series, 5 per cent developed epileptic seizures, and the mortality rate amongst those whose injury resulted in dural penetration was around 50 per cent. Death was almost always due to intracranial infection and cerebral abscess, and occurred in the great majority of cases within ten days of arrival at the hospital. The lucid report provides a vivid snapshot of the base hospital *modus operandi* and the challenges, and it was highly influential in dictating future policy, providing a valuable guide to the organisation of care in the Second World War.

In that conflict, a far more organised approach to the treatment of head-injured patients was devised, based on previous experience. Speed and specialisation were seen as crucial. A series of neurosurgical units dedicated to the management of head injury

---

[68] W. J. Adie and W. W. Wagstaffe, *A Note on a Series of 656 Cases of Gunshot Wound of the Head, with a Statistical Consideration of the Results Obtained*, Medical Research Committee Statistical Reports 1 (London: HMSO, 1918).

was established, of which the most celebrated – and the one with significant Queen Square input – was the Combined Services Hospital for Head Injuries in the grounds and buildings of St Hugh's College, Oxford. This opened in February 1940 and closed in September 1945, and was to have the most profound effect on British neurosurgery. It was led by Cairns, assisted by Symonds and Farquhar Buzzard, and was to a significant extent the result of planning by Riddoch. Many future neurosurgeons in Britain trained at St Hugh's during its five years of existence. Cairns applied the Cushing principles to surgery, peri-operative care and note-keeping. In this sense, the unit can perhaps be seen as a reincarnation, in wartime conditions, of what had been envisaged by the Rockefeller Foundation in awarding their grant to Queen Square, a plan that was thwarted by the declaration of war.

The origins of St Hugh's date back to the time of build-up towards war, in 1938. Jefferson described later how important had been the establishment of 'special neurosurgical centres' free from interference by physicians in determining improved outcome from head injury.

Jefferson quipped: 'We had early recognised that neurosurgery was a whole-time, and indeed a lifetime's work; we had outgrown our earlier, and the longer-surviving Continental, method whereby the professor of surgery did, when he had time, what the professor of neurology or the physician directed.'[69]

The British military authorities asked Cairns, Riddoch and Symonds to plan for the medical treatment of neurological casualties. This trio of surgeon and physicians knew that head injuries were treated most effectively in a designated neurosurgical unit with specifically trained staff. With the assistance of Farquhar Buzzard, who was by then the Regius Professor of Physic in Oxford, St Hugh's was requisitioned and the hospital established.

Riddoch and his colleagues also realised that neurosurgery for head injury should be carried out as soon as possible, and that early operation was key to good outcome. That was part of the reason for using St Hugh's, which was near the military airfield at Brize Norton, thereby minimising transit time for evacuated soldiers. The hospital treated around 13,000 patients in its 300 beds over the five-year period. Cairns was a supreme planner and, as director, he

was very much in charge.[70] As Peter Schurr, one of the next generation of British neurosurgeons who was trained at St Hugh's, wrote: 'Cairns enforced a regime of patient care involving meticulous accuracy, accurate examination, careful recording and attention to detail, which was to continue to be practised, even in the most adverse circumstances during the fighting and which produced a uniformly high standard of work.'[71]

Cairns followed the Cushing traditions of meticulous surgery and note-keeping, and this paid dividends. The unit not only developed protocols for treating head injury which were the most advanced in the world, but also focused on the consequences of head injury, including dysphasia, paralysis and epilepsy, and developed specialised rehabilitation facilities for the care of the head-injured after the acute phase. The influence of the techniques and specialisms employed at St Hugh's and by Cairns on the battlefield had a profound influence on the whole of postwar British neurology and neurosurgery.

Cairns made three additional wartime contributions to neurosurgery. First, he was involved with the initial clinical experiments with penicillin, developed and manufactured in Oxford, and travelled to North Africa in 1943 with Florey to initiate a trial of antibiotic treatment. They wrote a 'preliminary report', 114 pages in length, describing 23 cases of severe penetrating head injury treated with 15,000 units of penicillin instilled into the operative brain cavity. In 22 cases, the wound could be completely closed and 20 survived, the three deaths being unrelated to the infection. Since the mortality without penicillin was likely to be 30–40 per cent, these were startling results. The report was distributed in October 1943 to all the British forces and civilian medical services, and also to those of the Empire, USA and the Soviet Red Cross.

---

[69] G. Jefferson, 'Planning for Head Injuries', *British Medical Bulletin* 3 (1945): 5–9.

[70] Symonds, appointed as civilian consultant neurologist, noted: 'he and I got on happily together, though there were one or two collisions and sore heads before I learned that I served in Cairns' hospital'.

[71] It is recorded that when Peter Schurr was first taken on by Cairns in 1943, he had pulmonary TB, and Cairns suggested he rest and read – and for his reading matter Cairns suggested Gowers' *Manual*, etc.: 'You can't beat Gowers. Perhaps you should start with Gowers.' See G. J. Fraenkel, *Hugh Cairns* (Oxford University Press, 1991), and P. Schurr, 'The Contribution to Neurosurgery of the Combined Services Hospital for Head Injuries at St Hugh's College, Oxford, 1940–1945', *Journal of the Royal Army Medical Corps* 134 (1988): 146–8.

It was extremely influential. Clinical practice changed but a few die-hards were not impressed, including Sir Heneage Ogilvie, the celebrated consulting surgeon to the Army in Cairo, who wrote with remarkable venom that 'Penicillin under service conditions is totally impracticable and is being pushed by a group of interested parties.' Fortunately, this opinion was largely ignored. Cairns was so amused by this retort that he had it framed and displayed on the wall of his office. With Honor Smith, Dorothy Russell and Francis Schiller, Cairns also developed protocols for using penicillin in various clinical circumstances and this work, always practical and clinically oriented, must have saved countless lives.

A second contribution was the Cairns concept of the Mobile Neurosurgical Unit (MNSU). These six travelling neurosurgical theatres, set up in the battlefield, reflected his vision, determination and organisational genius. Cairns persuaded the Ministry to adopt the idea; enlisted the help of Lord Nuffield, who provided funds for the transport and some equipment for the first unit; and completed a trial run at RAF Benson, which showed that within one hour of arrival behind the lines, a team was ready to operate, fully equipped with facilities needed for many neurosurgical procedures.

The neurosurgeon William Robert Henderson was put in charge of the first MNSU. Tragically, however, the unit was captured more or less intact in the retreat to Dunkirk in France by the Germans, and Henderson was interned and, according to Symonds, he provided calm determination, surgical skill and patience in the prisoner-of-war camp in Obermassfeld, where he gained practical experience with peripheral nerve injuries. Later, he was transferred to Colditz Castle. Henderson's later career was spent developing neurosurgery in Leeds, where he had originally been appointed to the consultant staff in 1938.

The MNSUs were usually in ambulance trucks or, in one case, a 10-ton diesel motor-coach captured from the Italians. This MNSU (no. 4) was in the charge of Kenneth Eden, who was, as Cairns wrote: 'Able to excise and close the majority of the head wounds of the Eighth Army within 24 hours, and to obtain over 90% of primary healing, a great improvement on anything previously seen in this war, for on all fronts up to date the incidence of brain abscess after brain wounds has been high.'[72]

Head injuries constituted 5–10 per cent of all the British battle casualties evacuated from the front lines and these units treated the majority of cases – for instance, over 90 per cent of those injured in Normandy. Major Peter Ashcroft was in charge of MNSU no. 1 in North Africa, and wrote a detailed paper about treatment, reporting only a 15 per cent mortality.[73] Working in North Africa, Italy and Sicily, MNSU no. 4 treated 6,003 cases and operated upon 4,334, and no. 5 handled 4,600 casualties and performed 2,239 operations.[74] Whilst in many respects the principles that Cairns developed were those pioneered during the First World War and set out in Adie's report, as he explained at the end of the Second World War,[75] he and his teams in the MNSUs perfected the treatment of head injuries and laid the foundations for managing the increase in trauma that occurred in civilian practice after the war with the enormous increase in road traffic. In

---

[72] Cairns' initial plan was to staff each MNSU with one neurosurgeon, one neurologist, one anaesthetist, two general-duty RAMC officers, two Queen Alexandra sisters, four RAMC orderlies and two Royal Army Service Corps drivers. The original vehicles were converted ambulances, later replaced by 3-ton or 15-hundredweight trucks, with two sets of neurosurgical instruments, an electric generator, tents, a water tank, two operating tables, suction apparatus, diathermy and illumination – all that was needed for 200 operations without any replacements: see P. Schurr, 'The Evolution of Field Neurosurgery in the British Army', *Journal of the Royal Society of Medicine* **98** (2005): 423–7. There is also an interesting description of these units by Major Kenneth Eden, who was in charge of MNSU no. 4 in North Africa. He writes that the MNSUs were contained in the body of the vehicles, and comprised a scrub room, operating theatre with table and room for an anaesthetic machine, and a corridor to a tented 'pre-operation ward' which had room for 11 stretchers. There were a full set of neurosurgical instruments, diathermy, electric suction, and lighting provided by batteries charged by running the engine of the coach. Running water was provided from a water tank on the back of the vehicle. The whole formed a compact and dust-free operating theatre suite that could be packed up and moved within two hours. The vehicles shadowed the advancing forces just behind the front lines: see K. C. Eden, 'Mobile Neurosurgery in Warfare', *Lancet* **242** (1943): 689–92. Eden died in 1943 from poliomyelitis: see H. Cairns, 'Obituary: Kenneth Eden', *Lancet* **242** (1943): 653.

[73] P. B. Ashcroft, 'Treatment of Head Wounds Due to Missiles: Analysis of 500 Cases', *Lancet* **242** (1943): 211–18.

[74] J. T. Hughes, 'Hugh Cairns (1896–1952) and the Mobile Neurosurgical Unit of the Second World War', *Journal of Medical Biography* **12** (2004): 18–24.

[75] H. Cairns, 'The Organisation for Treatment of Head Wound in the British Army', *British Medical Bulletin* **3** (1945): 9–14.

that respect, his third contribution was also ahead of its time. Valentine Logue, the future professor of neurosurgery at Queen Square, commanded an MNSU in Burma.

Cairns had been present at the death of T. E. Lawrence (Lawrence of Arabia) following a head injury sustained in a motor-cycle accident in May 1935. Lawrence was not wearing any sort of crash helmet and Fraenkel believes this experience greatly affected Cairns, who recognised that an effective helmet would have saved his life. With the onset of war, he became passionate in his insistence that helmets should be compulsory for all service motor-cyclists. He suggested a new design.

It consists of an outer shell of some firm substance, shaped rather like an inverted pudding-bowl and quite smooth on its outer surface. This is supported by a lining consisting of a series of web slings fitting equally snugly on the rider's head and attached by its base to the base of the outer shell. The helmet is also retained in place by a chin-strap. Between the outer shell and the lining there is a gap which may with advantage contain some energy-absorbing material.[76]

Cairns made helmets out of vulcanised rubber and pulp (shredded jute rag, paper and wood) which were inexpensive, light, waterproof and extremely durable. They became compulsory in the forces and were the precursors of today's helmets. In November 1941, the Army Council made the wearing of helmets mandatory for all motor-cyclists, and they were adopted by the Royal Air Force in the following year. After 1945, Cairns became a strong advocate of crash helmets for all civilian motor-cyclists, a policy that was only adopted in 1973 in Britain, and one that has greatly reduced the mortality and morbidity of head injury. Evidence for the mitigating value of helmets with a soft padding, which cushions the brain by slowing up the deceleration forces of a blow resulting in closed head injury, was also provided in Oxford by Denny-Brown, Ritchie Russell and Solly Zuckerman in experiments on macaque monkeys[77] and the Oxford

physicist AHS Holbourne. They devised the percussion hammer model of brain injury in rodents (variants are still used today) and, using ingenious mechanical models made of gelatin and by correlating the shearing damage with pathological findings in human head injury, demonstrated the importance of rotational forces in causing concussion and contra-coup injury.[78] They concluded that concussion is due to sudden deceleration of the head, rather than force of the blow or a change in momentum, and made the distinction between head injury accompanying sudden acceleration and deceleration ('acceleration concussion') and that with crush or compression ('compression concussion') injuries. They found that by narrowing the point of impact, a penetrating injury could produce focal injury without concussion and that depressed skull fracture lessened the acceleration movement of the brain and lowered the incidence of concussion. They argued that concussion results from direct injury rather than vascular change, release of toxins or raised intracranial pressure.

After the war, Cairns became interested in psychiatry and the surgical treatment of mental disease, for which neurosurgery outside Queen Square eventually became notorious. He died young, but Symonds tells us that, first and foremost a doctor, Cairns' wish in retirement from surgery was to engage in general practice in the country.

Spinal Injury

Injuries of the spine and spinal cord are common on the battlefield, and many soldiers were so afflicted in each World War. They provided neurologists with an opportunity to study human physiology, confirming Sherrington's theories of spinal cord function, and, if the First World War provided new knowledge on the consequences of spinal cord injury, it was the Second

---

[76] H. Cairns, 'Head Injuries in Motorcyclists: The Importance of the Crash Helmet', *British Medical Journal* **2** (1941): 465–83.

[77] For example, D. Denny-Brown and W. R. Russell, 'Experimental Cerebral Concussion', *Brain* **64** (1941): 93–164. These studies were prematurely terminated by Denny-Brown's move to Harvard in 1941. Ritchie Russell served in the RAMC from 1940 to 1945, becoming officer in charge of the medical division of the Military Hospital for Head

Injuries in Oxford, and consultant neurologist to Middle East Forces. He kept a card index of patients, described by a colleague at the time as 'Russell's Folly'. This brought him into close touch with Cairns, who arranged his appointment as consultant neurologist in Oxford, where he was later elected professor of neurology.

[78] See A. H. S. Holbourn, 'Mechanics of Head Injuries', *Lancet* **242** (1943): 438–41; and H. Cairns and A. H. S. Holbourn, 'Head Injuries in Motorcyclists, with Special Reference to Crash Helmets', *British Medical Journal* **1** (1943): 592–8. Athelstan Hylas Stoughton Holbourn was a Scottish research physicist, recruited by Cairns to work in Oxford.

World War that advanced knowledge on improved care and treatment of the injured.

The key figures in the First World War were Gordon Holmes and his neurosurgical colleague Percy Sargent, Henry Head and George Riddoch. Holmes' experience was summarised in his Goulstonian lectures of 1915 at the Royal College of Physicians, in which the clinical features in about 300 cases of spinal injury were detailed and correlated with the histopathological changes obtained at post-mortem in 50 cases. He confirmed physiological phenomena in acute lesions previously observed by Sherrington in animals – for instance, spinal shock and reflex movements – but also described the neurological aspects of localised injury; trophic changes; autonomic features including effects on sweating, temperature and sexual function, including priapism; and altered function of the bladder.[79] Holmes concluded that injuries of the spinal cord seen in warfare are not sharply defined and the level of the lesion suggested by the clinical symptoms and signs corresponds poorly to the site of maximal damage, with late complications modifying clinical manifestations of the initial injury. Holmes returned to the neurology of altered bladder function in 1933 in work that anticipated many aspects of spinal cord injury experienced during and since the Second World War.[80]

Cushing had also described the situation in American expeditionary forces during the First World War:[81]

[Spinal cases] did very badly throughout, as was anticipated. Most of them were immediately evacuated to base hospitals and fully 80 per cent died in the first few weeks in consequence of infection from bed sores and catheterization. The conditions were such, owing to pressure of work, as to make it almost impossible to give these unfortunate men the care their condition required. No water beds were available, and each case demands the almost undivided attention of a nurse trained in the care of paralytics. Only those cases survived in which the spinal lesion was a partial one.

George Riddoch worked on spinal injury at the Empire Hospital for Officers. He was the only staff physician there, but was able to consult with visiting Queen Square physicians, who included Collier, Batten, Farquhar Buzzard and Wilson, and it was there also that he began a long association with Henry Head. They performed outstanding research into the effects of human spinal transection and injury, and published a series of landmark papers on reflex action and the consequences of spinal injuries;[82] 11 papers were published which established Riddoch as the authority in the area. After the war, he continued his research into spinal injury, especially sphincteric reflexes and phantom limb, and was one of the first neurologists to receive a grant from the MRC to support neurological research.

In 1941, Riddoch was commissioned as a brigadier and, with Cairns, was charged with devising the Army neurological services. He also was a key figure in the establishment of St Hugh's. At the start of the Second World War, the London Hospital unit was evacuated to Chase Farm Hospital, and Riddoch was appointed as the head of the EMS neurological services. He was also appointed to the War Office Medical Board. Under Riddoch's leadership, 12 specialised spinal units were set up during the course of the war, the first four being in Oswestry, Stanmore, Warrington

---

[79] G. Holmes, 'The Goulstonian Lectures on Spinal Injuries of Warfare. I. The Pathology of Acute Spinal Injuries. II. The Clinical Symptoms of Gunshot Injuries of the Spine. III. The Sensory Disturbances in Spinal Injuries', *British Medical Journal* 2 (1915): 769–74, 815–21, 855–61.

[80] G. Holmes, 'Observations on the Paralysed Bladder', *Brain* 56 (1933): 383–96. The same issue contained papers on the bladder by E. Graeme Robertson and Derek Denny-Brown, which were opaque – so much so that Walshe, encountering Denny-Brown in the corridors of Queen Square, told him that he was waiting for the English translation before reading them: see W. I. McDonald, 'Gordon Holmes Lecture: Gordon Holmes and Neurological Heritage', *Brain* **130** (2007): 288–98.

[81] H. Cushing, 'Neurosurgery', in M. W. Ireland, ed., *The Medical Department of the United States Army in the World War* (Washington, DC: US Government Printing Office, 1927), Vol. **XI**: *Surgery (Part 1)*, pp. 749–58.

[82] H. Head and G. Riddoch, 'The Automatic Bladder, Excessive Sweating and Some Other Reflex Conditions in Gross Injuries of the Spinal Cord', *Brain* 40 (1917): 188; G. Riddoch, 'Reflex Functions of the Completely Divided Spinal Cord in Man, Compared with Those Associated with Less Severe Lesions', *Brain* 60 (1917): 264–402; G. Riddoch and E. F. Buzzard, 'Reflex Movements and Postural Reactions in Quadriplegia and Hemiplegia, with Special Reference to Those of the Upper limb', *Brain* 44 (1921): 397–489; G. Riddoch, 'The Clinical Picture of Complete Transverse Division of the Spinal Cord', *Medical Science* 5 (1921): 44–52. For an excellent and scholarly appreciation of Riddoch and his publication list, see J. R. Silver and M.-F. Weiner, 'George Riddoch: The Man Who Found Ludwig Guttmann', *Spinal Cord* **50** (2012): 88–93.

and Bangour, with a total of around 700 casualties treated. Four of the units were for acute cases, and the others provided long-term rehabilitation. Riddoch's memorandum issued by the Nerve Injuries Committee, concerning therapy and care, covered bladder management with intermittent catheterisation, wash-outs, tidal drainage, the risks of infection, and ways of avoiding pressure sores. He warned against plaster beds and supra-pubic bladder drainage. Riddoch also devised systems for note-keeping and documentation, as did Cairns for head injury. He travelled around the country visiting the units, giving advice and instructions and setting himself a punishing regime of inspection, but, without his personal oversight, care lapsed in the face of the prevailing view that such cases were 'hopeless'.

It was Riddoch who appointed Ludwig ('Poppa') Guttmann to take charge of the hutted EMS spinal injuries unit at Stoke Mandeville (UK).[83] As a part-time medical orderly at a hospital in Königshütte, Poland, Guttmann had seen a miner with paraplegia from a fractured spine and was advised not to write any notes because the patient 'will be dead in a few weeks'. After medical studies in Breslau, Würzburg and Freiburg, Guttmann worked briefly as a neurosurgeon in Hamburg, before moving to Freiburg and rejoining Foerster, who had described the accepted orthodoxy of inevitable fatal outcome from bedsores and infection in those surviving the initial injury. Being Jewish, and realising that that he had to leave Germany, arrangements were made by the Council for Assisting Refugee Academics for Guttmann and his wife, son and daughter, aged nine and six years, to reach Harwich, England, in March 1939, with a grant on arrival of £250. Their reception from the immigration officer who sheltered the children from sleet and snow 'restored his faith in human nature'. Guttmann made his way to Oxford and, although he had hoped to practise as a neurosurgeon, was encouraged by Cairns to continue his work on sweating (and thereby

dubbed 'sweaty Guttmann') and peripheral nerve injuries. When he left for Stoke Mandeville, to take up the appointment of director of the Spinal Injuries Unit in 1944 (a post he held until 1966), the Oxford neurologists greeted his departure with some relief, because Guttmann was considered difficult as a colleague and his ideas on the management of paraplegia were not endorsed by others, especially Ritchie Russell.

It was at Stoke Mandeville that Guttman developed the programme that transformed the care of spinal injuries nationally and internationally. Initially, the unit had 26 beds, but it expanded to over 100 by the end of the war. His method was careful transportation, immediate transfer to a specialised unit, pillow packs, air mattresses (in opposition to plaster beds), regular turning, removal of pressure-sore sloughs, repeated dressings, closure of supra-pubic catheters with intermittent catheterisation, high output of acid urine from a clean bladder, tidal drainage, use of antibiotics, routine cystoscopy, reduction of the fracture, tendon lengthening, emphasis on nutrition and blood transfusion.[84] He set up systematic programmes of physiotherapy and transformed that specialty. Guttmann taught continuously, monitored the staff and patients in a determinedly autocratic way, and never let up – day or night. An inspirational and motivating man, Guttmann made it his job to counter the previously prevailing atmosphere of hopelessness. He introduced sport into his rehabilitation programmes in spinal units and organised the '1948 International Wheelchair Games' to coincide with the Olympics in London. This was repeated in 1952 and these 'Stoke Mandeville Games' evolved into the Paralympics, now a global sporting event.[85] Guttmann was knighted in 1966 and elected as Fellow of the Royal Society in 1976.

Peripheral Nerve Injury

Traumatic injuries to peripheral nerves were another medical consequence of the battlefield. Although these had been studied in the American Civil War by Silas Weir Mitchell,[86] there was little interest in

---

[83] The following details and much besides come from the affectionate and informed memoir written by Professor David Whitteridge in *Biographical Memoirs of Fellows of the Royal Society* **29** (1983): 226–44. Whitteridge worked with Guttmann at Stoke Mandeville from 1944, on the physiological basis for the viscerocutaneous reflex, and soon realised that 'to find out something about his patients that Guttmann did not already know was very rarely achieved'. Sir Roger Bannister, who was tutored by him at Oxford, recalls that Whitteridge was described by a colleague as 'a man of extremely high intelligence and very low pH'.

[84] J. R. Silver, *History of the Treatment of Spinal Injuries* (New York: Kluwer Academic, Plenum Publishers, 2003).
[85] The 2012 Paralympic games had 4,302 athletes from 164 countries, with 2.7 million tickets sold and broadcasting rights in 36 countries, with billions of viewers worldwide.
[86] S. W. Mitchell, *Injuries of Nerves and their Consequences* (Philadelphia: Lippincott, 1872).

the topic at the start of the First World War. It was recognised that suture of the two ends of severed nerves offered a chance of some recovery, but surgical treatment was rarely used.[87] Henry Head wrote on cases of nerve injury, some sustained in the Boer War, and he described in meticulous detail the pattern of recovery after having his own radial nerve sectioned and resutured by his colleague the surgeon James Sherren. The orthopaedic surgeon Robert Jones made important contributions in relation to rehabilitation and the treatment of weak limbs by musculotendinous transfer. Peripheral nerve injuries were documented in two monographs written from France during the First World War.[88] In his preface to one English edition, Farquhar Buzzard wrote:

> In no department of medical science has more valuable work been performed by our French colleagues since the commencement of the War than in the study of nerve injuries. The establishment of neurological centers throughout France has resulted in the addition of a number of interesting contributions to this subject, which testify to the zeal and industry shown by our allies in this as in other fields of activity.

War did, coincidentally, make one further contribution to neurology and the peripheral nervous system. George Guillain and Jean-Alexandre Barré first described their syndrome amongst the French forces at the front, and, interestingly, Cushing fell ill with what was almost certainly this condition in 1918 (and failed to diagnose it).[89] In 1919, Purves-Stewart and Evans wrote the first British book on peripheral nerve injury, describing 520 cases, and Hartley Sidney Carter published his papers on 1,000 cases of peripheral nerve injury.[90] In 1920, the Medical Research

Council published the *Diagnosis and Treatment of Peripheral Nerve Injuries*[91] under the chairmanship of Farquhar Buzzard, and this became the standard work until after the Second World War.

During the Second World War, these injuries were again the focus of attention, and a landmark was the now-famous short book prepared by the MRC Nerve Injuries Committee.[92] *Aids to the Investigation of Peripheral Nerve Injuries* was first published in 1942 as MRC War Memorandum No. 7, by His Majesty's Stationery Office, at a price of 2s 0d. It was designed to show doctors how to examine the limbs for peripheral nerve lesions. The illustrations, 74 figures on 48 pages, depicted normal anatomy, with photographic demonstrations of each muscle in action and, where appropriate, a guiding finger from the examiner pointing to a key tendon or muscle belly. Each group of illustrations was preceded by a diagram free from redundant anatomical information, which showed the main nerve trunk and the muscles innervated by its various branches. The atlas provided uniquely practical information and is still much in use by neurologists today. The 'MRC grade' suggested to record the state of each muscle has remained the standard clinical and research parlance for the semi-quantitation of muscle strength.[93] In addition to the spinal injuries centres, Riddoch also established five special units dedicated to the treatment of nerve injuries. These were usually

---

[87] H. C. Cameron, 'Lord Lister on Nerve Repair' (letter), *Lancet* 244 (1944): 833–4.

[88] C. Athanassio-Benistry, *Clinical Forms of Nerve Lesions* (London: University of London Press, 1918) (English translation with a preface by Farquhar Buzzard, based on the author's experience in the military wards at the Salpêtrière). See also J. Tinel, *Blessures des nerfs* (Paris: Masson, 1916), which was based on 628 peripheral nerve injuries.

[89] Walshe was at a meeting where Landry's ascending paralysis was linked to the Guillain–Barre syndrome. He recounted that Guillain was present, and, furious, stormed out shouting, 'Landry's patients die, my patients do not.'

[90] J. Purves-Stewart and A. Evans, *Nerve Injuries and Their Treatment* (London: Frowde, Hodder & Stoughton, 1919); H. S. Carter, 'On Causalgia and Allied Painful Conditions due to Lesions of the Peripheral Nerves', *Journal of Neurology and Psychopathology* 3 (1922): 1–38.

[91] Medical Research Council, *Diagnosis and Treatment of Peripheral Nerve Injuries*, Special Report Series 54 (London: HMSO, 1920).

[92] The committee was extremely effective, arranged with typical skill by Riddoch. Its members were leaders or future leaders in the field: W. Rowley Bristow, G. L. Brown, H. Cairns, E. A. Carmichael, M. Critchley, J. G. Greenfield, J. R. Learmonth, H. Platt, H. J. Seddon, C. P. Symonds, J. Z. Young and F. J. C. Herrald (Secretary).

[93] The figures were drawn by Mr Clifford Shepley. They were adapted from Pitres and Testut, *Les nerfs en schémas: anatomie et physiopathologie. Traité d'anatomie humaine* (Paris: Doin, 1925). The models used in the atlas were not selected for their muscularity. The organisation was top down: muscles of the shoulder innervated by nerves that do not arise from the brachial plexus; the plexus itself; and the five main nerves of the upper limb – circumflex, radial, musculocutaneous, median and ulnar. The leg follows the arm, first the nerves of its anterior, and then the posterior, aspect. The lumbar plexus is not illustrated. The atlas ends with charts of the approximate area within which sensory changes may be found in lesions of the brachial plexus, the peripheral nerves of the arm and leg, and their spinal segments. For a full history of this publication and subsequent editions, see *Brain* 133 (2010): 2838–44.

led by orthopaedic surgeons and, for instance in Oxford, Seddon and his colleagues carried out clinical research into nerve grafting, the rate of nerve regeneration, the effects of disuse and the regeneration of proprioceptors. This formed the basis for an extensive report on the clinical features, investigation, histology and surgical results of suture in nerve injuries, published on behalf of the MRC, and other important accounts of nerve injury.[94]

The special units for brain, spine and nerve injury, and especially St Hugh's in Oxford, strongly influenced the subsequent course of British neuroscience, and many of the younger doctors working there during the war went on to become leaders in their fields: Sir Herbert Seddon in orthopaedic surgery; Murray Falconer and Peter Schurr in neurosurgery; and, amongst the neurologists, Michael Ashby, Ken Heathfield, Maurice Parsonage, Hugh Garland, William Gooddy, Sean McArdle, Denis Williams and Michael Kremer.

Neurosurgery and War: The Dividend for Neuroscience Centres after 1948

Until the 1930s, neurosurgery was considered in Britain to be a subdivision of general surgery, a view promulgated by the physicians at Queen Square. This is partly why the discipline trod water in the interwar years. It was only through the efforts of the Cushing trainees – Cairns, Dott and Jefferson – that neurosurgery began to be accepted as a distinct specialty. Important landmarks were establishment of the British Society of Neurological Surgeons in 1926 (with work by Jefferson and Ballance), opening of the first dedicated neurosurgical unit at the London Hospital headed by Cairns in 1933 and Dott's dedicated neurosurgical ward in Edinburgh (ward 20) in 1938, and Jefferson's award of a personal chair in neurosurgery at Manchester University in 1939. These were external events, and at Queen Square little concrete progress was made in neurosurgery until the Rockefeller grant in 1938, the arrival of McKissock in 1946, and the academic appointments that followed in 1965. However, it was the experience of the war that became the main driver of the rapid evolution of the specialty of neurosurgery and the development of

regional neurosurgical units. Three wartime factors were of especial importance: Riddoch's efforts to establish neurosurgery as a distinct discipline within the military, Cairns' work at St Hugh's, the role of his hospital as a centre of neurosurgical training, and the success of the organisational structure of the EMS. Although it is clear that several members of the consultant staff of the National Hospital made substantial contributions to the war effort – including Horsley, Holmes and Sargent in the First World War, and Cairns, Jefferson, Riddoch, Williams and Symonds in the Second World War – the hospital as an institution played a passive role in each conflict and suffered as a result, with a re-run of threats to its survival as a national resource in the immediate postwar periods. The effective manner in which the practice of neurosurgery improved outcomes during the war had profound consequences for the organisation of services after 1948. As Jefferson wrote:

> We have reached a point when we can usefully enquire whether the plans that we made and put into action for the care of head-injured in war-time have been so beneficial that they should be prolonged and improved in time of peace ... There is something more than a hope, there is a very clear possibility, that under the new National Health Service ... regionalised schemes for the care of designated categories of illnesses and accidents will be established.[95]

Jefferson described a hub-and-spoke arrangement in regional centres for neurosurgery, linked to rehabilitation hospitals. With no mention of neurology, neurosurgery had firmly established its precedence in rural Britain, if not at Queen Square. In the postwar period, slowly but surely, regional centres were set up, with neurology and neurosurgery facilities combined and each covering a region, at large 'hub hospitals' linked to satellite (spoke) units, much as Jefferson proposed. Many of the MNSU neurosurgeons played a prominent part in these developments[96] in future years, and the Cairns–Jefferson (and Riddoch) vision of neurosurgery was put in place, external to and not dependent on Queen Square.

---

[94] See H. J. Seddon, *Peripheral Nerve Injuries*, Medical Research Council Special Report 282 (London: HMSO, 1954); and H. J. Seddon, 'Three Types of Nerve Injury', *Brain* **66** (1943): 237–88.

[95] Jefferson, 'Planning for Head Injuries', *British Medical Bulletin*, 3 (1945): 5–9.

[96] Including Johnson (MNSU no. 3), Jepson and Schorstein (MNSU no. 5) in Manchester, Gillingham (MNSU no. 4) in Edinburgh, Walpole Lewin (MNSU no. 1) in Cambridge, G. K. Tutton in Glasgow (MNSU no. 5) and Small in Birmingham (MNSU no. 6).

Chapter 10

Other Clinical Specialties at Queen Square

The National Hospital did not only provide clinical work in neurology and neurosurgery (despite its renaming in 1990), but psychiatry, neuro-otology and neuro-ophthalmology were also practiced, and the new speciality of neuro-anaesthesia arose.

Psychiatry

Psychiatry always had difficulties in establishing for itself a secure position at the National Hospital. Self-evidently, neurology and psychiatry share similar brain chemistry, pathways and mechanisms, their clinical features overlap, and boundaries between the two disciplines are distinctly blurred. That the relationship proved uneasy had much to do with the different attitudes, style and personalities of psychiatrists and neurologists of the British school, and the negative stigma and social attitudes towards psychiatric disease. For a brief period in the 1950s, the National Hospital did assume a position of prominence in psychiatry, but leadership was ceded with the departure of Eliot Slater to the Maudsley Hospital and Institute of Psychiatry. As with neurosurgery before the Second World War, the National Hospital's failure to nurture psychiatry, at various times in its history, resulted in lost opportunities.

The practice of psychiatry at Queen Square has in recent times been designated as 'neuropsychiatry', reflecting the emphasis on organic and biological mechanisms in preference to psychodynamic and social models of disease and psychoanalytical treatment. This neurological view of psychiatry results in an altogether different conceptualisation and management of mental health symptoms seen in a neurological setting, compared to the practice of general psychiatry. Many neurologists at the National Hospital, especially in the mid twentieth century, were disparaging of psychiatry and its practitioners. But, despite this negativity, the concept of neuropsychiatry, signifying abnormalities of mind with or without neurological symptoms from the perspective of altered brain structure and function, did gain support. One sign of this enlightened perspective was the title of the consultant positions appointed to the hospital – 'physicians in psychological medicine' rather than 'psychiatrists'. The approach to mental disorder grounded in a medical model of disease drew neurology and psychiatry together and, in time, allowed each to be advantaged by the applications of neuropathology, neurochemistry, neuroimaging, neurogenetics, neuroimmunology and quantitative psychology. As a result, psychiatric disorders were formulated in terms of altered brain structure and function. However, the concept of neuropsychiatry goes further, adding to these disciplines at least some consideration of social, psychodynamic, developmental and personality aspects which neurology completely ignores. In this respect, neuropsychiatry retains the link between mind and brain, a source of discussion for two millennia and which other branches of psychiatry have tended to ignore.

The psychiatric disturbances observed at Queen Square were usually seen in the context of organic conditions such as epilepsy, movement disorders, and genetic and degenerative disorders. The primary affective and psychotic conditions which, although considered now to be no less biological in origin, have no formal neurological connections remained areas with which psychiatrists at the National Hospital did not engage.

Another trend at the National Hospital in recent times has been to refer to the approach as 'biological psychiatry' or 'behavioural neurology'. Alwyn Lishman argued that biological psychiatry focuses on cellular chemical and microscopic defects, whereas behavioural neurology concerns abnormalities of behaviour derived from knowledge of brain organisation, and neuropsychiatry encompasses all these aspects but also deals with neural systems, pathology, anatomy, and psychodynamic and psychosocial aspects.[1] These distinctions are blurred in practice, and to some extent the use of the term 'behavioural neurology' reflects the wish of some neurologists to avoid any association with psychiatry.[2]

Perhaps rather surprisingly, there is one category of 'non-biological' conditions which did interest the neurologists and which loomed large at times in the history of the National Hospital. This is the category of 'somatoform conditions', notably hysteria and, during the First World War, shell-shock. These were topics with which the physicians did engage, making significant contributions.

Psychiatry at the National Hospital 1860–1914

Although, at the time of the foundation of the hospital, psychiatry was still relatively under-developed as a medical specialty in Britain – compared to Germany and France, for instance – it was still far more established than neurology. There was a widespread network of both public and private asylums which had grown up during the previous 50 years, a complex body of lunacy law and administration in place, and a professional association of asylum doctors founded in 1841 (the Association of Medical Officers of Asylums and Hospitals for the Insane). These asylums housed a mixed community of clinical cases, including many who would now fall firmly within the remit of neurology, such as individuals with dementia, movement disorders, general paralysis of the insane, epilepsy or one of the many neurogenetic and metabolic conditions affecting the brain, almost none of which was categorised at the time or differentiated from other conditions causing insanity. Institutionalised alongside others with primary psychiatric conditions, it was in this environment that the concepts emerged of the neuropathic trait and inherited degeneracy.

There was widespread public concern about the poor conditions in these hospitals. Nevertheless, the founders of the National Hospital sought to exclude those patients with epilepsy or paralysis who also had

psychiatric disturbance. Although eligible for outpatient treatment, the initial *Rules of the Charity* prohibited from admission as inpatients 'persons labouring under or liable to attacks of epileptic mania, or who are imbecile', epileptics who had at any time been certified inmates of lunatic asylums, and 'all other persons of unsound mind'. This policy was to some extent pragmatic since both the doctors and lay administrators, notably Burford Rawlings, considered acute psychiatric conditions such as 'epileptic mania' to be highly disruptive of good order, tranquility and a wholesome moral atmosphere on the wards. However, the major reason for the exclusion was surely the stigmatisation of psychiatric disease, widespread in Britain and other countries based partly on mystical and religious archetypes and fuelled by the concept of 'degeneration'. The administrative authorities, but less so the doctors, accordingly veered away from anything that associated the National Hospital with psychiatric care, considering this to be detrimental to the reputation, especially since this was likely to discourage philanthropic benefactors on whom the hospital's finances were largely dependent. These exclusions remained in force through each successive revision of the rules long into the twentieth century.

The minutes of the Board of Management, throughout the nineteenth century, reveal repeated attempts to hold the line against the admission of patients with 'borderline' psychiatric conditions or obvious mental deficiencies, and to resist any attempts by either the psychiatric profession or the Lunacy Commissioners to influence hospital policy and practice, or encroach on its independence. Thus, when, in 1884, the psychiatrist J. Mortimer Granville made discreet overtures to the Board suggesting that the National and the West End Hospitals should merge to create a single institution for the early treatment of 'nervous patients', the Board summarily rejected his proposal. Patients with psychiatric disturbance were, nevertheless sometimes admitted in error. The hospital records refer to outpatients said to have become insane while awaiting admission as inpatients, and to inpatients being summarily discharged after developing symptoms of acute mania during their stay in the hospital. Moreover, by claiming to act as a check on the growth of insanity, the National Hospital's own publicity in its early annual reports frequently drew attention to the close relations between nervous disease and insanity.

---

[1] A. Lishman, 'What is Neuropsychiatry?' *Journal of Neurology, Neurosurgery, and Psychiatry* **55** (1992): 983–5.
[2] Professor Michael Trimble notes that his senior lecturer position was designated as in behavioural neurology and not neuropsychiatry. Roger Gilliatt was not prepared to have psychiatry represented in his unit.

The physicians generally took a relaxed view of these distinctions and, ignoring the exclusion rules, admitted patients who interested them, even if these cases had marked psychiatric symptoms. This led to periodic clashes with Burford Rawlings and the Board of Management, but, in February 1890, after discussions with the Medical Committee, the Board agreed in principle 'to consider any special application in regard to the admission of a case where a member of the [medical] staff advises that some relaxation of [the] rules might be made with advantage'. However, this resolution solved little, and seemed only to contribute to the growing tension between lay managers and clinicians over control of admissions and discharges during the 1890s. An example was in May 1894, when the Board reluctantly agreed to a request by Hughlings Jackson to admit a male epileptic patient named Boddy 'who had been in a lunatic asylum'. On the day after admission, Boddy 'became extremely violent and attempted to stab the attendant with a dinner knife', whereupon Burford Rawlings ordered him to be discharged forthwith. The Board approved the secretary's action, 'and considered the case well illustrates the value of the rule which had been relaxed in this instance'. This and other clashes with Burford Rawlings over cases such as Olive Griffin and Grace Bridges were significant factors in the developing schism between the physicians and the administration that culminated in the events of 1901 and the Fry Commission.

However, as the century progressed and psychiatric disorders were increasingly considered likely to have an organic (neurological) basis, the relationship between neurological and psychiatric conditions became closer and the two disciplines started to converge. Indeed, leading continental psychiatrists such as Kraepelin and Meynert were trained in neuropathology, and the widely accepted hereditarian theories of the neurological taint and of degeneration increasingly placed neurological and psychiatric disorders within the same framework. Thus, maintaining the distinction between 'mental' and 'nervous' disease and the rigid admissions policy of the National Hospital became somewhat anachronistic.

Several of the early medical staff had begun to take an interest in aspects of psychiatric disturbance. Hughlings Jackson, as a member of the Medico-Psychological Association since 1866, wrote extensively on mind–brain issues, and his ideas on evolution and dissolution of the nervous system exerted much influence on the development of British psychiatric theory during the second half of the nineteenth century. Gowers also wrote on various psychological conditions (notably hysteria) as did other physicians, such as Joseph Ormerod and Risien Russell, and the ophthalmic surgeon Robert Brudenell Carter. Sir James Crichton-Browne, a leading British psychiatrist and patron of Hughlings Jackson and Ferrier's work in Wakefield, was for many years a governor and prominent public supporter of the National Hospital. Several house physicians and resident medical officers employed during the 1880s and 1890s, including William Stoddart, William Rivers and Frederick Golla, subsequently achieved distinction in British psychiatry.[3] For many young doctors interested in mental diseases, working at the National Hospital was as important a rite of passage for a career in psychiatry as it was in neurology.

In 1889–90, a notable episode in the history of British psychiatry occurred, in which the staff at Queen Square were deeply involved. This was the attempt, led by Robert Brudenell Carter, to persuade the newly formed London County Council to establish a hospital for the treatment of early cases of mental disorder. This proposal is interesting in that it shows how central the National Hospital had become in medical affairs, and also how psychiatric disease and asylum provision were viewed at the time.

The London County Council had recently assumed responsibility for asylums, at a time when there was considered to be a rapid increase in the number of cases of insanity in the community and much public debate about their management. Brudenell Carter, who had previously written a book on hysteria,[4] was one of the first elected members of the Council and vice-chairman of its Sanitary and General Purposes Committee. In response, in April 1889, the London County Council set up a committee to study his proposal, and Brudenell Carter was elected chair with 15 committee members, many distinguished figures in British medicine, including Clifford Allbutt, Sir John Banks, Thomas Bryant, John Marshall, Richard Quain, Thomas Whipham and Stephen MacKenzie. There were also five

---

[3] Two other leading British psychiatrists of the day, Henry Maudsley and Charles Mercier, had also both applied unsuccessfully for hospital appointments in the 1860s and 1870s.

[4] R. B. Carter, *On the Pathology and Treatment of Hysteria* (London: John Churchill, 1853).

members of staff from the National Hospital – Gowers, Ferrier, Bastian, Buzzard and Horsley – and two psychiatrists, Crighton-Browne and Batty Tuke. The committee took detailed evidence and also sent a questionnaire to the 65 medical superintendents of all the asylums around the country.[5]

The benefits of a medical hospital, in contrast to an asylum, were unanimously agreed by all committee members, a decision justified by the facts: that the study of insanity had lagged behind other fields of medicine, and especially neurology; that asylums could not treat patients in the contemporary medical manner, and patients were denied the benefit of modern investigatory and treatment facilities; that early cases of insanity might be curable; and that the establishment of a hospital along medical lines could 'scarcely fail to increase knowledge on the subject and consequently increases in prevention and cure'. In the committee's view, asylums provided treatments based on moral principles but which were not sufficiently scientific or medical. It was proposed that the new hospital should have 100 beds, be based in London and be staffed by visiting medical physicians. It seems very likely that the model of the National Hospital was in the minds of the committee, on the basis that its achievements in neurology could be reproduced in the field of psychiatry, and with the expectation that the visiting staff would be drawn from the National Hospital's own doctors.

Crichton-Browne offered an impression of asylum practice, emphasising that the medical superintendents were so weighed down with administration that medical study was virtually impossible. He mentioned a case of an asylum inpatient who thought the superintendent was the architect, as he only appeared 'when the chimney smokes or walls need repainting'. Crichton-Browne recalled that, when he was superintendent of the West Riding Lunatic Asylum:

> he had to sign cheques for £40,000 per year and [managed] a staff of 200 nurses and attendants, a large farm and butcher's shop, a bakery and a brewery and weaving sheds … that he was responsible to. The magistrates looked to me for the efficient management of all these departments, and it was with the

utmost difficulty that I succeeded in getting any time for medical or scientific work.

Ferrier pointed out that:

> until we are able to correlate mental disorders with their physical substrata, and this we are very far from being able to do, we cannot be said to possess any real knowledge on the subject and therefore investigations and means of research calculated to elucidate these problems are greatly to be desired … I have not the slightest doubt that a hospital for the insane, in which insanity shall be studied in the same manner, and with the same scientific methods as are applied to general diseases in our hospitals, will greatly enlarge our knowledge on this subject, and as a natural consequence, lead to more successful methods of dealing with this.

Clifford Allbutt gave his views on why psychiatry, based in asylum practice, could not hope to make progress. What was needed was

> to remove from such places the vast number of worn-out lunatics, chronic cases and wreckage of all kinds. These constitute really the great wet blanket which lies upon the whole thing. Worn-out old dements, imbeciles and aged people are shovelled in upon the asylums from the workhouses; and I think the first thing to be done is to get all the mere imbeciles back into the workhouses which is the proper place for them and where they are indeed much happier, for they are near their own friends and homes. And then the lunatic wreckage, or properly so-called for I certainly do not think that all people with failing memories ought to be called lunatics and sent to asylums as they are now; but the more hopeless cases of lunacy proper should be taken in larger number to places like Caterham and Leavesden where you would have a comparative small and inexpensive staff and where it would not be necessary to have a very accomplished medical superintendent to take charge of them. The place might be regarded as a special sort of workhouse.

There were 65 responses to the questionnaire from medical superintendents, and 75 per cent of respondents expressed dissatisfaction with the present system of investigation of disease in asylums, 63 per cent were dissatisfied with the facilities for careful treatment of individual cases, 32 per cent approved of the proposal to set up a medical hospital without qualification, and a further 26 per cent approved the proposals albeit with some qualifications. Only 23 per cent were opposed to the idea.

---

5 See *Report of the Committee of the London County Council on a Hospital for the Insane* (London, 1890), reproduced as Appendix A in H. C. Burdett, *Hospitals and Asylums of the World*, Vol. **II** (London: Churchill, 1891), pp. 159-247. Subsequent quotations from the various committee members are taken from this report.

The committee presented its report to the London County Council in March 1890 with the unanimous view that the Council should establish a 100-bed hospital 'for the study and curative treatment of insanity in pauper lunatics of both sexes'. This should be based in London, the honorary medical staff consisting of visiting physicians and surgeons who already held general hospital appointments, rather than specialists in 'psychological medicine', and with funding from the London County Council. The cost for admission might be 2–3 times that in an asylum but the gain for patients and the scientific study of lunacy would, in the committee's view, be great. A decision on the proposals was first postponed, and these were eventually rejected by the London County Council itself when the situation degenerated into a turf-war between alienists and physicians. Many alienists resented what they saw as a patronising attempt by neurologists to belittle their specialty and to take it over, and in July 1890, the Scottish psychiatrist David Yellowlees, the newly elected president of the Medico-Psychological Association, devoted much of his presidential address to denouncing the committee's report. During the heated discussion that followed, Dr David Bower, of the Springfield House private asylum near Bedford, alleged that 'What the [London County] Council Committee recommended as to the staff and situation [of the proposed new hospital] are suggestive of inspiration by certain witnesses who are on the staff of a certain hospital in a London square, the situation of which was by the Committee recommended for the proposed hospital.'[6]

In the face of hostility from the alienist establishment, the idea was dropped, but two prominent psychiatrists, Maudsley and Mott, were not to be dissuaded, and the debate was revived in 1907, in the Asylums Committee of the London County Council, and this led directly to the establishment of the Maudsley Hospital, exactly along the lines proposed by Brudenell Carter but by then with no link to Queen Square. The idea of a new type of asylum linked to the National Hospital presented an extraordinary opportunity, but regretfully it was not to be.

Brudenell Carter was not the only National Hospital staff member at the time to be involved with psychiatry. Risien Russell was also sympathetic

and, according to Macdonald Critchley,[7] had a practice comprising

> a large proportion of chronic psychotics and psychoneurotics ... he held strong views on the need for keeping such patients out of institutions ... for the insane, and he indubitably made himself unpopular among ... alienists by the force of his views which he never concealed. He often acted as an expert witness in the High Courts particularly upon psychiatric issues ... he became Chairman of the National Society for Lunacy Reform.

His psychiatric interest also resulted in a large and lucrative private practice.

The failure of Brudenell Carter's initiative seems to have signalled the end of any interaction between Queen Square and psychiatry over the next two decades at least. Furthermore, no psychiatrist was appointed to the staff at Queen Square until 1926, although other specialties, less relevant to neurology, were represented, such as gynaecology and orthopaedics. The hospital rules continued to exert a strong prejudice against the admission as inpatients of cases with definite symptoms of mental disorder or defect.

There were, however, two common conditions manifesting psychiatric symptoms that did concern the practice of neurology: hysteria and general paralysis of the insane. Gowers devoted 40 pages of the *Manual* to hysteria. He conceded that hysteria 'in its slighter forms ... is as much a temperament as a disease', but considered the condition, more generally, to have a strong component of inherited degeneracy comprising the neurological taint, for which an 'exciting cause' that might not necessarily be severe was needed. He believed that about 50 per cent of cases were associated with morbid conditions of the genital organs. The condition could be spread from one individual to another by 'moral contagion'. Although the symptoms often developed in the presence of organic disease, in the absence of anatomical or pathological findings, he considered hysteria to be

> A morbid state of the nervous system, which is far more common in women than in men. The primary derangement is in the higher cerebral centres, but the functions of the lower centres in the brain, of the spinal cord, and of the sympathetic system may be secondarily disordered ... [in contradistinction to the public

[6] D. Yellowlees, 'Presidential Address at the Medico-Psychological Association, held at the Royal Asylum, Gartnavel, Glasgow, July 24 1890'. *Journal of Mental Science* **36**: 473–489.

[7] Anon. (Macdonald Critchley), *Queen Square and the National Hospital 1860–1960* (London: Chartered Society of Queen Square, 1960).

view that the symptoms are simulated] in medicine it is now generally recognized that the malady is a real one, occasionally of great severity, and to a large extent beyond the direct influence of the patient's will ... Hysteria is probably the most perfect type of a functional malady. It not only consists in, but arises by, a functional disturbance, a loss of due balance between certain of the higher functions of the brain ... Our knowledge of the nature of the primary disturbance that constitutes the essential element in hysteria is too visionary to render its discussion of practical value ... In speaking of hysteria as a functional disease, it is not denied that changes in the finer nutrition of the nerve elements may underlie and result from it.

Another important ingredient of psychiatric theory at the time was the notion of inherited degeneration. Gowers fully subscribed to this concept and included hysteria within the group of conditions comprising the neurological trait (or taint). He then proceeded to give a masterly account of the clinical features of the condition, and its prognosis and treatment.[8]

Bastian made interesting contributions on the difference between organic and functional symptoms, and Kinnier Wilson devoted his Morison lectures to the topic, considering hysterical seizures to be perfect examples of Jackson's concept of 'highest level fits'. He also insisted that the distinction between functional and organic was

so far as I personally am concerned, an ancient platitude ... I date my awakening to a conversation with my old teacher, the late Dr. Charlton Bastian, who, when I told him a patient had been admitted under his care suffering from what I, with the dogmatism of the house-physician, described as 'functional fits,' replied: 'Did you ever see a fit that was not functional?'[9]

Hughlings Jackson, on the other hand, made almost no reference to hysteria, except to exclude it from a diagnosis of epilepsy. He did not consider it as a 'disease and preferred the adjectival use of the term hysterical to refer to an emotionally disturbed state usually encountered in unmarried females and closely linked to malingering'.

---

[8] Many symptoms and conditions were considered part of the neurological trait, and as Walshe rather pithily put it: 'There is ... no symptom-complex of somatic illness that may not have its hysterical "double".'
[9] S. A. K. Wilson, 'Morison Lectures on Nervous Semiology, with Special Reference to Epilepsy', *British Medical Journal* 2 (1930): 50–4.

Outside Queen Square, hysteria had also assumed great importance in neurological practice. Charcot devoted considerable attention to this disorder, which he considered to be organic. Widespread use of the term 'hystero-epilepsy' derives largely from Charcot's own confused appreciation of the condition, and his uncertainty about whether this was a form of true epilepsy or a psychological phenomenon. The confusion was intensified by the initial use of bromides, an effective therapy for epilepsy, in hysteroid cases. Romberg and other European authorities did, like Gowers, certainly consider hysteria to be an organic disease with both an 'invisible lesion' and psychological influences. Romberg noted the reflex hyperexcitability and uterine connections, and thought the condition had its origin in the sexual maturity of the female. He too was convinced of its heritability, but also concluded that it could be acquired by 'a luxurious and indolent mode of life'. Charcot believed that hysteria was largely inherited, but showed that paralysis in this context could result from psychological factors – it might be induced by shock, for instance – and could be treated by hypnosis. The French school of neurology and neurologists, including Babinski and Froment, were heavily influenced by Charcot, but his greatest legacy was the influence on Freud, who eventually placed hysteria firmly in the realm of the psychogenic.

By the end of the nineteenth century, psychiatry and neurology had converged more than at any previous time in history. The physicians at Queen Square did contribute to this enlightenment and, for a while, it seemed that the discipline of neuropsychiatry would flourish, but any optimism was misplaced. With the rise of psychoanalytical theory and of psychodynamic practice, a wedge was driven between the two disciplines, which diverged substantially over the next 50 years and, as the twentieth century progressed, the stigmatisation of psychiatric disease in both professional and public discourse increased.

Shell-shock and Psychiatry at the National Hospital 1914–1918

Although interest in routine psychiatry had diminished in the first decades of the twentieth century, the National Hospital and its physicians did play a significant role in the evolution of theory and treatment of what was to become known in the First World War as 'shell-shock'. These cases began to appear within a few months of the onset of hostilities in France. In

December 1914, William Aldren Turner, by then 50 years of age and one of the senior neurologists on the hospital staff, was dispatched by the War Office to France as a temporary lieutenant-colonel, to investigate what was emerging as an apparent epidemic of cases. There he met his younger colleague Gordon Holmes, already posted to the Western front, and also the physician-psychologist Charles Myers. Their discussions and decisions behind the lines in Boulogne were to play an important role in the story of 'shell-shock' and its treatment.

Initially, the universal military view was that the symptoms were 'pure funk', and the authorities were highly unsympathetic to the affected soldiers, who were generally considered to be 'scrim-shankers'. It is known that some were executed on the battlefield for cowardice. A similar strand of medical opinion was typified by Charles Wilson (later, Lord Moran), for instance, who viewed war neurosis as a form of degeneracy, linked to urbanisation, a throwback to the nineteenth-century theories of *dégénérescence*, and his views were a part of a growing eugenic tendency. Moran wrote: 'Such men went about plainly unable to stand this test of men. They had about them the marks known to our calling of the incomplete man, the stamp of degeneracy ... just a worthless chap, without shame, the worst product of the towns ... [sent to] a shell shock hospital with a rabble of mis-shapen creatures from the towns'.[10]

However, as the number of cases rapidly increased, medical interest was aroused. A debate then ensued about whether the condition was a form of blast injury or concussion (commotional injury), or psychoneurosis. The term 'shell-shock' first appeared in print in a paper by Charles Myers in the *Lancet* where he described three examples, concluding that the relationship of these cases to hysteria was 'close'.[11] Meanwhile, in 1915, the War Office established a 'shell-shock committee' which included as members the Bethlem psychiatrist Maurice Craig and the Queen Square neurologists Turner and Farquhar Buzzard. Craig and Buzzard, particularly, were said to have been instrumental in persuading the War Office to recognise shell-shock as a 'proper injury' that required specific treatment facilities. The situation was confused by the range of cases, some deemed simply to be cowardice, some functional neurotic conditions, and some genuinely post-concussional.

When Turner returned to London early in 1915, at his recommendation Myers was put in charge of the medical management of these cases on the Western front. Myers' initial plan was to repatriate affected soldiers to psychiatric hospitals being established for this purpose in various parts of the country. However, as the numbers rose, this proved impossible. By then Myers had furthermore formed the view that the longer the condition was left untreated the more it became a fixed idea and intractable, and so proposed a series of forward treatment centres, just behind the lines, to treat men promptly without evacuation. In August 1916, he was promoted to lieutenant-colonel, appointed psychological consultant to the Army and given responsibility for shell-shock along the entire front line. However, very quickly, the military authorities became concerned about the number of cases leaving the battlefield, and, in January 1917, Myers was relieved of his responsibilities and replaced by Gordon Holmes, who held radically different attitudes to the nature and treatment of the condition. Holmes had little patience with psychological approaches to shell-shock, and was contemptuous of hysterics. He was anxious, too, that transferring patients out of the battle zone would lead to a flood of copy-cat cases. In time, facilities close to the front were closed and Holmes seems to have dealt with the condition by denying its existence.

In the forward centres and the base (stationary) hospitals, a variety of treatment approaches was taken, the major aim of which was to get the soldiers back to a state where they could be returned to the front lines. Hypnosis was often tried for a quick result to demonstrate the 'false' nature of the neurological symptoms, and in one large centre, commanded by William Brown,[12] treatment involved

---

[10] C. Wilson, *The Anatomy of Courage* (London: Constable and Company Ltd, 1945).

[11] C. S. Myers, 'A Contribution to the Study of "Shell-Shock"', *Lancet* **183** (1914): 316–18. Later, he regretted using the term and suggested that it be dropped – a suggestion adopted in the Royal Commission report of 1922. Myers was a close associate of William Rivers and both were important figures in wartime neurology: see B. Shephard, *Headhunters: The Search for the Science of the Mind* (London: Bodley Head, 2014).

[12] Major William Brown commanded the centre for the Fourth Army on the Somme between November 1916 and 1918. He reportedly treated 2,000–3,000 soldiers with high success rates.

abreaction and hypnosis. Less psychological approaches were adopted by another ex-Queen Square trainee Dudley William Carmalt-Jones[13] in No. 4 Stationary Hospital in Arques. He eschewed hypnotism and treated his patients with rest, medication to induce sleep and a programme of graduated exercise, ending with route marches. William Johnson[14] followed Carmalt-Jones' therapeutic lines, supported by extensive massage, and did not believe that psychotherapy was either needed or beneficial. All recognised that the attitude of the physician towards the condition was an important factor in the success of the treatment.

The various shades of opinion about the cause and treatment of shell-shock were well represented in the special meeting of the sections on psychiatry and neurology of the Royal Society of Medicine held in January 1916. Julian Taylor was the president of the neurology section and Frederick Mott of the psychiatric section, and among the neurologists who expressed opinions were Collier, Fearnsides, Harris and Head. Collier believed that some of the cases were due to epilepsy, and Fearnsides presented his series of 70 cases admitted to Maida Vale 'arriving directly from France with special tickets', attributing some of the cases to syphilis. However, as the war proceeded, the Army and the neurological establishment increasingly agreed with Holmes that 'shell-shock' had no organic basis and was, in most instances, the consequence of mental trauma.

The soldiers who were returned to the UK were sent to a variety of specialist centres. The largest and most important was Maghull Hospital, which had been taken over by the military in 1914 to treat war neuroses, and became 'a centre for the study of abnormal psychology'. Those who spent time working there included the future Queen Square psychiatrist Bernard Hart, and also William Brown, W. H. R. Rivers and William McDougall. The staff at Craiglockhart, established in 1915 to deal with affected officers, included Rivers, Brown and

Major Ruggles (an American). Seale Hayne was a specialist rehabilitation unit for war neuroses staffed by physicians rather than psychiatrists. A special hospital for war neuroses run by Edward Mapother opened in Denmark Hill in August 1919, where Mott argued that psychotherapy could be harmful, preferring a quiet environment to allow diversion of the mind from the recollection of the terrifying experiences as essential for successful treatment commenting that: 'only common-sense and interest in the comfort, welfare and amusement of these neurotic patients are necessary for their recovery'.

The engagement of the National Hospital with shell-shock can be traced to a meeting of the Board of Management on 10 November 1914, at which an appeal from Lord Knutsford, chairman of the London Hospital House Committee, was discussed. This was published in the national press:

> There are a certain number of our gallant soldiers for whom no proper provision is at present obtainable but is sorely needed. They are suffering from very severe mental and nervous shock due to exposure, excessive strain, and tension. They can be cured if only they receive proper attention from physicians who have made a specialty of treating such conditions. These men are quite unsuitable patients for general hospitals, as their chance of recovery depends on absolute quiet and on the individual and prolonged attention of the physician. If not cured, these men will drift back to the world as wrecks, and miserable wrecks, for the rest of their lives.[15]

In response, on behalf of the staff of the hospital, Farquhar Buzzard drafted a letter to Lord Knutsford and the press pointing out that the hospital would make itself fully available to treat soldiers with nervous complaints, and, within a few days, Adolf S, a Belgian soldier, was admitted with a diagnosis of hysterical paraparesis. In December, a young private from the First Royal Dragoons with violent trembling of his legs and weakness, and an 18-year-old from the London Scottish Regiment suffering from mutism, were also accepted for treatment.

In 1915, Lord Beauchamp, the president of the National Hospital, announced in *The Times* that the War Office was 'arranging to send soldiers suffering

---

[13] *Dudley William Carmalt-Jones' Autobiography Entitled 'A Physician in Spite of Himself'* (London: Royal Society of Medicine Press, 2009): see A. Compston, 'From the Archives', *Brain* **136** (2013): 1681–6 for an account of Carmalt-Jones and his methods of treatment at Arques.

[14] Captain William Johnson was a neurologist posted to Passchendaele, and between August and October 1917 he treated 5,000 patients (1 per cent of all the troops engaged). He claimed a surprisingly high success rate.

[15] *Daily Mail*, 3 November 1914.

from shock to be treated at Queen Square in wards specially set apart for the purpose, and the cost of their maintenance would be met by the War Office and the Ministry of Pensions'. David Wire and John Back wards were both used for military casualties, and two adjoining houses in Guilford Street were fitted up to accommodate between 30 and 40 cases. At the request of the Minister of Pensions, many invalided sailors and soldiers were also investigated as outpatients.

A number of the hospital's physicians at the time focused on the condition. Aldren Turner chose the topic 'Neurosis and Psychosis of War' for his Bradshaw lecture delivered at the Royal College of Physicians in 1918. Frederick Batten, who had retired from clinical duties in 1908 to become the first dean of the medical school, resumed his clinical activities to deputise during Tooth's absence and, as physician to the forces in the Near East, took a particular interest in amnesia and psychasthenia. He employed the standard approach to the treatment of hysteria, which included physical exercise, rest, isolation, a change of surroundings, faradism and encouragement, but had to acknowledge that this had limited success.[16] Batten obtained a grant from the Medical Research Council to allow one of the residents at Queen Square, Francis Walshe, to determine whether shell-shock had a physical or psychological basis. Walshe, along with many of the staff physicians, was unsympathetic to this group of patients, and he used pejorative descriptive terms in the hospital case notes such as 'pale, effeminate youth ..., a typical hysteric, [who] makes the most of his illness'. Walshe was also not averse to using electrical therapy, as the following handwritten remarks in Batten's case notes indicate: 'a bumptious conceited young wiseacre' was given strong faradism until he completely recovered from his paralysis. In another severely depressed patient, a loss of sensation on the right foot was 'speedily and successfully exorcised by strong faradism and a day in bed and isolation. [The patient] remained however a neurotic creature never happy unless discussing his symptoms with some unwary fellow patient.' Although categorised as 'research', no publications emerged from this work.

In 1915, Lewis Yealland[17] was appointed to the post of resident medical officer at Queen Square, and he soon became the leading therapist for shell-shock at the hospital, working together with E. D. Adrian.[18] Yealland and Adrian devised an intensive treatment programme incorporating electrotherapy. Shocks to the head had been used occasionally before in the treatment of psychosis in the nineteenth century but this practice had largely vanished from the UK by the start of the twentieth century. At Queen Square, however, faradic and galvanic stimulation and sinusoidal baths were still being widely employed to treat a range of neurological conditions, and the National Hospital had gained a reputation for the excellence of its electrical therapy. This no doubt influenced the therapies developed by Yealland and Adrian.

At the time, neither were consultant-grade physicians, but they were given responsibility for the treatment of the patients admitted with 'shell-shock' on behalf of named consultants. In their view, patients with war neurosis had three unifying characteristics: weakness of the will, negativism (an active but not necessarily conscious resistance to the idea of recovery) and increased suggestibility. Previously, once the diagnosis of hysteria had been made at Queen Square, the patient was discharged with no serious attempt at rehabilitation, a situation that could not be allowed to

---

[16] F. Batten, 'Some Functional Nervous Affections Produced by the War', *Quarterly Journal of Medicine* 9 (1916): 73–82.

[17] Lewis Ralph Yealland was a Canadian who trained in medicine at the University of Western Ontario. In 1915, he worked at Queen Square, and was appointed after the war as a psychiatrist at the Prince of Wales' Hospital, Tottenham Green, and at the West End Hospital. His main postwar interest was in epilepsy (Anon., 'Obituary', *Lancet* 263 (1954): 577). His son Michael trained at Queen Square and worked as a consultant neurologist in Cambridge.

[18] Edgar Douglas (always known as 'E. D.') Adrian was born in Hampstead, educated at Westminster School and studied natural sciences at Trinity College Cambridge. During the war, Adrian served in the Royal Army Medical Corps and was neurologist to the Connaught Hospital, Aldershot. He also treated soldiers with nerve damage at St Bartholomew's Hospital. He returned to Cambridge in 1925, where he studied the electrical basis of activity in nerve cells, using electroencephalography to study Berger rhythms, and carried out work on sensation. He confirmed Berger's findings and this paved the way for the use of electroencephalography in epilepsy. He was appointed at the University of Cambridge, as Foulerton Professor in 1929 and then as Professor of Physiology in 1937. He received the Nobel Prize for physiology or medicine in 1932, jointly with Sir Charles Sherrington. He was elected FRS in 1923, and between 1950 and 1955 served as the Society's president.

continue in wartime when human resources were at a premium. At the National Hospital, these two young physicians treated over 250 cases with hysterical mutism, aphonia, deafness, blindness, paralysis, hysterical fits and gait disorder – each often of long duration. Their treatment was based on re-education and strong suggestion designed to convince the patient that he would certainly be cured. Yealland elected to use the term 'functional nervous disorder' rather than hysteria, and explained the soldier's handicaps in physical terms to avoid giving the erroneous impression that he considered him to be a malingerer. He adopted an authoritative manner and appealed to the serviceman's sense of honour and familial responsibility: 'if you recover quickly, then it is due to a disease, if you recover slowly … then I shall decide that your condition is due to malingering'. In 1917, they published an account of their approach. The key was to instill into the patient the belief that:

> the physician understands his case and is able to cure him. … The best attitude [for the physician to adopt] is one of mild boredom bred of perfect familiarity with the patient's disorder … it is better to avoid discussing the case … an argument in which the physician does not seem perfectly sure of his ground is likely to weaken his authority at the moment when it should be absolutely unquestioned … the patient is never allowed any say in the matter. He is not asked whether he can raise his paralysed arm or not; he is ordered to raise it, and told that he can do it perfectly if he tries. Rapidity and an authoritative manner are the chief factors in the re-educative process.[19]

Yealland provided greater detail about the methods in his book, published at the end of the war.[20] Whilst hypnosis and psychoanalysis might be employed, their preferred method of therapy for Yealland and Adrian was 'suggestive treatment and re-education', based on the principle that a disorder originating in suggestion could be alleviated by counter-suggestion, however made, provided that it was strong enough to persuade the patient of the likelihood of cure. The therapy usually included the use of a faradic current applied at increasing strengths to dysfunctional parts of the body until the pain was unbearable. For functional deafness, tuning forks of different frequencies were applied to the mastoid.

Occasionally, an electrical current was also applied to the scalp overlying the motor cortex, as, for example, in the case of an officer who had some knowledge of neuroanatomy and who recovered promptly after treatment. Re-education involved eliciting electrically induced or reflex activity in paralysed muscles to demonstrate that the affected parts could indeed function. An authoritarian and overbearing attitude was adopted so as to overawe the soldiers. The methods hovered between persuasion and punishment, and required the treating physician to appear confident, utterly familiar with this type of case, outwardly bored at having to deal with yet another case using faradism, and to adopt a patrician air of complete assurance rather than trifling with elaborate explanation: 'As soon as the least sign of recovery has appeared … the patient is given no time to collect his thoughts … but is hurried along … until the disordered function has completely recovered.'

The very first patient with shell-shock treated by Yealland was Solomon W, a 35-year-old private from the 9th Oxfordshire and Buckinghamshire Light Infantry who had worked as a waiter in the officer's mess in France and was admitted to Queen Square on 14 December 1915 complaining of intractable shooting pains in his neck and right arm. Yealland noted weakness of muscles around the shoulder girdle and proceeded to apply faradism to the right arm and leg with massage and radiant heat to the right shoulder. The case notes show that he was discharged 'improved' after 2½ months of inpatient therapy.

There is no doubt that fear of electrocution filled some of the soldiers with dread, forcing them to take their own discharge whereas the prospect of painful treatment led to a 'miraculous spontaneous recovery' in others. In his book 'Tales of the National', Godfrey Hamilton describes how, one morning, the matron, who called him each morning with an account of the previous day's activities, reported 'the fish was bad again yesterday and one of the soldiers hung himself in the stable'. A hand-written account by one of the residents, Dr Wilson, of a dream experienced by a 35-year-old private in the Army Service Corps, who had developed functional paraparesis after a shell explosion during the Battle of Ypres, appears in the hospital case notes of 1918:

> A fair-sized room painted white. In the centre of the room was a white enamelled table, and nearby two dressing trolleys. On the floor were yards and yards of

[19] L. R. Yealland and E. D. Adrian, 'The Treatment of Some Common War Neuroses', *Lancet* **189** (1917): 867–72.
[20] L. R. Yealland, *Hysterical Disorders of Warfare* (London: Macmillan & Co., 1918).

cable, which was strewn all over the place, and connected to a telegraph instrument placed upon an ordinary deal table. The room was crowded with nurses who were in white dresses and white aprons, they were all talking excitedly. A Doctor now enters in a white coat, he walks round the room, stepping over the coils of wire and is also excited and in a great hurry. He has a knife in his hand … The doctor was an exact representation of Dr. Yealland.

Many patients referred to Queen Square came from other military hospitals, for instance from Netley and the Maudsley wing at Denmark Hill, and also some from the American, Belgian, Canadian, Australian and South African military. Even the great authority on shell-shock, Frederick Mott, referred his most refractory cases for treatment to the National Hospital. Mott later wrote that he believed Yealland's success was attributable to his reputation for curing intractable cases, the impressive array of machines and coloured lights, and the power of suggestion. The greatest success with these methods occurred in the context of loss of function, such as in paralysis or mutism. A period of isolation was considered more successful for functional tremors, pseudoseizures and psychogenic jerks, because this rendered 'the patient's illness a dreary and unprofitable business'. Yealland also asked soldiers with functional fits to mimic these in an effort to demonstrate to the patient that there was an element of conscious control, and then taught them to inhibit the convulsion by re-education.

During the First World War, up to 100 of the hospital's 270 beds were occupied by wounded soldiers, and a total of 1,272 servicemen were treated. At least a third were considered to have chronic functional neurological disorders (and the others were largely spinal or head injury cases). The hospital case notes show that Yealland treated at least 196 of the 323 soldiers admitted with functional nervous disorders between 1915 and 1918, and he claimed full recovery in 88 cases and improvement in 84, with failure in 24. However, both he and Adrian conceded that their methods were not curative, nor did they permanently alter the soldier's mental state.[21] A relatively small number of soldiers returned to the front, and Yealland concluded that it would be unwise to send

even recovered cases back to the battlefield because relapse was highly probable.

The methods employed at Queen Square came under criticism from some, including Charles Myers, who wrote to the *Lancet*:

> During the war there were certain physicians who could explain to a patient suffering from functional hemiplegia that the cortical cells on one side of the brain were out of order … And they would proceed to tone up the disordered cells by painful faradism … I have always been convinced that such measures are not only needless, but also dangerous.[22]

The notion that punishment was a central part of the treatment at the National Hospital, and that Yealland was its most extreme advocate, is too harsh.[23] Although some criticism of Yealland's wartime approach to shell-shock may now seem justifiable, it was in line with the medical practice of the time, and aversion shock therapy continued to be used long into the second half of the twentieth century. Yealland's views on causation were not so very different from the modern somatic model. His methods also remain of more than historical interest as neurologists and psychiatrists continue to struggle to define a workable paradigm for functional neurological disease, and to develop effective treatment approaches for the many cases that continue to be seen at the National Hospital and elsewhere. Suggestion and persuasion probably play an important if unacknowledged role in many types of current technological or scientific therapies.

Yealland's obituarist hardly mentions his wartime work, highlighting his subsequent interest in epilepsy and his kindness and dedication to patients seen in civilian neurological practice. He remained interested in and involved with functional illness:

> Yealland would induce hysterical patients to produce fits at the clinic, and there only, with increasing

---

[21] S. Linden and E. Jones, '"Shell Shock" Revisited: An Examination of the Case Records of the National Hospital in London', *Medical History* 58 (2014): 519–45.

[22] C. S. Myers, 'The Justifiability of Therapeutic Lying', *Lancet* **194** (1919): 1213–14.

[23] Pat Barker's Booker Prize-winning *Regeneration* trilogy (1991–5) was partly responsible for this calumny. She characterised Yealland inaccurately and unfairly as a stern figure who punished shell-shocked soldiers with electrical torture, contrasting his allegedly callous approach with that of the more sympathetic Rivers, at Craiglockhart, who stressed the importance of empathy and adopted psychoanalytical techniques. See P. Barker, *Regeneration* (London: Viking, 1991), where whole tracts are copied directly from Yealland's own descriptions of his treatment approach.

periods of freedom from seizures at home. They were informed with absolute assurance that there could be no fits for a certain interval of time and he gravely wrote [that it was to be at] the next appointment at the clinic when the next fit, which would be milder, would be ready to take place. The final and last seizure was only partially induced. Thereby demonstrating to the patient that a cure was effected. The patient, purely as a matter of interest, was advised to come and have a talk with him in three months' time. In most cases the treatment was a complete success. He had a large consulting practice, and even when the patient was beyond effective treatment, he always left behind him an atmosphere of calm philosophy which was of great spiritual assistance to the household. In his later years he had few equals in the diagnosis of cerebral tumour. A non-smoker and teetotaller, L. R. Y. was a man of simple habits. His delightful personality will be missed by many both inside and outside the profession. His death is another instance of a lifetime of strenuous work in war and peace going unrewarded by any years of peaceful retirement.[24]

After the war, a Royal Commission,[25] chaired by Lord Southborough, was established, with the Queen Square physicians Aldren Turner and Birley among the members. The terms of reference of the committee were

> To consider the different types of hysteria and traumatic neuroses commonly called 'shell-shock'; to collate the expert knowledge derived by the service medical authorities and the medical profession from the experience of the war, with a view to recording for future use the ascertained facts as to its origin, nature and remedial treatment, and to advise whether by military training or education, some scientific method of guarding against its occurrence can be devised.

The committee had 41 sittings, with 59 witnesses.[26] The first was Gordon Holmes, whose

influence can clearly be seen in the committee's recommendations. The committee concluded that the term 'shell-shock' should be omitted from official nomenclature, and that no cases of mental breakdown should be classified as a battle casualty. It considered that the reported cases could be divided into three categories: (1) genuine concussion, without visible wound, as a result of shell explosion: all witnesses agreed that these cases were relatively few; (2) emotional shock, either acute in persons with neuropathic predisposition or developing slowly as a result of prolonged strain, the final breakdown being brought on by sometimes relatively trivial cause; and (3) nervous or mental exhaustion as a result of prolonged strain or hardship. In many cases, these categories were combined. The committee acknowledged the difficulty in differentiating cowardice from neurosis since fear was a causal factor in both. Following Holmes' line, treatment close to the front was preferred where possible, and every effort taken to prevent affected soldiers leaving the battalion or divisional area, with none allowed to think that loss of nervous or mental control could provide an honourable avenue of escape from the battlefield. When cases were sufficiently severe to necessitate more scientific or elaborate treatment, they should be sent to special neurological centres, under the care of an expert in nervous diseases, but no such patient should be allowed to accept the idea of nervous breakdown. Only in exceptional circumstances would individuals be returned to the UK. If this did prove necessary, treatment apart from other sick or wounded men was advised. It was recommended that

---

[24] Anon., 'Lewis Ralph Yealland: Obituary', *Lancet* **263** (1954): 577–8.

[25] *Report of the War Office Committee of Inquiry into 'Shell-shock'* (London: HMSO, 1922).

[26] Queen Square witnesses included Adie, Bernard Hart and Farquhar Buzzard. Buzzard's evidence is of interest, taking a more psychological view than that of Holmes, and partly reflecting the Jacksonian tradition of the hierarchical structure of the nervous system mixed in with Freudian elements. Shell-shock was, in his view, 'a failure on the part of soldiers to adapt themselves (or maintain their adaptation) to the stress of warfare. These manifestations do not differ in kind from those which characterise the failure of persons of either

sex to adapt themselves to the various forms of stress in civilian life. Failure of adaptation occurs when, for a variety of reasons, primitive instincts and emotions cease to be corrected or controlled by higher mental activities which, both from the individual and racial point of view, are a later development. In any individual therefore the liability to shell-shock must depend on the relative cogency of his primitive instincts and that of his higher mental activities.' Buzzard pointed out that shell-shock was more likely to occur during fatigue, intoxication, exposure to poisons or inadequate food or commotional disturbances of the brain due to injury, concussion etc. In his view, the soldier was usually exposed to more than one of these factors, and breakdown on the part of the higher mental activities could rarely be attributed to one factor alone. Hart was of the opinion that shell-shock was due to a multiplicity of factors, including the mental factors and personality, and he particularly emphasised the effects of secondary gain.

this policy should be widely known throughout the services.

Successful treatment depended much on the personality of the treating physician and his ability to create a curative atmosphere. Apart from physical methods such as baths, electricity and massage, the best results were obtained from simple psychotherapy involving explanation, persuasion and suggestion. Rest of mind and body was essential. In selected cases, hypnosis might be beneficial as a means of inducing suggestion or eliciting forgotten experiences, but usually proved unnecessary and might even aggravate symptoms. The committee did not recommend psychoanalysis in the Freudian sense. There was no mention of the approach to therapy used at Queen Square during the war, and it is notable that neither Yealland nor Adrian was invited to give evidence to the committee. Furthermore, there was no reference to Yealland's book or to his mode of therapy, which, presumably, was by then either diregarded or even discredited.

There was then little further discussion about shell-shock, until the late 1930s when the threat of a new war resulted in setting up the Horder Committee in July 1939 to devise a strategy for dealing with war neuroses. That committee comprised Holmes, Hart and Riddoch from Queen Square, and Mapother, Myers, McCurfy and T. A. Ross from elsewhere. It produced a new memorandum which advocated the psychological vetting of recruits, rapid therapy and a clear public statement that there would be no war pensions for psychological disorders.

Psychiatry at the National Hospital in the Inter-war Years

In the early interwar years, the physicians at the National Hospital seemed to have had little interest in nurturing the practice of psychiatry.

Quite why their engagement with psychiatry had diminished is not clear. In part, it may have been lack of affinity with the rising fashion for psychoanalytical theory, which was then very much in the ascendency, or disenchantment following the experiences with shell-shock, or simply due to the attitude and personalities of the physicians, who were generally more interested in physiology than in the patient as a person. It was, in contrast, a time when a first wave of physical therapies was developing in Europe –

malarial therapy for general paralysis of the insane in 1917, barbiturate-induced deep sleep for schizophrenia in 1920, insulin coma in 1933, and cardiazol shock in 1934. These interventions again seemed to have been largely overlooked at the National Hospital and there is no evidence that any were widely employed in the inter-war years. Equally, although the eugenic movement gathered considerable force elsewhere, there was no enthusiasm for this formulation of disease in clinical practice at Queen Square, despite the hospital physicians' earlier involvement with the concept of the neurological trait and interest in the hereditability of neurological disease.

Aldren Turner did propose the appointment of a 'psychotherapeutic officer' to the Medical Committee on several occasions, but, despite his seniority and influence, the idea was deferred and then finally rejected, largely it seems through the influence of Holmes. Eventually, in 1926, Bernard Hart was appointed as the first physician in psychological medicine at Queen Square, the title of the post itself emphasising the stigma of psychiatry and the view that the discipline should be seen as linked (and subservient) to medicine.[27] Hart was 46 at the time and, in addition to considerable experience in asylum practice, had been physician in psychological medicine at University College Hospital for several years, spending a formative period as a lecturer at Maghull during the war. Despite his intellect and the respect he

---

[27] Bernard Hart, a Londoner from an academic family, was educated at University College School and qualified in medicine from University College (1904). He was interested in philosophy but also in psychological measurement, and had worked with Spearman in measuring dementia by psychometric testing. In 1926, he gave the Goulstonian lectures on 'The Development of Psychopathology and its Place in Medicine', and these lectures formed the basis of a small book *Psychopathology*, which became a popular handbook at the time. He was a prominent London psychiatrist and had a large private practice in the 1920s. He was elected president of the medical section of the British Psychological Society in 1926, and in 1931 became president of the section of psychiatry of the Royal Society of Medicine. He lectured for many years at the Maudsley Hospital on psychotherapy. In retirement, Hart devoted himself to historical studies and was said to be disillusioned with the direction of psychiatry. One can speculate that he was a psychiatrist acceptable to the more hard-line Queen Square physicians because of his quiet nature, practical approach to his patients, disapproval of the wilder excesses of Freudian theory, and his scholarship and interest in history.

commanded, Hart's impact on psychiatry at Queen Square seems not to have been great, and there is little evidence that the subject impinged on hospital policy or practice in those years.

The *Journal of Neurology and Psychopathology*

Early in the twentieth century, in addition to journals devoted to either neurology or psychiatry, several publications attempted to embrace both disciplines. The *Review of Neurology and Psychiatry*, edited by Alexander Bruce and assisted by Byrom Bramwell, was founded in 1902. The first issue contained an article by Sir John Sibbald, the renowned Scottish psychiatrist, emphasising the 'essential unity of the two subjects [neurology and psychiatry]'.[28] When Bruce died in 1911, his son Ninian became the editor. The First World War brought this publishing enterprise to an end, along with many others, but in 1920, Kinnier Wilson, who was married to Ninian Bruce's sister, launched the *Journal of Neurology and Psychopathology* as a replacement, and he ran that journal until 1937. Wilson was one of the few National Hospital physicians in this period who took a sophisticated interest in psychiatry. He thought greatly about the interaction with neurology, and the journal provided a forum in which to express his views. In 'The Realm of Neurology', his unsigned editorial in the first issue, he delivered a warning to neurologists that they should not neglect the psychological and psychiatric aspects of their subject:

> Whither shall the nerve expert turn? Five years of war have led the psychotherapist or practising psychologist to give him a gentle hint that functional nervous disease is not for him; by way of consolation he can interest himself in chronic nervous degenerations, or classify myopathies and cerebellar aplasias to his heart's content. Let him beware, however, of the embryologist, the eugenist and the biometrician, who are hard on his heels ... the truth is, in reality, that the neurologist of today is he who pursues the study of either psychical or physical side, or both, and who has succeeded to an empire wherein is stored the accumulated wealth of knowledge derived and being derived from scientific and clinical research on the part of

many differing groups and fellowships of workers. The nervous system still stands as the very core, the hub, of ever-widening theoretical and practical interests. More than ever must the neurologist be a man of culture and of aspiration, a savant in the right sense of the word, who can see his subject whole, and appreciate contributions from whomsoever they come. He boldly takes its vegetative, sensorimotor, and psychical aspects alike for his province and will not relinquish any section of the field to deputies.

This was followed by another editorial entitled 'Present Position of Psychopathology', in which Wilson anticipated the rise of neuropsychiatry and the advances that would be likely to come in its wake:

> In this common ground the most fundamental principle is the recognition that psychological causes may produce disorder and that in the rectification of such disorder psychological methods of treatment – the methods of psychotherapy – must necessarily be employed ... The dispute which has long raged as to whether mental and so-called 'functional nervous' disorders are of psychical or physical origin – a dispute which is inevitably sterile – should be replaced by a careful taking into account of the material which every method of approach – chemical, physiological, anatomical, psychological – is able to offer, and an attempt to correlate this material into an harmonious whole. Perhaps the conception which promises the most fruitful line of advance in this direction is that of biological reaction, the view that the field of mental and 'nervous' disorders is one in which disease entities in the strict sense of the word cannot profitably be distinguished, but that the clinical pictures encountered are to be regarded as different types of reaction in a psychophysical organism to the environment in which it has to live. In the development of such a conception it may be hoped that all the facts ascertained, whether they be chemical, anatomical, physiological or psychological, will fall into place and be capable of correlation one with another. One of the chief objects of the JOURNAL is to help in this co-ordination and correlation.

Wilson's concept of disease and the marriage of neurology and psychiatry was further developed in the issue for August 1920, where he wrote on 'Conditionalism and Causalism'.

> The tendency either to take an extremely psychological or an extremely material view of certain forms of sickness is partly due to the old conception of causalism in the etiology of disease. Medicine has been cursed by a narrow outlook, which seeks to

---

[28] The journal was originally published by John Wright and Sons, Bristol, although three years later it was bought by William Heinemann (Medical Books), London, before being acquired by the British Medical Association in 1926. The first article was a brief case report: see W. R. Gowers, 'Local Panatrophy', *Review of Neurology and Psychiatry* **1** (1903): 3–4.

find one specific and definite thing as a cause for a most complicated condition such as insanity or neurotic sickness. A garden that has turned into a profusion of weeds has done so because of many factors in conjunction. In other words, the old conception of causalism needs to be replaced by the more modern and broader one of conditionalism … We are confident that once the full recognition of the importance of the psychological factor in some forms of illness is admitted, a reconciliation of the psychological and organic points of view in medicine would become possible through the conception of conditionalism.

These views clearly resonated more generally within the medical profession. In the issue of the *Lancet* for 24 July 1920, only two months after the *Journal of Neurology and Psychopathology* had first appeared, there was a comment under 'Annotations' entitled 'The Realm of Neurology and Psychopathology', referring to the Croonian lecture given by A. F. Hurst,[29] in which he discussed the concept of functional nervous disorder and endorsed the conditionalism argument, concluding: 'The most fruitful line of advance of the present time is that of biological reaction, mental and nervous disorders, not being distinguished as disease entities, but rather as different types of reaction to environment shown by a psychophysical organism.'

The 4 December issue of the *Lancet* in the same year carried an editorial, 'The Outlook in Neurology', taking Farquhar Buzzard's address as president of the psychiatric section of the Royal Society of Medicine to argue again that neurologists should recognise the importance of psychological factors in disease.

The initial editorial board was divided into neurology and psychopathology sections, although the distinction between these two in the journal frontispiece was dropped after only four years (1923–4).[30]

[29] Sir Arthur Hurst was a renowned figure at the interface of British medicine and psychiatry. He was appointed as physician at Guys Hospital, led the neurology department at Netley and Seale Hayne during the war and played an important role in the understanding and treatment of shell-shock; see A. F. Hurst, *Croonian Lectures: Psychology of the Special Senses and their Functional Disorders* (London: Oxford University Press, 1920).

[30] The Neurology board comprised Kinnier Wilson himself; T. Graham Brown, professor of physiology at the Welsh National School of Medicine; R. M. Stewart, deputy superintendent of Whittingham County Asylum and previous neurologist to the British Salonika Force; Charles Symonds, at that time assistant physician for nervous

When Kinnier Wilson died in 1937, Carmichael became editor and the following year the journal changed its name to the *Journal of Neurology and Psychiatry* with a major expansion in the editorial board, including several international members such as Denny-Brown. In 1944, the journal again changed its name to the *Journal of Neurology, Neurosurgery, and Psychiatry* and, in 1949, Carmichael stood down as editor and was replaced by Ritchie Russell. During Wilson's editorship, many Queen Square figures published in the journal, including Denny-Brown, Turner, Symonds, Greenfield, Adie, Stanley Cobb, Carmichael, Critchley and Yealland. Notably, however, Gordon Holmes, with whom Kinnier Wilson had a chronically hostile relationship and who was editor of *Brain*, older and more distinguished, never published in his colleague's journal.

Eliot Slater and Psychiatry at Queen Square 1939–1964

As far as can be ascertained, no acute unit for psychiatric cases was set up at Queen Square during the Second World War, and the discipline remained inactive at the hospital. Special psychoneurosis units were established in the outskirts of London – for instance, in Sutton, where Slater and Shorvon worked – organised in a centrifugal pattern that mirrored that of the neurosurgical units. Bernard Hart, although inactive at the National Hospital during the war, was appointed chief adviser to the Emergency Medical Service (EMS) on psychiatric matters, working in collaboration with Gordon Holmes, who, as in the First World War, remained antithetical to, and impatient with, psychiatric disease. This must have tested Hart's resolve, but he was compensated in 1945 by being appointed CBE for his work. Hart formally retired from his appointment at Queen Square in 1946, although for several years he had not featured on the consultant list in the annual reports. Nor was

diseases at Guy's Hospital, and soon to be appointed to Queen Square. The Psychopathology editorial board comprised Bernard Hart, who was physician for mental diseases at University College Hospital and at the National Hospital; Henry Devine, superintendent of the Borough Mental Hospital in Portsmouth; Maurice Nicoll who had worked with Carl Jung and subsequently at the Empire Hospital for injuries to the nervous system in Vincent Square; and Charles Stanford Read who was physician to the Fisherton House Mental Hospital.

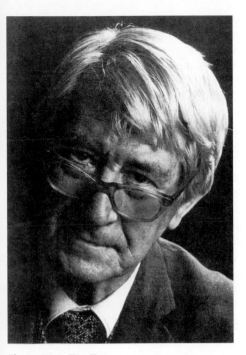

Figure 10.1 Eliot Slater.

Dr Aldwyn Stokes,[31] who was appointed as a temporary psychiatrist in 1945, serving for only 12 months, listed.

Hart's retirement, however, did trigger a seismic change in the fortunes of psychiatry at Queen Square, and, for the next 20 years, the hospital flirted with the opportunity of becoming a centre for advanced neuropsychiatry. This opportunity arose because of the appointment in 1946 of Eliot Slater, as physician in psychological medicine.[32] Slater was a remarkable

person and it is worth considering his career at Queen Square in detail for the light it sheds on the hospital's attitudes and process.

During the war, Slater had served as clinical director of the EMS Psychiatric Unit in Sutton, which became a centre for the reception of military psychiatric casualties (accepting around 20,000 admissions in total). He worked there with William Sargant, Martin Roth and Joe Shorvon, and it was during this period that his interests in the physical methods of therapy in psychiatry and its genetics were kindled.

On taking up his appointment in 1946, Slater managed to persuade the Queen Square Medical Committee to form a department of psychological medicine, and to provide beds, an outpatient clinic and junior staff. In all of this, Slater had the support of Carmichael, who recognised his academic potential. Slater approached his new post with energy and enthusiasm, and introduced into the hospital the new field of biological psychiatry. He was in the vanguard of this discipline, which was to become the predominant form of psychiatry worldwide. Slater assembled a group of very talented young research workers, including Malcolm Piercy, George Ettlinger (who restarted primate experimental work) and Oliver Zangwill (who moved from Cambridge to Queen Square to set up a research unit of clinical psychology within Slater's department). He also expanded the clinical NHS department by recruiting Joseph (Joe) Shorvon[33] as the second psychiatrist at

---

[31] Aldwyn Stokes was a distinguished figure in psychiatry. He was appointed physician at the Maudsley in 1935, then superintendent in charge of the psychiatric unit at Mill Hill during the war, and was awarded a CBE for his services to the EMS. In 1947, he emigrated to Canada to become professor of psychiatry in Toronto, and was a key figure in the foundation of the Canadian Psychiatric Association.

[32] Eliot Trevor Oakeshott Slater was born in London. His father was an historian, and later principal of Ruskin College Oxford. Eliot was educated in Leighton Park School and at Cambridge University and studied medicine at St Thomas' Hospital, qualifying in 1928. In 1934, he was awarded a Rockefeller Foundation Travelling Fellowship and studied psychiatric genetics under Bruno Schulz in Munich, at a time when racial hygiene was being promulgated. Slater met his first wife at a chess congress in Moscow. She was Jewish, and the sister of Boris Pasternak, and he detested the Nazi regime, but did have some sympathy with the scientific principles of eugenics and became vice-

chairman of the Eugenics Society. He viewed war neurosis as a breakdown caused by environmental stress, but dependent on polygenic risk. He also wrote extensively about eugenics, and had personally witnessed, during visits to Germany, the early Nazi forays into this area that were to have such dire consequences for mentally handicapped or epileptic patients. He was a brilliant intellect but thought by the neurologists to have a distant and detached personality and was not considered a good clinical psychiatrist. On leaving Queen Square, he took up a post at the Maudsley and the Institute of Psychiatry and was one of the most influential psychiatrists of his day.

[33] Hyam Joseph Shorvon was born in London, educated at the Jewish Free School and studied medicine at Kings College and St Thomas' Hospitals, qualifying in 1931. He trained and worked first as an anaesthetist and then switched to psychiatry, and in 1942 took the Diploma of Psychological Medicine. He worked with Slater and Sargant at the Belmont Hospital in Sutton, which nurtured a whole school of British psychiatry. After the war, he was appointed to the staff of St Thomas' Hospital, and to Queen Square initially as a clinical assistant, in 1946, and then as consultant psychiatrist, in 1948. He had an

the hospital in 1948, and then Patrick Tooley (1948),[34] R. F. T. Grace (1952),[35] Richard (Dick) Pratt (replacing Tooley in 1954)[36] and Alick Elithorn (1956).[37]

enormous practice – according to Sargant, the largest in London – and was a renowned clinician who specialised in abreaction and other treatments which mixed physical and psychodynamic approaches. He was a neurologist's psychiatrist and consulted by many of his colleagues. Shorvon died of colon cancer at the height of his powers at the age of only 54 years. According to Sargant, he 'had a very good intelligence, a tremendous capacity for work, a personal humility and affection for his fellow men', and these qualities underpinned his practice ('Obituary', *British Medical Journal* 1 (1961): 1546).

[34] Patrick Hocart Tooley was born in Guernsey, went to Mill Hill School and qualified in medicine from the London Hospital. He served in the Royal Navy and during this time took up psychiatry. He was appointed to the London Hospital and Maida Vale in 1948, resigning from the latter in 1952. In mid-career, he switched from clinical psychiatry to forensic psychiatry and medicine, and retired in 1976. He developed Alzheimer's disease in later life.

[35] Dr Richard Fairfax Tukine Grace was a New Zealander who came to England in 1914. During the First World War, he worked in the RAF on flying stress. He was more interested in psychotherapeutic approaches than physical psychiatry. He made little academic contribution to the hospital but was considered to be a good clinician. He retired in 1960.

[36] Richard Thomas Charles Pratt was educated at Cheltenham College and graduated in medicine from the Middlesex Hospital. In 1952, he was appointed senior registrar to Eliot Slater, and then in 1954 as consultant physician in psychological medicine, initially at Maida Vale and then, on Slater's departure to the Maudsley, at Queen Square. He specialised in physical treatments of depression and in the genetics of neurological disease. Pratt was a modest man with an interest in antiquarian books on sundials. He chose psychiatry and not neurology as a career because he suffered from brittle diabetes and was concerned about the risk of hypoglycaemic episodes whilst on-call and in emergency situations. His junior staff recognised occasional episodes of precipitate hypoglycaemia which, holding him in great affection and admiration, they managed by abruptly interrupting ward rounds with sweet tea and biscuits.

[37] Alick Cyril Elithorn was educated at Charterhouse and graduated in medicine from Cambridge University and University College Hospital. He trained at the Maudsley and at Queen Square and was appointed consultant in psychological medicine at Maida Vale in 1956, and at the same time became a member of the MRC external staff. In 1957, he became consultant psychiatrist at the Royal Free Hospital, and from 1956 to 1968 he was a lecturer in psychopathology at the University of Reading. His interest was in developing computer programs, psychological assessment and artificial intelligence. He did not develop a large clinical practice and retired in September 1986. Subsequently, he was involved in complex domestic legal disputes.

The position of physician in psychological medicine at Queen Square was no sinecure. Psychiatry was still seen very much as an inferior specialty, and psychiatrists as a group were still viewed with a fair degree of contempt by a significant number of neurologists. The psychiatrists, conversely, considered the neurologists to be cold and unkind to their patients. Slater negotiated these tricky waters and seems to have engendered the respect of his colleagues, at least initially. He was appointed to the Medical Committee early on, a favour not granted to consultants in other specialties.

Slater also began to play a central role in clinical research, at a time when most academic activities at Queen Square were minimal – for instance, he initiated genetic inquiry among all patients in the hospital. It is said that his opening gambit in consultations was 'Are you a twin?', and, to this day, the hospital outpatient notes still contain a section on the front page on 'family history', which Slater had designed. His works on the genetics of schizophrenia, manic–depressive illness and the nature of the neurotic constitution are enduring contributions to the growth of British neuropsychiatry. Apart from work on hysteria, Slater conducted seminal studies on leucotomy for intractable physical pain, including long-term follow-up of the effects of prefrontal leucotomy, and studies of the psychological and physiological effects of the procedure. By 1961, he was also focusing on the psychiatric associations of epilepsy, including fundamental work on epileptic psychosis, and the long-term follow-up of temporal lobectomy.

Slater spoke about his early experiences at Queen Square when, as a trainee, he was considering a career in neurology:

> I originally wanted to be a neurologist. I had seen wonderful demonstrations by James Collier at St George's Hospital, and I was fascinated by the crossword-like accuracy with which one could pinpoint lesions ... At that time there were three neurological hospitals in London, of which the National Hospital at Queen Square was sublime, the one at Maida Vale respectable and the West End despised. The reason for the contempt in which it [the West End Hospital] was held lay in the fact that, very sensibly, it had psychiatrists on its staff ... In due course a vacancy for a house physician at Queen Square was advertised. I made my application, and went the rounds of the doors in Harley Street, Wimpole Street, and Queen Anne Street calling on the demigods who had my fate in their hands. My reception was every

bit as forbidding as I could have feared. Both Kinnier Wilson and Gordon Holmes (names that were glittering with fame, in that little world) implied that it was really rather impudent on my part to be applying for such a wonderful job, and Gordon Holmes told me it was a senior appointment for which I was quite insufficiently prepared … Now, for the first time, it seemed to me that I ought to know something about psychiatry. Everyone knew that the neurologists drew most of their income from consulting on psychiatric patients, and it would be well then to have some understanding of them.[38]

He failed to obtain the position, and then applied to the Maudsley but, as there was no vacancy, Slater then took a job as assistant medical officer in a provincial mental hospital (Derby County Mental Hospital) and was paid the 'princely sum of £350 per annum'. This was, he discovered, disastrous for his chances of obtaining a post at Queen Square.

> In due course, another vacancy for a house physician at the National Hospital was advertised, and I applied. I might have spared my effort. It was for nothing that I invested in a short black jacket and waistcoat and pinstripe trousers, came up to London, and went from door to door in the Harley Street area. I had touched pitch and had now become defiled … [it is not clear whether he means by this the taking up of psychiatry or the accepting of a post in a peripheral hospital – perhaps both!]. I imagine that I was quite written off, and did not receive even that degree of consideration which had met my first application.[39]

Slater's appointment at Queen Square was opportune for it came at a time when rapid advances in psychiatric treatment were being made. As an alternative to psychoanalysis, a new wave of physical therapies and the first effective psychotropic drugs were being introduced into practice, and at the forefront of this revolution in therapy were the biological psychiatrists in London, including William Sargant, Slater and Shorvon. Indeed, psychiatry was threatening to overtake neurology as an emerging scientific discipline, and was attracting a great deal of interest. Newly introduced treatments included modified

electroconvulsive therapy (ECT) with short-acting anaesthetic and muscle relaxant introduced in 1951;[40] insulin coma which had become widely used in the 1940s and early 1950s; prolonged narcosis, with the patient put to sleep for weeks or months;[41] and, most controversial of all, prefrontal leucotomy.[42] Abreaction using methyl amphetamine, thiopental or inhalational drugs, a combination of physical and psychotherapeutic methods, was first used in 1948 and adopted at Queen Square in the 1950s, especially by Shorvon.[43] In 1952, the first psychoactive drug therapy, chlorpromazine, was reported to be effective in schizophrenia and licensed a year later. This was followed by imipramine in 1955 and then a range of tricyclic antidepressants, with the first monoamine oxide inhibitor (MAOI) and benzodiazepine (chlordiazepoxide) introduced from 1957. It was a time of tremendous optimism in psychiatry, in recognition that these physical and pharmacological methods were effective and would replace the long-winded, expensive and often ineffective psychoanalysis and psychotherapy. The fact that the physical and pharmacological therapies were sometimes so rapidly effective also encouraged psychiatrists to consider mental disorders as physico-chemical disorders of the brain, and the biological explanations of psychiatric disease rose into prominence. The distinction between psychiatric disorders, now considered to be organic, and neurological disease was becoming ever more blurred.

In 1944, Slater and Sargant wrote a short but influential book entitled *An Introduction to Physical Methods of Treatment in Psychiatry*, which laid out all the physical therapies then available in routine clinical practice. This was a high-water mark in physical therapy and the book went into five editions, but one

---

[38] 'In Conversation with Eliot Slater: Brian Barroclough Interviews Eliot Slater (February 1981)', *Psychiatric Bulletin* 5 (1981): 158–61.

[39] E. Slater, 'Autobiographical Sketch', in J. Shields and I. Gottesman, eds., *Man, Mind and Heredity: Selected Papers of Eliot Slater on Psychiatry and Genetics* (Baltimore, MD: The Johns Hopkins University Press, 1971).

[40] The induction of convulsions to treat schizophrenia was first introduced in 1937.

[41] In a 'Zombie ward' as an article in the *Daily Mail* put it (7 August 2013).

[42] First performed in 1935 under the direction of the Portuguese neurologist Antonio Egas Moniz. Moniz received the Nobel Prize for medicine in 1949 for 'discovery of the therapeutic value of leucotomy in certain psychoses'.

[43] Shorvon appeared, with Sargant, in the famous BBC documentary series *The Hurt Mind* (episode 4) in 1957, demonstrating the technique of ether abreaction at Queen Square: https://www.youtube.com/watch?v=2KxU3dPeink (in four sections). The series also shows ECT as it was performed then (by Dick Pratt, we think), and Geoffrey Knight discussing prefrontal leucotomy.

suspects that it reflected Sargant's massive enthusiasm more than Slater's more measured approach.[44] In 1954, Slater published the first edition of his *Textbook of Clinical Psychiatry* with his Maudsley colleagues Martin Roth and Willi Mayer-Gross. This was, in Denis Hill's words:

> A brilliantly written account of the subject … It became essential reading, and a valuable source of reference to every psychiatrist in training in the country. The neglect of the psychodynamic, and social determinants of personality, the study of personality itself, and – as some saw it – the savage and ill-informed attack on psychoanalysis could all be forgiven. The book contained the most comprehensive, brilliant account of the clinical phenomena of schizophrenia and other psychotic conditions which had yet been written in the English language. It was the epitome of a psychiatry based on the natural sciences.[45]

Slater's use of five beds at Queen Square was confirmed in the 1947 reorganisation, relocated to Hughlings Jackson ward on the seventh floor of the Queen Mary wing as originally intended. His salary was increased from £750 to £1,250 per annum[46] and,

in 1948, Slater was allowed to set up a genetics clinic. The hospital steadily increased its psychiatry practice, partially linked to St Thomas' Hospital. Slater was himself more interested in research, and responsibility for patients largely devolved to Shorvon, whose massive clinics often stretched long into the evening. Somewhat cold in his clinical manner and reluctant to treat patients himself, Slater relied on his colleagues to provide the empathy needed for a successful psychiatric service, and on Pratt particularly for ECT, Shorvon for abreaction, and Hunter for psychotherapy/psychoanalysis. But, towards the end of the 1950s, relationships between Slater and Queen Square soured. This was due to the age-old attitude of the neurologists to psychiatry and their disparagement of academic medicine. Slater's main ambition was to set up a professorial unit in psychiatry at Queen Square, but the physicians, led by Walshe, were not supportive, just as they were resistant to the establishment of professorial units in neurology and neurosurgery. Matters had not changed with respect to the scepticism concerning psychiatry expressed by the Medical Committee in its report to the Goodenough Committee in 1943.

> In respect of psychology, it can scarcely be denied that this branch of medicine has suffered from its isolation from other aspects of medicine, and particularly from what has been called organic neurology. This is seen in the exotic growth of psychological speculation, in the recent somewhat uncritical vogue of such drastic physical methods as convulsive therapy and amputation of the frontal lobes, and in general in the neglect of those principles of scientific control of observation so essential to the stable building of an ordered fabric of knowledge … It needs contact with biological scientific disciplines … Thus, advance in psychology cannot but be furthered by its study in an active school of neurology, while, on the other hand, neurology must widen its horizons by the introduction of psychology into its ambit.[47]

The last straw came in 1964 when an offer made by the Mental Health Foundation to fund a professorship of psychiatry for which Slater was earmarked was turned down by the Medical Committee on the grounds that a chair in neurosurgery should have

---

[44] W. Sargant and E. Slater, *An Introduction to Physical Methods of Treatment in Psychiatry* (Edinburgh: Livingstone, 1944). The book did not provide much in the way of outcome data for each therapy, a fact that Slater regretted, saying that it was brought out too quickly because of Sargant's impatience, and it was badly reviewed in *Brain* for the same reason. An indication of how excessive therapy was can be gathered from a few quotations from the book: 'Many patients unable to tolerate a long course of ECT, can do so when anxiety is relieved by narcosis … What is so valuable is that they generally have no memory about the actual length of the treatment or the numbers of ECT used … After 3 or 4 treatments they may ask for ECT to be discontinued because of an increasing dread of further treatments. Combining sleep with ECT avoids this'; and 'all sorts of treatment can be given while the patient is kept sleeping, including a variety of drugs and ECT [which] together generally induce considerable memory loss for the period under narcosis. As a rule the patient does not know how long he has been asleep, or what treatment, even including ECT, he has been given. Under sleep … one can now give many kinds of physical treatment, necessary, but often not easily tolerated. We may be seeing here a new exciting beginning in psychiatry and the possibility of a treatment era such as followed the introduction of anaesthesia in surgery.'
[45] W. Mayer-Gross, E. G. O. Slater and M. Roth, *Clinical Psychiatry* (London: Baillieres, Tindall and Cox, 1955).
[46] Medical Committee Minute 47/35. It seems strange how publicly this was minuted, since only rarely are the physicians' salaries mentioned in the minutes. The hospital was

to pay 50 per cent of the salary, and the medical school to pay the other 50 per cent.
[47] This report was anonymous but presumably written by either Greenfield or Purdon Martin, as deans of the medical school. The paper is appended to Medical Committee Minute, 19 August 1943.

precedence.[48] The rejection of the offer precipitated Slater's resignation from the National Hospital in 1964. His final letter to Macdonald Critchley, then chairman of the Medical Committee, includes a withering assessment of the neurologists' attitude to psychiatry:

> The neurologists at the National Hospital have followed policy with regard to psychiatric developments in the National Hospital which then turned increasingly counter to everything for which I have stood. As they will remember, I have consistently tried to persuade them of the need for an academic research organisation on the psychiatric side. When I first joined the staff eighteen years ago the prospects for this seemed favourable. As the years have passed the trend of opinion in the Medical Committee and in the Academic Board became less and less encouraging. After the episode of the proffered and rejected benefaction by the Mental Health Research Fund, it was borne in on me that there was nothing further to be achieved by continuing to serve the Hospital for another five years, and that my time and energies would be fruitfully spent in a more favourable environment. In my view the attitude toward psychiatry which now prevails in the Medical Committee of the National Hospital is one that is lacking in vision and is out of touch with the times. I wish my resignation of my post to be understood as the most energetic protest against that attitude which it is in my power to make …

He wrote later that:

> When I went to Queen Square as psychiatrist to the National Hospital, I was keen to pursue research there, which wasn't so easy. They didn't like it there. They wanted good clinical work and top level teaching. I started off at Queen Square with every sort of encouragement from people like Carmichael. But gradually things went wrong. I got at cross purposes with my colleagues. Looking back, I can't blame them. For instance, I refused the job of Dean. Of course that was very bad. If you are on board a ship and the captain says you will be the

officer who will receive the guests when we have our great gala day, you are then the officer who receives the guests, there is no help for it. I wasn't playing fair by the chaps. There were certain things I wasn't at all keen on that they wanted me to do. Lectures on psychiatry, for instance, struck me as a ghastly thing to have to do. What I really enjoyed was having teaching rounds or conferences on my own patients. The young housemen (not all that young, some of them were getting old) were wonderful people to teach, and to be taught by. The interesting thing was that the really bright, brightest of the bright, were the young house physicians who were going to be accomplished general physicians. These young people told me about everything that was going on in medicine, and were constantly keeping me up to the mark. What happened eventually was a sad storm. The Mental Health Research Fund had some money with which they wanted to endow an academic unit at one of the hospitals. I put in an application which they agreed. It was going to be an appointment for a senior lecturer, working in my department. It would have been the top of my ambition to make a small academic psychiatric unit at the National Hospital. This was battled in the hospital's Medical Committee for about a year, and they turned it down. I felt that was too much for me and I sent in my resignation. But I think if I hadn't blotted my copybook, neurologically speaking, I might have got their support … I think in a way, we were such different sorts of people, the more senior physicians and I. Another thing which must have irritated them very much was when I did a follow-up on National Hospital cases diagnosed as hysteria and found a big loading of organic disease had been missed. It was not a good thing.[49]

Slater's reference to 'blotting his copybook' refers to one of his most celebrated contributions, in which he showed that there were often occult neurological or medical conditions in patients in whom the diagnosis of hysteria had (thus, erroneously) been made by physicians at the hospital. Ironically, this research was the topic of the first Shorvon memorial lecture, which was scheduled on what turned out to be Slater's last day of employment at Queen Square (1 November 1964).[50]

Walshe's assault on psychiatry, in his 1959 lecture, perhaps sums up a viewpoint shared by some of the

---

[48] It was also said that the endowment was insufficient in the long term, and the university would not make up any shortfall. Slater was by then also at loggerheads with most of the neurologists, and Gautier-Smith recalls that, in the committee, only 'Helen Dimsdale supported the appointment and thought that the committee should listen to him sympathetically. Brinton was said to have replied that they had done so with greater patience than the man merited and that the item was closed and that if Slater didn't like it, he could always leave the room, which he promptly did' (unpublished papers).

[49] Draft letter dated 7 October 1964, from Eliot Slater, reproduced by kind permission of Dr Nicholas Slater.

[50] The lecture was published: E. Slater, 'The Diagnosis of "Hysteria"', *British Medical Journal* 1 (29 March 1965): 1395–9.

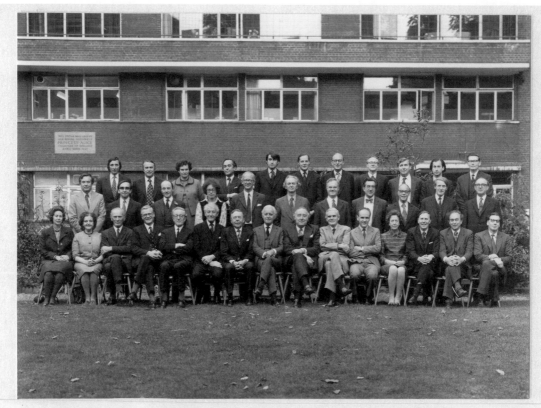

J.NEWSOM DAVIS N.GRANT D.JEWKES H.LUDMAN I.McDONALD M.SANDERS A.HALLIDAY B.KENDALL D.SUTTON R.KOCEN D.LANDON
A.DAVISON J.BLAU R.BARNARD E.WARRINGTON E.M.BRETT J.MARSHALL P.LASCELLES J.CAVANGH P.NATHAN R.ROSS RUSSELL W.MAIR
P.NORMAN M.DIX W.COBB L.SYMON W.BLACKWOOD J.BULL M.McARDLE D.WILLIAMS R.KELLY V.LOGUE P.GAUTIER-SMITH M.SMITH R.BANNISTER C.Du BOULAY A.ELITHORN
OCTOBER 1974

Figure 10.2 Consultant staff in 1974.

neurology staff – one that had hardened since the 1945 report of the Royal College of Physicians' Committee on Neurology, of which he was not a member:

A neurologist's discipline is primarily within the field of natural science, but the psychiatrist's lies within the field of historical science – much as the psychiatrist craves to shelter beneath the umbrella of natural science because of the prestige he supposes this lends to his discipline … [each has its own] criteria of evidence and of proof and these are not the same, and the two do not easily make a really happy marriage. You can be a good psychiatrist or a good neurologist, but the so-called neuro-psychiatrist is apt to be a synthetic schizophrenic trying to work with two quantitatively different disciplines conflicting in his mind, and the psychiatric trend always wins.[51]

Saying that a 'neuro-psychiatrist is apt to be a synthetic schizophrenic' was no doubt intended to wound and it must have hurt many feelings. Walshe also drew a distinction between the intellectual approach of psychiatrists and neurologists, and wrote in relation to neuropsychiatry that 'to straddle the wild horses of neurology and psychiatry is a gymnastic feat from which good rarely comes … neurology's real link is with internal medicine, from which, indeed, it is indivisible'.

The death of Shorvon in 1961 and Slater's move to direct the MRC Psychiatric Genetics Unit at the Maudsley Hospital in 1964 marked the end of academic neuropsychiatry at Queen Square for several decades.

Neuropsychology at Queen Square

The most notable dividend for Slater's colleagues was not in the field of clinical psychiatry, but in

---

[51] F. M. R. Walshe, 'The Present and Future of Neurology', *Archives of Neurology* **95** (1960): 83–8.

experimental and clinical psychology. This was led by Oliver Zangwill,[52] from 1947, and George Ettlinger, appointed as lecturer in the same year. Together they laid the foundations for the large corpus of distinguished research in clinical neuropsychology. This work was extended over the next several decades by Elizabeth Warrington, who joined the National Hospital in 1953, and Maria Wyke, who worked at Maida Vale from 1954. Relationships, however, were strained between Zangwill and Warrington, and also between the Queen Square and Maida Vale groups, with arguments over such matters as access to clinical data and post-mortem specimens. Studies were generally performed on post-surgical cases, or cases with focal lesions, and a range of cognitive functions investigated, with the emphasis on including speech, vision and memory.

Oliver Zangwill, to all intents and purposes, founded the science of neuropsychology during his time at Queen Square. Although Zangwill moved to Cambridge as professor of experimental psychology in 1952, where his trainees included Larry Weiskrantz and Richard Gregory. He continued as visiting psychologist at Queen Square until 1979, working on head injury and focal cerebral disease. Zangwill subscribed firmly to the Jacksonian view that the brain is organised in hierarchical modules, and wrote on many topics including aphasia, cerebral dominance, amnesia, dyslexia and Korsakoff's psychosis.[53] Ettlinger's work with Zangwill was on visual agnosia, showing that patients could suffer from severe sensory deficits but without agnosia or, conversely, could be agnosic and unable to recognise objects yet have only mild sensory deficits. After a year with Karl Pribram in Connecticut, Ettlinger turned his attention to studies in non-human primates. He used 'disconnection' techniques to demonstrate the crucial importance of a pathway for visual recognition connecting the monkey's primary visual cortex with the temporal lobe. He also carried out extensive work on the role of the corpus callosum, the effects of epilepsy on memory, and on tactile recognition. Initially, clinical neuropsychology was based within the department of psychiatry, in part because of the neurologists' concern that a separate group of neuropsychologists would not be appropriate. Independence was granted much later after a working party, established to consider the issue of merging the departments of psychology and psychiatry at Maida Vale and Queen Square, concluded that psychology should be independent of psychiatry, but that there should be a single head of psychology for the two hospitals. Elizabeth Warrington was recommended to lead this new department and, in 1982, she was appointed professor of clinical neuropsychology.

Tria juncta in uno

On 25 September 1970, Sir Charles Symonds gave the sixth Hugh Cairns memorial lecture, during the 81st meeting of the Society of British Neurological Surgeons. Symonds, who was 80 years old at the time and a senior statesman of British neurology, provided an interesting insight into a line of thinking in the middle years of the century among those neurologists at Queen Square who were sympathetic to psychiatry. Symonds believed that the future of neurology should be the coming together of its 'three divisions – medical, surgical and psychiatric' – *Tria juncta in uno*.[54] He argued that the emergence of dynamic psychopathology had resulted in the separation of neurology and psychiatry in the 1930s and 1940s, and that most neurologists in Britain had 'stayed apart, letting their academic stake in the psychiatric field go by default'. Symonds had been an intern under Alfred Meyer and considered himself an exception to this trend. Indeed, he saw large numbers of patients in private practice who had primarily psychological symptoms and was said regularly to use hypnosis. In 1941, he had served as president of the

---

[52] Oliver Zangwill was a leading world figure in neuropsychology, elected president of the British Psychological Society in 1974 and FRS in 1977. He was an important figure at Queen Square where, even during his Cambridge years, he conducted much of his work. His book *Amnesia* (1966) was an important influence on neurology at Queen Square, where he was respected by the neurologists. The difficult relationship between Zangwill and Warrrington (see below) was noted by the dean of the Institute to cause many problems and to inhibit the potential for psychology at Queen Square.

[53] Richard Gregory recalls that, when seeing a patient with Korsakoff's syndrome each week, Zangwill would take a pen out of his pocket and ask: 'Have you seen this before?' The patient always said 'no'. At the final session, Zangwill duly asked: 'Have you seen this before?' The patient replied: 'Are you the man with all those pens?' R. Gregory, 'Oliver Zangwill', *Biographical Memoirs of the Royal Society* **47** (2001): 515–24.

[54] Charles Symonds, *Tria Juncta in Uno: Addressed to the Society of British Neurological Surgeons at its 81st Meeting in Hull on 25 September 1970*, Hugh Cairns memorial lecture (Cambridge: Seacourt Press, 1970).

section of psychiatry at the Royal Society of Medicine and had given his presidential address on 'The Neurological Approach to Mental Disorder', advocating that psychiatrists and neurologists should unite to form departments of neuropsychiatry in general hospitals – a plea that had fallen on deaf ears. In 1944, he and Riddoch submitted a memorandum to the RCP Committee on Psychological Medicine, of which both were members, in which it was suggested that the psychiatrist should be based in a neuropsychiatric clinic working alongside neurologists and neurosurgeons: 'In view of the wide overlap between these subjects, their common use of specialised techniques and the interweaving of their research techniques, this development seems highly desirable.' They also suggested much greater integration of training. The memorandum was rejected by the Committee on Psychiatry and also subsequently discussed and overwhelmingly rejected by the Association of British Neurologists. The Royal College of Physicians' Committee on Neurology, of which Riddoch and Symonds were members, had in 1945 also considered

the memorandum and agreed that all neurology trainees should have one year's training in psychiatry, six months in a psychiatric teaching hospital, and six months studying mental deficiency.

This idea was not followed though, nor was it again mentioned in subsequent committee reports, and joint departments of neuropsychiatry were not developed. Even in 1970, Symonds still believed that the three disciplines of medical and surgical neurology and psychiatry could provide joint clinical services, under the umbrella of neuropsychiatry. The flame lit by Symonds flickered but was not fully extinguished, and neuropsychiatry did flourish at Queen Square from the 1980s, although always as a somewhat marginalised activity.

Psychiatry at Queen Square after 1964

In 1964, Richard (Dick) Pratt became the senior psychiatrist in the National Hospitals. Grace had retired in 1960, and was replaced in the same year by Richard Hunter, and Alick Elithorn had largely withdrawn

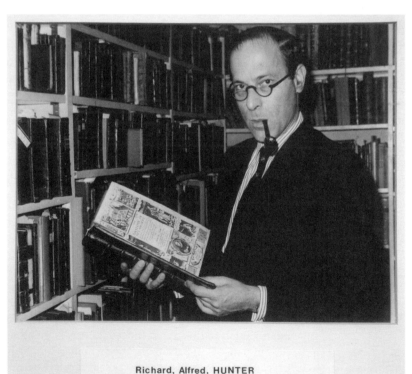

Figure 10.3 Richard Hunter (in this illustration he has open the 1632 edition of Robert Burton's *Anatomy of Melancholia* with its famous engraved title-page – one of the many treasures in his collection).

Richard, Alfred, HUNTER
[11.11.23. ~ 25.11.81.]
"An impeccable scholar, he gave pleasure to thousands through his writings. He wore his learning with a light touch and shared it generously with his many friends."

from clinical work. Pratt was highly respected as a clinical psychiatrist and well liked by his patients and colleagues. He was very much aligned with the school of physical treatments and specialised particularly in unilateral ECT, holding long and busy sessions in a corner of the medical outpatients' waiting room with an anaesthetist and nurse, shielded from the gaze of the other patients waiting for their neurological appointments by a portable curtain screen.

Richard Hunter[55] was another gifted and highly intelligent psychiatrist, with many interests. He wrote on various neuropsychiatric topics but did not undertake much clinical research, and was essentially a dilettante whose heart was never in the routine practice of psychiatry. His mother, Ida Macalpine, was a formidable psychoanalyst and it has been remarked that her shadow looked over Hunter's shoulder at all his consultations. She attended all his lectures, and together they published a celebrated book proposing that the madness of George III was due to porphyria, an idea that still causes controversy.[56] Hunter was an avid book collector and historian of psychiatry who, with his mother, built up a renowned library of several thousand historical psychiatric volumes, which was dispersed on his death, many of the books going to Cambridge University Library.[57] Hunter had been

appointed by Slater as a psychotherapist, but very soon did a *volte-face*, adopting an organic position with respect to psychiatric illness. He described the first cases of tardive dyskinesia as a secondary effect of treatment with phenothiazines.

The appointments of Elithorn and Hunter must initially have promised much from the academic point of view, but everything lapsed with Slater's resignation, and their lasting contributions to psychiatry were slight. Slater was replaced on the staff of the National Hospital by Alwyn Lishman,[58] who stayed a year but then also moved to the Institute of Psychiatry, at the invitation of Denis Hill, to take up a position as neuropsychiatrist, where he had a distinguished academic career. Lishman was replaced at Queen Square by Harold Merskey in 1967. He worked largely in the field of chronic pain, and left in 1976 to take up a professorship in Canada. This rapid turnover of staff resulted in failure of the department of psychological medicine to gather momentum and make an impact on the rest of the hospital. Research was largely inactive, and leadership in British neuropsychiatry moved definitively to the Institute of Psychiatry and Maudsley Hospital in Camberwell, led by Slater and consolidated by the arrival of Lishman a year later.[59] These institutions continued to attract others interested in psychiatry, including many who attended Queen Square for periods of training and research. This situation was regretted by some of the physicians at the National Hospital who were sympathetic to psychiatry, but the antithesis to mental illness persisted and psychiatry failed to prosper in this atmosphere.

In 1976, Merskey was replaced by Michael Trimble and, in 1984, Maria Ron joined him as the second psychiatrist, supported by Ray Dolan from 1986 (all three were later awarded personal chairs).

---

[55] Richard Alfred Hunter was born in Nurenberg and fled to England with his family on the rise of the Nazi party. He was educated at St Paul's, and graduated in medicine from St Bartholemew's Hospital. He served in the RAMC from 1948 to 1950, and was appointed senior registrar in psychiatry at Queen Square in 1957, and consultant in psychological medicine in 1960, and at Friern Barnet Hospital in 1963. His mother was an overwhelming influence and, when she died in 1974, he was released from her spell. He then married Thea Bostick, superintendent radiographer at Queen Square, and they lived a more relaxed domestic life until Hunter's death seven years later from complications of surgery.

[56] R. Hunter and I. Macalpine, *Three Hundred Years of Psychiatry, 1555–1860* (Oxford University Press, 1963) is a compendium of extracts from contemporary works, with excellent commentaries and annotations by Hunter and Macalpine. The work on George III was first published, also in collaboration with his mother, in the *British Medical Journal* 1 (1966): 65–71.

[57] On one occasion, Hunter walked into the offices of a small publisher close to Queen Square and asked idly whether they knew of a second-hand copy of an extremely rare and much sought-after book which had been published by that firm in the nineteenth century that he lacked for his collection: 'Yes, sir', came the reply, 'we still have half a dozen new copies available for sale.'

[58] Alwyn Lishman initially trained as a neurologist but found psychiatry more interesting. Slater advised him to 'Go there [Queen Square], have a wonderful time but don't stay more than a couple of years, because they'll do to you what they did to me.' Lishman found some of the neurologists extremely hostile to psychiatry (notably Walshe), in his view treating psychiatric patients as 'specimens'. Others, such as Critchley, Williams and Symonds, were very welcoming: interview with Alwyn Lishman (http://pb .rcpsych.org/content/37/10/343).

[59] This is all the more ironic since the Maudsley Hospital can be said, in part at least, to owe its existence to the failed attempt of Queen Square to create a psychiatric hospital in 1890.

In 1988, the family of Mr Raymond Way gave a donation to establish a research unit in neuropsychiatry in the Institute of Neurology. This was named 'the Raymond Way Unit', with Trimble as director.[60] The unit specialised in epilepsy, movement disorders and somatiform disorders. The research was very much in the tradition of behavioural neurology and a number of young trainees moved through the department who later developed distinguished careers in the field of neuropsychiatry. Trimble and Ron had substantive appointments as part of the university department of clinical neurology as well as the hospital, and Trimble also held an appointment at the Chalfont Centre for Epilepsy. Dolan initially had a post in the hospital, with linked sessions at the MRC Cyclotron Unit at the Hammersmith Hospital.[61] After the Wellcome department of cognitive neurology was formed, in association with the Leopold Muller Functional Imaging Laboratory, research again flourished in the field of neuropsychiatry, focused on the nature and treatment of the behavioural effects of neurological disease, and the behavioural adverse effects from treating neurological disease (especially epilepsy and movement disorders), and using fMRI to study human behaviour.

Neuropsychiatry at Queen Square: A Perspective

Throughout the life of the hospital, a number of fundamental questions arose in the field of neuropsychiatry. First was the relationship of mind to brain. Hughlings Jackson took an extreme view with his doctrine of 'concomitance' (as outlined most clearly in his Croonian lectures of 1884). Taking a materialist view of the brain as a sensorimotor machine, Jackson's position was that physical and psychical activities run in parallel but are unconnected. Thought and mentation are 'concomitant' with neural activity. He did accept that some psychiatric symptoms of disease are due to disturbances of the brain and consequent upon dissolution of one structure resulting in loss of higher function and release of lower, subservient, properties, but emphasised the separation of mind and brain in his aphorism that 'there is no physiology of the mind any more than there is a psychology of the nervous system'. Others showed no interest in exploring this issue and, for Gowers, 'with the much disputed relation of mind to brain, the physician has nothing to do'.[62] By this, he meant that a sensible neurologist would not meddle with phenomena beyond the realm of physiological investigation. The debate took on a new perspective with Freudian psychiatrists considering many mental and neurological symptoms to be symbolic and psychological in nature. The findings of biochemical changes in mental disorders, even without any physiological or visible pathological abnormalities, and, particularly, the success of psychotropic drugs and physical therapies in the 1950s and 1960s provided evidence that mind is a function of neural activity although by mechanisms which are still completely unknown. Advances in single cell physiology showed quite conclusively the link between aspects of perception and some mental and brain functions, and Russell Brain, for instance, held that events in the brain are 'simultaneously mental and physiological'.[63]

A second question that concerned the physicians at Queen Square from the time of Jackson, also a source of much disagreement, was the extent to which mental functions could be localised to one area of the brain. In recent times, theories of localisation have been ferociously pursued by many working in the field of functional imaging, where regional changes in cerebral blood flow are considered to indicate the seat of many brain functions, including perception, memory, mood and emotion (the 'love centre', 'pleasure centre', 'art centre' are extreme examples). The over-interpretation and over-simplification of functional imaging findings has led to much critical reaction, and to some extent is

---

[60] Raymond Way was a self-made man who founded 'The Raymond Way Motor Company', selling cars and motorcycles. In a vivid obituary (by Andrew English, *Daily Telegraph*, 18 August 2001), entitled 'Death of a Salesman', Ray is described as 'sharp as a needle, but as straight as a gun barrel'. He was a consummate salesman, a bit of a huckster and full of chutzpah – part-exchanging cars for pianos, parrots in cages, dray horses or radiograms. The company had lots of good mottos, including 'Don't delay, buy your car the Raymond Way'. His press advertisements were described as minor works of literature, and he was full of 'mysterious catch phrases to inspire and motivate his staff'.
[61] Thus, the Institute ended up with three separate departments of psychiatry, just as it had two departments of neurosurgery. Such separations were one way of dealing with the inevitable personality clashes which characterise academic medicine.

[62] *A Manual of Diseases of the Nervous System* (London: J. & A. Churchill, 1886).
[63] Lord Brain, 'Some Reflections on Brain and Mind', *Brain* **86** (1963): 381–402, based on his Hughlings Jackson's lecture at the Montreal Neurological Institute.

mollified by the neuropsychiatric approach. Accusations of 'neuromythology' (the first reference we can find to this term comes, perhaps not surprisingly, from Walshe), 'neuromania' and 'cerebral photography' are all made, and the findings are condemned by some as modern phrenology. At a more sophisticated level, Jackson's view that psychosis and serious mental disorders are due to 'dissolution' of orderly structures has something in common with the current emphasis on networks and brain systems. In this, as in the mind–brain debate, the pendulum swings.

From the clinical point of view, over the course of its history, the main focus of psychiatry for doctors at the National Hospital has been on the mental changes associated with neurological conditions, notably epilepsy and movement disorders, rather than the primary psychotic or affective disorders. The physicians published definitive descriptions of these phenomena, and in the second half of the twentieth century have at times played a significant role in the treatment of the psychological disturbances in these neurological conditions. Perhaps the greatest clinical contribution to clinical psychiatry in the twentieth century has been the introduction of psychotropic drugs. Although psychiatrists at the National Hospital played almost no part in the discovery of these therapies, they did have an important role in assessing and refining the therapies in clinical practice, and in moving the emphasis of psychiatry from psychoanalytical to pharmaceutical therapies.[64]

In making this switch, psychiatrists might have hoped for a more sympathetic hearing from colleagues working in neurology and that this change in emphasis would have brought psychiatrists and neurologists at Queen Square closer together. However, the old tensions never entirely disappeared. The reasons are complex and had much to do with personalities and style of practice, but as a result psychiatry has never flourished at Queen Square to its full potential. In not adopting a more welcoming attitude to psychiatry, either in the decades after its foundation, or especially when Slater was offered funding

for the professorship of psychiatry, the potential of the hospital to advance the topic of neuropsychiatry, clinically and experimentally, remained a grievous lost opportunity.

Neuro-ophthalmology at Queen Square

It was not only the nervous system, as defined anatomically, that attracted the attention of doctors at Queen Square. From the time of its foundation, there was also an interest in the sensory organs, and particularly the eye, the ear and the throat. In large measure, the subspecialties of neuro-ophthalmology and neuro-otology were pioneered at Queen Square. Crucial to these developments was a series of significant appointments to the hospital staff, prominent amongst whom were surgeons. Despite their background, neither ophthalmic nor otological surgery has ever been much performed at the National Hospital, and these surgeons tended to work on the development of medical, rather than surgical, aspects of the topics. Enabled by the large number of patients with neurological disease, the most significant advances made at Queen Square were in relation to visual, auditory or vestibular function in neurological disease. Working at the interface with neurology, this medical focus has been the defining characteristic of the Queen Square contribution and the opportunity was exploited to good effect. In few other institutions in Britain was this the case.

John Zachariah Laurence[65] was one of the four medical staff appointed at the National Hospital in 1860, and the first of a distinguished line of ophthalmic surgeons. He was a philanthropist whose first involvement was as a member of the Board of Management, but he was appointed to the staff when it was decided that a visiting surgeon would be advantageous. It is his signature on the telegram sent on behalf of the Board, informing Brown-Séquard of his

---

[64] Dick Pratt used to teach his medical students that the abnormal mood of depressed patients was due to their perspective (using the analogy of looking at life through a telescope, focused selectively on negative aspects). This perspective he considered to have a chemical–physiological basis.

[65] John Zachariah Laurence graduated at University College Hospital. He became the leading surgical ophthalmologist of his day and founded the first ophthalmological journal, the *Ophthalmic Review*. He invented a number of ophthalmological instruments. He is best remembered for describing the Laurence–Moon–Biedl syndrome. Laurence made a significant contribution to ophthalmology but not to neurology: see A. Sorsby, 'John Zachariah Laurence: A Belated Tribute', *British Journal of Ophthalmology* **16** (1932): 727–40.

appointment to the National Hospital. Laurence soon resigned from Queen Square as his interest in ophthalmology grew, and he went on to establish the Southern Ophthalmic Hospital (which later became the Royal Eye Hospital and then the Medical Eye Unit at St Thomas' Hospital). His association with the National Hospital was brief, but he was a scholarly and wise man, and his intelligence and versatility served the hospital well at its inception. He may have helped to introduce the ophthalmoscope, developed by Hermann von Helmholtz (1851), at Queen Square.

The next contributor to medical ophthalmology was Hughlings Jackson. On coming to London, one of his first duties was to accompany his sponsor and mentor Jonathan Hutchinson to the Royal London Ophthalmic Hospital,[66] where Jackson became skilled at using the ophthalmoscope. He maintained an interest in medical ophthalmology throughout his career but saw these cases at both the London Hospital and Queen Square. Jackson wrote extensively on neuro-ophthalmological topics, including optic neuritis, the eye sign in tabes dorsalis, and ocular nerve palsies, and when he gave the William Bowman lecture to the Ophthalmological Society of the United Kingdom in 1885, he stated that the topic of ophthalmology was 'pervaded with Spencerian ideas'.[67] His contributions to ophthalmology were recognised early in authoritative reviews by Taylor and Burton Chance.[68]

William Gowers was also an expert ophthalmoscopist. One of the referees for his application to the post of assistant physician to the National Hospital (1872) was the celebrated German ophthalmic surgeon, and later painter and sculptor, Richard

Liebreich, who had been appointed as an ophthalmic surgeon at St Thomas' Hospital in 1870:

> I have had the opportunity of examining a great number of patients together with Dr Gowers and I am very glad to express the opinion that he is not only thoroughly acquainted with Ophthalmoscopy in general but that he is a very practiced diagnostician observing the minutest details and representing them in drawings of remarkable correctness to nature and also to interpreting very accurately their clinical significance in relation to diseases of the nervous system.[69]

Hughlings Jackson also paid tribute to his younger colleague's skills:

> I would draw the attention both of ophthalmic surgeons and physicians to some minute ophthalmic observations by Dr Gowers in certain cases of Bright's disease. Dr Gowers is so good an ophthalmoscopist, and, above all knows so thoroughly well the varied healthy appearances of the normal fundus oculi, that I should accept these minute observations of his as being as precise and as exact as it is possible for such difficult observations to be.[70]

Early ophthalmoscopes consisted of a set of lenses suitable for bringing into focus parts of the eyeball and retina. Illumination was provided by an independent, non-electrical source. Gowers persuaded a London manufacturer named Pillischer to produce a smaller, more manageable instrument in which the lens disc could be moved between two pivot positions, the weaker lenses arranged more centrally in the rotating disc with the stronger and less often used ones on the periphery. In the same year, he designed a triple-wick candle to allow use of the ophthalmoscope in poorly lit homes. When all three wicks were lit, the candle provided a stable and uniform source of light for examining the retina. Gowers' interest in neuro-ophthalmology led to him being one of the founders of the Ophthalmic Society of the United Kingdom. Together with Hughlings Jackson, Laurence and (Sir Thomas) Clifford Allbutt, Gowers also helped to popularise the ophthalmoscope in the UK and, importantly, to provide a bridge between medicine and the otherwise somewhat isolated specialty of ophthalmology.

---

[66] The hospital was founded in 1804 as the Dispensary for Curing Diseases of the Eye and Ear. It was then renamed the London Ophthalmic Infirmary in 1822, the Royal London Ophthalmic Hospital in 1837, the Moorfields, Westminster and Central London Ophthalmic hospital in 1947, and finally the Mooorfields Eye Hospital.

[67] Cited in M. Critchley and E. Critchley, *John Hughlings Jackson: Father of English Neurology* (Oxford University Press, 1998).

[68] J. Taylor, 'The Ophthalmological Observations of Hughlings Jackson and Their Bearing on Nervous and Other Diseases', *Brain* 38 (1915): 418–46; B. Chance, 'Hughlings Jackson, the Neurologic Ophthalmologist, with a Summary of his Works', *Journal of the American Medical Association* 17 (1937): 241–89.

[69] Letter to the National Hospital dated 7 November 1872.

[70] Letter to the National Hospital dated 11 November 1872.

Gowers published *A Manual and Atlas of Medical Ophthalmoscopy* (1879) based on his experience at University College Hospital and Queen Square. The first edition included 125 pages devoted to 50 case histories. The main body of the text contained detailed discussion of the types of pathological appearance of the optic disc, the surrounding retina and the retinal blood vessels; and an account of the appearances associated with neurological and general medical disease encountered in Gowers' own practice and supported by the existing literature. The book proved popular among the profession and was serially revised (1882, 1890 and 1904), the last two editions being written with Marcus Gunn, providing an early example of collaboration between physician and ophthalmic surgeon in the field of medical ophthalmology, thereby sowing the seeds for what eventually became the defining characteristic of the specialty of neuro-ophthalmology. Many linked appointments were maintained throughout the twentieth century between the National Hospital, Moorfields Eye Hospital and the specialist eye hospitals in south London.

Robert Marcus Gunn[71] was appointed assistant surgeon at the Royal London Ophthalmic Hospital in 1883, and ophthalmic surgeon to the National Hospital and the Hospital for Sick Children, Great Ormond Street, from 1886. He was a close neighbour of Gowers in Queen Anne Street and both had an interest in disorders of the optic nerve. Gunn is remembered through several eponyms: the Marcus Gunn phenomenon (synkinetic lifting of a ptosis on jaw opening or lateral jaw movements, sometimes called 'jaw winking'); the Marcus Gunn pupil (now usually referred to as a relative afferent papillary defect); Gunn's sign (arteriovenous nipping in hypertension); and Gunn's dots (glistening non-pathological Muller's foot cell plates close to the macula seen in young people on oblique bright illumination). These provide lasting testimony to his clinical prowess. In his presidential address to the section of ophthalmology of the British Medical Association on 'Certain Affections of the Optic Nerve' in 1906, Gunn was the first to propose that disc oedema in cases of cerebral tumour is due to pressure on the small veins of the pial sheath by fluid in the interstitial space.

Gunn was appointed to the staff at the National Hospital on the same day as Robert Brudenell Carter.[72] Only one post had been

---

[71] Robert Marcus Gunn was a Scottish Presbyterian from Viking stock, born in Golspie, and educated at the universities of St Andrews and Edinburgh where his teachers included Douglas Argyll Robertson and Lord Lister. Whilst in residence at the Perth District Asylum (1875), Gunn spent time examining the 'fundus oculorum' of lunatics, having been attracted to the subject by the published work of Clifford Allbutt. Gunn found them precisely like those of the sane. He enjoyed this work but was once set upon, his assailant being an old melancholic woman from whom he was saved by another inmate. Gunn carried out eye research with Jager in Vienna and Professor Schäfer at University College London. He went to Australia (1879) to collect the eyes of marsupials and the *Monotremata* with a view to microscopic examination. On his return, Gunn worked under Sir William Bowman on zoological specimens collected by the *Challenger* expedition, and gave the Arris and Gale lectures (1888) on this topic. His obituarist in *Plarr's Lives* noted that 'eulogists unite in bearing witness to his charm, his simplicity, his sense of humour, and his lofty character, and his many pursuits being a botanist, a marine zoologist, and a keen geologist and with a collection of fossils from the Jurassic and old red sandstone, which crops out in his own native district of Scotland, being exceptionally fine': https://livesonline.rcseng.ac.uk/biogs/E002074b.htm.

[72] Robert Brudenell Carter was one of the most celebrated medical men of his generation. Born into a well-connected Berkshire family, he trained at the London Hospital and worked first as assistant in a country practice, during which time he wrote his first two books – *The Pathology and Treatment of Hysteria* (1853) and *The Influence of Education and Training in Preventing Diseases of the Nervous System* (1855). At the start of the Crimean War, he joined the Turkish Army as a staff surgeon and met Sir W. H. Russell, a journalist for *The Times*. Carter sent back reports from the front line and continued to work as a correspondent for *The Times* over many years, and was said to be the first *Times* journalist to use a typewriter. He wrote widely on a number of topics and provided an insight into medicine and the medical professional for the general public. On his return to England, Carter developed a special interest in ophthalmology, being considered one of the most accomplished surgeons of his day, and helped set up eye infirmaries in Nottingham and Gloucester. He entered London politics as a member of the Moderate party, and was elected to the London County Council where he set up the special committee proposing establishment of a hospital for the insane based on medical, not asylum, lines, which he hoped would be linked to the National Hospital. During this time, he published further books including: *The Artificial Production of Stupidity* (1859); *The theory of ocular defects and of spectacles* (1869); *The Ophthalmoscope: Its Varieties and its Use* (1864); *A Practical Treatise on Diseases of the Eye* (1875): *Eyesight, Good and Bad; a Treatise on the Exercise and Preservation of Vision* (1880); *Our Homes, and How to*

advertised and the medical staff all strongly favoured the appointment of Gunn, but Burford Rawlings argued that the political and financial influence of Brudenell Carter would be advantageous for future growth of the hospital. A compromise was reached, with Brudenell Carter being appointed to the senior post and Gunn to a second but junior position. Carter was known for his heroic optic nerve decompressions for visual loss due to chronic papilloedema. His work for *The Times* was described as:

> Eloquent, incisive, more than occasionally bitter, he was also a generous writer, and few members of the Medical Profession have wielded greater power with the pen, while he possessed the equally valuable gift of being able to speak in public with the same command of language and high level of literary style. Carter's 'leaders' belong to an older day; he used the Latin 'period' and a rotund full-dress method; but any appearance of pomposity thus given to his writings was purely superficial; no writer of to-day is more fastidious than was Carter in his choice of language, or more resolutely averse from the use of 'stale metaphors, trite tags and obvious morals'.[73]

This literary prowess was something Burford Rawlings came to rue, because Brudenell Carter proved a powerful adversary, and his letters to *The Times* were crucial in destroying the reputation of the

hospital's administration in the run-up to the Fry Commission's deliberations.

As neurology and ophthalmology both became more specialised in the twentieth century, the two disciplines drifted apart. Ophthalmic surgeons were still appointed to the staff of the National Hospital, but it is not clear how often, if at all, ophthalmic surgery was performed at the hospital, although refraction clinics continued until the 1940s and medical eye clinics were held throughout the century. Leslie Paton[74] was ophthalmic surgeon to the National Hospital between 1907 and 1937, and was joined by Frederick Williamson-Noble[75] in 1925. Williamson-Noble seems to have been the more active of the two in the hospital and he was also an assiduous member of the Medical Committee after the

---

Make Them Healthy (1883); *Ophthalmic Surgery* (1887); and *Doctors and Their Work, or, Medicine, Quackery and Disease* (1903). He worked at the Royal Eye Hospital set up in Southwark by Laurence, and then at St George's Hospital Medical School. He traced his family to the fifteenth century and held his own Arms. He was awarded the Crimea Medal and made Knight of Justice of the Order of the Hospital of Saint John of Jerusalem. At Queen Square, Carter was appointed ophthalmic surgeon in 1886 and consulting ophthalmic surgeon on his retirement in 1899; from 1887 to 1900, he was a member of the General Medical Council. His views on the administration of the National Hospital, as expounded in the letter pages of *The Times*, carried great weight. Curiously, the portrait by Stuff in *Vanity Fair* shows him using two eye glasses – said to be a personal affectation, but possibly also a reference to his wisdom (or perfidy – this is for the reader to decide): see R. R. James, 'Robert Brudenell Carter', *British Journal of Ophthalmology* 7 (1941): 330–9.

[73] Anon., 'Obituary: Robert Brudenell Carter FRCS', *Lancet* **192** (1918): 607.

[74] Leslie Johnson Paton was born in Edinburgh, educated at Glasgow High School, Cambridge University and St Mary's Hospital, qualifying in 1897. His junior appointments were in London, with time spent in Bonn, and he then served as clinical assistant to Marcus Gunn at Moorfields before being appointed assistant ophthalmic surgeon to St Mary's in 1902, and ophthalmologist to the National Hospital from 1907. A tall and imposing figure, with a large private practice in Harley Street, Paton served as president of the Ophthalmological Society of the United Kingdom, the section of neurology at the Royal Society of Medicine, the section of ophthalmology at the British Medical Association's annual meetings, and as chairman of the Council of British Ophthalmologists. He carried out important early research with Gordon Holmes on papilloedema and intracranial tumours, and described what later became known as the Foster–Kennedy syndrome (*Archives of Ophthalmology* **28** (1942): 704–10). He edited the *British Journal of Ophthalmology* and was involved in the International Congresses of Ophthalmology. Paton retired from the hospital in 1937 and was elected consulting ophthalmic surgeon.

[75] Frederick Arnold Williamson-Noble was educated at Oundle and qualified in medicine from Cambridge and at St Mary's Hospital Medical School in 1914. He had active service in the Navy in the First World War, and was appointed supernumerary ophthalmic surgeon at St Mary's Hospital (1924), surgeon to Maida Vale Hospital (1921–36) and, from 1925, the National Hospital, the Central London Ophthalmic Hospital and the Royal National Throat, Nose and Ear Hospital. He worked as civilian consultant in ophthalmology to the Royal Navy from 1943. Various surgical instruments have his name attached, and he was joint author of *A Handbook of Ophthalmology*, which was a popular undergraduate text (1927). He was a well-known and highly respected opinion in London medicine who continued in practice until his death.

introduction of the NHS, and, like Walshe, worked without taking a salary. In 1937, Keith Lyle was appointed assistant ophthalmic surgeon,[76] in place of Paton, and he was the first surgeon to have a paid position at both the National Hospital and Moorfields. In 1955, Stephen Miller[77] was appointed and served until 1980. When Maida Vale merged with the National Hospital, Henry Edwin Hobbs[78] was on the Maida Vale staff but it is not clear whether he ever contributed to ophthalmological clinical practice at Queen Square, and the Maida Vale department closed on his retirement in 1975. He was also attached to the Institute of Neurology and researched new methods of stereo-campimetry. At the core of research into ocular disorders at Queen Square was an emphasis on new technologies. Lyle and Miller were both heads of the department of ophthalmology at the National Hospital in the 1960s. Lyle, who retired in 1968,

mainly worked on long-term follow-up of clinical cases. In the 1960s, Miller set up the first facility in the country for fluorescein angiography at the National Hospital and carried out research, particularly with Michael Sanders and Ralph Ross-Russell as research fellows, which more than anything else established the pre-eminence of the department of medical ophthalmology at Queen Square. Sanders was then appointed to a consultant position on 1 January 1969 in place of Lyle, and both he and Miller also had honorary positions in the Institute of Neurology from 1969.[79] In the early 1970s, their research focused on new techniques, especially fluorescein angiography, electronystagmography, ocular electromyography and, after 1975, 'EMI-scanning'. The research was clinical in nature and they applied these new techniques to the retinal, optic nerve and ocular muscle disorders that occurred in the context of neurological disorders. Their research depended on access to the large number of neurological patients. In 1979, Sanders took over the department and his main interests initially were in ischaemic and inflammatory retinal and optic nerve diseases, and in papilloedema, a condition of which he collected and published an enormous series of 500 cases. Over the next decade, the focus of research changed to oculomotor disorders on which Sanders worked with the Sobell department of neurophysiology. David Taylor was appointed in 1979, based mainly at Great Ormond Street, and his research focused on congenital disorders of the eye and ocular development. He retired in 1989/90. Elizabeth Graham was appointed in 1990 when John Elston, appointed in 1988, moved to Oxford. A full-time senior registrar was appointed for the first time in 1991, and Paul Riordan-Eva joined as a consultant ophthalmologist in 1995/6. In August 1992, James Acheson joined as a consultant ophthalmologist and became head of department in 1999 on Sanders' retirement. Over the Miller and Sanders years, the National Hospital had become a leading centre for neuro-ophthalmology, active clinically and in research that had moved from the physiology of fluid dynamics, the pupil and eye movements to genetic disorders and inflammatory eye conditions.

In addition to the ophthalmologists and ophthalmic surgeons (who, despite being surgeons, had an entirely

---

[76] Thomas Keith Selfe Lyle was educated at Dulwich College, and graduated from Cambridge University and King's College Hospital. He was appointed surgeon to Moorfields Eye Hospital, King's College Hospital and the National Hospital, and served as dean of the Institute of Ophthalmology. In the Second World War, he was mentioned in dispatches and reached the rank of air commodore. He became a knight grand cross of the Order of St John in 1981 and was a knight of the Holy Sepulchre, retiring from the Queen Square staff in December 1968.

[77] Sir Stephen James Hamilton Miller was born and educated in Arbroath and qualified in medicine from Aberdeen University in 1937. After the war, he was appointed consultant ophthalmologist at Hull, but resigned after only six weeks, returning to junior positions in London before being appointed consultant at St George's Hospital in 1952, and then Moorfields Eye Hospital and the National Hospital in 1955. He was soon recognised as a pre-eminent ophthalmologist and a world expert in the management of glaucoma. In 1974, he was appointed surgeon oculist to the Queen. He resigned from the NHS in 1980, he said because of the proliferating bureaucracy, and became hospitaller to the St John Ophthalmic Hospital, Jerusalem, in succession to Sir Stewart Duke-Elder and Keith Lyle. He was appointed KCVO in 1979.

[78] Henry Edwin Hobbs was born in London, educated in Canada and at Tottenham Boys' Junior Technical School and graduated in medicine from the London Hospital in 1938. He was appointed to the consultant staff of Maida Vale Hospital in 1946, and also the Metropolitan Hospital, the Royal Free Hospital and the Royal Northern Hospital. Like Brudenell Carter, Lyle, Williamson-Noble and Miller, he was involved with the Order of St John, and was elected as a Commander of the Most Venerable Order of the Hospital of St John of Jerusalem in 1970. He retired from the National Hospitals in 1975.

[79] Lyle and Miller had only one session each at Queen Square, and when Sanders was appointed, he was given four sessions. All contributed greatly to the hospital despite their limited contracts.

medical practice at Queen Square), some of the neurologists also developed a deep interest in ophthalmology, following the example of Jackson and Gowers. In the post-Second World War period, Swithin Meadows, Ralph Ross-Russell, Christopher Earl and Ian McDonald all became renowned in the field of neuro-ophthalmology and each held a joint appointment at Moorfields. The links between Queen Square and Moorfields were strengthened in this period, with shared junior appointments. Meadows did not publish much but had a formidable reputation in the field of neuro-ophthalmology, focusing mainly on optic nerve, pituitary and occipital lobe disease. Ross-Russell was the first to observe the cholesterol embolus as a cause of amaurosis fugax. Earl was an all-rounder but had a particular interest in the central visual pathways, and McDonald made major contributions to optic neuritis, especially in relation to pathogenesis and prognosis, and its relationship to multiple sclerosis. All four were excellent clinical opinions on any aspect of neuro-ophthalmology. Williamson-Noble, Lyle, Critchley, Miller, Meadows, Jefferson and McDonald were all invited to give the Doyne memorial lecture, the leading named lecture in British ophthalmology, and a sign of the high esteem of Queen Square in British, and indeed international, ophthalmological circles.

Neuro-otology at Queen Square

Clinical examination of the throat and vocal cords was not possible until invention of the laryngoscope in 1855 by the Parisian singer and music teacher Manuel Garcia. He adapted a dental mirror and used sunlight reflected from another mirror to visualise the throat. This new technique was taken up by Sir Morell Mackenzie, who founded the Free Dispensary for Diseases of the Throat and Loss of Voice at 5 King Street (now Kingly Street), London, in 1862. Mackenzie's brainchild was a success and his specialist institution moved in 1865 to new premises at 32 Golden Square, the former home of the London Homoeopathic Hospital, with enough room for 16 beds. This was renamed the Hospital for Diseases of the Throat and, in the same year, Mackenzie published his first textbook, *Use of Laryngology in Diseases of the Throat*. At the time, laryngoscopy was not considered important in general hospitals and delegated to a junior physician or surgeon. The young Hughlings Jackson was put in charge of the throat department at the London Hospital and, despite his protestations, the pathologist W. S. Greenfield was obliged to look after the service at St Thomas'. Queen Square took an early interest in the neural connections of the vocal cord, with the work of A. E. Cumberbatch,[80] who served as the first aural surgeon between 1886 and 1907. However, the most significant appointment was that of Felix Semon in 1887.[81] He became the most prominent laryngologist in Britain,[82] a remarkable achievement at the time for a Prussian Jewish émigré.

---

[80] Alfonso Elkin Cumberbatch resigned his post at Queen Square to become consulting aural surgeon at St Bartholomew's Hospital. He wrote little in the medical literature, but was a founder member and treasurer of the Otological Society of the United Kingdom. His few contributions to otology at Queen Square were outclassed by Ballance in securing the interface between aural and neurological surgery in the early years of the hospital.

[81] Sir Felix Semon was born in Prussia, and graduated in medicine from Berlin. He was introduced to laryngology by Störk and von Schrötter in Vienna, and then moved to London in 1874. He was appointed by Mackenzie as physician at Golden Square and St Thomas' Hospital (1882), and then as laryngologist to the National Hospital (1888). In 1893, he founded the Laryngological Society of London, and was given the title of Royal Prussian Professor (1894). He soon had a very large clinical practice. He was consulted by Queen Victoria, knighted in 1897, and formed part of the social circle around the Prince of Wales, who appointed Semon as his physician when he became King Edward VII in 1901. In *The Sands of Time* (1939), Sir James Purves-Stewart provides a vivid description of Semon as 'a picturesque figure … a bright, restless, energetic little man with a bristling moustache and attractive German accent. Even now I can hear him saying to a patient: "open your mouse, and breeze qvite quietly".' Semon courted controversy in a famous row in which he (and others) claimed that Morell Mackenzie had mismanaged the laryngeal cancer of Frederick III, Emperor of Germany and King of Prussia, leading to the emperor's premature death 99 days after his assumption to the throne – an event that changed the course of European history. Rightly or wrongly, Mackenzie's career was ruined, and Semon benefitted. *The Autobiography of Sir Felix Semon* (1926), written in German but edited and translated posthumously by his son Henry, has been criticised for its egotism and incessant name-dropping. Although undoubtedly an essay in self-aggrandisement, the criticism smacks of sour grapes because it is clear that Semon was very popular socially and had a large and successful clinical practice.

[82] The banquet marking his retirement at the Whitehall Rooms of the Hotel Metropole was held just before Semon left on a world cruise, and was described as 'a formal banquet as has never to our knowledge been accorded to a member of the medical profession'. Anon., 'A Complimentary Dinner to Sir Felix Semon', *Lancet* **174** (1909): 102; and Anon., 'Banquet to Sir Felix Semon', *British Medical Journal* **2** (1909): 88–9.

Semon conducted a series of definitive animal experiments with Victor Horsley at the Brown Institute on the cerebral localisation of speech articulation, leading him to the conclusion that unilateral paralysis of a vocal cord adductor is due either to psychogenic or to neuromuscular causes such as myasthenia gravis. He showed that the abductor fibres are always involved before the adductors in central nervous system damage, an observation that was designated Semon's Law.[83] In a clinical lecture at the National Hospital (16 November 1897), at which he presented cases where central organic affections had led to unilateral or bilateral laryngeal abductor paralysis, Semon concluded:

> The multitude of possibilities which ought to occur to your minds when discovering paralysis of both and even more so of one Abductor is so great that unless there be plain collateral evidence of a definite form of organic disease, you ought to look upon that symptom as a silent storm signal, hoisted for the benefit of the physician, but not justifying you in pronouncing the death warrant of the patient.[84]

Semon's skill with the laryngoscope allowed him to discern that laryngeal cancer always begins on one vocal fold and is commonly associated with nerve paralysis. He developed the modern operation of laryngo-fissure for early cancer; and introduced the treatment of vocal rest for laryngeal tuberculosis, which became universal therapy in sanatoria throughout the world. Despite the fact that he was not a neurologist, Semon seems to have engaged fully with hospital life, being a regular attendee at the Medical Committee, and later serving on the Board of Management. His importance to Queen Square resided not only in his experimental, clinical and administrative work, but also in the reflected glory of his reputation, and with Semon the hospital demonstrated again its ability to attract high-profile and well-regarded doctors onto its staff, a significant factor in its rising reputation.

The next figure in the field of oto-laryngology who was appointed to the hospital, Charles Alfred

Ballance,[85] proved to be another example of the hospital's auspicious choice of staff. He was a close friend of Horsley from their medical school days, and it was Ballance who assisted Horsley in the first removal of an extradural tumour from one of Gowers' patients (1887), an operation that is a landmark in the history of neurosurgery. Through detailed knowledge of the relationship between the vertebrae and spinal cord segments, Ballance encouraged his friend to remove one more lamina just as Horsley was on the verge of aborting the famous operation. Ballance was much more engaged with the general developments in neurology and neurosurgery than Semon, and his appointment as surgeon at the National Hospital in 1891, to join Horsley, was generally welcomed. Regarded as a 'slow, gentle and painstaking operator', Ballance complemented perfectly the more mercurial style of Horsley. In his reminiscences, he recalled that he and Horsley 'had only a kitchen to operate in at the National Hospital ... but following Listerian doctrines I do not think we ever had sepsis supervening on an operation. In those early days very few operations on

---

[83] F. Semon, 'On the Proclivity of the Abductor Fibres of the Recurrent Laryngeal Nerve to Become Affected Sooner than the Adductor Fibres', *Archives of Laryngology* 2 (1881): 197–215.

[84] F. Semon, 'The Clinical Significance of Laryngeal Abductor Paralysis', *British Medical Journal* 1 (1898): 1.

[85] Sir Charles Alfred Ballance was born in London, educated privately and trained at St Thomas' Hospital where he was awarded one of two gold medals at the final surgery examination in 1882, the other being won by Horsley. In addition to his post at Queen Square, he also held staff appointments at Great Ormond Street and the West London Hospital and was appointed chief surgeon to the Metropolitan Police from 1912 to 1926. He served as vice-president of the Royal College of Surgeons, and was the founding president of the Society of British Neurological Surgeons and a leading figure in London surgical circles who was notable for his interest in experimental research throughout his career. Purves-Stewart worked with Ballance at the Brown Institute and also at Queen Square, and recalls 'A dark-haired man of fine presence with a solemn, deliberate manner, a widely read scholar and philosopher, with an erudite literary style and a great fondness for Shakespearean quotations. He was a man of deep religious convictions, possibly associated with his Huguenot ancestry. Had he entered the church, I feel sure he would have attained and adorned the episcopal bench.' His obituarist in the *British Medical Journal* ('HGT') noted that 'he was a little alarming until one got past the first contact, and his natural dignity made one think sometimes of Aristotle's "magnificent man"; but this first impression quickly melted, and the full warmth of his kindly nature soon shone through'. Amongst his writings were *The Healing of Nerves* (1901, with Sir James Purves-Stewart), *Some Points on the Surgery of the Brain and its Membranes* (1907), *Essays on the Surgery of the Temporal Bone* (1919, with Charles Green) and *A Glimpse into the History of the Brain* (1922).

the nervous system were performed – probably not more than one a month, if so many.'[86]

Ballance resigned his National Hospital position to take up an appointment at St Thomas' Hospital in 1908, but retained close connections with Queen Square and, during the First World War, served with Holmes and Charles Symonds in France. He was also instrumental in organising emergency hospital services in Gallipoli. Ballance was decorated for his work and appointed KCMG in 1918. His main achievements in civilian practice were the standardisation of an effective approach for the drainage of temporal lobe abscesses; the instigation of skull base approaches to deal with sinus thrombosis; radical mastoidectomy for chronic middle-ear disease with ligation of the jugular vein; section of cranial nerve VIII in intractable vertigo; first successful removal of an acoustic neuroma (1894); and first to perform anastomosis of the facial to the spinal accessory nerve for facial palsy.

After retirement, Ballance remained involved in medicine and chaired the meeting at the Athenaeum when the Society of British Neurological Surgeons was founded (2 December 1926). Jefferson felt that a generation of young neurosurgeons in Britain owed Ballance a great debt and he was an important link to their surgical past: 'He was a Victorian who held the men of that time in the greatest veneration, and was proud that he had worked and moved among them.'[87]

Thus, the specialty of laryngology had, from its fragile start, become well established at Queen Square, as indeed it had done elsewhere, to the extent that, by 1904, there were five specialist ear, nose and throat hospitals in London. Later, the King's Fund proposed that they should merge but, as with neurological hospitals, this attempt was to fail.

In 1909, on Ballance's retirement, Sidney Scott[88] was appointed aural surgeon and he remained in

post until 1939, and thereafter as consulting aural surgeon. He was joined at Queen Square by Theodore Just, another graduate from St Bartholomew's Hospital.[89] Both were renowned aural surgeons, and, also much admired as people, they seem to have provided an excellent clinical service at Queen Square. Just and Ballance no doubt enhanced the *esprit de corps* and elite nature of the medical establishment at the National Hospital, but most of their work was based at St Bartholomew's Hospital and Golden Square, and, academically, otology at Queen Square trod water during these inter-war years.

This was to change completely with the appointment in 1936 of Terence Cawthorne[90] and, in 1939,

---

[86] C. B. Ballance, 'Remarks and Reminiscences', *British Medical Journal* 1 (8 January 1927): 64–7.

[87] Jefferson's 'brief eulogium' is in the *British Medical Journal* 1 (1936): 340.

[88] Sydney Richard Scott was born in Shrewsbury and qualified from St Bartholomew's Hospital in 1899. He then signed up immediately to serve in the South African Field Force during the Boer War, and for his bravery and military work was decorated with the Queen's Medal with three clasps. He returned to London in 1902 and passed the London MB BS with a

gold medal. In 1908, he was appointed assistant surgeon to the ear department at St Bartholomew's Hospital, and in 1909 published a textbook (*The Operations of Aural Surgery*). He served with the RAMC in France (for which he was awarded the 1914 Star [also known as the Mons Star]) and and later worked with the MRC on the problems of vertigo in flying. In 1921, he became senior surgeon to the ear department at St Bartholomew's Hospital retiring in 1940.

[89] Theodore Hartman Just was another remarkable figure. He was born in Bristol, the son of Sir Hartman Just, legal adviser to the Colonial Office, and educated at St Paul's School, where he had a brilliant career as a scholar, obtaining an honours degree in zoology at London University whilst still at school. He then obtained a first in natural science in Cambridge and qualified in medicine at St Bartholomew's Hospital. He was a notable athlete, president of the Cambridge Athletic Club where he completed the Great Court run at Trinity College (made famous in *Chariots of Fire*) in 55 seconds, and then ran in the 1908 Olympiad, finishing fifth in the 800 metres. He saw active service in France from 1915 to 1919, and was mentioned in despatches for conspicuous devotion to duty. In 1921, he was elected aural surgeon at St Bartholomew's Hospital, and in 1921 as assistant aural surgeon to Scott at the National Hospital, and also as surgeon at Golden Square. He was, as his obituary put it, a good aural surgeon, a very fine athlete and a great gentleman.

[90] Terence Cawthorne was born in Aberdeen, and educated at Denstone College and King's College Hospital, from where he qualified in 1924. He was appointed consultant ENT surgeon at King's in 1932, and at the National Hospital in 1936, where he remained until retirement in 1967. He developed an interest in neuro-otology, and with Dix and Hallpike was one of the founders of the discipline. Cawthorne was a renowned lecturer, in rather a grand manner, and was in great demand nationally and internationally. In the Second World War, he carried out distinguished work for the EMS, and was also appointed clinical director of the MRC Wernher Research Unit on deafness at

Charles Hallpike,[91] after Theodore Just developed pancreatitis, from which he died in 1937 after some months of illness. Cawthorne replaced Just as assistant aural surgeon to Sidney Scott, and when Scott retired in 1939 was promoted to the position of aural surgeon, with the assistant post left unfilled since very little surgery was carried out at the National Hospital during the war. As a young man, Cawthorne had carried out experimental work with Ballance at The Royal College of Surgeons and had been appointed as a consultant aural surgeon at King's College Hospital in 1932, where he had a distinguished clinical career and developed an academic interest in neuro-otology. He was a charming and urbane man and an excellent teacher, who fitted in well at Queen Square, contributing greatly to the life of the hospital, not only surgically but also administratively, taking an active role in the Medical Committee. Cawthorne also was instrumental in providing a career path for the younger Hallpike. The two promoted research, and, although Hallpike was said to be a difficult colleague and their relationship was at times strained, this proved a very productive collaboration.

King's. He worked seven days a week and became renowned as a pioneer in ENT surgery, and especially for his work on otosclerosis, stapedectomy (which he could complete in 15–20 minutes) and surgery of the labyrinth. He also carried out facial nerve decompression in Bell's palsy, which was the subject of the 5th Gowers memorial lecture at Queen Square in 1968. He was appointed dean of the Medical School of King's College Hospital, and awarded the Dalby and W. J. Harrison prizes of the Royal Society of Medicine. He was knighted in 1964 for his services to medicine. He was of the old school, arriving at Queen Square in his chauffeur-driven primrose-and-black Rolls Royce, and immaculate in dress and manners. He was a popular figure amongst the neurologists and a long-serving and active member of the Medical Committee.

[91] Charles Hallpike was born in India into a colonial family, although his grandmother was a Rajput and Charles had a dark complexion himself, about which he remained sensitive. At the age of 12, he developed Perthes' disease of the hip after a minor injury playing soccer at school, and as a result spent long periods confined to bed with his leg suspended by weights. Nevertheless, he was an excellent student, a classics scholar at St Paul's School, and in 1919 entered Guy's Hospital where he qualified in 1924. He trained initially in ENT surgery at Guy's Hospital and in Cheltenham, and then took the post of research fellow at the Ferens Institute of the Middlesex Hospital, where he established the first temporal bone microscopy unit in England. After ten years in the Ferens Institute, he moved to Queen Square.

Charles Hallpike published his first articles on hearing, including a paper in *Nature*, in 1934, and then a celebrated account with Hugh Cairns on the histopathology of Ménière's disease in 1938.[92] He was prevented from military service by Perthes' disease, and in 1939 Sir Edward Mellanby, secretary of the MRC, recognising Hallpike's academic ability, suggested to Carmichael that he be offered a post in the MRC unit at Queen Square. Cawthorne backed the proposal and Hallpike was appointed to the scientific staff in Carmichael's unit in 1940, supported by the MRC. His rise within the hospital was rapid. In December 1940, he was appointed as clinical assistant to Cawthorne and, in 1942. made 'temporary assistant surgeon for diseases of the throat and ear', with the position of aural physician added in 1943. Hallpike quickly established himself as a researcher, and there followed an important series of three papers by Hallpike, Cawthorne and their research fellow Gerald Fitzgerald, in 1942, describing directional preponderance and the clinical features of caloric testing in Ménière's disease.[93] His potential to advance the field, and the quality of his work, were clear, and on 20 January 1944, Carmichael, with the support of the Medical Committee, wrote to the Board of Management requesting the establishment of a neuro-otological research unit, with Hallpike as director and with a full complement of beds and clinics in appreciation of 'the importance to neurology and to medicine and the value of the research work being carried out in the Hospital Laboratories and Clinics by Mr Hallpike, working in collaboration with Mr Cawthorne, and of the desirability of ensuring that such work be facilitated and promoted'.

---

[92] C. S. Hallpike and H. Cairns, 'Observations on the Pathology of Meniere's Syndrome', *Journal of Laryngology and Otology* 53 (1938): 625–54.

[93] Studies in human vestibular function: G. Fitzgerald and C. S. Hallpike, 'Observations on the Directional Preponderance of Caloric Nystagmus ("Nystagmusbereitschaft") Resulting from Cerebral Lesions', *Brain* 65 (1942): 115–37; T. E. Cawthorne, G. Fitzgerald and C. S. Hallpike, 'Observations on the Directional Preponderance of Caloric Nystagmus ("Nystagmus-bereitschaft") Resulting from Unilateral Labyrinthectomy', *Brain* 65 (1942): 138–60; T. E. Cawthorne, G. Fitzgerald and C. S. Hallpike, 'Observations on the Clinical Features of "Ménière's Disease": with Especial Reference to the Results of the Caloric Tests', *Brain* 65 (1942): 161–80. See also A. Compston, 'From the Archives', *Brain* 128 (2005): 1475–7.

This position was equivalent to Carmichael's own as director of the neurological research unit, and was a generous gesture. The Board agreed, and Hallpike was provided with four beds (shared with Cawthorne), annual funds of £600 for five years towards the expenses of the unit, and a house officer for clinical work and research. The unit was situated in the basement under David Wire ward and, although periodically promised more space, seems to have remained there for many years.

The establishment of the neuro-otological research unit was to prove an important development in the academic contribution of Queen Square. Hallpike applied scientific principles to the clinical problems in otology with ingenuity and energy, and in 1946 described vestibular neuronitis and benign positional vertigo, and made further contributions to the study of Ménière's disease.[94] According to Baloh, when Hallpike arrived at Queen Square in 1940, he was fortunate to find two young technicians, Best in histology and Bolum as a mechanic, who stayed with him throughout his career. Technical challenges were met through improvisation and Hallpike's laboratories were filled with ingenious home-made devices.[95]

Among these was the famous rotational chair, which Bolum helped to build, and a new form of microtome. With Fitzgerald, in 1942, Hallpike also devised the bi-thermal caloric test, showing that this could provide information about central as well as peripheral lesions. In 1948, with Margaret Dix and Derrick Hood, Hallpike demonstrated that loudness recruitment is the result of damage to cochlear nerve endings.

Hallpike's elegance and perfect manners were rivalled only by Macdonald Critchley. This helped him to secure and maintain high standing among his illustrious neurological colleagues. Not for him was membership of the 'baggy trousers brigade', a derogatory term used by Roger Gilliatt for scientists and provincial doctors. Nor was Hallpike content to be relegated as 'one of our men in the basement', a designation favoured by Denis Williams. His 'D-room' neuro-otology clinic became world renowned,

and Hallpike received many referrals from physicians and surgeons. He was said to be difficult at times, and very determined, and his friend and great supporter Wylie McKissock remarked: 'Woe betide any resident who allowed a patient with an eighth nerve tumour to come to surgery without having had his Hallpikery!' When Hallpike was elected FRS in 1956, Critchley commented: 'Well, Charles, we will have to take you seriously now.' Certainly, the unit gained worldwide recognition, and Queen Square remains a centre for neuro-otology, a specialty that owes its existence in large part to his work. He retired from his position at Queen Square in July 1965.

In 1940, Hallpike was joined by another remarkable figure, Margaret Dix.[96] She was employed first to assist the many soldiers who sustained loss of hearing in active service, seeing over 2,000 such cases. Encouraged as a researcher by Hallpike, she became a pioneer in the emerging specialty of neuro-otology. With Hallpike, Dix published a series of landmark papers describing the main causes of vertigo, including the condition known as benign positional vertigo, and she devised the Dix–Hallpike test in which vertigo and nystagmus are induced by rapid lowering of the patient's head into a supine position. Dix was appointed consultant at Queen Square in 1965 until her retirement in 1976, although she continued to work in a locum capacity at Queen Square until the age of 70. From 1944, she was assisted in her work by the scientist J. D. ('Derrick') Hood.[97]

---

[94] M. R. Dix and C. S. Hallpike, 'The Pathology, Symptomatology and Diagnosis of Certain Common Disorders of the Vestibular System', *Proceedings of the Royal Society of Medicine* 45 (1952): 341–54.

[95] R. W. Baloh, 'Charles Skinner Hallpike and the Beginnings of Neurotology', *Neurology* 54 (2000): 2138–46.

[96] Margaret Ruth Dix was born in Shropshire, the daughter of a rector, and educated at Sherborne School and the Royal Free Hospital Medical School, from where she qualified in 1937. She was destined for a career as an ENT surgeon when, in an air raid in the blitz in 1940, she suffered severe facial injuries and glass fragments damaged her vision. Sir Archibald McIndoe restored her facial appearance, but the loss of vision prevented her from continuing a surgical career and, in 1945, she joined Hallpike as a research assistant. She received many national and international honours for her work, including the W. J. Harrison prize in otology in 1954, the Dalby prize of the Royal Society of Medicine in 1958, and the Norman Gamble research prize in 1980: see 'Margaret Ruth Dix' in *Plarr's Lives*, and annual report of the Institute of Neurology 1991–2.

[97] J. D. ('Derrick') Hood was the best-known British scientist in the field of neuro-otology of his generation. He graduated in physics from Durham University in 1944 and joined the MRC Otological Research Unit in the same year, where he collaborated with Dix and Hallpike for many years. In 1965, he was appointed honorary consultant physicist to the National Hospital and, on the basis of his

In 1970, the Otological Research Unit became the MRC Hearing and Balance Unit with Hood as director. In 1980, the work at the Institute of Laryngology[98] was transferred to Queen Square, and the unit again changed its name to the MRC Neuro-otology Unit. On Hood's retirement in 1989, it was absorbed into the MRC Human Movement and Balance Unit under the directorship of David Marsden. Hood's main research work was on the eighth cranial nerve and its central connections, and the vestibular system – focusing on habituation, adaptation and fatigue and optokinetic mechanisms – and vestibular migraine. In 1974, the consultant neurologist Peter Rudge joined the department and provided the main link between the hospital patients and the unit. When this was dissolved, Rudge remained attached to the neuro-otology department of the hospital.

In addition to the neuro-otological research unit of the Institute of Neurology (in its various incarnations), there remained also a neuro-otology department in the hospital, providing a clinical service. After the retirement of Cawthorne in 1967, Mr Spencer Harrison was appointed as aural surgeon and he was joined by Harold Ludman. Spencer Harrison had earlier worked with Hallpike and was an authority on Ménière's disease. He retired in 1973 and was replaced by W. McKenzie (who had retired from Maida Vale that year) and A. D. Cheeseman, initially as locum appointments, and then in 1977 by W. F. R. Gibson. Ten years later, in 1987, Gerald Brooks replaced Gibson as the second aural surgeon working with Ludman, and they provided the service until Ludman's retirement in February 2000. Having retired from his position at Charing Cross and the Eastman Hospital, Anthony Cheeseman was then appointed, 20 years after his temporary appointment in the 1970s, when he had started the development of skull-base surgery with Logue and worked on clinical uses for the rotating swing with the Hearing and Balance Unit. During this intervening period, Cheeseman had continued his developmental work on skull base surgery with the neurosurgeons Symon, Thomas, Powell and Crockard, as an

honorary senior lecturer. In 1981, expansion occurred on the medical side also with the appointment of Linda Luxon[99] and, in 1989, Rosalyn Davies, as consultant audiological physicians.

Neuro-anaesthetics

Neuro-anaesthetics at the National Hospital was always closely aligned to general anaesthetics, and therefore had little academic impact on neurology. Despite this separation, it played a vital clinical role in the advance of neurosurgery and intensive care at the hospital.[100]

The first surgical anaesthetic given anywhere in the world was the administration of diethyl ether by Willam T. G. Morton during an operation on 16 October 1846 in the surgical amphitheatre of the Massachusetts General Hospital (which has come to be known as the Ether Dome). Less than ten weeks later, on 21 December 1846, William Squire, a medical student at University College Hospital, administered the first ether anaesthetic in Britain, during a leg amputation by the professor of clinical surgery Robert Liston. In the following year, James Young Simpson, professor of medicine and midwifery in Edinburgh, performed the first chloroform anaesthetic. Horsley, who was aware of these events, became deeply interested in anaesthesia and experimented with chloroform himself. It became his preferred anaesthetic agent for experimental work on primates and his clinical operations at Queen Square. By then, chloroform had gained the reputation as a dangerous form of anaesthesia, and the London anaesthetists replaced Simpson's method of dripping chloroform onto a cloth with the introduction of inhalers ensuring regulated exposure. Horsley was directly involved in the design and development of this technique. A series of chloroform committees and commissions were set up internationally, the first in London in 1862. Horsley was appointed to the British Medical

---

research work, won many awards, including the Medallion of the Royal National Institute for the Deaf ((https://www.ucl.ac.uk/ion/education/alumnusassociation/archivenewsletterspdfs/issue28).

[98] The Institute of Laryngology and Otology was closed down as a result of the Flowers report.

[99] Linda Luxon was awarded a personal chair and on Ludman's retirement in 2000 took over the headship of the department.

[100] This survey is based largely on the annual reports and archival material, published works and obituaries of key figures, and the website entry 'History of the Anaesthetic Department at The National Hospital for Neurology & Neurosurgery, Queen Square' by Dr Gordon Bond (https://www.uclh.nhs.uk/ourservices/servicea-z/neuro/anae/Pages/Historyqsnancc.aspx).

Association's 1901 committee and it was he who proposed that the committee should 'determine what is the minimal dose of the drug which would secure adequate anaesthesia for operations and at the same time not endanger life'.[101] The dosage of 2 per cent was agreed and this regimen became standard practice.

The first anaesthetist appointed to Queen Square was J. Frederick W. Silk,[102] who worked at the hospital between 1888 and 1891, when he was succeeded by his friend and colleague Dudley W. Buxton.[103] In 1896, Buxton was appointed consulting anaesthetist and Robert T. Bakewell succeeded him as anaethetist. Bakewell retired in 1905 and was replaced by

Llewellyn Powell,[104] who worked at the National, the Samaritan and Queen Charlotte's Hospitals. In the famous 1906 photograph of Horsley in the operating theatre, it is Llewellyn Powell administering chloroform using the Vernon–Harcourt chloroform inhaler.

Powell was joined in 1911 by perhaps the most celebrated of the early anaesthetists, Dr Zebulon Mennell.[105] Just as Horsley was dubbed the father of neurosurgery, so Mennell was known as the 'father' of British neurosurgical anaesthesia. He worked at St Thomas' and the National Hospital, in close association for many years with Percy Sargent, and was renowned for the skill and speed with which he induced anaesthesia, developing new techniques in neuro-anaesthesia and recognising the specific challenges that neurosurgery posed for the discipline of anaesthetics. The introduction of hedonal and the intra-tracheal insufflation of ether were his most important academic contributions.

Thus, by the end of the First World War, there were two honorary anaesthetists at Queen Square, Mennell and Llewellyn Powell. In 1922/3, Llewellyn Powell retired and was replaced by J. F. Ryan who retained his honorary post until 1935. When Ryan retired, three replacement appointments were made, and unlike the other senior medical staff, the appointees were remunerated for their work.[106] Two were the first female consultants appointed to the hospital staff, Olive Jones[107] and

---

[101] The committee also included as members Vernon-Harcourt, Sherrington and Buxton, and concluded that the Vernon-Harcourt regulating inhaler was the preferred type, 'having the advantages of simplicity exactness and portability', with a maximum of 2 per cent on its scale ('Report of the Special Chloroform Committee', *British Medical Journal* **324** supplement 2 (9 July 1910): 47–72.

[102] J. Frederick W. Silk was a qualified surgeon, appointed as anaesthetist at King's College Hospital as well as Queen Square. He was a renowned and fashionable London practitioner. His early work included a book, a *Manual of Nitrous Oxide Anaesthesia* (1888), and he also played an important and public role in pressing for systematic teaching, writing frequently in the medical journals on this topic. During the First World War, he served as lieutenant-colonel in the RAMC and consulting anaesthetist in the Malta and Home Commands. In this capacity, he visited over 1,000 war hospitals and wrote influential papers on the administration of anaesthesia in wartime. He was an advocate for professionalisation of the discipline, and was instrumental in the foundation of the Society of Anaesthetists (1893), which, in 1908, became the section on anaesthetics of the Royal Society of Medicine.

[103] Dudley Wilmot Buxton was another well-known figure, whose book *Anaesthetics: Their Uses and Administration* (1888) remained in print for 35 years and went through a number of editions. He pioneered the use of nitrous oxide for minor surgery by continuous nasal infusion, and also contributed to the advisory work on chloroform (as secretary to the 1901 committee with Vernon Harcourt and Victor Horsley – both lifelong friends – as members). He also worked to raise anaesthetic standards, and it was he who proposed that final-year medical students should observe 50 anaesthetic procedures, resulting, in 1912, in addition by the GMC of anaesthesia as the last subject to be studied in the medical curriculum. Buxton designed his own mouth-gag and props, and modified the Junker chloroform inhaler, but neither he nor Silk seems to have made much specific contribution to neuro-anaesthesia.

[104] Llewellyn Powell was a renowned London anaesthetist, with a large private practice, who played a prominent part with Silk and Buxton in the affairs of the section of anaesthetics at the Royal Society of Medicine, of which he was at times secretary and president. But he also did not contribute academically to neuro-anaesthesia.

[105] Zebulon ('Zeb') Mennell was anaesthetist to St Thomas' Hospital and the National Hospital (1911–45) and was the first to focus on the problems of neuro-anaesthesia. His reputation was such that he lectured around the world at a time when few anaesthetists travelled; and he held many professional offices, including presidency of the section of anaesthetics at the Royal Society of Medicine and treasurer and president of the Association of Anaesthetists of Great Britain and Ireland – the AAGBI – which awarded him the Snow Medal in 1948.

[106] The remuneration was a guinea per hour, with a minimum of £3.3.0 per session.

[107] Cairns persuaded the Rockefeller Foundation to fund a specialist neuro-anaesthetist, and Dr Olive Jones was appointed, and she then followed him when he moved to Oxford. Cairns' insistence on specialised neuro-anaesthesia

Edith Margaret Taylor,[108] and the third was V. F. Hall. A year later, Olive Jones retired and was replaced by R. A. Beaver and, thus, when the new theatres were opened in the Queen Mary wing, there were four active anaesthetists at Queen Square – Mennell, Hall, Beaver and Taylor. During the Second World War, each was relocated and a general practitioner, David Aserman, provided whatever anaesthetic work was needed. In 1945, Mennell retired and became the hospital's consulting anaesthetist. By January 1947, the subcommittee on 'surgical assistants' had become concerned about the *ad-hoc* nature of anaesthesia at Queen Square. On their return to the hospital after the war, the medical committee recommended that salary levels for the anaesthetists be set at pre-war levels, but 'the panel of anaesthetists [should] be strengthened by recognition of Dr Aserman[109] and

___

was a legacy of his training with Cushing, who had been profoundly influenced by an experience as a medical student when he was called from the 'benches' to administer ether. The patient vomited, aspirated and died and the surgeons told him 'Don't worry. This happens all the time' (P. Farling, 'The History of the NACCSGBI', http://naccsgbi.org.uk/about-nasgbi/history-of-the-society).

[108] Edith Margaret Taylor (née Ross-Johnson) was a famous figure in London medicine. Her flaming red hair, beauty and engaging and attractive personality ('gay and gracious', according to her obituarist) and the high standards of her work made her a popular figure in the Elizabeth Garrett Anderson Hospital where her primary appointment was based. She married Julian Taylor in 1926, and when he was appointed consultant neurosurgeon at the National Hospital in 1931 and she as consultant anaesthetist in 1935, they were the first man-and-wife team on the hospital consulting staff. During the war the anaesthetists were dispersed: Edith Taylor was posted to Haywards Heath and Julian, although 50 years old, volunteered for active service and was captured by the Japanese at the fall of Singapore, enduring an extremely traumatic period as prisoner for the remainder of the war. Edith Taylor's obituaries speak of her courage in this period, her grace and steadfastness.

[109] David Aserman, born in Rhodesia, was one of the last general practitioners to hold a part-time post in anaesthesia in a London hospital in the pre-war years. With the coming of the Second World War, he became a full-time anaesthetist with the EMS at the evacuated Great Ormond Street and National Hospitals and, after the war, was appointed consultant anaesthetist to both, and to the Atkinson Morley Hospital, where he acted as anaesthetist to Wylie McKissock. He made a notable contribution to the medical literature in a paper describing a series of patients treated with procaine amide and hexamethonium to lower the blood pressure and intracranial pressure in order to provide a bloodless field for neurosurgery. He outlined the risk of

Dr Cobb[110] as official anaesthetists and their terms of appointment be investigated so that the position may be regularized for the future'. In January 1948, the subcommittee reported again, complaining that the current situation regarding anaesthetists remained unsatisfactory since 'no one person was responsible for the direction and co-ordination of their duties'. It was recommended that an honorary anaesthetist be appointed who could direct the three assistants, each of whom was appointed yearly and paid on a sessional basis. In fact, with the introduction of the NHS, salaried posts were introduced, and no honorary staff were then retained, but the 'panel' expanded quickly so that, within five years, there were six anaesthetists on the staff – Beaver, Aserman and Wylie[111] at Queen Square, and Hewer (Logue's initial anaesthetist), Trapps and Roberts at Maida Vale. The fortunes of anaesthetics mirrored closely the trajectory of neurosurgery and, with an increase in the scope and range of neurosurgery after the war, the number and quality of the anaesthetists also rose, with more consultants appointed in anaesthetics in the postwar decades at Queen Square than in any other specialty except neurology, reflecting a similar trend in most hospitals throughout Britain.

Whilst neurosurgery after the Second World War grew in stature at Queen Square, and significant clinical and experimental neurosurgical research was being conducted, the academic area in which the anaesthetists made the greatest impact was not in the operating theatre but in the intensive care unit. Intensive care was a new development and the Batten

___

thrombosis, reactionary haemorrhage and 'retractor anaemia', the last of which complications he described in detail (there were three deaths in his series of 90 patients – considered reasonable for neurosurgery at the time). He was a modest and humble man, with great personal charm and an engaging personality that attracted many friendships.

[110] Cobb and Aserman were duly appointed, but Cobb quickly devoted his attentions to electroencephalography, at the recommendation of a subcommittee in the department of applied electrophysiology, at a salary of £1,000 per annum, rising by £60 each year.

[111] W. Derek Wylie was a leading figure in the world of London medicine. In addition to his post as anaesthetist at the National Hospitals (1950–67), he was consultant anaesthetist at St Thomas' Hospital (1948–79), dean of the Faculty of anaesthesia of the Royal College of Surgeons (1967–9), president of the Association of Anaesthetists of Great Britain and Ireland (1980–2), dean of St Thomas' Hospital Medical School (1974–9) and president of the Medical Defence Union (1982–8).

Unit at Queen Square, opened in 1953 in response to the postwar polio epidemics, was one of the world's only dedicated intensive care units and the first devoted entirely to neurological cases. It was jointly run by a physician and an anaesthetist, in a way which was to become a model for future neurological intensive care. R. Atwood Beaver[112] was consultant anaesthetist to the National Hospital between 1936 and 1971, and he was the founding anaesthetist on the unit. He served as house physician to James Birley at St Thomas' Hospital, where he attained considerable understanding of neurophysiology. Beaver used this, together with his anaesthetic experience and natural engineering skills, to construct one of the first mechanical ventilators, the 'Beaver respirator', in 1953. This machine was employed in Oxford and Queen Square for many years and went into commercial production. He also designed a tubular laryngoscope, made at Queen Square, which facilitated the intubation of patients within box respirators. Beaver pioneered the use of an optional negative phase during expiration, became an expert on the management of acute respiratory failure in neurological patients, and wrote influential papers on specification of the burgeoning numbers of mechanical respirators. On retirement, he was replaced as anaesthetist to the Batten Unit by Laurie Loh, who was equally physiologically minded and, with John Newsom-Davis who acted as neurologist to the Batten Unit, carried out distinguished work on the physiology of respiration. In 1986, the unit was extended and modernised with a donation from the Harris family, to become the Harris Medical Intensive Care Unit, and relocated to the first floor of the Queen Mary wing. When Newsom-Davis and Loh moved from Queen Square to Oxford in 1988, Nicholas Hirsch was appointed anaesthetist to the unit with Mark Wiles as neurologist. In 1990, the first dedicated neurosurgical intensive care unit, the Tavistock unit, comprising seven beds, was opened at Queen Square, funded by a donation from the Tavistock family, and led by the anaesthetist Martin Smith. It was initially based on the seventh floor of the Queen Mary wing, but moved as a nine-bedded unit into the newly built Chandler wing in 1995.

Between 1948 and 1980, 14 consultant anaesthetists were appointed to the National Hospitals. Throughout this period, five consultants were based at Maida Vale (providing around 600 anaesthetic procedures each year) and 6–8 at Queen Square. Most were part-time, with joint appointments at other London teaching hospitals. From around 1977, the two departments, which had previously functioned separately, were merged administratively. At Queen Square, Beaver was head of the anaesthetic department until his retirement when this role was taken on by David Coleman, and then Nicholas Hirsch. At Maida Vale, T. B. L. Roberts led the service until merger of the two departments. Those who worked only at Maida Vale were A. Hewer,[113] Trapps and Roberts. Derek Wylie was an early joint appointee, and those who worked only at Queen Square were Beaver, Aserman, Coleman, Howell-Jones and McDonald. Thereafter, Ellis, Painter, Loh and Jewkes[114] worked at both hospitals.

---

[112] Robert Atwood Beaver was a gregarious man who attracted many loyal friends. He was educated at Winchester and Oxford, and was appointed consultant anaesthetist at the National Hospital, the London Chest Hospital and the Queen Elizabeth Hospital for Children, and worked also during the Second World War on the management of burns with Archibald McIndoe in East Grinstead. He joined the RAMC and served in the thoracic unit in North Africa, attaining the rank of lieutenant-colonel. He returned to Queen Square in 1946 to work one day a week as anaesthetist to Harvey Jackson and Wyllie McKissock. A man of many talents, he was an Oxford half-blue in athletics and, as a young man, a motor-racing driver who acted as reserve for the great teams of the inter-war years, competing in the Mille Miglia in Italy in 1933. In his later years, he acted as medical adviser to racing drivers and, when the days of amateur racing were at an end, he took up sailing, and oil painting, exhibiting at the Royal Academy.

[113] A. L. H. ('Jan') Hewer was well known internationally, especially for his advocacy of induced hypotension and he introduced the antigravity suit for patients being operated on in the sitting position. He was the UK representative of neuro-anaesthesia at the World Federation of Neurology. He was also one of the first to introduce nerve blocks for chronic pain, and he was interested in clinical measurement and helped form a department of clinical measurement at the Middlesex Hospital, to which he was subsequently appointed director when he had to give up anaesthesia following an injury to his hand (*British Medical Journal* **299** (29 April 1989): 298).

[114] Doreen Jewkes was consultant anaesthetist at Queen Square from 1967 to 1995, and worked for a further five years at King's College Hospital after her retirement. She dedicated much time to charitable work and assisted in the establishment of the first neurosurgical centre in Nepal, work for which she was awarded the Order of Gorka Dakshina Bahu in 2002 by the King of Nepal. She also volunteered for many years with the Crossroads Charity (Caring for Carers) in Lewisham, serving as chair of the board and for 18 months as chief executive. Her final years

The subsequent appointees – Ingram, Salt, Hirsch, Calder, Bowen-Wright – were based exclusively or largely at Queen Square.[115] A pain service was established at Queen Square in 1989 by M. R. Bowen-Wright and, with the appointment of the anaesthetists Frank Kurer and then Paul Nandi, Mary Newton and Lena A. Anagnostopoulou-Ladas, pain was managed through a multidisciplinary arrangement including anaesthetists, neurologists and psychiatrists.

In its early years, anaesthetics was considered a marginal specialty in medicine and it struggled to gain recognition and status. In the nineteenth century, anaesthetics were usually administered by amateurs with little training, sometimes general practitioners, medical students or even members of the public. Queen Square was unusual in having staff who were well trained, and the first anaesthetists at the hospital were leading figures in their field, although the tradition of 'amateur' anaesthetists persisted up to the Second World War (Aserman was perhaps the last of these). In these years, and particularly because of the growing recognition of the dangers of chloroform, there were strenuous efforts to provide proper training, to form professional associations and to add anaesthesia onto the medical student curriculum. The Queen Square anaesthetists Silk, Buxton and Powell were instrumental in these efforts, but formal qualifications and professional status were slow to arrive. The first postgraduate qualification in anaesthesia, the Diploma in Anaesthetics,[116] which

required one year of supervised clinical experience, was introduced only in 1935, and the discipline remained close to the bottom of the steep hierarchical pyramid of British medicine. At Queen Square, the fact that anaesthetists were remunerated from 1935, in contrast to the physicians and surgeons whose appointments were honorary, was perhaps a sign of their lowly status as surgical assistants, and, even in 1948, the anaesthetists at Queen Square were not included as members of the Medical Committee. At the time of the introduction of the NHS, when all medical staff were to became salaried, there were long and contentious negotiations at a national level about the conditions of service and remuneration of anaesthetists (and those in other 'minor specialties') who fought hard for the principle that all specialties should be treated equally.[117] This was accepted finally, and proved instrumental in raising the status of anaesthetics, leading to a rapid increase in the number of doctors entering the specialty nationwide.[118] Its standing within medicine improved, and, as a result, a faculty of Anaesthetists was established within the Royal College of Surgeons of England in 1948, which evolved into the College of Anaesthetists within the Royal College of Surgeons in 1988, and then into an independent Royal College of Anaesthetists in 1992. The Diploma became a Fellowship with establishment of the College and, at the time of writing, requires training over six years. Parallel developments occurred in intensive care, and the Intensive Care Society, the first in the world, was founded in 1970.

Subspecialisation in anaesthetics, as in many of the medical disciplines after the war, soon followed, with neuro-anaesthesia one of the first subspecialties to develop. The Neuroanaesthesia Society was founded

---

were blighted by osteoporosis and resulting fractures, and she died following pulmonary embolus.

[115] The dates of appointment and retirement of the anaesthetists at the National Hospitals are shown here (the post-1948 dates have in part been ascertained from the annual reports, which cover academic not calendar years, and so are given as a date range): J. Silk 1888–91; D. Buxton 1891–6; R. Bakewell 1896–1905; Llewellyn Powell 1905–23; Z. Mennell 1911–45; R. Ryan 1925–35; V. Hall 1934/5–1947/8; O. Jones 1935–8; E. Taylor 1939–48/50; R. Beaver 1937–72; D. Aserman 1947–72; A. Hewer 1948/50–1967; W. (Derek) Wylie 1950–67; M. Trapps 1952/3–1974/5; T. Roberts 1952/3–1979/80; H. Howell-Jones 1955/6–1965/6; D. Coleman 1964/5–1987/8; J. McDonald 1965/6–1967/8; D. Jewkes 1967–95; P. Painter 1968–90; D. Ellis 1966/7–1974/5; L. Loh 1972–88; G. Ingram 1975/6–1991; I. Calder 1979–2010; N. Hirsch 1988–2015; F. Kurer 1988/9–1994/5; M. Bowen-Wright 1989/90–1993; M. Smith 1991–2017; P. Nandi 1990/1–present; S. Wilson 1994/5–present; M. Newton 1995/6– ; AVL Agastopoulou-Ladas 1996/7–2001/2.

[116] The Diploma (the DA) later evolved into the FFARCS and then, in 1989, the FCA.

[117] The anaesthetists were perceived up to this point largely as 'surgical assistants' and it is noticeable that it was the president of the Royal College of Surgeons, Sir (later Lord) Alfred Webb-Johnson, who particularly pressed for equal pay and status for anaesthetists. In 1948, the Spens Committee Report on the remuneration of consultants and specialists recommended a consultant pay scale of nine equal annual increments from £1,500 to £2,500 to be applied equally to physicians, surgeons and anaesthetists.

[118] The numbers of specialist anaesthetists country-wide increased from 76 in 1938/9 (4.7 per cent of all specialists) to 906 in 1964 (11.4 per cent of all specialists) (R. Stevens, *Medical Practice in Modern England* (New Haven: Yale University Press, 2003)).

in 1965, with Dr Olive Jones as a founding member, and Jan Hewer presenting the first paper (on hypothermia in neurosurgical anaesthesia) at the inaugural meeting. The setting up of a new society was not welcomed by the AAGBI, and so the society changed its name to the Neurosurgical Anaesthetists Travelling Club. Over the years, several further attempts were made to give the 'travelling club' a more formal status, and eventually, in 1987, the Queen Square anaesthetist Stuart Ingram was instrumental in its evolution into the Neuroanaesthesia Society of Great Britain & Ireland (NASGBI).[119]

Notwithstanding the vicissitudes of the specialty more generally, the National Hospital was successful in its choice of anaesthetic doctors, almost all of whom were at the forefront of their specialty. The unique features of the work and clinical material at the National Hospitals allowed niche areas of anaesthetics and intensive care medicine to flourish after inception of the NHS. There were a number of firsts, especially in the field of intensive care. The most celebrated anaesthetists at the National Hospital were all physiologically minded and this shaped the style of their work. With time, a recognisable programme of academic work in neuro-anaesthetics began to be undertaken, especially in the fields of neurological respiratory failure, intensive care and neurophysiological monitoring during anaesthesia, and some significant and important papers were published. In the final analysis, though, in contrast to other subspecialties in the postwar years at Queen Square, anaesthetics remained a largely hospital-based specialty, with few formal connections to the Institute of Neurology or University College London, and with no academic preferment for its practitioners. It was the provision of unique and specialised clinical services, not academic research, that characterised neuro-anaesthesia at Queen Square.

---

[119] The NASGBI became the voice of neuroanaesthesia in Britain, and then as the specialty of neuro-intensive care (neuro-critical care) developed, the society again changed its name, in 2015, to the Neuroanaesthesia and Critical Care Society of Great Britain and Ireland (NACCSGBI).

The Investigatory Specialties at Queen Square

Three investigational specialties – neuropathology, neuroradiology and neurophysiology – flourished at Queen Square in parallel with the mainstream clinical disciplines. Each earned widespread recognition for its clinical work, teaching and research.

Neuropathology

Neuropathology as we know it today first emerged in Great Britain about ten years after the opening of the National Hospital, although its evolution can be traced back to the end of the eighteenth and early nineteenth centuries through the pioneering studies in morbid anatomy of individuals such as Mathew Baillie, Robert Hooper, John Abercrombie, Robert Carswell, Richard Bright and James Hope. Each published written accounts of the morbid anatomy of diseases affecting the brain and spinal cord, some as part of more general works on pathology. With the exception of Abercrombie, these were illustrated by engravings or chromolithographs. But not one of these authors attempted more than the description of macroscopic appearances of disease. It was advances in the field of microscopic pathology that moved the discipline forward, following the conclusion of Virchow in 1858[1] that: 'the cell is "the ultimate irreducible form of every living element, and … from it emanate all the activities of life both in health and in sickness"'. This led to the search for microscopic changes of disease, and amongst the first in Britain to grasp the scientific potential of the new brain staining techniques was James Crichton-Browne, who appointed Bevin Lewis in 1871 as pathologist at the West Riding Lunatic Asylum. Lewis devised and published

detailed accounts of new neurological staining and post-mortem techniques in the 1870s and 1880s, and his work helped to broaden the scope of neuropathology.[2]

Neuropathology at the National Hospital 1889–1950

Despite these developments elsewhere, there were no facilities for microscopic studies and no dedicated pathologist in post at the National Hospital for the first 30 years of its existence. This was partly because morbid anatomy and pathology were a fundamental part of the training and work of the physicians, who were expected routinely to examine brain specimens. As a result, they became highly proficient in morbid anatomy and the naked-eye diagnosis of abnormalities. The first recorded post-mortem at Queen Square, in Buzzard's case notes for 1870–7, was a case of tuberculous leptomeningitis. Hughlings Jackson informed the section of pathology at the annual meeting of the British Medical Association in 1882 that all clinicians should perform their own post-mortem examinations. We know that William Gowers routinely adopted this practice after 1870, and he summarised the prevailing view in stating that 'A practitioner must not be a pathologist only, although unless he be a pathologist

---

[1] *Vorlesungen über Cellularpathologie in ihrer Begründung auf physiologischer und pathologischer Gewebelehre. Zwanzig Vorlesungen Gehalten Während der Monate Februar, März und April 1858 im Pathologischen Institute zu Berlin*, (1858), translated by Frank Chance as *Cellular Pathology as Based upon Physiological and Pathological Histology* (1860).

[2] B. Lewis, 'A New Process of Preparing and Staining Fresh Brain for Microscopic Examination', *The Monthly Microscopical Journal* (1 September 1876), and his paper in four parts published in *Brain* between 1880 and 1882 entitled 'Methods of Preparing, Demonstrating, and Examining Cerebral Structure in Health and Disease' (**3** (1880): 314–36; **4** (1881): 82–99; **4** (1881): 351–60; **4** (1882): 441–66). His papers exploited the rapid developments of the period, including the use of carmine in 1858, chronic acid fixation in 1872, and haematoxylin and eosin in 1884. Paraffin embedding was used first in 1868, and Bevin Lewis' freezing microtome in 1877; and new staining techniques revealed detailed cellular structures – for instance, by Nissl in 1885, Marchi in 1886, Golgi in 1887 and Cajal in 1888.

he cannot be a good practitioner.' The bye-laws of the National Hospital in 1885 explained that the 'Senior House Physician and Registrar shall conduct all Post-Mortem Examinations and make records of the results.'[3] In the 1885 building project, a post-mortem room (measuring 15 feet × 16.5 feet), with an adjoining but wholly separate mortuary (13 feet × 10 feet) and a 'pathology' laboratory (11 feet × 9 feet), were provided in the basement of the outpatient Powis Place pavilion, on the west side of the hospital.[4]

However, as special staining techniques developed, neuropathology began to change and to be seen as a specialty in its own right, allied more closely with neurology than general medicine. In 1889, Walter Colman[5] became the first doctor to be appointed formally with specified duties as pathologist to the National Hospital, and, for the next 25 years, the post was seen as a stepping stone to, and training for, appointment as physician (to which post Colman was duly appointed in 1896). As the pathologists tended to be young physicians, anxious to move onto the staff, they were treated like the resident medical officers, from whose ranks they often came. They were not allowed to absent themselves from the premises without the express approval of the secretary-director (Burford Rawlings). This and other restrictions were presumably tolerated in the expectation of preferment. Microscopy was introduced in the 1890s, and by 1900 the complex histological techniques involved in cerebral microscopy had led to a reluctance amongst general pathologists to be involved in neuropathology. This left the responsibility for moving the field forward in the UK to the pathology staff at Queen Square. The period after 1880 was indeed a golden age for neuropathology at the hospital. Although no new techniques had been introduced, the physicians were able to align their clinical and pathological findings and this method of 'clinico-pathological correlation' produced a most important series of neurological discoveries. Several classical papers were published by members of the staff using this approach, often in *Brain*. These included the thesis by Tooth on what came to be known as 'Charcot–Marie–Tooth' disease and his later papers on cerebral glioma, Batten on diseases of muscle, Jackson and Colman on temporal lobe epilepsy, and Collier on cerebral diplegia. Gordon Holmes published extensively on a range of pathological topics including traumatic brain and spinal disease, the cerebellum, the origin of the pyramidal tracts, amyotropic lateral sclerosis and the pathology of papilloedema. Perhaps the pinnacle of achievement in this respect was Wilson's 213-page paper on progressive lenticular degeneration (Wilson's disease), which has the dubious accolade of being the longest paper ever published in *Brain*[6] and occupied almost the whole of the quarterly issue in which it appeared. Experimental pathology also flourished but this was usually elsewhere, for instance at the Brown Institution or University College London, through the work of Victor Horsley (who was a practising microscopist), Beevor, Semon and Ferrier.

In 1908 the Board of Management re-created rules for the office of pathologist, which stated that the holder of the post should be held responsible for the efficient and prompt carrying out of post-mortem examinations on all cases dying at the National Hospital, and, if required, at Finchley Convalescent Home. Full details of the findings were recorded in the 'post mortem register' and presented to the Medical Committee. An abstract was provided to the registrar and appended to the clinical case notes. The pathologist was also responsible for the safe-keeping and preservation of the pathological collections, including macroscopic and microscopic material, lantern slides and photographs. It was also agreed that the director of the Nervous Disease Research Fund should be in charge of the laboratory.[7]

---

[3] 'National Hospital for the Paralysed and Epileptic Bye-laws 1885', para. 17, on p. 18.

[4] The mortuary had its own separate pedestrian access from the street by a flight of steps down, but it is interesting to note that there is no sign of any vehicular access to deliver and receive corpses. The conditions in the mortuary were far from ideal and, four years earlier, the Board of Management minutes recorded that the architect Michael Manning and the contractor had opened up the drains of 23 and 24 Queen Square and discovered that the efflux ran into a large cesspit under the post-mortem room, which had no connection with any sewer or main drain.

[5] Coleman was an Edinburgh graduate and student of Professor William Smith Greenfield, the father of J. G. Greenfield. He appears to have acted as hospital pathologist on two different occasions. A full list of the junior staff pathologists is given in Appendix 1.

[6] S. A. K. Wilson, 'Progressive Lenticular Degeneration: A Familial Nervous Disease Associated with Cirrhosis of the Liver', *Brain* 34 (1912): 295–507.

[7] All was not plain sailing though, and the Board of Management minutes record that the young James Collier was rapped on the knuckles by the Board for conducting a post-mortem examination on a Mr Earl after permission

Interestingly, in 1909 it was the refusal by the lay governors to accede to a request from the physicians to appoint a pathologist at the Chalfont Colony for Epileptics which resulted in the mass resignation of the medical staff, and the de-medicalisation of the colony.

Kinnier Wilson was perhaps the greatest of the physician-pathologists, but he was also the last. In *Tales of the National*, Godfrey Heathcote Hamilton describes how Wilson, during his tenure as pathologist, and prior to his appointment as physician, used to spend odd hours at the hospital and, as a diversion from his post-mortem examinations, would break off to build specimen cabinets and autopsy tables using the hospital carpenter's tools. The carpenter objected to his brace and bit going missing and started to lock his door at night. One evening the night stoker heard crashing noises caused by Wilson breaking in through the skylight, only to become trapped inside.

One event of great importance was the 17th International Congress of Medicine, held at University College London in August 1913. A number of physicians from the Naational Hospital played a prominent role, including Sir David Ferrier, who served as chairman of the section of neuropathology, and Henry Head and Frederick Batten as secretaries of the congress. The meeting began on 7 August at the Plant Physiology Laboratory of Imperial College, South Kensington, with Wilson, Tooth and Collier also in attendance. The Board of Management allowed the section of neuropathology to visit the National Hospital in the afternoon, 'at which will be exhibited patients illustrating various forms of family and hereditary diseases of the nervous system. There will also be an exhibition of pathological specimens. Tea will be provided in the Quadrangle of the hospital at 5 p.m., when it is hoped that ladies will be present.'[8]

There was to be no re-run of the controversies of the Goltz–Ferrier debate in 1881. The event was 'well attended' and went off smoothly, if unexceptionally. Many of the great international neurologists of the day led the discussions, and may have visited the hospital, including Joseph Babinski, André Thomas,

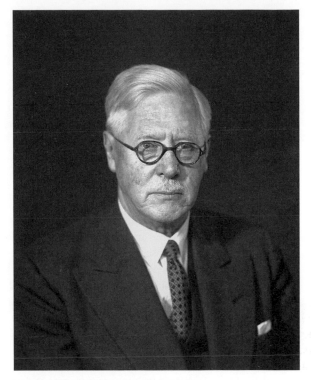

Figure 11.1 Joseph Godwin Greenfield.

Joseph Déjerine, Robert Bárány, Hermann Oppenheim and Hugo Liepmann.

When Wilson announced his intention of not reapplying for the post of pathologist in 1912, Batten wrote to Joseph Godwin Greenfield, who had worked as house physician at the National Hospital in 1910 and subsequently in Leeds, urging him to apply. He did so, and on 29 January 1914 Greenfield was appointed as the first 'professional' pathologist employed full-time at the National Hospital. He remained in post until retirement in 1949 and it was he who first brought great distinction to the neuropathological work and academic reputation of the National Hospital.

When Greenfield[9] moved to Queen Square, his post was one of only three salaried medical positions at the National Hospital (all other consultant-level posts, bar

---

to do so had been expressly refused by the deceased's relatives. Burford Rawlings was instructed to point out to Dr Collier the grave error of judgement that he had committed but, despite this, two months later, in January 1899, Collier was appointed senior house physician to the hospital.

[8] *British Medical Journal* **1** (28 June 1913): 1375–6.

---

[9] Joseph Godwin Greenfield was born in Edinburgh in 1884, the son of W. S. Greenfield, professor of pathology and clinical medicine at the University of Edinburgh. He qualified in medicine from Edinburgh in 1908 and worked in Leeds before moving to the National Hospital. His career at the hospital lasted over 30 years and, by the end of this period, he was the undisputed leader of the specialty in Britain (dubbed the 'father of neuropathology') and a well-known figure internationally.

those of the anaesthesists, were honorary). It offered little security of tenure or financial security, and the incumbent was expected to reapply for renewal on an annual basis. Almost immediately after his appointment, Greenfield was enlisted and served in the RAMC in France and Belgium, returning full-time to the National Hospital in 1919, and it was then that his career in neuropathology began to flourish. In that year, he wrote a paper with Buzzard on von Economo's encephalitis which was becoming epidemic at the time, and, two years later, his first book, a textbook of pathology of the nervous system with Buzzard, appeared.[10]

As a salaried member of the hospital staff, Greenfield was initially precluded from attending the Medical Committee, and yet progressively his role and authority in the hospital rose. He served as dean of the medical school between 1923 and 1946 and, in due course, as chairman of the Medical Committee. Universally admired, even after compulsory retirement at the age of 65, Greenfield continued to visit the hospital, working in his old room four times each week.

In the early years, there were only around 35 postmortem examinations to perform each year but, according to Critchley, with 'meagre equipment and little in the way of technical facilities, Greenfield steadily and quietly amassed a formidable experience in neuropathology'. His laboratory was in the operating theatre assigned to Horsley but not used as such – a spartan room with a high ceiling, where the working conditions were vividly described by McMenemy:

A visitor to his department in the mid-thirties would traverse a dismal underground corridor roofed in by a mass of dusty pipes and conduits and pass into the main laboratory – a chilly, somewhat dreary and sparsely equipped room of lofty proportions – and enquire whether the Doctor was in. 'Yes, he's inside', the lab-boy would answer casually, and one entered a small dimly lit inner room to find Greenfield surrounded by mountainous boxes of slides in no very great order and volumes of reports all written in long-hand. No secretary guarded his door and no one was ever announced. The London grime adhered to the outside of the window. On the walls was a series of photographs revealing him as the acknowledged patron of the exclusive postgraduate students' club.[11]

Symonds wrote in Greenfield's obituary:

Greenfield in the midst of all his own activities was always generous of his time. Often a colleague would consult him on some problem arising from a case or in the preparation of a paper and pose what might seem to him a simple question. Greenfield would put aside his own work, look up reprints, refer to post-mortem data, bring out microscope slides, and give all he knew, frequently revealing the question to be far more complex than it had appeared.[12]

Greenfield enjoyed the visits of his clinical colleagues, and any serious expression on their arrival would soon be replaced by an engaging chuckle and an encouraging 'Let's take a look at it then.' When the slides had been carefully scrutinised under the light microscope, tea would be provided and the discussion of the case and others he had recently been asked to review would continue, often in the presence of his technician, a Yorkshireman and ex-miner, J. Anderson, who would also sometimes express his own opinion on the case.[13] When Greenfield and Cumings conducted post-mortems, a double buzz on the hospital bell system signalled that one was about to take place, encouraging the junior physicians and surgeons to attend, and these were popular teaching events.

In these exchanges, McMenemy always felt that Greenfield's mind was at the bedside as if he were trying to visualise the patient's handicaps in life and reveal the truth. Greenfield's laboratory became a popular meeting place and the focal point for most of the hospital's investigational work. In his later years, equipment in his department improved, not least with 'splendid wooden cabinets' that Greenfield had personally designed.[14]

Under his leadership, a period at Queen Square became an essential training requirement for all training neuropathologists, and Greenfield was a beloved

---

[10] J. G. Greenfield and F. Buzzard, *Pathology of the Nervous System* (London: Constable, 1921). This was the forerunner of Greenfield's *Neuropathology* discussed in more detail below.

[11] W. McMenemy, 'Obituary Notice of Joseph Godwin Greenfield, 24th May 1884–2nd March 1958', *Journal of Pathology and Bacteriology* **78** (1959): 577–92.
[12] C. Symonds, 'Joseph Godwin Greenfield: Obituary', *British Medical Journal* **1** (8 March 1958): 585–6.
[13] J. Anderson later was the author of a highly commended book entitled *How to Stain the Nervous System: A Laboratory Handbook for Students and Technicians* (London: E. and S. Livingston, 1929). As Schiller and Haymaker put it: 'There is little doubt about Greenfield's major role in the book's modestly camouflaged joint authorship': W. Haymaker and F. Schiller, eds., *Founders of Neurology* (Springfield: Charles C. Thomas, 1970).
[14] Haymaker and Schiller, eds., *Founders of Neurology* (1960).

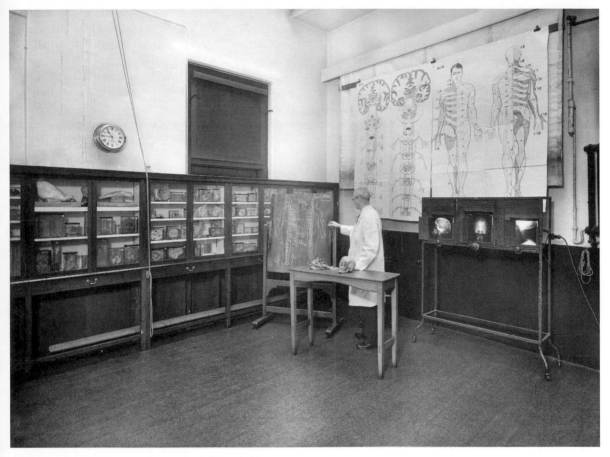

Figure 11.2 Greenfield teaching in the pathology teaching rooms.

mentor to a whole generation of British and foreign neuropathologists and also neurologists. Indeed, it was said that there was 'hardly any British neurologist of repute who failed to spend some time in this small laboratory of Greenfield'.

All wrote of Greenfield's modesty and warmth, his impeccable manners, and his kindness and generosity. Despite the reservations concerning professorships at Queen Square, it was a cause of regret amongst his friends that London University never offered him that title. Greenfield served as president of the section of neurology of the Royal Society of Medicine (1938) and of the Association of British Neurologists (1954–6). He helped to found the Neuropathology Club in 1950, which started with just 28 founding members, eventually growing to become the British Neuropathological Society in 1962. Greenfield took part in the First International Congress of Neuropathology in Rome (1952), a meeting about which Walshe commented that separate

international meetings for neuropathologists 'tore the seamless garment of neurology'. Greenfield delivered the Oliver Sharpey lecture at the Royal College of Physicians (1938) and the Hughlings Jackson lecture of the Royal Society of Medicine (1949).

In the last three years of his life, he took up a post at the National Institute of Neurological Disorders and Stroke (NINDS) in America for part of each year, where he was regarded as the 'dean of neuropathologists'. With all the facilities of the National Institutes of Health at his disposal, the optimism of America must have been a great contrast with the dreary postwar austerity of Britain, but he died suddenly in 1958 from myocardial infarction in Bethesda, before he could fully exploit the opportunity.

Greenfield worked on the whole range of clinical neuropathological topics, but never did any experimental work. Many of his 125 papers were case reports, and all his writing was firmly embedded in clinical neurology. Between 1919 and 1940, he published a series of important papers on a very wide range of neuropathological topics – sometimes with colleagues – which included spinal disease such as syringomyelia, subacute combined degeneration of the spinal cord and subacute necrotic myelitis; muscle disease such as myotonic dystrophy; degenerative diseases such as Schilder's disease, metachromatic leucodystrophy (which came to be known as 'Greenfield's disease'), and spinocerebellar degeneration; anatomical studies of pituitary adenoma and lesions of the corpus Luysii; vascular disease and cerebral oedema; intracranial tumours; and other neurological conditions such as disseminated sclerosis, subacute sclerosing panencephalitis and post-encephalitic Parkinsonism. He clarified the pathology of the encephalitides and made classical descriptions of the neuropathology of measles encephalomyelitis, metachromatic leucodystrophy and the spinocerebellar degenerations which have hardly been bettered.

Of equal importance were the five monographs that Greenfield wrote, each showing his enormous breadth of knowledge. *The Cerebrospinal Fluid in Clinical Diagnosis* (1925) was written with E. A. Carmichael, and other books included *The Spinocerebellar Degenerations* (1954) and the *Atlas of Muscular Pathology in Neuromuscular Disease* (1957, with Shy, Alvord and Berg). However, his most famous publication, extending the book from 1921 with Buzzard, was the textbook of neuropathology the first edition of which was published in 1958 with Greenfield assisted by co-authors Blackwood, McMenemey, Alfred Meyer, and Robert Norman from Bristol. *Neuropathology* was 640 pages in length, containing around 200 black-and-white photographs and diagrams, with seven of the 13 chapters written by Greenfield himself. The book covered the whole of the topic with the exception of tumour pathology[15] and was an instant success, demonstrating with its strong Queen Square style, the predominance of the National Hospital in anglophone neuropathology over that period. The book was definitive, didactic and authoritative, just as was the practice of neuropathology at the National Hospital. As the subject grew, so too did the book. The second edition was published in 1963 (five years after Greenfield's death) and was appropriately renamed *Greenfield's Neuropathology*. It took a very

similar format and style to the first edition, but had expanded to 679 pages and now listed Blackwood, McMenemey, Meyer, Norman and Dorothy Russell as authors.[16] The forward march of *Greenfield's Neuropathology* after this can be seen as a further metaphor for the role of Queen Square in the evolution of neuropathology in Britain.[17] It is now in its ninth edition and, although the name of Greenfield is still attached, he would barely recognise the style, text or format of this lasting tribute to the greatest British neuropathologist of the twentieth century.

Neuropathology at Queen Square After 1950

In 1946, Greenfield separated neuropathology into two departments – histopathology and clinical pathology. He also ensured that the discipline of neuropathology retained its academic position by placing both under the administration of the newly formed Institute of Neurology, but with part-funding from the hospital, and from 1950 onwards, therefore, the two

---

[15] The pathology of tumours was not included as the first edition of Dorothy Russell and Lucien Rubinstein's *Pathology of Tumours of Nervous System* was also scheduled for publication in 1959.

[16] The copy in the Queen Square archive was Blackwood's own edition, and he made a number of hand-written corrections on the book. These make it clear that the seven chapters by Greenfield were 'revised', not authored, by Meyer, as the table of content implies. It is interesting, too, to see Blackwood also change the spelling of 'neurones' to 'neurons' wherever this appears.

[17] The third edition, published in 1976, extended to 946 pages and 20 chapters, now with some colour plates. It was edited by Blackwood and Corsellis and all the authors were British. The fourth edition of 1,136 pages and 20 chapters was edited by Hume Adams from Glasgow, Corsellis from the Maudsley, and Duchen. There were 24 authors, of whom 23 were British (with Larroche from Paris as the only outsider), but only five were from Queen Square. Corsellis dropped out of the fifth edition of 1992, but, otherwise, it was very similar in size and scope to the fourth, with again only 5 of 27 authors from Queen Square. The sixth edition of 1997 was a complete rewrite and change in style. It was now a multi-authored and international production, with two volumes, 2,200 pages, 27 chapters and 64 authors (29 from Britain and only four from Queen Square; and tumours were now included with a self-justifying note in the preface). Both editors were from Britain, but neither from Queen Square (David Graham and Peter Lantos). Since then, three further editions have been published and the book has become truly international. The ninth edition is now just under 2,000 pages in length, in two volumes and with 4,000 illustrations, many in colour. Of the 78 authors, 45 are from the UK but only five are from Queen Square. Nevertheless the book continues to be entitled *Greenfield's Neuropathology* and it remains the world-leading neuropathology text.

neuropathology departments received facilities and support from both the National Hospital and the Institute of Neurology, and worked to the mutual benefit of both.

In 1947, Greenfield chose William ('Beachey') Blackwood[18] as his assistant pathologist and, in 1949, on Greenfield's retirement, Blackwood was appointed consultant neuropathologist in charge of the department of histopathology (the name of which was changed again in October 1958 to the university department of neuropathology with Blackwood as the first professor of neuropathology). Although he worked in a university department, Blackwood's first priority was to provide a clinical service dealing with biopsies and autopsies and, as with Greenfield, he liked to interpret clinical signs in the light of their pathology. His laboratory was on the first floor of the Queen Mary wing, four small rooms lined with cupboards packed with boxes of slides. This was a huge display of neuropathological material which duly impressed visitors. Downstairs in the basement, freezing in the winter, was the post-mortem room and mortuary, where specimens were stored in formalin-filled bottles, and blocks of brain tissue embedded in celloidin preserved in alcohol. On the Queen Square House site, there existed a small museum and lecture theatre where Blackwood conducted a weekly clinico-pathological conference. The department moved to Alexandra House in 1963, to make way for the new department of clinical neurology, and remained there until 1978. Blackwood was a reluctant academic: 'I did not want to be a professor, I just wanted to look down the microscope and report the tumours and brains.'[19] Such investigative work as he did focused initially on the effects of prolonged immersion in sea-water (usually seamen torpedoed during the war) and on the peripheral nerve system, and he contributed to *Neuropathology* (1958), writing the chapter on cerebrovascular disease, and was co-editor of the *Atlas of Neuropathology* (1949). He trained

many pathologists from all over the world, and served as president of the British Neuropathological Society from 1965 to 1967. In retirement, he helped found the department of neuropathology at the Charing Cross Hospital. Bill Mair[20] was appointed consultant neuropathologist in 1958 and assisted Blackwood for the next 18 years. Mair specialised particularly in neuromuscular diseases, and he introduced electron microscopy to the Institute.

Anthony Dayan was also appointed in 1965 jointly with Great Ormond Street, moving from the Wessex Neurological Centre in Southampton, where he had founded the neuropathology department. He was the most academic of the neuropathologists at this time, specialising in a wide range of areas, including the pathology of old age. He did not find the Great Ormond Street appointment fulfilling and in 1972 was recruited to become a principal scientist in the Wellcome Research Laboratory, where he specialised in toxicology.[21]

During the 1950s and 1960s, the focus of the department was on clinical service, and the demand for pathological services increased. In 1950, there

---

[18] William Blackwood was born in Cornwall, educated at Cheltenham College and qualified from Edinburgh University in 1934. He retired in 1976 after more than 30 years at Queen Square. The origin of his nickname is obscure and is sometimes spelt 'Beechey'. He was a popular head of department who was supportive and helpful to all his colleagues. He was renowned for his teaching, rather than his research, and he and Mair were responsible for the training of many neuropathologists from around the world.

[19] 'Dean's Report', annual report of the Institute of Neurology, 1990.

[20] William George Parker (Bill) Mair graduated in medicine from Aberdeen University, and trained in pathology in Glasgow and Berlin. He served in the RAMC and then, after the war, joined the pathology department at the National Hospital under the guidance of Greenfield, and was appointed senior hospital medical officer in the department in 1953 and consultant neuropathologist there in 1958, retiring in 1978. In the early 1960s, he spent time in Uppsala to learn electron microscopy on the Siemens Emisscope 1 microscope, and brought back this skill to Queen Square, where Cumings installed one of these machines to study the ultrastructure of muscle. Mair worked in this area for many years, making a number of important contributions, and trained many postgraduate students. He co-authored the *Atlas of the Ultrastructure of Normal and Diseased Human Muscle* (Edinburgh: Churchill Livingston, 1972). He was renowned for his teaching and counselling of students, and for his integrity, modesty, humility and generosity of character. A lecture was given in his honour at the VIth European Congress of Neuropathology in 1999. Mair died from pneumonia on 8 July 2002.

[21] Dayan published a number of seminal papers on encephalitis, subacute sclerosing panencephalitis, carcinomatous neuromyopathy, and comparative studies of the neuropathology of 47 species of aged vertebrates with specimens sent to him from London Zoo (*Brain* **94** (1971): 31–42). On moving to the Wellcome research unit, he focused on toxicology, and later returned to academia as professor of toxicology at St Bartholomew's Hospital.

were 111 post-mortem examinations, and 400 surgical biopsies. By then, the department functioned as a centre for second opinions, and an additional 57 specimens of brain or spine were sent from other institutions. Ten years later, there were around 135 post-mortems and 450 surgical specimens examined, and the amount of material received from external sources had risen to 120 a year. In 1971, there were 57 post-mortems, 499 biopsies and 207 specimens from other sources. However, over this period, only 5–10 papers were published annually, reflecting the low level of research activity.

On Blackwood's retirement in 1976, Professor Leo Duchen[22] was appointed as head of department. He was previously professor of experimental neuropathology at the Institute of Psychiatry where he worked with a stimulating group of pathologists, including Corsellis, Strick and Bignami, and was renowned for his work on the pathological effects of botulinum toxin, which opened the way for its later clinical use, and also his development of mutant animal models of human diseases. When he moved to Queen Square he set about a large-scale reorganisation and, in 1978, the department moved to a floor of Queen Square House, and took on the form of a modern clinical and experimental neuropathological unit. He was quickly joined by Jean Jacobs and Francisco Scaravilli. Duchen's achievement was to develop research as well as managing an increasing clinical load, and the reputation of the group, for both the quality of clinical work and its teaching and research, grew. Students came from many parts of the world, and a number of trainee neurologists also became proficient in neuropathological method under his tutelage. Duchen retired early in 1992 to care for his wife when she fell seriously ill.

Other consultant pathologists also worked in the university department at various times. Marion Smith, employed as a member of the MRC external staff, also held a consultant post from 1970 to 1973, and then, in 1974, Magda Erdohazi was appointed as consultant neuropathologist, a post she held until 1983. She was born in Komarom in Hungary and fled to Palestine in 1939, and then to England with her husband Hugo, and was a specialist in the neuropathology of childhood metabolic conditions, working at Great Ormond Street as well as the National Hospital. Dr Brian Harding took over the joint post with Great Ormond Street on Erdohazi's retirement in 1983,[23] and Francisco Scaravilli was also promoted to senior lecturer in October 1978, and in 1992 he was awarded a personal chair and appointed acting head of the department of neuropathology on Leo Duchen's retirement, and then confirmed as established head of the department in 1995. Tamas Revesz was then appointed as senior lecturer in 1991, and Maria Thom in 1996 (both later being awarded personal chairs).

The department of clinical pathology, created in 1946, was directed by John Nathanial Cumings.[24] He had arrived at Queen Square in 1933, five years after qualifying from King's, and was a close friend of Greenfield, who did his best to promote the career of his junior colleague. Cumings was one of the first to recognise the importance of biochemistry in neurology, and his new department focused on this aspect of pathology in parallel to Greenfield's expertise in histology and microscopic anatomy. This engagement

---

[22] Leo Wilfred Duchen was born in South Africa and completed his medical training at the University of Witwatersrand in Johannesburg in 1950. He spent a year of training at the Hammersmith Hospital in 1953, and, as an opponent of apartheid, he found the political situation in South Africa on his return intolerable, and moved permanently back to London in 1958, where he took up an appointment as research assistant (1959), then lecturer (1964), senior lecturer (1965) and reader (1970) in the department of neuropathology at the Institute of Psychiatry, where in 1975 he was appointed professor of experimental neuropathology. He was devoted to his family and wife and when she fell ill in 1986, and died in 1994 of renal cancer, he was profoundly affected. He himself developed bowel cancer shortly afterwards, and died in 1996.

[23] Harding gave up his appointment at Queen Square and moved to Great Ormond Street full-time in 1994 (and on retirement in 2008 moved as professor of pathology and laboratory medicine to the Perlman School of Medicine at the University of Pennsylvania and as consultant neuropathologist at the Children's Hospital of Pennsylvania).

[24] John Nathanial Cumings was educated at Ealing County School and qualified from King's College in 1927. He had a distinguished career, serving at various times as chairman of the Medical Committee, treasurer of the Association of British Neurologists, foundation fellow of the Royal College of Pathologists, president of the Association of Clinical Pathologists and the section of neurology of the Royal Society of Medicine, and on the editorial board of *Brain*. A devout Christian, Cumings held high office in the Baptist Union and the Baptist Missionary Society, and also worked to assist Jewish physicians displaced from central Europe: *British Medical Journal* **3** (1974): 632; *Lancet* **304** (1974): 603; *The Times*, 26 August 1974; and *Munk's Roll* (http://munksroll.rcplondon.ac.uk/Biography/Details/1101).

with chemical pathology was the stimulus that caused Walshe, at the end of his career, to come to the conclusion that the study of chemistry of the brain would supersede neurophysiology as the most important and relevant branch of science in neurology. Cumings' work in neurochemistry was ahead of his time, as no such specialty existed, and, on 1 October 1958, he was appointed to the professorship of clinical pathology (in parallel to Blackwood's appointment as professor in neuropathology), and these were the first two chairs to be established at Queen Square. Cumings was a pioneer in exploring the potential for analysis of lipid chemistry and its application to neuropathology. His research focused initially on the properties and constituents of cerebrospinal fluid, another topic that Greenfield had promoted, and on enzymes in cerebral tumours and biochemical tests for multiple sclerosis. He studied cerebral oedema and lipid and protein disorders in degenerative familial disease, especially the lipidoses and demyelinating leucodystrophies. His best-known work was on the chemistry of trace metals in the brain, the role of heavy-metal metabolism in disease, and the efficacy of chelating agents in Wilson's disease. Cumings gave the Hughlings Jackson lecture in 1971 on 'Inborn Errors of Metabolism of the Brain', and wrote a monograph entitled *Heavy Metals and the Brain* (1959). He also edited, with Kremer, three volumes of *Biochemical Aspects of Neurological Disorders* (1959, 1965 and 1968) that recorded the course of advanced lectures held in the Institute of Neurology. Cumings established a research group focusing on muscular dystrophy, and retained an interest in migraine, contributing much to the lay charities in both conditions. The department grew under his leadership so that, at the time of his retirement, there were 23 academic staff, much larger than its sister department of neuropathology. Cumings also worked tirelessly in administration and played a pivotal role in the project to rebuild Queen Square House, which was still in the final stages of construction when he retired in September 1971, and there was widely expressed sadness that he could not see this through to completion.

On Cumings' retirement in 1971, the department was first renamed the 'department of chemical pathology and neurochemistry' and split into two sections (chemical pathology supervised by Peter Lascelles, and neurochemistry supervised by Gerald Curzon who was then reader in neurochemistry). In 1972 the neurochemistry section was renamed the Miriam Marks

department of neurochemistry, after large donations to promote neurochemistry by the Miriam Marks Foundation,[25] the Worshipful Company of Pewterers and the Nuffield Foundation, and Alan N. Davison[26] was appointed as its first director and Curzon as his deputy. Davison had been recruited by Kelly and Gilliatt in 1971 and became the first professor of a neurochemistry department in Britain, and the first non-clinician to head an Institute department. Davison worked on multiple sclerosis, Alzheimer's disease, taurine as a possible neurotransmitter, and on experimental models of phenylketonuria. Always optimistic, at a time in academic life of the country when enthusiasm was in short supply, he was influential in the Multiple Sclerosis Society where, as the scientist responsible for academic advice on funding, he enabled several large and ambitious centre grants, including that made to Ian McDonald, which paid dividends in terms of new discoveries relating to aetiology, mechanisms and treatment. Under Davison's leadership, neurochemistry rapidly expanded and, by 1981, comprised 63 academic staff publishing around 100 scientific papers each year and was, as the Institute's annual report proclaimed, one of the largest centres in the world for research in neurochemistry. This investment was ahead of its time and, since then, neurochemistry has become integrated with molecular biology and permeates the research methods of many and disparate university departments. David Bowen[27] was a non-clinical scientist who joined Davison's department as lecturer in 1970.

---

[25] Miriam Marks was the sister of Lord Sieff, owner of Marks and Spencer. She died of Alzheimer's disease and Sieff, through the agency of Denis Williams, donated £250,000 to set up the department and research in this area.

[26] Alan Davison was born in Leigh on Sea, and obtained a degree in pharmacy from the University of Nottingham in 1946, before moving from London University to the MRC Toxicology Labs at Carshalton. His PhD, written in 1954 during the Cold War, was on the topic of the effects of organophosphates on cholinesterases in the central nervous system. Between 1957 and 1965, Davison worked at Guy's Hospital Medical School and achieved an international reputation for his work on myelin lipid and protein metabolism. In 1965, he was appointed as professor and head of the department of biochemistry at Charing Cross Hospital Medical School. He was a modest and generous person, a francophile always pleased to arrange exchanges with the Sorbonne. He died of a glioma in 1993, three years after retirement.

[27] David Bowen was educated at Reading University and spent his formative training years in Pittsburgh before

It is recorded that he met Tony Dayan who introduced him to the neuropathology of tangles in Alzheimer's disease, and this began a distinguished research career in which he was particularly noted for his work on the decline in cholinergic neurones in this condition, and the reduction in a range of enzymes including choline acetyl transferase, which led to a range of therapeutic trials. The work on his 'cholinergic hypothesis' led to the establishment of the Astra research unit within the Institute of Neurology based in Hunter Street.

In 1979, haematological and microbiological work left the university department of chemical pathology to become administered by the hospital, and then, in 1982, the department underwent further large-scale reorganisation when the section on chemical pathology moved under the administrative control of the National Hospital, due, it was stated, to concern from the hospital over its lack of accountability for clinical work in laboratories. Peter Lascelles, who was previously senior lecturer in the university department, and had been in charge of the chemical pathology section, was appointed as its head.

Davison retired in 1990 at the age of 65 years, and was succeeded by Professor John B. Clarke,[28] whose interest was mainly in energy metabolism of the brain and muscle. He collaborated with John Morgan Hughes, and Queen Square quickly became a pioneering centre for clinical and biochemical studies on mitochondrial disease. Clarke particularly worked on oxidative and nitrosative stress as the cause of the mitochondrial dysfunction associated with neurodegeneration, the characterisation of glial and neuronal energy metabolism, and the trafficking of antioxidants between glia and neurones. Under his direction, the department

remained one of the largest in the institute, employing 53 academic staff and publishing 80 papers in 1991. He contributed greatly to administration of the institute, and to various national bodies, was deputy editor of *Brain* between 1990 and 1997, and chairman of Portland Press at the Biochemical Society between 2004 and 2010.

Under Peter Lascelles, the hospital department of chemical pathology focused particularly on measurement of anticonvulsant levels. Lascelles took early retirement in 1989 under the euphemistic NHS scheme known as 'Achieving a balance', after 23 years of service, and Dr Ed Thompson was appointed, on an acting basis, as his successor. In 1991, yet another name change created the National Hospital department of clinical chemistry. By then, academic work had largely ceased and chemical pathology activity in the hospital was focused on providing a clinical service. However, Thompson was awarded a personal professorship in 1993 and moved to John Clarke's university department of neurochemistry, with clinical chemistry in the hospital taken over by John Land. Philip Patsalos, who had worked with Peter Lascelles, supervised the serum anticonvulsant monitoring service, and as Land and he clashed almost continuously, the anticonvulsant laboratory returned under the control of the Institute, this time in the university department of clinical neurology.

Three other pathologists deserve mention. In 1964, Professor John Cavanagh was appointed head of the MRC research group in applied neurobiology, which was housed at Queen Square on the understanding that the university would take over long-term funding. This was productive but, in the climate of severe financial restriction, MRC funding came to an end in 1967 and the group was dissolved. Cavanagh stayed on at Queen Square outside any departmental structure until his retirement in 1982. He was an experimentalist who studied cellular and biological mechanisms of neurological disease and, especially, the toxic effects of chemical agents on the nervous system. Cavanagh also founded *Neuropathology and Applied Neurobiology* as the official journal of the British Neuropathological Society, and this remains a core journal in the field of neuropathology.[29]

Gerald Curzon joined Cumings' department of chemical pathology in 1953, moving to the Miriam Marks department of neurochemistry in 1971, where

---

returning to work for Unilever. He left industry to return to academia in 1970 when appointed to the Institute of Neurology. He won many international prizes for his 'cholinergic hypothesis' of Alzheimer's disease. He was also central to the identification and characterisation of frontotemporal dementia. Papers from his festschrift in 1996 were published in a special issue of *Neurodegeneration* (5 (1996)). He had a myocardial infarction in 1993, leading to his premature retirement in 1995.

[28] John Clarke was born in Essex, educated at Southend High School for Boys, and then at University College London. After completing his PhD at UCL, he spent time in Philadelphia, then returned to the department of biochemistry at St Bartholomew's Hospital, and moved to Queen Square in 1990. In the later years, neurochemistry was rather overtaken by molecular neuroscience and, on Clarke's retirement in 2013, the department of neurochemistry ceased to exist.

[29] The inaugural paper in the journal was by Cavanagh with Neil Carmichael and Jean Jacobs, on the pathological effects of experimental mercury poisoning.

he worked on 5-hydroxytryptamine. He was awarded a personal professorship in neurochemistry in 1975 and retired from the Institute of Neurology in 1994.

William McMenemey[30] was pathologist to Maida Vale Hospital and was awarded a personal professorship in pathology at the Institute of Neurology in 1965. He had worked as a registrar in neurology at the Maida Vale Hospital, and then was appointed assistant pathologist to W. E. Carnegie Dickson at the West End Hospital for Nervous Diseases, from where, in 1933, he wrote his first paper, on familial presenile dementia, with Charles Worster-Drought. Having trained in neurology, psychiatry and pathology, McMenemy was one of the very few fellows of three Royal Colleges (Physicians, Pathologists and Psychiatrists). He worked first in Oxford and Worcester as a general pathologist, before returning to Maida Vale Hospital as neuropathologist in 1949. He was an expert on cerebral degenerative diseases, but his most memorable contributions were in teaching and training. As his obituarist in the *Lancet* explained, 'There are many neuropathologists throughout the world who owe their initial interest in their subject and their first-class basic training that has helped them to establish their own departments, to him. They will miss him, and the intense interest he always showed in them, just as much as those of us at home.'

McMenemey served as president of various organisations, including the International Society of Clinical Pathology, the Association of Clinical Pathologists, and the sections of neurology and the history of medicine of the Royal Society of Medicine. He was one of the old school, immaculate and with charming manners, much like his successor as pathologist at Maida Vale, the equally elegant and dapper Robin Barnard.[31] Barnard

continued to run the pathology service at Maida Vale until the hospital's closure and he retired in 1991. During this time, the Maida Vale department provided a clinical service, but little research.

In addition to routine clinical roles within the National Hospitals, it is worth emphasising two other important aspects of the neuropathological work at Queen Square and Maida Vale, which were to prove vital in ensuring the survival of the hospital in the second half of the twentieth century. The departments of pathology at both Queen Square and Maida Vale acted as referral centres for difficult pathological diagnoses and, throughout this period, between a quarter and a half of all specimens examined were sent in from other hospitals, some within Britain and some from abroad. The departments also had a vital training function and almost all the neuropathologists in Britain, at least up until the 1970s, had spent significant training periods at Queen Square or Maida Vale. Neurology and neurosurgery at Queen Square shared similar tertiary centre and training roles, but in a small specialty like neuropathology these functions were of even more importance in enhancing the reputation of the National Hospital, and remain so to this day.

Neuropathology at Queen Square: A Perspective

Two great tensions played out in the twentieth century in relation to the organisation of neuropathology and these can be clearly seen in the evolution of the subject at Queen Square. First was the extent to which the subject should be pursued as a service to clinical medicine rather than an academic discipline, and with the constant threat that the clinical work would overwhelm research. In Britain, as it evolved in the early part of the twentieth century, neuropathology remained largely embedded in clinical practice. The two dominant figures in this period were J. G. Greenfield at Queen Square and Dorothy Russell in Oxford and then the

---

[30] William Henry McMenemey was educated in Birkenhead School and trained at Oxford and St Bartholomew's Hospital. With an interest in medical history, he wrote a history of the Worcester Royal Infirmary (1947), and a biography of James Parkinson in the commemorative volume edited by Macdonald Critchley (*James Parkinson (1755–1824): A Bicentenary Volume of Papers Dealing with Parkinson's Disease, Incorporating the Original 'Essay on the Shaking Palsy'* (London: Macmillan, 1955)); see also the annual report of the Institute of Neurology 1978; *Munk's Roll*, Vol. **VII**, pp. 368–70; *Who Was Who*; and notices in the *British Medical Journal* **2** (1977): 1551 and *Lancet* **310** (1977): 1239.

[31] Robin Osler Barnard, born in London and qualified at St Thomas' Hospital in 1956, was appointed pathologist to

Maida Vale Hospital in 1964. He was a dependable neuropathologist who did not carry out much research or writing. His passion was restoring classic motor cars, of which he had 12, including a 1924 Rolls Royce which seemed to complement Barnard's style and sartorial elegance. Even in the 1980s, he ia remembered for his impeccable style, arriving at work in Maida Vale in his bowler hat, morning suit and briefcase. He suffered from severe diabetes, which eventually led to blindness, and died of a coronary thrombosis.

London Hospital.[32] Both encouraged the close working relationship of pathologists with physicians – neurologists in the case of Greenfield, who indeed dressed and behaved like a neurologist. Conversely, Russell developed strong ties with neurosurgery, facilitated by her close working relationship with Cairns. Both emphasised what was undoubtedly the strongest quality in British neuropathology, its practical nature and links to clinical medicine. British pathologists were renowned internationally for their clinical skills, and, reflecting this reputation, Greenfield's *Neuropathology*, as well as Russell and Rubinstein's *Pathology of Tumours of the Nervous System*, became the standard neuropathology textbooks in the English-speaking world. With the arrival of the NHS, regional neuropathology units developed as part of the expansion in specialist services for neurosurgery, and these also were dominated by clinical work. Growth in the demand for expert surgical pathology since the Second World War can be gauged by the number of surgical biopsies at Queen Square, which exceeded 1,000 per year by 1991, and the complexity of the tasks required for their analysis.

Greenfield recognised the danger of being flooded by clinical work, and locating the department within a university setting rendered this problem less acute at Queen Square than in many regional centres. However, Blackwood, his successor, was essentially a teacher and clinician and not an academic researcher. Although research in the field of the pathology of old age did flourish, both on the pathological and neurochemical sides, as did research into metabolic and toxic conditions, but the main thrust of the department in the middle years of the century was on training and clinical service. McMenemey understood that neuropathology might become entirely subservient to clinical requirements and suffer from lack of investment. As he wrote in 1972, when considering the future of pathology in the NHS:

The fact remains that we medical practitioners are dependent now for our livelihood on the good-will of Parliament ... it is certain that, through shortage of money, pathologists will for many years to come be restricted in space, equipment and personnel ... we mostly work in antiquated and overcrowded premises and in fact after eleven years still await the first of the post-war hospitals. We are near the end of a long and expensive queue.

By any analysis, the research contribution of British neuropathology had hit a low point in the mid-century, with most work confined to clinical description and case reports. Experimental neuropathology was sidelined in Britain generally, and at Queen Square between and during the two World Wars. Although he recognised this problem, McMenemey felt that separating experimental and clinical neuropathology would be a mistake. Each had flowered independently on the continent and in the USA, and although pathological research in the UK has flourished belatedly in recent years, many still consider that, by comparison with continental Europe, the appropriate balance of clinical and research work has never been achieved in the UK. Much came down to resources, and at Queen Square the area within neuropathology that remained most prominent in the post-war years was neurochemistry, and this flourished as it was heavily supported by the philanthropy of the Miriam Marks Foundation and the Pewterers' company.

Embedding neuropathology in the university also allowed easier access to research funding and stimulated collaborative work with the basic science departments at University College. Since the 1980s, the pathologists have become more closely aligned to the basic sciences of the university than any other grouping at Queen Square. From this time onwards, experimental neuropathology has blossomed, with input from molecular biology, immunology and molecular genetics, which envigorated the subject and galvanised the university departments.

The second tension played out in the twentieth century was that caused by differing opinions on whether neuropathology should be retained within general pathology or allowed to develop as a specialty in its own right. The old arguments with respect to the relationship of neurology to general medicine, and neurosurgery to general surgery, were replayed. Greenfield, McMenemey and Dorothy Russell saw risks in isolating neuropathology from pathology, and

---

[32] Dorothy Russell was professor of morbid anatomy at the London Hospital between 1946 and 1960. Previously she had worked at the London with Cairns and then moved with him to Oxford, where she succeeded Pio del Rio-Hortega as neuropathologist at the Radcliffe Infirmary. Her interest was the importance of neuropathology for neurosurgery, with contributions to the study of hydrocephalus and brain tumours which still remain important. She was also the first woman to become head of a department of pathology in the Western world (and was always known as 'The Lady').

argued for leaving the discipline firmly embedded within general pathology. However, this was a losing battle, and as time passed there was an increasing tendency to treat neuropathology separately, not least because of the special techniques involved in staining and interpreting abnormalities in nervous tissue. After Greenfield's departure, there was a rapid move to specialisation, and the links with general pathology at University College Hospital became tenuous. Subspecialisation within neuropathology also developed, especially from the 1970s, with different groups focusing on increasingly narrow areas. Linked to this was the tendency to separate clinical chemistry from general clinical pathology, which happened at Queen Square and was not a success. Neurochemistry though, divorced from routine clinical work, flourished, and the Miriam Marks department of chemical pathology was, for a time, the largest and most celebrated of its kind in the world.

Neuroradiology at Queen Square

Arguably the most important step forward in the practice of neurology and neurosurgery in the twentieth century was the introduction of neuroimaging. Until then, clinical diagnosis was based entirely on clinical observation educated by clinico-pathological correlation, but, during the course of the twentieth century, a succession of new 'imaging' technologies completely restructured the practice of medicine. CT and MRI were applied first in disease of the brain and spinal cord, and had their most immediate benefits for neurology and neurosurgery. The application of imaging in neurology led theoretical advance, demonstrating the overwhelming extent to which clinical neurology became an empirical discipline as the twentieth century progressed, in contrast to the focus on theory in nineteenth century. It was physics, engineering and computing that underpinned these developments, not emerging concepts on how the nervous system works. The National Hospital physicians recognised the importance of the new technologies, and their insistence on the early acquisition of X-ray, EEG, electromyography (EMG) and methods for nerve conduction measurement, CT (after a wobbly start) and MRI for the National Hospital was one element in keeping it at the head of the pack.[33]

The first human X-ray picture was published by Roentgen in December 1895, and his discovery attracted immediate public interest. In Britain, the *Standard* recorded on Tuesday 7 January 1896:

> A very important scientific discovery has recently been made by Professor Rontgen of Wurzburg University … it has become possible to photograph the bones without the flesh surrounding the bones appearing on the plate … ghastly enough in appearance, but from a scientific point of view, they open up a wide field … The Press assures its readers that there is no joke or humbug in the matter. It is a serious discovery by a serious German professor![34]

The medical applications were quickly foreseen, and such was the rapid impact of this discovery that, within months, X-ray machines were being produced commercially, the first textbook of radiology was published (1896), the Roentgen Society was founded in Britain (1897), and Roentgen was awarded his Nobel Prize (1901).

Radiology at the National Hospital 1903–1946

Private X-ray laboratories opened in London in 1896, but it was the military that led the implementation of radiology in medicine in Britain. The Army installed its first X-ray machine at the Netley Military Hospital in 1896, and soon after in other military base hospitals and mobile units on the battlefields – including, for instance, the 1897 Graeco-Turkish and Boer Wars. Civilian hospital practice then followed suit. In October 1903, Gowers urged the hospital to purchase an X-ray machine and, in January 1904, this request was approved by the Medical Committee and the Board of Governors.[35] The equipment was located within the electrical department, and the registrar was responsible for examinations, interpretation and maintenance of the X-ray equipment. The minutes record that 'a limited number of X Ray photos can be taken if the Registrar can find time for the work'. It was, however, obviously

---

[33] Although the National Hospital was slow in utilising ventriculography, angiography or myelography during the inter-war years, due to the fact that neurosurgery was somewhat inactive during those years. Radiology did not really reach its full potential at the hospital until Wyllie

McKissock was appointed as consultant neurosurgeon in 1946.

[34] Articles then appeared from the January 1896 editions of *Nature*, the *British Medical Journal* and the *Lancet* onwards, initially treating the discovery as a Dickensian joke but soon becoming enthusiastic.

[35] Exactly when the first X-ray machine was installed is not clear, but in the 1908 management minutes there was mention of the purchase of X-ray plates.

a service in demand because, in 1910, the Medical Committee noted that physicians were bringing their private patients to Queen Square for X-rays, thereby increasing the workload. The Electrical Sub-committee was by then reporting every year to the Medical Committee of the hospital and requests for X-ray equipment were made periodically.[36] There are no records of how many X-rays were taken but it is clear that, particularly in the wartime, demand did increase rapidly.

X-rays had an immediate application for many branches of medicine, but their initial effect on the practice of neurology was compromised by the inability to differentiate cerebral soft tissues from fluid and other non-bony structures. For the while, the brain remained largely 'a dark continent'.[37] The first mention of the nervous system in the *Archives of Radiology and Electrotherapy*, the main journal in the field of radiology, was in 1916, and nothing was published in *Brain* until 1924, when the contemporary uses of plain X-rays in neurology were listed by the young Geoffrey Jefferson to detect general changes in the skull (sutural diastasis in hydrocephalus, ribbing of the skull or convolutional atrophy in raised intracranial pressure, and imaging of the sella turcica in pituitary lesions and hydrocephalus); local changes in bone (hyperostosis in an endothelial or meningeal tumour); and shadows cast by cerebral tumours (due to calcification, which he recognised to be an uncommon event).[38]

Interest in the radiology of the nervous system much increased when, in 1918, Walter Dandy devised air ventriculography, a technique that, for the first time, provided sufficient contrast differentiation to outline the ventricles.[39] A year later, he introduced the air via lumbar puncture and, with ventriculography and air encephalography, concluded that 'It is difficult to see how intracranial tumours can escape localization.' Despite their utility, ventriculography and air encephalography were risky procedures in those days, and both were unpleasant for patients. In 1925, there was, for the first time, a session on neuroradiology at the International Congress of Radiology held in London (with no lectures by British radiologists). Dandy's radiologist, Dr J. W. Pierson, referred to ventriculography as 'dangerous and complicated, but in competent hands it should not be nearly so dangerous as an exploratory craniotomy and it frequently yields more information than the latter operation. Dandy reported three deaths, which had occurred very early in the series of at least 500 cases.'[40]

Dandy also experimented with air myelography in 1918, but did not publish his work. The first published air myelogram was by Jacobaeus from Sweden in 1921, who concluded – as presumably Dandy also had done – that the radiographs were too difficult to read to be of value. Then, also in 1921 the technique of lipiodol myelography was described by Jean-Athanase Sicard and Jacques Forestier in Paris. Sicard and Forestier were instilling lipiodol into the epidural space for the treatment of pain, and by mistake injected some of the contrast medium into the subarachnoid space. When taking the X-ray they recognised immediately its utility in outlining the spinal cord. The procedure was thought to be effective and non-toxic and soon attracted worldwide attention. It was this technique that Percy Sargent saw in his visit to Paris and which was introduced into British practice in the early 1920s.

In 1927, Egas Moniz in Lisbon introduced cerebral angiography into clinical neurology. Inspired by the use

---

[36] Risien Russell seems to have been a particular supporter of X-rays and, in 1914, it is recorded that he allocated a donation of £25 received from a patient for the purchase of X-ray equipment.

[37] Britain, and Queen Square, lagged behind. The pioneer of practical neuroradiology was undoubtedly Arthur Schüller from Brünn in Moravia. He published his landmark book *Röntgen-Diagnostik der Erkrankungen des Kopfes* (Vienna and Leipzig: Hölder) in 1912 (translated into English in 1918). His sad life is documented by Erwin Schindler in 'Arthur Schüller, Pioneer of Neuroradiology', *American Journal of Neuroradiology* **18** (1997): 1297–302.

[38] This was a report of a meeting at the Royal Society of Medicine with Wilfred Harris in the chair: W. Harris, 'Discussion of the Value of X-rays in the Localisation of Cerebral and Spinal Tumours, with Special Reference to Ventriculography and Lipiodol Injections', *Brain* **47** (1924): 77–382.

[39] A case was published by Dr Gilbert Scott in the *Archives of Radiology and Electrotherapy* in 1917, in which air introduced into the ventricular system after surgery on a skull tumour was demonstrated by X-ray outlining the ventricular system: see J. W. Bull and H. Fischgold, 'A Short History of Neuroradiology', in E. Cabanis, ed., *Contribution à l'histoire de la neuroradiologie européenne* (Paris: Éditions Pradel, 1989). This and another paper (W. H. Lockett, 'Air in the Ventricles of the Brain Following a Fracture of the Skull: Report of a Case', *Surgery, Gynaecology & Obstetrics* **17** (1913): 237–40) were to some extent precursors of air ventriculography, although it is not clear whether Dandy was aware of them.

[40] Cited in J. W. D. Bull, 'History of Neuroradiology. The Presidential Address, Delivered at the British Institute of Radiology on October 20, 1960', *British Journal of Radiology* **34** (1960): 69–84.

of lipiodol in myelography, Moniz explored the intra-arterial injection of contrast media. As an oil, lipiodol was unsuitable and so he experimented with water-soluble salts of bromide, strontium, lithium and iodine, looking for a medium which would not be diluted by the blood flow to such an extent that it was invisible to X-rays and yet was non-toxic. He eventually selected a 25 per cent solution of sodium iodide. Using a surgical cut-down to the carotid artery, the iodide was injected directly into the artery and Moniz presented the first human angiogram to a neurological meeting in 1927. Sodium iodide, however, proved toxic and difficult to image, and in 1929 he replaced this with thorium dioxide (marketed as Thorotrast[41]).

For a number of years, there was heated discussion on whether angiography or pneumography was the superior technique. Cushing expressed a preference for angiography and wrote in strongly disparaging terms about ventriculography. On the other hand, Dandy, in 1932, stated: 'since ventriculography can accurately localize all intracranial tumors causing pressure and without danger or after-effect, it is difficult to believe that there can be a place for arterial encephalography in the diagnosis or localization of brain tumors'. To some extent, this disagreement reflected the strong personal enmity between these two American neurosurgeons, but it nevertheless exposed the general uncertainty about the relative merits of the two procedures.

Over succeeding years, there were progressive incremental improvements in the technologies and methods of radiology, with investigation becoming safer and the radiographs more detailed and clearly defined. Queen Square, it seems, remained very much on the sidelines of these advances during the inter-war years and played little part in the controversies surrounding advanced neuroradiology, no doubt largely because of the lack of engagement of the hospital or its physicians with neurosurgery.

It is possible to gain a flavour of the role of radiology in neurological and neurosurgical practice in London and at Queen Square from the proceedings of the meeting of the section of neurology held in 1924 at the Royal Society of Medicine, and mentioned above. This meeting was focused on the topic of lipiodol myelography and air ventriculography. Geoffrey

Jefferson spoke about his own series of 13 cases of ventriculography (two of whom died immediately, due to the procedure). Sir Percy Sargent lectured on his favourable impressions of lipiodol myelography during a recent visit to Paris, and described his first experience of using this method. Others who were familiar with the techniques were Sir James Purves-Stewart, Wilfred Harris, L. Bathe Rawling and Lancelot Bromley from London, and Adam McConnell from Ireland. The young Charles Symonds, a few years before his appointment to Queen Square, mentioned the diagnostic importance of the protein content of the cerebrospinal fluid obtained during the procedure. There is no mention, however, of the purchase of lipiodol or of ventriculography or myelography in any of the Queen Square documents at that time.

The speakers at the Royal Society of Medicine were neurosurgeons or neurologists, and not radiologists. Radiology as a specialty had developed strongly in the 1910s and 1920s, but neuroradiology remained a topic too specialised for most general radiologists. However, as soon as angiography was introduced into British practice, an inevitable turf war developed between radiologists and neurosurgeons about who should lead in these investigations. Surgeons were needed to cut-down on arteries for angiography and so retained the upper hand initially, but when this was replaced by percutaneous and catheter angiography, the specialty of neuroradiology began to develop.

Russell John Reynolds was a Londoner, educated at Westminster School and qualified from Guy's Hospital Medical School. He was appointed to the National Hospital in 1919, as its first radiologist. The post, proposed by Risien Russell, had been agreed a year earlier but the appointment was delayed until after demobilisation, so that the field might be as strong as possible. In the event, there were three candidates – Reynolds, Kempster[42] and Williams. Russell Reynolds was to become one of the great British pioneers of radiology. As a child, in the same year as Roentgen's discovery, he and his father had constructed a home-made X-ray apparatus,[43] and as a result of his interest and his

---

[41] Thorium, however, accumulates in the body, and is an isotope with a very long half-life (10^{10} years); 30 years after its introduction, it was found to produce malignant tumours and its use then abandoned – by which time, no doubt, thousands of patients had been affected.

[42] Christopher Kempster became a distinguished radiologist, with appointments in the London hospitals specialising in skin, cancer and military medicine.

[43] The machine is now in the science museum, and details of it were published in the *English Mechanic* of 11 February 1898. It was a primitive coil used to activate an early Watson X-ray tube on a wooden retort stand and housed in a cardboard box. He then made a barium platinocyanide screen, and noticed that the backs of his hand

inventions Reynolds was, in 1901, elected to the Roentgen Society.[44] He qualified in medicine in 1907 and within two years had specialised in radiology. During the First World War, he served in India as 'electrical specialist to the Karachi Brigade', and on his return was appointed consultant radiologist to both Charing Cross Hospital and the National Hospital. He acted as adviser in radiology to the Ministries of Pensions and Supply, and was elected president of the section on radiology of the Royal Society of Medicine in 1927, and was rewarded with a CBE in 1932. The Roentgen Society amalgamated with the British Institute of Radiology and, in 1937, Reynolds was elected president of the joint society.[45] In 1936, he was appointed Hunterian Professor at the Royal College of Surgeons, where he pioneered methods for cine-radiology. This research contribution, produced relatively late in his career, was the development for which he received many international awards.

Reynolds was, however, very much a general radiologist and seems to have published nothing on the radiology of the nervous system. His appointment at the National Hospital in 1919 was for two days a week. It was agreed at the time that the radiological unit be managed separately from the 'Electrical Department' although this was where the X-ray equipment was located. He seems to have been reasonably well supported, because, in November 1920, £400 was spent buying a high-tension transformer, but the terms of his appointment appear rather harsh,[46] and it seems

clear that the neurologists did not consider the radiologist, even one as celebrated as Reynolds, as their equal. When Aldren Turner proposed, in 1923, that Reynolds be elected to the Medical Committee, the minutes record that 'after some discussion, Dr Turner decided not to pursue the proposal'.[47] Radiation was by then also being used widely for therapy in skin and cancer, and there is an interesting reference to the use of radium in glioma in the Medical Committee Minutes in 1924.[48]

Reynolds resigned from his position at the National Hospital in 1939 and was succeeded by Hugh Davies, the second radiologist appointed to the hospital. Davies was educated at Marlborough, obtained a scholarship to Oxford University to read Medicine, took up radiology in 1929, and in 1931 he was awarded the Cambridge diploma (DMRE), which was one of the few radiological qualifications existing at the time. He then was appointed consultant radiologist to King's College Hospital, consultant radiotherapist to the National Hospital in 1931 (at a very young age), and, in 1939, consultant radiologist. Davies went on to have a distinguished career as a radiologist, becoming president of the British Institute of Radiology in 1948 and Mackenzie Davidson Lecturer in 1965. He had a large private practice run from his home in Queen Anne Street, and neither published nor contributed to academic debate. He retired from King's College Hospital in 1948 and worked entirely thereafter at the National Hospital, retiring in 1966, and he died a year later from a glioma. He was said to be an excellent administrator

---

became red and sore when using the machine and so coated the outside of the box with lead paint.

[44] The Roentgen Society was an important group in the development of British radiology, and it is interesting to see that David Ferrier was one of the six vice-presidents appointed at its inaugural meeting in 1897.

[45] Subsequent Queen Square presidents were Hugh Davies in 1948, J. W. D. Bull in 1961 and E. P. G. du Boulay in 1977.

[46] At the meeting of a subcommittee of the Medical Committee, 5 January 1919 (comprising Colonel Armour and Dr Grainger Stewart), convened for this purpose, the duties of the newly appointed consultant radiologist were defined. The appointee was personally to superintend the X-ray department and its efficient work; attend the hospital at least twice a week at regular times; take any X-ray photographs that may be required and be available for consultation with physicians and surgeons; be available for any emergency case; and have personal charge of the apparatus and be responsible for it. The hospital should assign to him a sister or nurse who should be especially attached to the department to assist him, and he should be allowed a holiday when he wished, provided he nominated a substitute who was not

a member of the executive staff of the hospital and had been approved. It was also noted that, if he intended to be absent for more than one week, he should inform the chairman of the Board and name his substitute. On the appointment of the radiologist, the registrar would relinquish his role in relation to the taking of X-rays.

[47] Minutes of the Medical Committee, 5 February 1923.

[48] Minutes of the Medical Committee, 11 February 1924. It was reported that Dr Russell Reynolds had employed 15 mg of radium in the treatment of glioma with promising results, and the Committee was asked to explore the possibility of using this as a therapy. This dose of radium could be bought for £800. An alternative was to hire 'radium emanations' from the Radium Institute at a cost of 3 guineas for the equivalent of 50 mg. However, the surgeons felt that the efficacy of this 'emanation' was inferior to the actual substance and were not prepared to experiment with this if radium could not be obtained. Dr Russell Reynolds, it seems, also had ownership of a personal quantity of radium, and it was suggested that he should be paid 4 guineas for the hire of 50 mg for 24 hours. It was noted to be unlikely this would be used more than a dozen times a year.

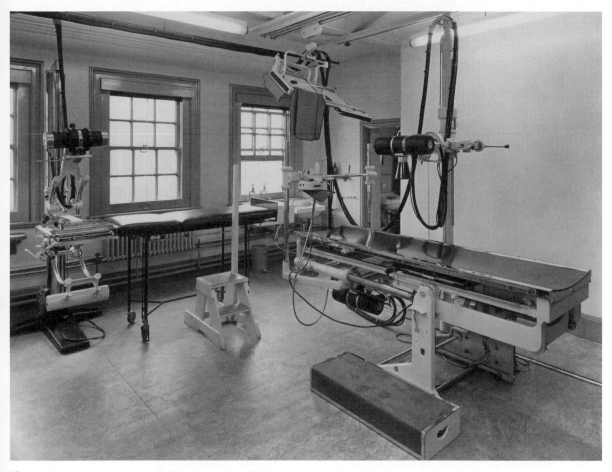

Figure 11.3 X-ray room no. 1, radiology department, 1949.

and chaired the Medical Committee just before he retired.

It was the work of the next two radiologists appointed to the National Hospital, James Bull and George du Boulay, that raised the profile of radiology at Queen Square and propelled the hospital into a world-leading position in the burgeoning specialty of neuroradiology.

Neuroradiology at Queen Square After 1946

James William Douglas Bull was born in Buckinghamshire, educated at Repton and qualified in medicine from Cambridge and St George's Hospital Medical School. He was the third radiologist appointed to the hospital in 1948, and worked there until retirement in 1975. Bull had become interested in neuroradiology in the 1930s and, encouraged by Wyllie McKissock, won a Rockefeller Travelling

Scholarship to Stockholm to work with Erik Lysholm in 1938, with whom he cemented a great friendship.[49]

Major technical developments in radiology were taking place in Stockholm at the time, under the leadership of Lysholm. He developed what came to be known as 'precision radiology'. This was made possible by the development of a head unit allowing radiographs to be taken from a range of projections. The machinery was developed by Lysholm and his engineer Georg Schonander, who also designed a skull table separated from the body table enabling the head to be moved around and aligned to the planned projections. Lysholm and his successor Lindgren developed close connections

---

49 See E. Lindgren and T. Greitz, 'The Stockholm School of Neuroradiology', *American Journal of Neuroradiology* 6 (1995): 351–60.

with the neuroradiologists at Queen Square, notably James Bull and George du Boulay, and the Lysholm techniques of precision radiology and of percutaneous angiography became deeply embedded in subsequent years into the local approach to radiology.

Bull was appointed radiologist at Maida Vale in 1939, but joined the RAMC in 1940 and was transferred to serve in the Far East. In 1942, he was interned by the Japanese following the fall of Singapore and, as a prisoner of war for 3½ years, was treated with appalling brutality.[50] On his release, he spent a further period in Stockholm with Lysholm and then Erik Lindgren (who subsequently took over the department after Lysholm's death in 1947) and was appointed consultant radiologist at Atkinson Morley Hospital, working with McKissock, in 1946; assistant radiologist at the National Hospital in 1947, joining Hugh Davies; and consultant radiologist in 1948. He assumed the directorship of the department in 1966. Bull introduced Lysholm and Lindgren's work to Britain, notably precision radiography and percutaneous angiography – of which he is said to have been the first British practitioner – and also air encephalography using the Swedish method.

When Bull was appointed to Queen Square, the X-ray department was on two sites: in the outpatients department and next to the theatre. Under his guidance, it was relocated into a single site on the third floor of the old hospital in 1947. The design and the layout were based on plans given to the hospital by Lindgren, and the unit was re-equipped partly with gifts from Sweden by Lysholm and Lindgren. Schönander donated one of his skull stands and provided three others at a much-discounted price. In 1947, it was agreed that the new department should be named after Lysholm. Activity increased after the war and, in 1950, 398 cerebral angiograms, 221 air encephalograms, 207 ventriculograms and 27 myelograms were carried out. In the same year, Bull was experimenting with vertebral angiography and had initiated the use of myodil for ventriculography, which was to prove much less problematic than lipiodol. He refused to use water-soluble contrast agents for myelography, and his concerns were justified later

when the dangers of metrizamide became recognised. Later, it was said to be Bull who convinced Zena Powell, the wife of the managing director of EMI, whom he had met at a reception, of the importance of the new imaging method of computerised axial tomography (CAT), and as a result of this meeting she persuaded her husband to invest in the technology. Bull was a 'quintessential English gentleman', described by a neurologist who did not know him well, as 'such a very grand man'. He brought together colleagues and raised the profile of radiology at the National Hospital. His generous support for colleagues, especially younger ones, is in contrast with his public presence: splendid, dominating, English yet austere. In what must have seemed inevitable natural steps, he was appointed foundation president of the British Society of Neuroradiologists and the European Society of Neuroradiology. Under Bull's directorship, radiology at the National Hospital rose to international prominence for its advanced clinical work, and under his mentorship a whole generation of neuroradiologists around the world were trained at Queen Square, using a scheme that was very much Bull's creation. He suffered a coronary thrombosis in 1975 and retired from Queen Square, but remained active. He was appointed CBE in 1978, and died in 1987 following a road traffic accident, in which he sustained severe brain damage, diagnosed on CT scanning.

Edward Philip George Houssemayne du Boulay was born in Alexandra into a Huguenot family, and his father was a major in the Egyptian Labour Corps and Egyptian Government Service. He was schooled at Christ's Hospital, Horsham, and trained in medicine at the Charing Cross Hospital Medical School, from where he qualified in 1947. His early general radiological training was at the Middlesex and St Bartholomew's Hospitals, and at Atkinson Morley Hospital where, like James Bull, he was attracted to neuroradiology by Wyllie McKissock. Du Boulay was appointed consultant radiologist at Maida Vale and St Bartholomew's Hospital in 1954, and moved to Queen Square in 1968. There, with no office provided, he erected a garden shed on the roof of the radiology department, which remained in place for over 20 years. He took over the directorship of the Lysholm Department in 1975 on the retirement of James Bull, and held this position until his own retirement in 1984. In 1976, du Boulay was also awarded a personal professorship in neuroradiology, the first in Britain, at the Institute of Neurology. George du

---

[50] A memoir of his time in Changi is in the Imperial War Museum. His affidavit reporting Japanese war crimes and the Japanese massacre of troops in the military hospital in Singapore is in the National Archives of UK, File Reference WO 325/88.

Boulay's arrival in the radiology department increased its research activity. He already had a distinguished record in veterinary radiology, and had become *de facto* head of radiology at London Zoo. At Queen Square, he was initially interested in angiography, working not only on patients but also, with Lyndsay Symon, on arterial spasm in baboons. Over the next few years, they carried out extensive research on spasm after subarachnoid haemorrhage, and also other aspects of stroke. Du Boulay worked on metabolic effects on the cerebral vessels and showed that hyperventilation could greatly improve image quality, allowing visualisation of arterial, capillary and venous phases of the arteriogram. The department also was notable for developing new techniques and, for instance, collaborated on studies of isotope brain scanning with zenon and Hg 197 chlormerodrin, a gamma-ray emitter. Du Boulay initiated early investigations into the value of carotid ultrasound. In 1973, a second experimental 'B' mode scanner was installed and subsequently used for measuring arterial wall thickness. He was awarded the Barclay Medal by the British Institute of Radiology in 1968, and became its president in 1976. He was editor-in-chief of *Neuroradiology* and, in 1990, was elected president of the XIVth Symposium Neuroradiologicum, held in London. He published over 150 scientific papers and several books,[51] and was a successful fund-raiser both for the British Institute of Radiology and the National Hospital Development Foundation, for which he raised several million pounds. He was appointed CBE in 1985.

Queen Square radiologists played a significant role in the development of imaging using radioactive isotopes (nuclear medicine). This technology became feasible as a clinical method in neuroradiology with the development of collimators in the 1950s. Wyllie McKissock was an early pioneer in the development of isotope encephalography as a non-invasive method for imaging the ventricular system. Geiger counters were replaced by scintillation counters, and in the mid-1960s brain scintography with collimated

detectors in two planes was introduced into clinical practice. An isotope brain scanner was installed in Queen Square in 1963, one of the first sites in Britain, and research using this technique was carried out by du Boulay and Bull. In 1972, Bull concluded that the technique 'had revolutionized the field of neuroradiology', pointing out that its introduction at Queen Square had reduced dramatically the number of venticulograms.

The introduction of CT scanning then rendered isotope technology almost redundant, but it nevertheless was much used at the National Hospital throughout the 1960s and remained in general use elsewhere for bone scanning. Single Proton Emission Computer Tomography (SPECT scanning) was another radio-isotope technique, first used in 1972 to track cerebral blood flow as a measure of brain function. Colour was introduced into the computer-reconstructed images, giving them a spectacular appearance but with no physiological basis, and tending to exaggerate the differences in flow. Nevertheless, the technology caught on and SPECT scanning, in all its technicolour glory, continues to be used, albeit now mainly in the field of epilepsy to localise seizures (which were shown to be accompanied by increased blood flow by Hughlings Jackson). No SPECT scanner was ever installed at Queen Square, although access to equipment at University College Hospital made the technology available for patients in the hospital.

As was soon to become clear, however, the game-changer of the period was neither ultrasound nor isotope brain scanning, but CAT (CT) scanning. This technology was a paradigm shift for radiology and its introduction and that of MRI were to change completely the way neurology was practised thereafter. The general history of CT scanning has been well rehearsed elsewhere, but it had an early impact on neuroradiology in London and at Queen Square. In 1960, Godfrey Hounsfield, an engineer without a university education, was working on computer memory with the British company EMI, based at Hayes in the western suburbs of London. He developed a mathematical method for depicting the shape of an object by reconstructing an iterative series of X-ray scans taken from different angles, and displaying these as a series of 'slices' (tomograms). The first experimental scans were made in 1968, on a lathe using inanimate objects of varying shapes. The results were promising, and Hounsfield applied to the British Department of Health and Medical

---

[51] The list includes: *Principles of X-ray Diagnosis of the Skull* (1965), *Cranial Arteries of Mammals* (1973, with P. M. Verity), *Atlas of Normal Vertebral Angiography* (1976), *Computerised Axial Tomography in Clinical Practice: The First European Seminar* (1977, with I. F. Moseley), *A Textbook of Radiological Diagnosis*, Vol. **I**: *The Central Nervous System* (1984); *Magnetic Resonance Imaging in Multiple Sclerosis* (1989, with I. E. Ormerod, W. I. McDonald and D. Miller).

Research Councils for support. In the transition of the work to human subjects, three London neuroradiologists were chosen to work closely with him – Frank Doyle from the Hammersmith Hospital, Louis Kreel from the Royal Free Hospital, and James Ambrose from Atkinson Morley Hospital. There was governmental vacillation about the value of such an experimental project, but somehow (and unusually) funding was committed. It is said that James Bull at Queen Square was initially approached to collaborate with Hounsfield, but was lukewarm, despite his enthusiasm for the idea, and suggested Ambrose. Certainly, when the first experimental clinical scanner was constructed, it was placed at the Atkinson Morley Hospital (in October 1971) and not at Queen Square, which was later considered a grievous blow to the hospital's pride. However, the radiology department at Atkinson Morley Hospital, under the leadership of Ambrose and with the support of Wyllie McKissock, was then the busiest unit in London and a natural home for the scanner. McKissock did most of his operating there and not at Queen Square, and both he and Ambrose were said to have rather disliked the invasive practice of percutaneous angiography in the Lysholm manner, which was favoured at Queen Square. They were actively investigating alternative techniques, such as ultrasound and isotope scanning, but when CT arrived all other methods were dropped as the potential of the new technology was appreciated. The prototype scanner took 4 minutes to capture images for each slice collected at 1 cm thicknesses and, as the scanner had no inbuilt computer, the data had to be collected on magnetic tape and sent by road to the EMI laboratories for analysis. The first patient scanned, on 1 October 1971, was a woman in whom a cystic frontal tumour was clearly visualised. The results were presented at the 32nd Annual Congress of the British Institute of Radiology, at Imperial College, London, with George du Boulay in the chair. The presentation was a sensation, not unlike the first demonstration of X-ray, and was reported in the international press. In 1972, the EMI Mark 1 scanner was presented at the November meeting of the Radiological Society of North America by Ambrose, after which interest in CT rapidly proliferated. The Mark 1 scanner imaged only the head, and a series of neurological papers was then published as CT scanning moved into clinical neurological practice. The scanners were known then as 'EMI Scanners' (and the scans as 'EMI scans') and by the summer of 1973, five scanners had been installed at Queen Square (funded largely by a donation from Mr Basil Samuel[52]), Manchester, Glasgow, the Mayo Clinic and Massachusetts General Hospital. In 1979, Hounsfield was awarded the Nobel Prize for medicine or physiology.

Amends were being made at Queen Square for the initial disinterest and, within a year of its installation in late 1972, the CT scanner was being used for a broad range of research projects in various neurological diseases. In 1973, Hounsfield was appointed honorary physicist to the department and, in 1975, a second CT1000 scanner was installed, funded by the Department of Health and Social Security R&D fund, thereby doubling the scanning capacity. By 1976, 17 research projects were in progress and Queen Square was again amongst the leading neuroradiological centres internationally.[53] EMI also funded research fellows who worked on many of these projects,[54] and many doctors and technicians became attached to the department for periods of training. Within a few years, CT was the predominant and undisputed investigatory imaging technology in neurology. As an editorial in the *New England Journal of Medicine* in 1976 put it: 'CAT fever has reached epidemic proportions and continues to spread among physicians, manufacturers, entrepreneurs and regulatory agencies. A cursory review of any radiologic or neuroscience journal attests to the virulence of this new disease. Within the United States alone the costs of this epidemic are staggering.'[55]

Imaging became a big business and, as EMI became engulfed in attacks on its patents, US companies took over manufacture so that, by 1981, there were 1,300 CT scanners in the USA, whereas, at a time of national financial decline, their distribution was restricted to regional neurological centres in the UK, with local hospitals resorting to appeals in order to acquire equipment. Technology continued to improve with the

---

[52] Mr Basil Samuel was a member of the Board of Governors of the National Hospital, and a generous philanthropist who funded many developments. The outpatients hall in the new wing of the rebuilt hospital was named after him in 1996.

[53] The international interest of the department is shown by the fact that, of the 13 postgraduate clinical students attached in 1976, nine were from other countries – USA, Brazil, Greece, Dominican Republic, Denmark, Spain, Venezuela, Cyprus and Israel.

[54] Early fellows were Eric Claveria, E.-W. Radu, Patrick Pullicino and Jeff Gawler.

[55] S. H. Shapiro and S. M. Wyman, 'CAT Fever', *New England Journal of Medicine* **296**. 17 (1976): 954–6.

introduction of body scanning – first at the Royal Free Hospital directed by Kreel – and then other innovations such as spiral scanning, CT angiography and multislice scanning, becoming possible as computing power increased. Within a few years, air encephalography at Queen Square was consigned to history, with the suite formally dedicated for this purpose laying idle, and the use of percutaneous angiography also declined.

The Lysholm department continued to expand. In 1975, when du Boulay became director, Ivan Moseley, previously senior registrar, was appointed to the staff and the two radiologists at Maida Vale, Brian Kendall and David Sutton,[56] also started working at Queen Square.

Brian Kendall[57] had been appointed as consultant radiologist to Maida Vale Hospital in 1967, and moved to Queen Square and Great Ormond Street in 1975. He was appointed director of the Lysholm department in 1984 on the retirement of du Boulay. In the same year, John Stevens joined the staff and, in 1985, Derek Kingsley became the fourth member of a team which became renowned for its advanced neuroradiology and its training. In the 1970s, Kendall devised techniques for treating cerebral haemorrhage by inserting small home-made balloons into blood vessels to occlude aneurysmal dilatations, a novel method at the time. Kendall was awarded the Barclay Medal in 1988 and became president of the British Society of Neuroradiology in 1992. He was one of the new breed of radiologists with a brilliant

capacity to interpret subtle changes on MRI scanning, using his extensive knowledge of neuroanatomy and its variation, and his intuitive understanding of MRI physics. He also excelled in interventional treatment of vascular anomalies, and published many clinical and technical articles. He retired from the National Hospital in 1994, as was then the contractual obligation on reaching the age of 65 years, but continued to work without payment as radiologist to the National Society for Epilepsy and remained active on a sessional basis at the Royal Free Wellington and Princess Grace Hospitals in London, as well as building up a busy medico-legal practice, highly regarded by many lawyers, until his death in 2015.

After the 1970s, the Lysholm department became much busier, as the potential for neuroimaging impacted more and more on the practice of neurology. The radiologists were now recognised to be international experts but the clinical demand was such that very little experimental or basic science work was carried out in these years. In 1980, a third CT scanner was installed, the EMI CT5005, and, in 1983, a CT9800 was funded through research grants. New applications for ultrasound and isotope scanning were identified and these technologies were sometimes used in combination with CT, for example in studies of cerebral blood flow using stable xenon on the CT9800 scanner, in stroke and epilepsy.

Then, in the 1980s, a totally new technique arrived, which was to overshadow the unique place of CT imaging in clinical neurology and, for the second time in less than 20 years, another huge step forward was taken by neuroimaging. This technology was known initially as Nuclear Magnetic Resonance scanning (NMR). This time, Queen Square was quickly in on the act. After the first images of a human finger were shown in 1974, EMI built a head scanner in 1978 and installed the first clinical instrument at the Hammersmith Hospital in 1980, based in the unit directed by Professor Graeme Bydder.[58]

---

[56] David Sutton was born into a poor Jewish immigrant family in Manchester, and qualified in medicine in 1942 from Manchester University. He served in the RAMC in Burma and there became interested in radiology. He trained with Bull and became the second person in the UK to practise percutaneous angiography. He was appointed consultant radiologist at Maida Vale in 1950 and moved to Queen Square in 1975. He was also head of the radiology department at St Mary's Hospital. He edited the *Textbook of Radiology* (Edinburgh: Churchill Livingstone, 1969) and published *Angiography* (Edinburgh: Churchill Livingstone, 1962). He retired in 1984, later developed Parkinson's disease, and died from a coronary thrombosis.

[57] Brian Ernest Kendall was born in Bolton and lived as a child in Limerick, qualifying in medicine from Trinity College Dublin. He moved to London in 1954 and his intention was to specialise in paediatrics, but he developed pulmonary tuberculosis and had to avoid contact with patients for two years. He then switched to radiology and obtained his first consultant post at the London Chest Hospital. He then moved to the Middlesex Hospital where he specialised in neuroradiology. He was a humorous person, well liked by everyone and a superb teacher.

[58] NMR was entering a world which was becoming intensely commercialised. In 1977, General Electric Company had also begun to develop NMR imaging and, in April 1981, acquired the Picker Corporation and the rights to MRI from EMI, including their programme at the Hammersmith Hospital. Other companies involved at this stage included M and D Technology from Aberdeen, led by Professor Mallard, who installed a machine in St Bartholomew's Hospital, and Oxford Instruments, who produced the magnets. These and many other companies soon became involved in manufacture. Aggressive recruitment of scientists from Britain, in what was an NMR brain

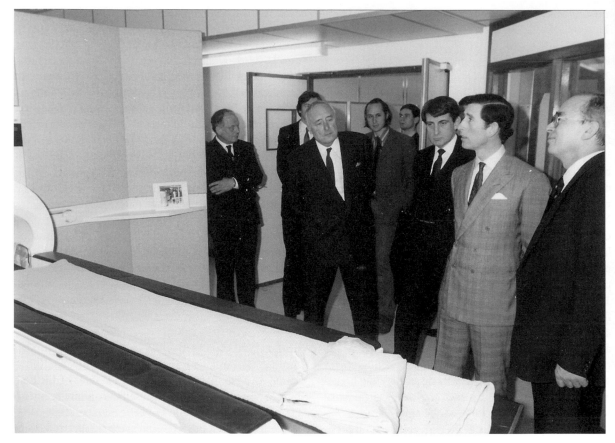

Figure 11.4 Opening of the NMR scanner by HRH Prince Charles (right), with Reginald Kelly (left) and Ian McDonald (centre), and George du Boulay (far right) (collection of Alastair Compston).

Within a year, Bydder and colleagues had demonstrated that NMR could identify the lesions of multiple sclerosis.[59] NMR was soon rapidly applied to other neurological fields and quickly usurped CT imaging in many of these.

---

drain, included William (Bill) Edelstein from Aberdeen, who was instrumental in the development of GE's famous Sigma range of scanners. Protected by the US government, these companies began a series of take-overs which destroyed the British manufacturing effort, and GE became the predominant manufacturer by the mid-1980s, with only Siemens and Phillips competing in Europe.

[59] I. R. Young *et al.*, 'Nuclear Magnetic Resonance Imaging of the Brain in Multiple Sclerosis', *Lancet* **317** (1981): 1063–6; S. A. Lukes *et al.*, 'Nuclear Magnetic Resonance Imaging in Multiple Sclerosis', *Annals of Neurology* **13** (1983): 592–601; E. S. Sears, 'Nuclear Magnetic Resonance versus Computerized Tomographic Enhancement Imaging in Multiple Sclerosis: An Apples and Oranges Comparison?' *Annals of Neurology* **15**. 3 (1984): 309–10.

Ian McDonald recognised the potential for NMR in the study of the pathogenesis of multiple sclerosis and persuaded the Multiple Sclerosis Society to fund a 'Multiple Sclerosis NMR Unit' at Queen Square, the first imaging unit in the world dedicated to research into multiple sclerosis. The Society provided a grant of £1 million, an enormous award for the time that reflected confidence in McDonald and Queen Square. They were not to be disappointed. The unit was opened in 1984 by Prince Charles and had a Picker superconducting NMR imaging system, initially at 0.25 Tesla. Dr Reginald Kelly, physician at Maida Vale and dean of the Institute of Neurology, was chairman of the Medical Advisory Board of the MS Society and no doubt an important influence on this decision. The first published report from the unit was a letter in the *Lancet* published in December 1984 in which the diagnostic value of NMR was demonstrated in 60 patients with MS, of whom 59 had lesions revealed by NMR.[60] The original scanner was upgraded to 0.5 Tesla in January 1986, and a GE 1.5 Tesla scanner and Philips 3 Tesla scanner were installed in 1991 and 2008, respectively, each improvement being funded by grants from the MS Society, who also provided a succession of five-year programme grants to sustain the research. Under McDonald's leadership, the focus of the research was diagnosis and understanding of the pathogenesis of MS and on MR physics, but his successors moved towards developing outcomes for clinical trials. Other grants were also received from the Wellcome Trust, the MRC, the NHS and from the pharmaceutical industry for studies of the effects of drugs in reducing the accumulation of MS lesions. Over 100 fellows, from many parts of the world, worked on the unit over the period of its MS Society grant income, and over 1,000 papers were published. Another important feature of the unit was its emphasis on MR physics, and, in parallel with the clinical studies, a programme of applied physics research was also prosecuted, with an emphasis on finding new sequences and improved scanning techniques.[61]

For a time, the MS Society scanner was the only MR machine at Queen Square, but, before long, NMR was applied to many other neurological conditions. Although CT continued to be an important clinical tool in the acutely ill patient, in bone pathology, and for its ease of co-registration with other technologies, the advantages of NMR were quickly appreciated. The MS scanning unit at the hospital provided an example of what could be achieved through research funds. Although commonplace in many American universities, this was a new departure for the National Hospital. But, as the demand for MRI increased exponentially in the 1980s and 1990s, the hospital had difficulty managing the enormous clinical pressure for scans even when, in 1985, another machine was bought by the Queen Square Imaging Centre.[62] At times, the waiting list for routine scans reached 12–18 months. The NHS simply could not afford to provide MRI scanners to public hospitals in sufficient quantity. That situation improved in later years but, with the relentless increase in requests, mobile MRI scanners placed on lorries and parked outside the hospital, hired from private suppliers on a temporary basis and creating a rather sinister presence with large power cables leading from the hospital and emitting loud thumping sounds as the scans proceeded, became a common sight.

Scanning technology also improved rapidly, inspired by the massive global market for radiological equipment, which at the time of writing is around $12 billion. Industry stepped in, and regular international meetings of radiology have enormous commercial exhibitions with companies showing new hardware and software. For a hospital to choose equipment and compete in the race to equip proved difficult, and so it was at Queen Square.

In 1964, at the Hammersmith Hospital, a radionucleotide scanning method was developed, which was designated Positron Emission Tomographic (PET) scanning. This technology provided images of the distribution of radioactive-tagged molecules, and required the presence not only of a scanner but also of a cyclotron to produce the radioactive ligands. A PET scanner was installed in the Functional Imaging Laboratory at Queen Square for a number of years and then decommissioned. The major clinical use of PET scanning has proved to be as an adjunct for the detection of metastases from malignant tumours, and it has greater value in non-neurological indications. Arising out of developments in the field of imaging using PET scanning at the Royal Postgraduate Medical School, Hammersmith Hospital, a Functional Imaging Laboratory was created in 1995, directed by Professor Richard Frackowiak, which evolved into the Leopold Muller Functional Imaging Laboratory and Wellcome department of imaging neuroscience, based in the refurbished St John's House. Functional imaging attracted a great deal of attention and its scientists became amongst the most cited in the world. A particular contribution was the introduction of

---

[60] I. E. Ormerod *et al.*, 'NMR in Multiple Sclerosis and Cerebral Vascular Disease', *Lancet* **324** (1984): 1334–5.

[61] As mentioned earlier, Nuclear Magnetic Resonance (NMR) was the original term for the scanners, but the word 'nuclear' was thought by some to hold too many negative connotations in the post-Cold War period, and so the technique began to be universally known as Magnetic Resonance Imaging (MRI). At Queen Square, the designation 'NMR' stuck, and the facility continued to be known as the MS NMR unit.

[62] The Queen Square Imaging Centre, based at Queen Square, was a non-profit private company providing scanning in the private medical sector. Its profits were donated in their entirety to the National Hospital and it remains one of the few examples of a social enterprise working for the direct benefit of the NHS.

statistical parametric mapping (SPM) which became a gold standard for analysis of functioning imaging data.[63]

In 1993, the National Society for Epilepsy raised £3 million to establish an Epilepsy Research MRI unit, closely modelled on the MS NMR unit. The money raised included £1.2 million from Glaxo. Initially, it was hoped that an epilepsy scanner could be placed at Queen Square, but the dean opposed this idea (for reasons that were never made clear). It was therefore decided to site the purpose-built unit at the Chalfont Centre for Epilepsy. This was a radical step and propelled the Chalfont Centre to the forefront of the international research arena. A major decision had to be made about whether to purchase an off-the-shelf commercial machine, or to link up with Peter Mansfield from the University of Nottingham and acquire a prototype of the advanced echo-planar research scanner being developed there.[64] The latter option promised innovative research at Chalfont, and the former a safer but less exciting prospect of routine MRI. After much agonising, a GE 1.5 Tesla scanner was purchased and installed in 1994. The Queen Square–Chalfont research link became firmly established, and, over the next 20 years, the unit remained in the vanguard of MRI research in epilepsy.

Following the example of multiple sclerosis and epilepsy, the dementia group at Queen Square also purchased dedicated research time on a hospital scanner and used MRI to detect atrophy as a surrogate for disease progression in neurodegenerative disease. Thus, by investing in brain imaging as research technology and dedicating facilities to specific clinical conditions, Queen Square consolidated its position as an internationally renowned centre for imaging research.

The technological advances in radiology since 1970 were not confined to CT and MRI. Of great importance also was the introduction of digital imaging, made possible by advances in computing power. Digital subtraction angiography (DSA), in which computing systems converted analogue fluoroscopic images into digital data, was implemented at Queen Square in the late 1980s, although in later years it was largely superseded by CT-based angiography.

Initially, physicians and surgeons looked at X-ray plates and made their own decisions about what these showed. It was only in about 1920 that reporting became the function of the radiologist and, at the same time, radiographers and physicists and others were excluded from this role. By the 1930s, there were agreed formats for the systematic reporting of X-ray images, and so it remained until the 1980s. However, with the advent of digital slice images, physicians and surgeons assumed an increasingly large role in interpreting the scans, although the official 'report' still remained with the radiologist.

In the 1990s, interventional radiology became a major part of the hospital's radiological service. This focused on the endovascular treatment of cerebral aneurysms and arteriovenous malformations (AVMs) and soon displaced neurosurgery in the treatment of uncomplicated cases, and became an adjunct to surgery in other vascular lesions and tumours. This major change in practice was led especially by Brian Kendall, who became internationally known for his skill in this area. A new angiographic suite devoted to interventional studies was opened by the Minister of Health, Frank Dobson, in 1997. A new radiologist, Wendy Taylor, was appointed in December 1993, and she specialised in this area. Links were made with Professor Lasjaunias, a Parisian radiologist and anatomist who visited London on a regular basis, attending the vascular meetings to discuss the treatment of difficult cases (and, in 2010, interventional radiology was granted subspecialty status with its own training curriculum). The interventional radiographic therapy and vascular radiology at Queen Square expanded, and the number of operations on aneurysms, previously a major activity of the neurosurgical department, reduced to a trickle over the period of only a few years. A small turf war has been conducted ever since the 1990s about who 'owned' patients treated by endovascular means. On several occasions, the Medical Committee debated the proposal that a patient should be admitted directly under a radiologist, and not a neurologist or neurosurgeon. This was turned down in a manner reminiscent of the earlier arguments about ownership of 'beds', which had recurred regularly since the foundation of the hospital.

Another problem arising from the proliferation of imaging technologies and capabilities was the troubling tendency to over-investigate and order multiple

---

[63] The technique was invented and developed by Professor Karl Friston FRS who, based at Queen Square, became one of the most influential theoretical neuroscientists of his generation.

[64] Sir Peter Mansfield had introduced magnetic resonance imaging, work for which he received the Nobel Prize for physiology or medicine in 2003, jointly with Paul Lauterbur.

screening investigations, without considering what individual tests might contribute. There was an urgent need to assess the specificity and sensitivity of each investigation, and their relative utility in specific clinical situations. This was recognised within the hospital and often discussed. Radiologists challenged clinicians on the value of so many tests and requested prior discussion on the schedule, but in the rush of clinics this was seldom achieved. The number of scans carried out rapidly increased, causing repeated logistic problems.

A profound change was initiated in 1996, when the Hammersmith Hospital opened a film-less radiological unit. This experience was invaluable in assisting University College Hospital to trial a Picture Archiving and Communication System (PACS), and the National Hospital was nominated as the trial location. This led, within ten years, to the complete termination of the practice of presenting radiology in the form of films. The previously common sight of doctors carrying around A3 sized packages of radiographic images came to an end and the X-ray viewing boxes, which had proliferated on all wards and offices, became obsolete as imaging moved to digital viewing. The experience of the Hammersmith Hospital was invaluable in assisting UCLH to set up the system at the National Hospital. However, PACS was only fully implemented at Queen Square by the year 2000. In parallel, a massive programme was initiated for retrospectively digitising existing patients' radiological films, and the huge stores of radiology films and reports completely disappeared.

Clinical Neurophysiology at Queen Square

In the nineteenth century, physicians at the National Hospital laid great emphasis on pathology and morbid anatomy. Jackson considered that all diseases must have a pathological basis, even if microscopic and invisible. To be familiar with the anatomical and pathological basis of neurological disease was an essential requirement for all neurologists. By contrast, although modern neurophysiology had its origins in the early nineteenth century, physiological ideas were not easily linked to neurological disease, and the contribution of physiology was less valued. Studies of reflex action were initiated in the nineteenth century, pioneered by Marshall Hall and taken up by Brown-Séquard, but the most important step in the advance of neurophysiology – and one with which Ferrier and Horsley were intimately involved –

was its utility in asserting the doctrine of cerebral localisation. Experiments were carried out by electrical stimulation (and lesioning), and electricity was also adopted as a therapy. However, electrical measurements for diagnostic purposes were not considered – or, indeed, possible.[65]

In the early twentieth century, understanding of the physiological basis of neural activity and neurological symptoms advanced greatly through the experimental work of Sherrington on decerebrate rigidity, reflex function, spinal cord and brain stem function, and the reciprocal innervation of agonist and antagonist muscles. He defined the word 'synapse' and recognised the importance and inter-dependence of neural facilitation and inhibition. Under Sherrington's influence, British neurophysiology came to the forefront of biological science, and his laboratories in Cambridge and also the work in the universities of Liverpool and Oxford, gave Britain unrivalled prominence in contemporary science. Amongst those who contributed to the rapid development of neurophysiology in the first half of the twentieth century were Lucas, Head, Rivers, Adrian, Hodgkin and Huxley – the latter three, with Sherrington, receiving Nobel Prizes for their physiological discoveries. This work, however, remained experimental, and had remarkably little translational impact on the day-to-day practice of neurology, at Queen Square or elsewhere. Indeed, Walshe, in his celebrated lecture on 'The Present and the Future of Neurology', given as late as 1959, had a point when he deprecated the contribution of neurophysiology as an abstraction which had contributed nothing to 'the age-old burning problems of the etiology, pathogenesis or treatment of the many chronic and killing affections of the nervous system'. As he put it in

---

[65] Interestingly, the role of 'electricity' in diagnosis had been the subject of *A Practical Treatise on Electro-diagnosis in Diseases of the Nervous System* (1882) by Alexander Hughes Bennett, a physician at the Hospital for Epilepsy and Paralysis in Regent's Park. He believed that research into electricity in neurology had been discredited by unscrupulous practitioners using electrotherapy, and was falling into disrepute. He claimed that the diagnostic potential of electricity was underestimated: 'there are already enough facts to indicate the great practical importance of the subject, and to point to a vast field of research, which will doubtless lead to future profit'. Of course, in those days, the technologies were not sensitive enough to record electric potentials from the human nervous system, but his predictions about the diagnostic value of 'electricity' were to prove correct.

a lecture at Columbia, he considered that the upsurge of interest in the electroencephalogram (EEG) was getting 'out of hand with its bloodless dance of action potentials'.[66] It is interesting that he did not include 'diagnosis' as one of the age-old burning problems, for it was in the field of neurological diagnosis that physiology was beginning, in the period after the Second World War, to have an impact – a role in which the National Hospital played an important part. Walshe's dismissal of neurophysiology chimed with the emerging view that the EEG had its limitations, at a time when neurophysiology of the peripheral nervous system had yet to flourish. Nevertheless, it was in this period that clinical neurophysiology began to make its mark.

Electroencephalography at the National Hospital 1936–1948

The EEG was the technology that, in the late 1930s and 1940s, launched the discipline of clinical neurophysiology. The story is well known. In 1875, Richard Caton in Liverpool had shown that the exposed hemispheres of rabbits and monkeys exhibited electrical activity. Other research followed and Hans Berger recorded the first human EEG in 1924 and named this the *Elektrenkephalogramm*.[67] His discovery was largely overlooked until E. D. Adrian and B. H. C. Matthews published a paper in 1934,[68] confirming the findings and bringing them to the attention of the wider community. The first clinical EEG department (the electroencephalographic laboratory) opened in 1936 at the Massachusetts General Hospital. The importance of EEG in human disease, and especially in epilepsy, began to be explored. In Boston, the leading figures were Frederick and Erna Gibbs, Stanley Cobb, Hallowell and Pauline Davis, and William Lennox. At the same time, in London, a series of clever, young, physiologically minded scientists and physicians also became involved in EEG, although the Second World War temporarily suspended their efforts. The National Hospital, was a magnet and amongst those involved who worked either at Queen Square or Maida Vale were E. D. Adrian, Denis Hill, Frederick Golla, William Grey Walter, William Cobb,[69] George Dawson and Denis Williams. Herbert Jasper visited Queen Square before setting up his own renowned EEG department in Montréal, and in the immediate postwar period, London was, for a short time, with Boston, the epicentre of the EEG world. Organised by Grey Walter, chaired by E. D. Adrian, who was then president of the EEG Society, and with 80 participants from 16 countries, the first international EEG congress was held in London at the National Hospital on 14–16 July 1947.[70] In Britain, in these early years, EEG studies were centred at Queen Square with Cobb, Dawson and Williams, at the Maudsley with Hill, Golla and Grey Walter and, after their move, in Bristol at the Burden Institute with Golla and Grey Walter.

Cobb pointed out that the first one-channel EEG at Queen Square was carried out in 1935 by Frederick Lemere,[71] a year after the publication of Adrian and

[66] Cited in F. C. Rose, *History of British Neurology* (London: Imperial College Press, 2011). Rose also cites Walshe's remark that students 'must not think that physiology began with the introduction of electroencephalography; it didn't, any more than civilisation began with the Declaration of Independence'.

[67] H. Berger, 'Über das Elektrenkephalogramm des Menschen', *Archive für Psychiatrie und Nervenkrankheiten* **87**. 1 (1929): 527–70.

[68] E. D. Adrian and B. H. C. Matthews, 'The Interpretation of Potential Waves in the Cortex', *Journal of Physiology* **81** (1 December 1934): 440–71.

[69] William Albert Cobb was born in Margate, educated at Dauntsey's School (as was Martin Halliday), and qualified in medicine from St Bartholomew's Hospital in 1936. In addition to his work at Queen Square, he was a founder member and later president of the EEG Society (1974–6) and subsequently the Association of British Clinical Neurophysiologists. He served as president of the International Federation of Societies for Electroencephalography and Clinical Neurophysiology (IFSECN) and as editor of *Electroencephalography and Clinical Neurophysiology* (known by all as 'the EEG journal') for many years.

[70] The EEG Society in Britain was founded in 1943, the first in the world (the American EEG Society was not formed until 1947). Adrian's opening address is a most interesting document, reproduced in M. R. Nuwer and C. H. Lucking, 'Wave Length and Action Potentials: History of the IFCN', *Clinical Neurophysiology* **51** (supp.) (2010): 3–10, which includes a photograph of the delegates in the lecture theatre at Queen Square. Even by then, the limitations of EEG were beginning to be recognised: as Adrian put it, 'some of the dreams of the adolescent have been abandoned: the EEG is not the sure guide to the state of the brain that we may have hoped it would become, but we now know far better what it can show and what it cannot and the physician and surgeon have far better reason to trust the advice you can give them'.

[71] Lemere was visiting Adrian on a Rockefeller Foundation scholarship and recorded patients with disseminated sclerosis at Queen Square: see F. Lemere, 'The Significance of

Matthew's paper, but this was merely a prelude to the more systematic work on EEG at Queen Square started by Denis Williams. As a young training neurologist in the mid-1930s, Williams had been awarded a Rockefeller Travelling Scholarship to Harvard, where he found himself working with William Lennox and Stanley Cobb at the time they were exploring the potential of electroencephalography in epilepsy. The newly applied technology was headline news and Williams was in the right place at the right time.[72] It must have been with a sense of optimism that he returned to Britain in 1936 by ship, with an electroencephalograph machine (probably a 3-channel early Grass machine) that he installed at Queen Square – in all likelihood, the first in Europe. On his return, Williams began his work on electroencephalography at the National Hospital but, unfortunately for the hospital, the war intervened and Williams was enlisted in the Royal Air Force and moved with his machine to Oxford, where he carried out notable studies of flying stress with Charles Symonds in the head injury unit at St Hugh's.

Another important strand in the rise of EEG and clinical neurophysiology at Queen Square was work in the MRC neurological research unit, directed by Carmichael. Towards the end of the war, Carmichael actively recruited the technician Bert Morton and the clinical scientist George Dawson[73] to his unit. Morton had recently served in the Army as a radar sergeant, and, as Gilliatt pointed out, the technologies of radar, developed because of war, accelerated the growth of electronic engineering, which created dividends for British clinical neurophysiology. Furthermore, and fundamentally, war also forced basic scientists to focus on immediate and practical applications of their work.[74] Although the war had prevented the National Hospital from implementing EEG and rivalling the Massachusetts General Hospital in the mid-1930s, the very British skill in devising practical yet advanced technology was stimulated by the war and was to stand the National Hospital in good stead in the post-war years.

The minutes of the Medical Committee for 28 June 1943 record that the Air Ministry had offered to return the hospital's electroencephalograph machine but had refused Arnold Carmichael's request for the services of Squadron Leader Denis Williams to interpret the findings. Following this refusal to release Williams, in July 1943 Denis Hill, who was then working at the Maudsley, was approached by the National Hospital to enquire whether he would report on encephalograms.[75]

Individual Differences in the Berger Rhythm', *Brain* **59** (1936): 366–75.

[72] Denis Williams was born in Bangor, where his father was a Presbyterian minister. He trained in medicine at Manchester. Williams was 'clever, articulate and amusing, nimble of mind and elegant in dress'. He was unusual in not having worked as resident medical officer before becoming a consultant at Queen Square, as one of the physicians appointed just before the introduction of the National Health Service (in a post held jointly with St George's Hospital). His interest in epilepsy developed during his time in Boston and remained his focus within neurology but, although a popular teacher, he did not carry out much research after his move to Queen Square. The striking characteristic of his clinical work was interest in the lives of his patients, not just their diseases. He combined a very sound understanding of neurology, and an air of authority, with genuine kindness and sensitivity. Williams had a very large private practice attracting the rich and famous from all over the world (one of his favourite questions to aspiring colleagues was 'How many kings have you treated?') and was the only doctor at the time to hire a suite of rooms at Queen Square for the purpose. His secretary, Betty Osborne, ran his schedule and his practice. He founded the Brain Research Trust for which he raised several millions, in an utterly selfless manner, for the benefit of others at the National Hospital. He served on numerous bodies and committees, as treasurer of the International League Against Epilepsy, editor of *Brain* and second vice-president of the Royal College of Physicians of London. He was appointed CBE in 1955.

[73] George Dawson trained in medicine in Manchester and, after reading Adrian and Matthew's paper, built his own 1-channel EEG machine (there were less than half a dozen in the world at that time) and used this in Geoffrey Jefferson's unit there. He served in the RAF Volunteer Reserve as a doctor at the beginning of the war but was then invalided out because of tuberculosis and became the medical officer at the David Lewis Epileptic Colony. There, he recorded myoclonic epilepsy and discovered the giant central EEG potential accompanying a myoclonic jerk, and then moved to Carmichael's MRC unit at Queen Square: see M. Merton and H. Morton, 'Obituary: George Dawson (1912–1983) and the Invention of Averaging Techniques in Physiology', *Trends in Neurosciences* **7** (1984): 371–4.

[74] Golla also worked on radar in the Second World War.

[75] Sir John Denis Nelson Hill was educated at Shrewsbury School and graduated in medicine from St Thomas' Hospital. Whilst working as house physician to Russell Brain at Maida Vale in 1936, he saw Grey Walter's home-made electroencephalograph, and realised its potential for psychiatry and epilepsy. He joined the staff at the Maudsley Hospital in 1938 and worked during the war at Sutton Emergency Hospital. He was appointed to Queen Square in 1946 as physician in applied electrophysiology, as physician in psychological medicine at King's College Hospital in 1947, and as senior lecturer in neurophysiology at the Institute of Psychiatry in 1948. He was appointed to

Terms for the sessional work were a fee of 2 guineas for the examination, with 50 per cent paid to the reporting physician. The hospital engineers, under the supervision of Dawson and Hill, were constructing a 4-channel EEG machine. By 1945, work had increased to such an extent that Hill told the Medical Committee it was no longer possible for him to carry on using the existing facilities, and reporting on so many recordings in the time available. Denis Williams was approached again and, immediately after demobilisation at the end of 1945, he was appointed registrar at Queen Square and promoted to assistant physician in 1946.

In 1945, the Medical Committee made a number of important decisions which were to influence the development of electroencephalography at the National Hospital over the next few decades. Charles Symonds wrote to the Board of Management asking them to consider purchasing, presumably as a second machine, 'a modern 6-channel EEG apparatus now on order from the USA, with the object of installing it in the hospital'. Notwithstanding Walshe's criticisms, the development of neurophysiology as a distinctive feature of work in the hospital was endorsed. The minute recorded that:

> Considerable discussion took place. Dr Carmichael pointed out that instruments were being built in the hospital workshops and which were of superior quality as well as lower cost than those which could be purchased from America or outside instrument firms … To provide an adequate service in the hospital it was essential that at least two instruments each with its technician should be in use in the hospital, quite apart from the research instrument in use in the Research Unit. This would necessitate the rehousing of the department elsewhere.[76]

In the event, the Board agreed to purchase Williams' EEG machine, authorised construction of another instrument under the direction of George Dawson, took on further technicians, invited Drs Williams and Hill to assist with the reporting, and

---

a professorship at the Institute of Psychiatry in 1966, remaining there until retirement in 1979, and in that post was profoundly influential on the development of psychiatry in Britain. Hill recruited Slater and Alwyn Lishman to the Maudsley from Queen Square. He was knighted in 1966.
[76] The minutes confirmed that 'one such four-channel instrument was already being assembled and should be ready in March 1945; assuming that further technical assistance is provided, it should be possible to produce a second instrument of similar design fairly soon thereafter … the hospital would save a considerable sum of money'.

appointed Williams with responsibility for the general administration of the department based, at least for the first year, in David Wire ward. Clearly the hospital was prepared to invest heavily, as it did later in relation to magnetic resonance imaging, and, in both instances, although stretching the finances, the backing of new technologies and new disciplines proved to be of great importance for the hospital's reputation. Carmichael was asked to oversee the interests of the Medical Committee in the deployment of EEG, liaise with Hill, Williams, Cobb, Dawson and Morton, and not to ignore the need to provide adequate electroencephalography services for private patients. A newly established department of applied electrophysiology was duly established, with Williams as its temporary head. Williams also set up a special clinic for epileptics in 1946, modelled on the epilepsy unit in Harvard created by Lennox. In that respect, however, due largely to lack of resources, the clinical electroencephalographic work at Queen Square did not match that in Lennox's clinic; nor, at that time, did it nurture epilepsy research to the level achieved in Boston. Over time, Williams' involvement in EEG waned and his interests turned more to clinical neurology, and especially epilepsy.

Whether, thus placed at the forefront of hospital activities, electroencephalography actually fulfilled the promise of those years is arguable (as Adrian recognised in his 1947 address), but neurophysiology of the brain and peripheral nervous system assumed much prominence at Queen Square in subsequent years. By 1951, 12-channel machines were in routine use, and, in 1951, Dawson published his first paper on averaging, which transformed the whole field of neurophysiology. Dawson was medically trained but at heart more of a physiologist, and he was recruited by Carmichael to join the MRC unit after the Second World War to work on EEG. He built EEG machines and devised ingenious methods for averaging over many readings, producing recordings that were more sensitive than those obtained using conventional methods. He invented a method for reducing the signal-to-noise ratio and, in 1951, built electronic averaging equipment that was in advance of any previous machine and used this to record evoked potentials to study peripheral nerve and muscle. A subsequent version of the averaging system, using a barrier grid storage tube, was used in Gilliatt's laboratory in the 1960s to record the amplitudes of sensory and motor nerve conduction.

The Departments of Applied Neurophysiology at the National Hospitals 1948–1969

When the National Health Service was founded in 1948, there were two independent departments of applied neurophysiology, at Queen Square (since 1946) and at Maida Vale. The main focus was on EEG; indeed, the Queen Square department was generally known as the electroencephalographic department, although, by the mid-1950s, studies of the peripheral nervous system were also beginning to become established. William (Bill) Cobb was appointed as the only senior full-time staff member at Queen Square, with Denis Williams and Denis Hill as visiting physicians to the department. Sam Nevin had responsibility for neurophysiology at Maida Vale.

EEG was by then being used in the routine investigation of diverse neurological and psychiatric conditions, and the number of examinations carried out each year was rapidly escalating. By 1950, for instance, 3,657 EEGs (with activation methods), 75 electrocardiograms (ECGs) and 86 EMGs were performed, and the first annual report of the Institute of Neurology (1950/1) noted that the provision of service to the hospital allowed little time for research. Cobb was also keenly interested in training and teaching and he ran three annual courses with around 22 students each year, many of whom subsequently established their own units around the world. These training courses were a key factor in the high reputation that the unit had achieved. In that respect, Cobb's role at Queen Square was similar to that of George du Boulay in radiology, and, by 1953–4, he had impressed the Medical Committee to the extent that he was granted the title of physician; and this was a sign that he, and his department, were now recognised as indispensable.

Staffing then increased. Tom Sears was appointed as physiologist in 1954/5, and took an academic title as lecturer in 1955/6. But, despite the growing interest in research, the demand for clinical work continued to expand in these early years, and, although some clinical studies were undertaken, most developments were technological rather than providing insights into the pathophysiological theory. Dawson, Merton and Bert Morton were all physiologically minded and, by 1955 for instance, Merton had devised a 16-channel EEG machine, built in the department. Measurements of nerve conduction were also being introduced, using equipment designed by Morton and Sears. As the number of examinations continued to increase, with 4,423 in 1957/8, the vast majority of which were standard EEGs, the unit was then provided with purpose-built facilities on the mezzanine floor. In 1955, Roger Gilliatt was given the responsibility for electromyographic examinations as these also had increased in number, with 1,417 examinations performed in 1960. In that year, Denis Hill resigned as visiting physician and Cobb was joined by John Bates, who held two consultant sessions in the department, spending the rest of his time working as a member of the MRC external staff. An academic registrar was appointed (half-time) and a research assistant (initially Dr Graham Wakefield[77]), with four hospital registrars and one senior registrar. The number of examinations now was around 5,000 - per year but, with the increase in staffing, research was being pursued more actively.

Gilliatt was joined by Robin Willison[78] to work on peripheral nerve and muscle in 1964 and, in the same year, Tom Sears was appointed senior lecturer, and then, in 1968/9, reader. Martin Halliday, another member of the MRC external staff, joined Bates as a part-time worker in the neurophysiology department in 1965/6. In the following year, Wing

---

[77] He was subsequently appointed consultant neurologist in Bath.

[78] Robin Willison was educated at Highgate School, and qualified in medicine from Oxford and the Middlesex Hospital. He served with the RAMC at Wheatley and in Oxford, working with Ritchie Russell and Charles Whitty and using the new artificial ventilators on paralysed patients. It was in Oxford that Willison's interest in neurology and neurophysiology developed. Initially, he was appointed to the Middlesex Hospital as an MRC research fellow, working on analysis of peripheral nerve and muscle activity with Roger Gilliatt. In 1962, he moved to the National Hospital and the Institute of Neurology as a neurophysiologist based in the new university department of clinical neurology, also working under Roger Gilliatt, and then progressively increasing his hospital sessions to became a full-time NHS neurophysiologist in the department of clinical neurophysiology. On Cobb's retirement in 1980, Willison became head of department, a post he held until his own retirement in 1990. He was a pioneer of electromyography and a crucial collaborator and supporter of Roger Gilliatt. They held each other in mutual respect, and when he attended ward rounds, Gilliatt would often address Willison to the exclusion of all others present. Robin's son, Hugh Willison, became professor of neurology at Glasgow University and is an expert on the neurobiology and immunology of peripheral nerve disease.

neurophysiology. This was perhaps a reflection of rising interest in experimental neurophysiology which emanated from the clinical studies. Tom Sears was appointed as head of the new department, with a personal professorship. This was initially a small group with Sears, one lecturer (D. T. Stagg) and two research workers (P. Kirkwood and C. Bainton, the latter visiting from the USA). To begin with, the research focused on anatomical localisation of respiratory neurones in the medulla. In 1974, Hugh Bostock joined the department and, in June 1975, the University of London established the Sobell department of neurophysiology, as the fifth university department at the Institute of Neurology,[84] with Sears as the first established professor. By 1977, Kirkwood, Stagg and Bostock had been appointed as lecturers and there were three visiting research fellows from abroad and two attached workers. The research interest remained the physiology of respiration, cardiovascular reflexes and nerve conduction. In 1978, Stagg retired and was replaced by Anthony Pullen as lecturer. Research activities increased over time so that, by 1980, there were seven attached workers and two PhD students, in addition to Sears, Bostock, Pullen and Kirkwood. In 1990, Pullen was appointed senior lecturer and Bostock as reader. The research portfolio widened and became less focused, and in the 1991/2 annual report, Sears described the Sobell department: 'Although nominally dedicated to neurophysiology, work in the Sobell Department has a wide brief, encompassing systems neurophysiology, membrane biophysics, neuroanatomy and cell biology, and utilises electrophysiological, ultrastructural, immunocytochemical, and tissue culture techniques. The research is predominantly basic and directed towards fundamental problems of direct relevance to neurological disease.' This having been said, the department did not expand at the same rate as others in the Institute of Neurology and its style was for few but careful publications (around 7–10 in most years).[85] However, at a time when all consultant neurologists had to learn some neurophysiology and many were required to provide that service

to district general and regional centres in the United Kingdom, the Sobell department served also a training role. Indeed, the dual training at Queen Square in clinical and basic neurophysiology contributed to the scientific qualities and reputation of British clinical neurology in that period.

In 1993, Sears retired after 20 years as head of department, and a three-day symposium was held in his honour. He was replaced by Professor Roger Lemon who moved from Cambridge to Queen Square in December 1993. The grant income of the department increased rapidly, with Lemon, Kirkwood and Pullen supported by the Wellcome Trust for studies of the pathways and mechanisms by which the cerebral cortex controls voluntary movement, and studies of the cerebral control of hand and finger movements. The research direction of the department was now more aligned with the studies in the university department of clinical neurology of movement and its disorders, introduced by David Marsden when he transferred to Queen Square, and the linking of clinical and basic research led to a rapidly rising reputation in this area, a model of interdisciplinarity which was to characterise much of the subsequent research at Queen Square. Lemon reintroduced primate research (with macaque monkeys), making him, in subsequent years, a target for animal rights activists. He became dean and director of the Institute of Neurology in 2002, and, in July 1995, Daniel Wolpert joined him as lecturer. His work with Lemon was supported by the MRC, with a large grant to study motor planning in primates.[86] In 1996, Bostock was awarded a personal chair, and elected FRS in 2001; his interest in biophysics and ion-channels took the work of the department into another area where Queen Square was able to make important contributions in understanding the pathogenesis of epilepsy and neuromuscular disease. Research in these years attracted collaboration with groups in Germany, France, Finland, Japan, the USA and Canada.

The appointments of Marsden to the university department of clinical neurology and Lemon to the Sobell department, after the retirements of Gilliatt and Sears respectively, signalled a change in style and momentum at the Institute at a time when, for better or worse, biometrics were becoming increasingly important and the success of a university department

---

[84] The other university departments were in clinical neurology, neurosurgery, neuropathology, and chemical pathology and neurochemistry.
[85] In 1984/5, for instance, the department of neurology published 205 papers, neurosurgery 83, neurochemistry 64, neuropathology 49 and the Sobell department 27. In 1989/90 the figures were: neurology 461 articles, neurosurgery 44, neuropathology 33, neurochemistry 58 and the Sobell department 18.

[86] Daniel Wolpert subsequently became professor of engineering in Cambridge, specialising in bioengineering and the robotics of movement. He was elected FRS in 2012.

was increasingly measured in grant income, publications and number of PhD students, and the establishment of large-scale groups and international collaborations. This was the beginning of a rapid and escalating change in the culture and ethos of university science and, in contrast to former years, Queen Square did not stand aside.

There was a further significance in the work of the Sobell department. Over the previous long period in which Queen Square did not invest in basic science – a deficit which came close to tripping up the institution when neurobiology, immunology and molecular biology began to make their impact – the Institute of Neurology could now turn to its experimental and clinical neurophysiology portfolio and rightly claim to be highly successful in basic, translational and clinical research.[87]

Clinical Neurophysiology at the National Hospital After 1969

When Nevin retired in 1969, the independent hospital departments at Maida Vale and Queen Square were merged under the leadership of Bill Cobb. By then, there were six other part-time consultant neurophysiologists in the merged department – Halliday, Bates, MacGillivray,[88] Willison, Wynn Parry and Kocen –

and also Pat Merton[89] joining in an honorary capacity.

A key technological development was the introduction of computers, moving neurophysiological studies from the analogue to the digital age. In 1969, a PD12 computer was installed at Queen Square, and this stimulated development of evoked potential measurements and new analytic techniques for recording the EEG, and these became the focus of clinical practice and of research. It was the time too when Marsden, Morton and Merton were conducting their first experiments within the department on the stretch reflex and servo mechanisms, using the PD12 computer, which had a significant effect on the study of movement and its disorders.

William Cobb retired in 1980 after more than 30 years in charge of the hospital department. He was a leading figure in the world of clinical neurophysiology and the department had flourished under his leadership. During the Second World War, he had worked as an anaesthetist with the Emergency Medical Service at Hurstwood Park, and, whilst there, he was guided to an interest in EEG by Harvey Jackson. At the end of the war, he transferred to the National Hospital, with the return of the neurosurgical unit, as a part-time anaesthetist and a part-time researcher in Carmichael's MRC unit. There, he collaborated with George Dawson and Bert Morton in constructing EEG machines, and with Denis Williams in setting up the clinical EEG service with a 3-channel EEG machine. Initially, Cobb was employed as a class II officer

---

[87] As mentioned throughout this book, our policy of not describing the work of living persons makes for all too brief a description of contemporary work at Queen Square. This is particularly true in the field of neurophysiology, which expanded greatly in and beyond the period where our narrative stops and where much illustrious work was carried out.

[88] Barron Bruce MacGillivray was born in Durban, South Africa, and educated at King Edward VII School, Johannesburg, entering medical school at the University of Witwatersrand. He was a vocal opponent of apartheid, and, because of the political situation, moved to Britain in 1951. He qualified in 1955 from Manchester, gained the MRCP in 1959 and moved to Maida Vale, initially as a registrar and then as a senior registrar. In 1962, he graduated MB BS (a rare example of obtaining the MRCP before qualifying MB) as an external student. He was appointed as a consultant clinical neurophysiologist and neurologist at the Royal Free Hospital in 1964, spent a year in research at UCLA, and in 1971 was appointed consultant neurophysiologist at the National Hospital. He retired in 1992. MacGillivray worked on EEG and its automatic analysis, and had a special interest in metabolic disorders and computer-aided EEG diagnosis. From 1975 until 1989, he served as dean of the Royal Free Hospital School of Medicine and this role (in the era of several green papers and the Todd and Flowers reports) consumed much of his energies. He had a longstanding

interest in medical education and made important contributions to this field, in addition to clinical neurophysiology. He died after a long, complex and debilitating illness.

[89] Patrick Anthony Merton was born in Kent, educated at Ampleforth and Beaumont, and graduated from Cambridge and St Thomas' in 1946. Eschewing clinical medicine and deciding on a career in science, immediately on graduation he applied for and was appointed to the staff of Carmichael's unit. He remained there from 1946 until 1957, when he became lecturer in physiology at Cambridge, and he was awarded a personal chair in human physiology there in 1984. He was elected FRS in 1979, and in the same year appointed as an honorary consultant neurophysiologist at the National Hospital. Even while at Cambridge, his experiments, where they involved patients, were conducted at the National Hospital, and he there carried out a series of profoundly important studies of human muscle, muscle spindles, the stretch reflex, the control of movement and muscle fatigue and also pioneering work on transcranial magnetic stimulation which was to have an important clinical role in later years.

seconded from the Ministry of Health (with a salary of £800 a year), but when the department of applied neurophysiology was established in 1948, Cobb was appointed as consultant in charge and gave up his work as an anaesthetist. In addition to EEG, he also became interested in evoked potentials and made original observations on pattern reversal stimulation, including the first successful recording of half-field visual evoked potentials (VEPs) (following a suggestion from Adrian) but leaving Martin Halliday to exploit this clinically. Cobb wrote papers on many aspects of clinical neurophysiology, including on EEG in Creutzfeldt-Jakob disease. This led him, in 1970, to visit the highlands of New Guinea, with Susan Sanders, his technician, performing EEGs on tribesmen with Kuru, in collaboration with R. W. (Dick) Hornabrook, and was disappointed to find that the EEG changes proved rather non-specific.

When the university established the Sobell department in 1975, the hospital department underwent a name change to become the department for clinical neurophysiology. Cobb was replaced in 1980 as head of department by Robin Willison who had by then moved all his sessions from the university department of clinical neurology to a full-time hospital position. There were now eight part- or full-time consultant neurophysiologists: Bates, Halliday, Kocen, MacGillivray, Merton, Small, C. E. Storey[90] (as a locum until March 1980) and Horace R. Townsend (from January 1980). The clinical load continued to expand as neurophysiological testing entered routine clinical practice (exactly as CT scanning had done) and the department became an important facility in the two hospitals, with, by 1982, over 10,000 diagnostic examinations carried out at Queen Square and 3,000 at Maida Vale.

Clinical research also expanded under Willison's leadership with work on quantitative assessment of EEG and processing of EEG signals, EMG, evoked potentials (EPs) and autonomic function. In 1982, Nick Murray was appointed as a full-time consultant neurophysiologist, so that the department then had three full-time consultant neurophysiologists (Willison, Townsend and Murray), four part-time consultants with other positions in the hospital or university (Bates, Halliday, Kocen and MacGillivray) and five

attached workers, and a steady stream of research papers were published.

In August 1989, Willison retired and Horace Townsend was appointed head of the department. New appointees in that year included David Fish, Clare Fowler and Shelagh Smith. Townsend, Fish and Smith focused on EEG in epilepsy, reflecting the rapidly growing resurgence of interest and renewed commitment of the hospital to the condition that had first inspired the Chandler siblings. An epilepsy surgery programme was initiated, centred around the new EEG telemetry unit and the utilisation of novel recording hardware and analytical software developed in-house. The departmental research expanded into transcutaneous electrical and magnetic stimulation, magnetoencephalography, sleep studies, brain mapping and epilepsy. Academic work flourished and, in terms of publications and training, the hospital department was more active than the university Sobell department, which continued to focus on basic research. MacGillivray retired in 1992, having served as a consultant at the National Hospital for over 20 years, and he was replaced, in 1993, by Bryan Youl. When Horace Townsend retired in 1994, Nick Murray took over the headship of the department. Dr G. L. Sheean briefly joined the department in a linked consultant appointment with St Mary's in April 1996, but left for the United States in December 1997.

In the 1990s, the departmental research concentrated on epilepsy, evoked potentials and electromyographic techniques. Murray carried out early studies of single-fibre EMG in myasthenia gravis (and also experimental EMG in mice with induced myasthenia) with John Newsom-Davis, and on human transcutaneous magnetic cerebral electrical stimulation.

One particular characteristic of the hospital department was its strong collaboration with physiological work taking place in other units, particularly within the university department of clinical neurology, the MRC unit, and the units of uro-neurology, autonomic disease and neuro-otology. The neurophysiological research of MRC external staff included the work of Bates, Nathan and Halliday, and when the MRC unit closed on Halliday's retirement in 1991, 50 years after it was established by Carmichael, a large body of important physiological work had been achieved. Physiological research in the field of neuro-otology was undertaken initially in collaboration with the neuro-otological research unit headed by Hallpike, which evolved into the MRC Hearing and Balance

---

[90] Catherine (Kate) Storey spent some years in London and worked particularly on evoked potentials with David Small before returning to Sydney.

Unit headed by Hood, and then was incorporated into the MRC Human Movement and Balance Unit under the directorship of David Marsden in 1989. Bannister[91] founded a unit dedicated to the investigation of autonomic function, one of the first in the world, supported by the appointment of Christopher Matthias as senior lecturer and honorary consultant in 1988. Bannister's textbook, a pioneering work that stimulated interest worldwide in autonomic disease and inspired the

establishment of autonomic investigation units along the lines of that at Queen Square in many other countries, is a classic in the field.[92] Clare Fowler created a uro-neurology unit which soon moved from the hospital department to the university department of clinical neurology, led by David Marsden, and carried out pioneering studies of the neurogenic bladder, detrusor innervation, and intra-vesicular techniques for managing urinary dysfunction. She defined a new eponymous syndrome of urinary retention in young women, and characterised previously unknown abnormalities of unmyelinated bladder wall nerve fibres in tropical spastic parapareisis.

A Perspective on the Role of Neuroradiology and Clinical Neurophysiology at Queen Square

The phenomenal rise of technologies of neuroradiology and neurophysiology is a remarkable story. Prior to their introduction, diagnostic neurology was confined to the evaluation of clinical symptoms and the physical examination. Indeed, the high reputation of the National Hospital was largely due to the development of a system for clinical history-taking and examination which spread around the world. Pathological examination helped confirm the diagnosis but not usually in life. All this was to change with the introduction of radiology and clinical neurophysiology, as complementary methods for revealing structure and function in neurological disease. These were supplemented by neurochemistry, recognised by Walshe in his 1959 lecture, and only fully realised with the advent of molecular biology and genetics, developments which largely postdate our history.

Radiology and neurophysiology share certain characteristics. Both depend on technologies derived from physics, engineering and computing. In the case of radiology, the technologies were developed largely elsewhere and subsequently introduced at Queen Square. The uptake of the earliest ancillary investigations – angiography, encephalography and myelography – was slow, but lessons had been learned, and the introduction of MRI (and, after a stuttering start, CT) was rapid and altogether more decisive. It was explicitly recognised then that early investment in new technology was a vital priority for the National Hospital in

---

[91] Roger Bannister was born in Harrow in 1929, attended University College school and studied medicine in Oxford and St Mary's. As a young man, he was Britain's leading mile and 1500-metre runner, representing his country in the 1952 Olympics, the British Empire Games and European Games, and, a few months before qualifying in medicine in 1954, he became the first man to run the mile in under 4 minutes (3 min 59.4 seconds, a feat then thought almost impossible). The 4-minute mile was voted the greatest sporting achievement of the twentieth century. That said, Denis Williams, on seeing Sherrington's film demonstrating a decerebrate dog running on a treadmill, shown at an ABN meeting, remarked: 'You will see, Dr Bannister, it is not necessary to have a brain in order to run fast'. In conversation, Bannister attributed his outstanding ability as an athlete to the favourable distribution of muscle fibre types that gave him an advantage over others for acute anaerobic exercise. But he decided to pursue a career in medicine rather than in athletics and continued his training in Oxford and London, and then, after National Service in the Army, moved as a registrar to the National Hospital in 1959. In 1962, he spent a year in Harvard, having been awarded a Radcliffe travelling fellowship, and in 1963 was appointed consultant neurologist at the Western Ophthalmic (now Eye) Hospital, St Mary's Hospital and the National Hospital. It was here that he developed his lifelong research interest in diseases of the autonomic nervous system. In 1974, he was badly injured in a road traffic accident, which caused problems with walking for the rest of his life, and then gave up his private practice to continue his autonomic research. He worked first on the Shy–Drager Syndrome (multiple system atrophy) and made a number of important contributions to the field. He founded the Autonomic Research Society, and published the first edition of his celebrated textbook in 1982. He was knighted in 1975, and in 1985 returned to Oxford as master of Pembroke College. He served as chairman of the Sports Council (1971–4) and president of the International Council for Sport and Physical Recreation (1976–83), and on many other committees in the fields of health and sport. He died from complications of Parkinson's disease in 2018. Although seen as somewhat aloof by colleagues and trainees at Queen Square, Bannister was greatly admired and well liked by sportsmen of all ages and those with whom he interacted in Oxford. Several anecdotes that demonstrated his attractive personality and human qualities appeared in the national newspapers after his death.

[92] R. Bannister, ed., *Autonomic Failure: A Textbook of Clinical Disorders of the Autonomic Nervous System* (Oxford University Press, 1982).

order to stay ahead of the pack. In the case of neurophysiology, innovation often occurred inside the National Hospital, partly because the technologies were simpler and cheaper, but also because new ideas came more easily to the physiologically minded physicians and scientists. Thus, the initial recording equipment for EEG, electromyography, evoked potentials and nerve conduction was made in-house. Later, instrument manufacture was ceded to industry, and domestic apparatus appeared increasingly amateur. The last homemade appliance was the EEG telemetry equipment, but even this was soon replaced by commercial off-the-shelf apparatus. The hospital's real contribution was therefore not in the manufacture of these diagnostic tools, or even in contributing to the theoretical basis, but, rather, in working out the indications and limitations of the technologies and their application to its huge and diverse patient base. This translation was achieved with great skill, and it ensured a surge of reputation for many of the hospital staff. It reaffirmed the close relationship of clinical and experimental medicine, and the fact that medicine is, at its core, an applied science.

Another striking aspect relating to the development of these specialties at Queen Square was the strong interaction between the Institute and hospital departments. This applied particularly to the close relationship between members of the university department of clinical neurology and the hospital department of applied neurophysiology (later clinical neurophysiology). The university provided clinical and technical support and the hospital supplied well-characterised clinical material, and this was a powerful and mutually beneficial arrangement. These links in physiology were stronger perhaps than in any other area of work at Queen Square and serve as a model for future development.

The trajectory of the new technologies in radiology and neurophysiology, such as EEG, CT and MRI, followed a very similar pattern. There was a very rapid take-up as soon as they were available for clinical practice. The technologies then inevitably strained the capacity of the hospital departments to cope with demand and waiting lists grew, with pressure to increase staffing and resources an inevitable consequence. The size of both departments of radiology and neurophysiology did increase rapidly and each became central to hospital practice, but the enthusiasm engendered by the new non-invasive diagnostic technologies led invariably to over-use, and attempts to rein in unnecessary referral by guidelines or rules were often ineffective. However, as their novelty waned, the usage of the new technologies became more refined and more appropriate. EEG, for instance, was used initially to investigate a wide range of psychiatric and neurological conditions, but by the 1970s its limitations were fully recognised and its usage became confined mainly and more appropriately to the investigation of epilepsy and management of patients in the ITU. The same reduction occurred in use of CT scanning, although this was largely the result of introducing MRI, which has shown no sign of reduction despite large numbers of normal investigations. The waxing and waning of the demand for new and expensive technologies, and the tendency to over-use, did at times put enormous pressure on the hospital finances, sometimes relieved only by appeals for philanthropic and research grant support.

Another noticeable trend, as new technologies became embedded into clinical practice, was for researchers to introduce novel technological variants, only some of which proved to be of clinical utility, and an overall strategy often proved lacking. In EEG, for instance, newer methods such as computerised analysis, brain mapping and power spectrum analysis all failed to make an impact, despite the investment of considerable time and energy. In radiology, similarly, a number of new MRI and CT sequences and new post-processing tools were developed or applied at Queen Square, but only a few proved of lasting clinical benefit. Whether a more thoughtful appraisal or strategy could be applied to such developments is not clear.

In such fast-moving technological fields, redundancy of equipment became another recurring issue, and in both radiology and neurophysiology, a pattern developed in which whole technologies were rendered obsolete by the next advance. It proved difficult and expensive to respond by reinvesting in new instruments in the clinical setting, but this was vitally necessary if the National Hospital was to remain in a leading position. At times, the decision to abandon a redundant technology was made too slowly, much to the frustration of those involved.

The focus of physiological investigation also has changed over time. Clinical neurophysiology began with the EEG and an emphasis on the central nervous system, but this changed over time to be dominated by the physiology of peripheral nerve and muscle. In relation to diseases of brain and spine, the demonstration of structure had more utility than that of function, and, like EEG, newer technologies for studying central nervous system physiology – transcutaneous electrical (and subsequently magnetic) stimulation, brain mapping and evoked potentials – proved of only limited value. Perhaps function is too complex, involves too many brain structures and is too subtle to be dissected by the tools being applied.

As neuroradiology and neurophysiology developed, training became an important function of the hospital departments. Both developed excellent schemes and most of Britain's future neuroradiologists and clinical neurophysiologists, and many from abroad, benefited from attachments or full-time posts in the hospital. This contributed significantly to the rising reputation of Queen Square in this period. The small number of clinical neurophysiologists in Britain in the mid to late twentieth century meant that clinical neurologists often had to perform their own studies, and the training of neurologists in this period often included an attachment to clinical neurophysiology at the National Hospital. Senior department staff in radiology and neurophysiology were prominent in the national and international societies, ensuring further influence of Queen Square on the development of both specialties.

The evolution of radiology and clinical neurophysiology reflects in many ways the general trends in development of the National Hospital in the postwar years. These included the inexorable rise in costs and the constant squeeze on resources, the growing reliance of the clinical service on academic and research activity, the need to remain flexible and manage change, and the importance of introducing new technologies in maintaining the position of Queen Square as a leading national and international centre. Rapid growth from the 1980s transformed the hospital, physically and in terms of its style and reputation in the modern age. Large areas of the basements of the Queen Mary and Powis Place wings, Queen Square House and 8–11 Queen Square became devoted to radiology, with, by 1997, four large MRI scanning units, angiography and CT, and an interventional suite. Radiology had become by far the largest of the diagnostic departments and occupied a central place in the life of the hospital. The scale of these developments has made for the largest change in the organisation within the hospital over the past three decades. However, Queen Square, through introducing technology and nurturing academic work, remains at the forefront of both specialties and, seen from the perspective of a hospital founded in 1859, these two specialties have moved diagnostic neurology forward at a considerable pace and over a relatively short time. Their success provides a template for implementing technologies that will follow – for instance, in the field of molecular biology and genetics – and the new fields would do well to learn from the experience of the old.

Chapter

12

The Medical School and the Institute of Neurology

Almost from the start, medical education was one of the National Hospital's objectives. As early as 1861, Brown-Séquard and Ramskill lectured at the hospital on anatomy and physiology, and on the diagnosis and treatment of epilepsy and other nervous disorders. The Board of Governors expected the physicians to give such lectures and this requirement was subsequently written into their contracts and the bye-laws, explanation being needed if they failed to comply. In due course, lectures were delivered at Queen Square, and published along with books and papers, by most physicians appointed to the hospital, including Radcliffe, Buzzard, Reynolds, Bastian, Jackson and Gowers. Lectures were delivered in the late afternoon, probably in one of the outpatient rooms, and, from 1890, also in the operating theatre. Then, as now, some of the staff were also invited to deliver prestigious lectures in the medical calendar, including the Croonian lectures of the Royal Society and the Royal College of Physicians, and the College's Goulstonian lecture and Harveian Oration.[1] This worked to the advantage of both the hospital and the medical staff, with publicity attracting wealthy and influential subscribers and patrons, and enhancing professional reputations.

In 1880, the importance of medical education in the work of the hospital became more formally acknowledged by the appointment of James Ormerod as the first dean of medicine. Soon after, the physicians' rota of regular attendances for

teaching was fixed and it became customary to offer practical clinical teaching for the junior staff in the outpatients' clinic on three or four days each week. In 1888, a notice was first published that students and all medical practitioners were invited to attend. The first sessions were offered by Gowers, as assistant physician, and became extremely popular, contributing to the reputation of the hospital. Formal teaching on inpatients was initially discouraged but, from 1902, special tickets began to be issued for students to accompany Gowers and some of the other physicians around the wards. Although these were at first less popular than outpatient teaching, eventually large crowds attended the bedside rounds, and, after a few years, these lectures and teaching clinics were prized by students from all over the world. The more prestigious visitors to the hospital, including Jean-Martin Charcot, were themselves also invited to lecture. As one delegate to the London International Medical Congress (1881) wrote:

> The National Hospital ... has become an authority on the treatment of nervous disease, not only in the United Kingdom but in every land where English is read or spoken. Men skilled in the medical profession come to it from all parts, in order to see the treatment employed for the amelioration and cure of those mysterious maladies with which it deals. As many as 2000 such visits were paid last year.

In 1902, the house physician, Dr Goldwin Howland (a Canadian who returned to Toronto to become a leading neurologist), similarly observed:

> This hospital holds an important position as the centre for the study and treatment of nervous disease in Great Britain – indeed for all English-speaking countries ... professional men of almost every nationality daily visit [the] hospital, in order to gain an acquaintance with the various forms of nervous disease and their treatment, and to carry the knowledge obtained to all parts of the world.

---

[1] Between 1860 and 1902, Queen Square consultants who gave the Goulstonian (before the end of the 19th Century, the spelling was often Gulstonian) lectures were Radcliffe (1860), Brown-Séquard (1861), Jackson (1869), Ferrier (1878), Tooth (1889) and Rose Bradford (1898); the Croonian lectures (Royal College of Physicians) were given by Sieveking (1866), Radcliffe (1873), Jackson (1884) and Ferrier (1890); and the Harveian Orations were delivered by Sieveking (1877), Russell Reynolds (1884) and Ferrier (1902). The Croonian lectures at the Royal Society were delivered by Brown-Séquard (1861), Ferrier (1874, 1875) and Horsley (1891).

According to a later estimate, 2,500 qualified doctors attended clinical lectures or ward rounds between 1887 and 1896. The intensity of teaching was not, however, without its detractors, and in the 1890s Burford Rawlings began to ask whether neurological education and research were being pursued at the expense of care for patients, but the lay managers and supporters were content to bask in the reflected glory of the reputation of the medical staff. Over time, Burford Rawlings increasingly felt that there was too little regard for the philanthropic ethos and original purpose of the hospital, and became convinced that the institution was being corrupted by excessive medicalisation. He recruited the more conservative Board members onto his side, and this issue was one of the major factors leading to the showdown and appointment of the Fry Commission in 1901. After Rawlings' departure and the overthrow of the old regime in the hospital, teaching and research were fully endorsed and supported, at least in principle.

The Medical School 1895–1950

Although the relatively informal arrangements for postgraduate medical education were quite adequate in the early years of the National Hospital, by the 1890s there was a need for much greater organisation in order to keep pace with the growth in complexity of medical practice and changes to the training of both doctors and nurses. At the same time, the increasing prestige of the staff seemed to call for more explicit acknowledgement of the hospital's educational role. Inevitably, there arose a growing demand for formal recognition, by professional bodies and London University, of the hospital's status as a teaching institution within the orbit of London postgraduate medical education. But the university demurred, and its failure formally to recognise the medical school in the first half of the twentieth century was a recurring bone of contention. Given the intransigence of the university, in May 1895, Beevor[2]

suggested seeking approval from the Royal Colleges of Physicians and of Surgeons for formal recognition as a teaching institution. The Board agreed to pursue this, and Burford Rawlings approached the Conjoint Board. In November 1895, he was able to notify the Medical Committee that he had succeeded, and the annual report for 1895 duly announced 'That the Conjoint Board of the Royal College of Physicians and the Royal College of Surgeons have granted ... official recognition to the Hospital in its teaching capacity ... arrangements are now completed ... for the establishment of a [Medical] School, and for carrying out ... regular courses of clinical instruction with Lectures and Demonstrations.'

The Colleges' recognition of the medical school was an important step and, notwithstanding the university's refusal to accredit the School, education at the National Hospital was now put on a more official footing. Beevor was appointed dean of the medical school (1896) and, for the first time, a formalised system of teaching was introduced, including lectures and instruction in pathology. The central position of education at Queen Square was reinforced when, in 1903, the hospital was granted a Royal Charter which included the stipulation that a medical school should be an integral part of its activity.

The hospital was now the only institution in the capital providing postgraduate instruction in neurology. Nevertheless, despite this privileged position, its teaching activities were plagued with difficulties over the next 35 years, including: concerns about finance and student numbers; the crisis produced by the First World War; unwelcome meddling (as it was seen) by government attempting to improve the provision of postgraduate education in London; continued lack of recognition by the University of London; and, finally, the threat in the 1930s posed by creation of the British Postgraduate Medical School. These issues loomed like dark shadows.

---

[2] Charles Edward Beevor was born in London, the son of a surgeon, and educated at Blackheath Proprietary School and University College London. He was appointed resident medical officer at the National Hospital (1880), assistant physician (1882) and physician (1883–1908). He carried out experimental work with Horsley on the representation of movements in the primate cortex (published in the *Proceedings of the Royal Society*). His best research was on the morphology and distribution of the arteries of the brain, using coloured dyes injected via the great vessels, in the laboratory – an important conceptual advance that contributed to the development of angiography and to the concept of cerebral infarction. His Croonian lectures at the Royal College of Physicians (1903) on the cortical representation of movement stated that 'the condition of the antagonists acting before the principal movers begin, I have never seen in any other conditions besides those of so-called hysterical or functional paralysis'. This is the basis for Beevor's sign of upward umbilical movement in paralysis of the lower abdominal muscles and legs. He described the jaw jerk, and stated the axiom that 'the brain does not know muscles, only movements'. Beevor died suddenly from a coronary thrombosis, after the annual dinner at the Royal Society of Medicine.

The medical school was surprisingly active, considering its lack of dedicated premises and minimal finances. Thus, in 1903, 732 medical graduates from Australia, Canada, India, the Cape Colony, Ceylon, the USA, Germany, Italy, Greece, Sweden, Denmark, Switzerland, Bulgaria and South America, as well as every part of Great Britain and Ireland, made nearly 3,700 attendances, and corresponding numbers for the next few years were broadly similar. In the first decade of the twentieth century, three courses of 20 lectures were given in the spring, summer and autumn sessions, each attended by around 20 fee-paying students, with further special courses of lectures, clinical demonstrations and pathological laboratory work given in the summer. Clinical clerkships were available for postgraduates holding the 'yellow tickets' of the London Postgraduate Association, both in outpatients and on the wards. James Collier[3] is said to have been the first to instigate the form of public clinical demonstration at the National Hospital, held on Wednesdays and Saturdays, in which the patient's signs were demonstrated in front of the audience (although demonstrations had been performed since the time of Gowers). Dressed in black coat and striped trousers, he used every trick of display, exaggerated gesture and emphasis to capture his audience's attention. Flights of fancy scandalised some of Collier's more sober colleagues, and postgraduate students were regaled with his repertoire of incredible fishing yarns. At the inception of each demonstration, the resident medical officer was advised not to attend because 'sometimes', Collier explained, 'I am tempted to take liberties with the clinical history and I might be rather embarrassed if I realised that you were listening.' For many years, until shared out amongst the staff, these clinical demonstrations remained Collier's sole responsibility.

Whilst appreciating benefits brought by the medical school to the hospital's reputation, the Board of Management was clearly concerned by the drain on financial resources, and, in July 1911, asked the school to pay a fixed annual sum to cover the costs of rent, rates, water, heating and lighting. Partly for this reason, a new comprehensive scale of fees was adopted in 1911. Ordinary students were charged 1 guinea for three months, or 3 guineas for 12 months, to cover the privileges of attending outpatient and inpatient teaching and clinical lectures, and the opportunity to clerk patients and attend operations. A further fee of 2 guineas was levied for a trimester of inpatient clerking, and 5 guineas for a 'perpetual ticket'. Doctors visiting from overseas and local practitioners attending the teaching were requested to hand their visiting card to the hall porter for presentation to the dean of the medical school, and those holding the membership card of the London Postgraduate Association were admitted without additional charge. In 1913, 81 students 'subscribed to the hospital practice' in this way, of whom six clerked on the wards and one worked in the pathology department. A further 54 subscribed between January and July 1914, of whom six were based in the wards and one in the laboratory.

Postgraduate medical training in London at the time lacked any coordination and this began to cause widespread disquiet. The concern was strongly articulated, at the International Medical Conference in London in 1913, when Dr C. O. Hawthorne, chairman of the Medical Graduates College and Polyclinic in London, addressed a special symposium on postgraduate education. Hawthorne pointed to the lack of

---

[3] James Stansfield Collier, the son of a Cranford doctor, trained at St Mary's Hospital. He was appointed assistant physician to Thomas Buzzard at the National Hospital Queen Square in 1902 and worked in the pathological laboratory before he became assistant physician and finally staff physician in 1921. At St George's Hospital, where he also held a staff appointment, Collier acquired the nickname of 'Truthful James' because he sometimes consciously exaggerated the number of cases of uncommon disorders he had seen, when teaching the students. For a time he shared consulting rooms with Charles Symonds, where Collier would seek to impress his younger colleague with delightful but invented case histories. Collier was one of the first to recognise subarachnoid haemorrhage, but is best remembered for his paper on subacute combined degeneration of the cord with Risien Russell and Batten, and the sign of lid retraction in midbrain lesions. He also introduced the terms 'false localizing sign' and probably 'motor neurone disease' into neurology. Collier gave the Lumleian lectures on epilepsy (1928), the Fitzpatrick lectures on the history of neurology (1931–2) and the Harveian Oration (1934) on 'Inventions and the Outlook in Neurology' at the Royal College of Physicians. His unorthodox approach was not constrained by convention, and Collier was famous at hospital soirées for attending in fancy dress and performing violent gyrations on the dance floor. His interests outside work included archeology, philately and fly-fishing. His most damning indictment of a person of whom he did not approve was that he was 'the kind of man who has never caught a fish'.

coordination in London of the various educative efforts and what he perceived as a lost opportunity: 'It is notorious that as a centre of postgraduate medical education, London, in proportion to her opportunities and responsibilities, can hardly boast a mere minimum of success.'[4]

He proposed three steps to improve the situation: the establishment of a bureau to act as a central office supporting students; the encouragement of cooperation and coordination between institutions engaged in similar types of work; and the development of a new hospital devoted to postgraduate education. The last proposal was the most far-reaching, for it contained the kernel of an idea that eventually germinated as the Royal Postgraduate Medical School at the Hammersmith Hospital.

> By the development of some such organisation London might well become the centre of post-graduation study for all English-speaking practitioners, while within the borders of the plan could easily be preserved the opportunities which already exist for practitioners resident in the metropolitan district and able to devote only a limited amount of time weekly to the cultivation of some selected branch of clinical or laboratory practice. So long as London is something less than this it is living below the height of its opportunity.

Hawthorne drew unfavourable comparisons with the situation in Berlin,[5] where postgraduate education was better organised but, within a year of the conference, Britain was at war with the country singled out as the model for postgraduate education, and no further progress was made on these points until the Athlone Committee reported in 1921.

During the First World War, as the supply of students largely dried up and most of the younger lecturers were away on military service, activity at the medical school sank to a very low level. By 1917–18, members of the Medical Committee had to meet the operational deficit from their own pockets, and, had it not been for an unexpected request from University College Hospital in May 1918 to allow clinical clerking for medical students in the wards of the National Hospital, the school might have been forced to close. The arrangement proved relatively short-lived but,

starting in 1919, a longer-lasting and more financially beneficial relationship was formed with the London Royal Free Hospital School of Medicine for Women. The question of educating female doctors had long been a contentious issue. Initially, they were excluded from Queen Square but, in April 1891, the Board of Management voted to allow lady practitioners to attend postgraduate lectures given in the hospital. This met with strong resistance on the part of the medical staff, and when, in June 1896, the dean of the School of Medicine for Women again asked the National Hospital to admit female undergraduate students to clinical lectures, the Board reflected the Medical Committee's reluctance, answering 'that it is impossible for the Board to reconsider at the present time their decision of some years ago'. Not until December 1903 did the Medical Committee finally agree to allow women of all grades to be admitted to lectures, but, even in 1916, there was a discussion in the committee about whether women students should be allowed to observe the electrical treatment of male patients. Only in 1919 were a certain number of women from the London Royal Free Hospital School of Medicine permitted to attend ward rounds and clinics at Queen Square on a regular basis.

After 1918, the hospital turned its attention to devising measures which it was hoped would protect it from the fragility of the finances of the medical school exposed during the First World War. A 'Memorandum as to the New Medical School' was adopted in 1919 by both the Board and the Medical Committee, which reconstituted the school as an independent body administratively and financially separate from the National Hospital. The school was to have a new governing body formed from the Medical Committee together with two lay representatives from the Board of Management, and with the dean serving as chairman, but in practice most day-to-day decisions were made by the three-man management subcommittee that was soon established.

The Board's over-riding concern was that the school should be financially self-sufficient and not a burden on general funds, which were by then severely stretched. Clinical and pathology teaching were further systematised, and regular courses of lectures on the anatomy and physiology of the nervous system, pathological demonstrations and lectures, exposure to neurosurgery, and instruction in clinical examination were offered during each university

[4] C. O. Hawthorne, 'An Address on the Position of Post-graduate Medical Education in the United Kingdom', Lancet **182** (1913): 707–8.

[5] Anon., 'Post-graduate Study', Lancet **182** (1913): 745–6.

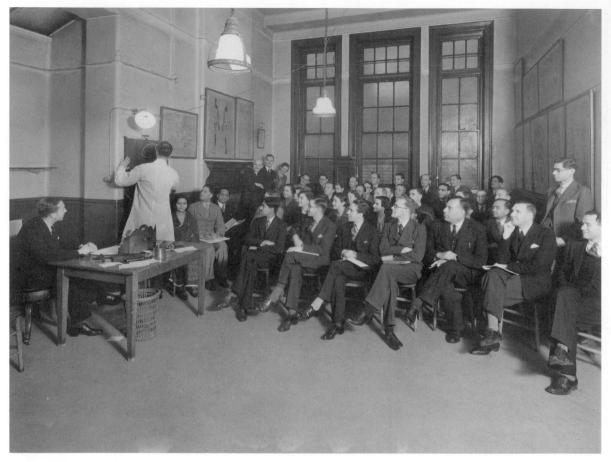

Figure 12.1 Teaching a group of postgraduate medical students.

term. Consideration was given to coordinating teaching with three other special hospitals,[6] but this did not prove feasible. Despite its new autonomous administrative structure, the school continued to rely on the National Hospital for staff and access to clinical material, and space was rented at a cost of £100 per year. In 1924, the school's assets were valued by the Finance Committee of the University of London at only £1,102 and its income at £641. Without property or endowment of its own, until the 1930s income was derived almost entirely from graduate student fees. In 1927, for example, all but £43 of the net income of £589 11s 2d came from this source; and in 1930 fees provided £967 9s 0d out of a total net income of £1,015 3s 1d. Much was being achieved on this relatively modest

budget, and the school managed to run at a surplus in most years.

Despite its precarious financial base, the school had achieved an excellent reputation in neurological circles, both nationally and internationally. Between 1922 and 1938, 250–500 students made around 2,500–4,000 visits to the hospital each year. In addition, there were usually 10–20 clinical clerks from many countries of the British Empire, but also Europe and America, as well as around 50 appointed from the Royal Free Hospital. Much as before the war, medical students paid for tickets which entitled them to attend lectures and take part in ward rounds and bedside clinical teaching on specified days, though there were frequent complaints about unauthorised attendances without tickets and the inaccurate registers of attendance.

These numbers were maintained throughout the inter-war years but, as many of the students were from overseas, in these times of international conflict the

---

[6] These were the Royal London Ophthalmic Hospital, the Hospital for Consumption and Diseases of the Chest, and the Hospital for Sick Children.

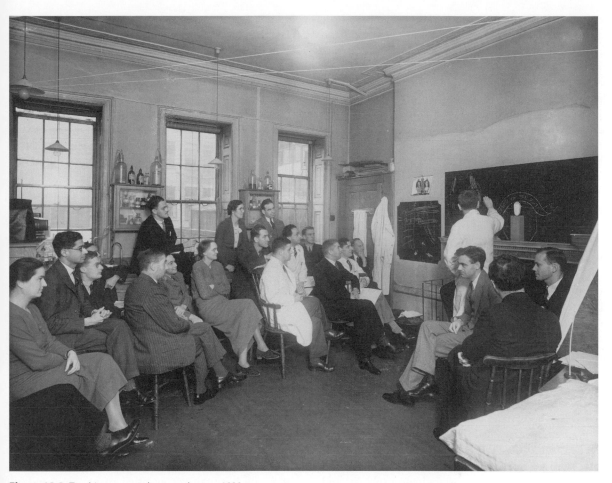

Figure 12.2 Teaching postgraduate students, c. 1930.

supply was vulnerable. Greenfield as dean recognised this threat and in 1930 wrote:

> This school is at present dependent on students from America and the Dominions to such an extent that if for any reason this support from outside Great Britain were withdrawn, it would be unable to continue active teaching ... in order to attract ... students, it is necessary to keep the standard of teaching high ... indeed probably rather too high for the needs of the average undergraduate, but it is well suited to the needs of those who are proceeding to the higher University degrees.[7]

He was right, and, during both World Wars, the student stream became a trickle, and, as many of the teaching staff also became unavailable, activities virtually ceased.

[7] Letter to the Academic Council of the University of London, May 1930.

The British Postgraduate Medical School and Relations with the University of London

After the end of the First World War, the broader issues of postgraduate medicine in London were debated repeatedly. A profusion of reports emerged from various committees, university bodies, government agencies and pressure groups, each offering their own sometimes contradictory recommendations, but all agreed that the provision of postgraduate education in London was chaotic, uncoordinated and failing to realise its potential.[8] Furthermore, in the

[8] These included the Fellowship of Medicine, the Association for Co-operation in Medicine amongst English-speaking Nations, the Emergency Postgraduate Courses Committee, and the Inter-allied Fellowship of Medicine, Postgraduate Medical Association: see G. C. Cook, *John MacAlister's Other Vision* (Oxford: Radcliffe Publishing, 2005).

immediate aftermath of the war, there had been pressure to provide short courses for the many doctors released by the British, American and Empire Armed Forces, and this had highlighted the inadequate arrangements. Although postgraduate educational activities had developed in a number of hospitals in London, including Queen Square, these were neither coordinated, as Hawthorne had earlier noted, nor regulated by any central authority. Furthermore, they were not directly linked to the university. This situation was considered unsatisfactory then, as it had been decades earlier, but what had now changed was the much greater role that central government felt it could take in the organisation of education. Thus, in 1920, the Minister of Health had appointed a committee, led by the Earl of Athlone, chairman of the Middlesex Hospital, to investigate the requirements and structure of postgraduate medical education in London. It reported in May 1921 and reiterated the suggestion made by Hawthorne that a new school of London University, attached to a large hospital of 300 beds, devoted entirely to advanced postgraduate education, should be established, and that the special hospitals with their medical schools should be closely associated with this school. The financial crises of the early 1920s effectively prevented any action on this report but, in 1925, the Minister of Health, Neville Chamberlain, began to take steps to form such a school. He set up a new committee to 'solve the postgraduate problem' and, after much political manoeuvring, the Athlone Committee's vision was realised in 1930 with the establishment, by Act of Parliament, of a new postgraduate school at the Hammersmith Hospital. The London Voluntary Hospitals Committee objected, not least because the Hammersmith was a municipal hospital – in fact (horror of horrors), formerly a workhouse infirmary. They pointed out that, staffed by experienced and knowledgeable clinicians, the voluntary hospitals had traditionally carried out teaching to a high standard, and, furthermore, were concerned also that the new hospital staff would be whole-time university employees, thereby undermining the role of 'famous doctors' and threatening their private practices. The National Hospital, as a member of the committee, strongly supported these objections. Their views were ignored and the government pressed on, and the British Postgraduate Medical School (BPMS) obtained a Royal Charter in 1931 and opened in 1935, with Sir

Francis Fraser appointed professor of medicine. He was able to ensure that the consultant staff of the Hammersmith Hospital were, in large part, full-time academics, a principle that was a break from the past and no doubt ensured the subsequent success of the school.

It is interesting to reflect on the impotence of the voluntary hospitals, including Queen Square, in failing to stop these London-wide developments. In previous times, the opinions of the voluntaries would have held sway but, by the 1920s, central government was taking an increasing role in decisions on health and education, and there was a perception that the voluntary hospitals were out of touch with the pulse of the nation at a time when, increasingly, they were financially dependent on state subsidy. In any event, the logic behind strengthening postgraduate training was irrefutable and this development presented many opportunities for improving medical education. However, achieving the cooperation and collaboration of existing providers, and engendering a greater sense of shared purpose, proved very difficult to achieve in practice, as the hospitals raised objections at every stage.

The National Hospital was insulated from this otherwise risky strategy of obstruction because student and staff numbers in peacetime were relatively stable, but this was to change in the Second World War, much as Greenfield had feared. In the autumn of 1939, the hospital was emptied of patients, and all clinical teaching in the wards and outpatients suspended. Later that winter, the question of restarting some outpatient teaching was raised but the shortage of medical staff made this impossible. Francis Walshe offered to resume the Wednesday demonstrations and these became popular and well attended during the war. Then, as clinical activity in the hospital increased, outpatient teaching was restarted on each day except Saturday (the fee was 2 guineas for three months, but free to members of HM Forces) and a limited number of clinical clerks were appointed. A 'course of wartime neurology' was also agreed,[9] which was so well attended that another, less advanced in nature, was approved for the following winter. Before long, however, the depleted consultant staffing could not maintain these lectures. An indication of how badly hit

[9] This would consist of 12 lectures on neurology and six on psychoneurosis. Dr Hart turned down the invitation to participate and the tuition was provided by Dr T. A. Ross, who was paid 2 guineas per lecture.

financially the medical school now was can be seen from the accounts showing income and expenditure to be matched at £1,057 in 1935, but reduced to £95 and £99, respectively, in 1942.

In 1941, Sir George Broadbridge joined the Medical School Committee. He was also chairman of the Board of Management and, throughout the war, stressed the importance of maintaining as much activity as possible. Broadbridge was the embodiment of the 'Keep Calm and Carry On' campaign initiated by the Ministry of Information in August 1939. He was not one to give in and, despite depleted student numbers, lack of consultant staff and a disastrous financial situation, he emphasised that teaching should continue in anticipation of the hospital reorganisation that he predicted would take place at the end of the war. It was therefore agreed that there should be a course of clinical presentations at Christmas 1941, and another early in 1942. The dean pointed out that staff numbers at the National Hospital were so reduced that it would be necessary to seek help from neurologists not on the consultant staff, and this heretical step was agreed, with requests going first to the undergraduate teaching hospitals. Additional help was obtained from former residents at the National Hospital engaged on EMS duties near London, and the lectures did go ahead, but the impression was that they were 'attended by many who were not interested in systematic lectures', and so it was agreed to focus thereafter on clinical demonstrations as the best form of instruction.

After the BPMS opened in 1935, it had as predicted soon begun to attract postgraduate students who otherwise might have paid fees to the National Hospital medical school. The fledgling BPMS tried to engage constructively with the other London schools but met with continued resistance. In the autumn of 1935, following an invitation from Colonel Proctor, the BPMS dean, the National Hospital medical school did agree to offer 'refresher courses' in neurology for qualified GPs (which must have seemed a calculated insult by the hospital to the BPMS, and a similar suggestion was later made to Maida Vale), and to allow postgraduate students at the Hammersmith Hospital to attend ward rounds at Queen Square. When Colonel Proctor proposed a more comprehensive scheme of collaboration between the two institutions, the National Hospital hastily rejected these proposals as 'impracticable'.

The competition from the BPMS for students was no doubt one reason for rejecting the proposal, but more pressing was the view held by the senior physicians at Queen Square that collaboration would result in take-over. This threat of domination by 'Du Cane Road' preoccupied the minds of the Medical School Committee throughout the 1930s. An olive branch was offered in June 1937 when Greenfield was invited to represent the National Hospital medical school on the Council of the BPMS, one of only three special hospital medical schools given this opportunity. Greenfield saw the benefits of collaboration, mainly in terms of university recognition, but he was unable to persuade his colleagues.

It did not help that Greenfield was handicapped by a long history of failed attempts to achieve university recognition. That saga had rumbled on since the foundation of the medical school at the end of the nineteenth century and had flared up in 1913 when the principal of the university asked Queen Square to delete the phrase 'this hospital is a school of medicine of the University of London' from its documents. A renewed application to the University of London for recognition, made in February 1925, was declined 'owing to the financial position of the Medical School', specifically its meagre assets and dependence on income from fees. Subsequent applications made in 1926–7 and 1930 were again refused on the grounds that the medical school provided almost no undergraduate teaching in neurology, and had no internal students studying for medical degrees in the University of London. Indeed, in 1929, the University had only narrowly refrained from adopting a proposal no longer to recognise clinical teachers attached to the National Hospital unless they were also on the staff of another teaching hospital.

In 1931–2, the medical school reorganised its programme and timetable into a single systematic course of lectures in neurology lasting for 20 weeks, so as to meet requirements of the university and, in 1940, the School again applied for university recognition. That application document provided a summary of facilities and activities which sheds light on the school in these pre-war years.

The National Hospital desires recognition by the University: (i) As providing courses of instruction in neurology for internal students for the degree of MB and MD, and for the DPM; (ii) As providing unique facilities for the study in neurology, both in its clinical and scientific aspects; and (iii) As an institute for research in neurology ... the medical school, with the 'Institute', is housed in new buildings opened in 1938, made possible through the Rockefeller grant ... these new buildings contain a lecture theatre for 120 students, out-patient theatre and a practical classroom, a common room, library, and cloakroom facilities. There are also X-Ray viewing apparatus, an epidiascope, and a large number of wall diagrams.[10]

The application mentioned that the library subscribed to most of the current neurological journals and had many textbooks and monographs. It emphasised that the student body consisted mainly of graduates in medicine, with the occasional scientist or final-year medical student. Supported by travelling fellowships from their universities or the Rockefeller and Commonwealth funds, most were from Canada, Australia and India or the USA, with a few from European countries, South America, Egypt, Iraq and other parts of the world. It was pointed out that, in 1938–9, 203 students had attended, of whom a quarter to a third were studying for an MD degree. Their days were spent in the wards, outpatients, attending lectures or demonstrations, reading in the library, working in the laboratories, dissecting or examining pathological material, or attending post-mortem examinations, and they were encouraged to form clubs for scientific discussion and to support their social life. The document stated that teaching was provided by the honorary medical and surgical staff of the National Hospital, as well as Carmichael and Hallpike, who were employed full-time by the MRC.[11] Laboratories of the medical school and National Hospital were shared, and provided for histology, biochemistry, serology, bacteriology and electrophysiology. There were also nine smaller rooms for individual researchers, and a darkroom. The top floor of the new building, accessible only by a special lift, contained large and small animal rooms, and operating and post-mortem facilities. Two endowed research posts (the Halley Stewart and Kathleen Schlesinger Fellowships) were administered by the MRC, and others were supported by research funds and occasional private donations. Despite this impressive list, the School's application to the university was again refused.

Greenfield realised that the major advantage to the National Hospital of collaboration with the BPMS would be formal recognition of the medical school by the University of London, as this would very likely follow any substantial collaborative agreement. In February 1943, Greenfield reported to the Medical Committee that he had attended three further meetings of the Council of the BPMS, at which incorporation of the National Hospital medical school into an enlarged BPMS grouping had again been under discussion. He had agreed to consider the proposal, provided that 'it was as an equal partner, had financial autonomy and did not lower the standard of teaching given at Queen Square'. He explained to his colleagues that recognition of the National Hospital as a postgraduate medical school in neurology by the University of London would follow as a natural consequence of its association with other postgraduate teaching hospitals in the enlarged British Postgraduate Medical School, but his position was still not supported by the senior physicians at Queen Square, who remained fiercely opposed to any form of amalgamation. In a similar vein, the eight small voluntary hospitals which were most concerned about the risk of domination by Du Cane Road held separate meetings, at which it was agreed that they should cooperate in resisting this threat.[12] In May 1943, a further paper was received from the BPMS, making a plea for more vision and cooperation from these special hospitals.

> London should be the most important medical centre in the world. That it is not is due to 'lack of organization and cohesion' (*Osler Quarterly Review* 1931). After the War, a great opportunity will occur to make London such a medical centre. Large numbers of medical officers of the allied nations will be passing through London. A proportion of these will wish to stay for postgraduate instruction and will be disappointed if it is not available on a generous scale.

---

[10] This document was undated and unsigned, but was presumably written by Greenfield. The School Committee in those days comprised: Greenfield, Carmichael, Denny-Brown, Elkington, Harvey Jackson, Purdon Martin, Grainger Stewart and Julian Taylor.

[11] Greenfield was full-time pathologist and dean of the medical school (receiving an annual salary of £750 from the National Hospital and £150 from the medical school). A list of publications by medical and surgical teaching staff and students was appended to the application to the university, but unfortunately this is not included in the archived copy.

[12] The National Hospital; Great Ormond Street; Royal National Ear, Nose and Throat Hospital; Moorfields Eye Hospital; Maudsley Hospital; Royal London Ophthalmic Hospital; St John's Hospital for Diseases of the Skin; and the London County Council Hospital for Fever: minutes of the meeting of the Medical School Committee, 16 March 1943.

As a result, London's reputation as a postgraduate teaching centre will be made or marred. The medical officers of some forty nations will either recommend London or the reverse.

The document pointed out that, when the BPMS was founded by Royal Charter, one of its roles was the coordination of teaching. In the event, little progress had been made since 1935, and this lack of organised postgraduate medical teaching of university standard had prevented London from becoming as great a world centre of medical education as its facilities justified. Even in those places that did have a high standard of teaching, there was a total absence of any integration. Resolution required the university to provide instruction in all specialties. The BPMS had to be more than just the Hammersmith Hospital and, rather, an organisation that encompassed postgraduate education in all the special hospitals.

To make London the Medical Centre of the world should be easier than 30 years ago when Osler considered that the only obstacles were those 'whom the fear of changes not only perplexes but appals'. All that is required is finance, good will and determination. We hope Governments will provide the first. Is it too much to hope that the Medical Profession of London will provide the rest?

The impassioned plea fell on deaf ears and, despite Greenfield's more conciliatory stance, the National Hospital medical school continued to show little inclination to concede autonomy. The hospital replied:

The Medical School of the National Hospital has considered the memorandum sympathetically, and with interest, but that as several members of the medical staff of the National Hospital were absent on War service, the hospital did not feel able to commit itself at present to co-operation with the British Postgraduate Medical School, and in view of this did not feel justified in accepting the invitation to discuss the terms of co-operation.

The BPMS responded in June 1943 that it was not 'the Du Cane Rd Hospital but an organisation which could span London', that the Hammersmith Hospital would not control the special hospital medical schools nor interfere with them, and that its governing body was concerned with the advancement of postgraduate medical education and not the development of one school at the expense of others. Greenfield then wrote a further paper on 'Teaching at the National Hospital after the War', which was presumably sent to the BPMS. He pointed out that the National Hospital had two main functions as an institution teaching neurology: (1) the education of neurologists and those who wish to combine a sound knowledge of neurology with work as general medical specialists or psychiatrists, as well as of neurosurgeons and surgeons with neurological leanings; and (2) education in research methods, for a smaller number of students. He recognised too that, after the war, the numbers from the USA would probably decrease ('as there were good schools there'), but engagement by the British Empire and Dominions would likely increase as the demand for neurologists expanded. He went on to say that the school should provide a thorough training in the scientific basis of neurology, including anatomy, pathology and physiology, and also ophthalmology, otology and radiology, and in psychiatry matching the standard of the Diploma of Psychological Medicine. After six months of intensive study, students should then work as clinical assistants, with more time spent in outpatients and the wards, and carrying greater responsibility than in the past. Careful selection of students was therefore important. Trainees in neurosurgery should have a good grounding in neurology.

At this point, Greenfield resigned as dean. It was recorded that this was not because of the attitude of his committee to the BPMS, but because he did not have enough time to devote to plans for the future of the medical school. More likely, the highly negative responses from colleagues were partly responsible. Purdon Martin was elected dean, initially on a temporary basis but, in the event, he remained in post until 1948, and was immediately invited onto the council of the BPMS in March 1944. He and Walshe were nominated 'to negotiate with the BPMS'. As the war drew to a close, the need to achieve formal recognition of teaching hospital status became the dominant concern, as it was then realised that, once the hospital was absorbed into the NHS system, this would provide special status and relative independence of management and finances. Greenfield's foresight was beginning to be understood and his position vindicated.

In retrospect, it is clear that the lack of vision shown by the senior medical establishment had, not for the first time, exposed the vulnerability of the National Hospital and its medical school, and led once more to the threat of closure. The entrenched position reflected a sentimental and deeply conservative attitude that neurology was a specialty above all others in its intellectual approach and that the neurologists at Queen Square were endowed with an elite status. A more progressive, insightful and collaborative approach might well have changed the course of neurology at the time. However, subsequent events forced the hospital's hand.

The Goodenough Report and the British Postgraduate Medical Federation

Government was irritated by failure of the special hospitals to engage with the BPMS and, in 1942, had set up a new committee, the Inter-Departmental Committee on Medical Schools, chaired by Sir William Goodenough, deputy chairman of Barclays Bank. The committee was tasked with advising on the future organisation of medical education, and its report was published in 1944.[13] The committee was asked to examine specifically the position of postgraduate medical education in London but at the same time to achieve some form of amalgamation amongst the smaller clinical schools. It was clear from the beginning that the Goodenough committee was to act as the government's executioner, that its main conclusions were determined before the committee met, and that the National Hospital medical school had no chance of survival as an independent entity. It is notable that, amongst almost 300 people invited to give oral evidence, there was not a single nominated representative from the hospital (although Farquhar Buzzard and Bernard Hart were listed as 'independent witnesses'). The hospital did submit a lengthy document, passionately argued and again parading the role, facilities and position of the medical school:

(a) The National Hospital Medical School has a high reputation; (b) recognized by Rockefeller and MRC grants, and has a modern research institute and is 'the obvious centre for the development of a modern postgraduate school of neurology adequate to the needs of

the future'; (c) the scope of neurology is increasing; (d) the National Hospital Medical School is aware of the nature of these problems; (e) it is believed that the hospital and its school can best meet these needs by preserving an independent existence; and (f) its traditions and opportunities would be greatly enhanced by University recognition, by a scheme of control similar to those of the undergraduate teaching hospitals, and by methods of staff appointment likely to become operative in these schools.

The submission made clear the view of the medical staff that the hospital was:

The chief training centre for neurologists, not only of the English-speaking world, but for postgraduates from all the continental countries ... in the present war, the research had been very fruitfully diverted to maintaining the physiological efficiency in fighting man (but the nature of the work 'cannot be divulged') ... it is a quite remarkable achievement, in that what was primarily a neurological research unit within the medical school of the hospital, should have been able to turn over without delay to a field of work directly and greatly serving fighting men ... in the recent past, the view has been expressed that the day of the special hospital and attached medical school is over, and that both should be replaced by the special department in the general hospital ... increased specialization in medicine is inevitable, critical mass of people essential, collocation allows interchange of ideas, this should be a growing point of knowledge, concentration of clinical material and facilities, intellectual isolation is profoundly detrimental ... throughout Europe and America the reverse trend is occurring ... there are three neurological hospitals in London – West End Hospital, Maida Vale Hospital and the National Hospital – and of these, the National Hospital is the largest and the oldest, and the only one of the three which has a modern surgical department, and research institute. It is also the only one in which hitherto research and serious postgraduate teaching have been uninterruptedly conducted. Occasional refresher courses for general practitioners constitute the only teaching formally carried out by the other hospitals, and they have no modern research facilities whatever.

The Goodenough Committee seems completely to have ignored these various points and concluded, as had all other previous reviews, that, despite the establishment of the BPMS, training 'remained insufficient' and the exceptional resources of London as a centre for postgraduate education for medical practitioners from all over the world were under-utilised. Recognising the obstacles to achieving an integrated

---

[13] *Report of the Inter-Departmental Committee on Medical Schools* (London: HMSO, 1944) (the 'Goodenough report'). Published at the time of the Normandy landings, this attracted little attention but was to prove highly influential. The solution for the special hospitals was part of the overall plan to link every hospital to a university teaching centre. Goodenough also considered that, in managing teaching hospitals, equal weight should be placed on clinical care, research and teaching. This was a vision for the future NHS that played to the strengths of the National Hospital in relation to teaching and clinical care.

system, Goodenough proposed that special hospitals constitute institutes for teaching and research in their specialist areas, and that the BPMS be reconstituted as a federal organisation, with the Hammersmith Hospital and the institutes in the special hospitals managed as 'units'. One can sense the frustration of the committee: 'In spite of the size of the task, it is believed that, with support from public funds and the enthusiastic cooperation and goodwill of all concerned, the scheme can result in the building up in London of a great world centre for post-graduate medical education and research.'

Neither neurology nor Queen Square received more than very brief mention in the 313-page report, but it was stated that the Royal London Ophthalmic Hospital, the Hospital for Sick Children and the National Hospital for Diseases of the Nervous System should be among the first of the special hospitals to form institutes and federate them within the new structure, the British Postgraduate Medical Federation (BPMF). The report noted that negotiations along these lines were already under way and it was to be hoped that 'these will be pursued, with mutual understanding, for a successful conclusion'.

As before, during these arduous debates on proposals for a merger between the National Hospital and other London neurological hospitals and the incorporation of the medical school in the larger structures, the lay members of the Board were generally in favour but deferred to the opposing view of the Medical Committee. However, the time for prevarication had passed and it was quite clear that incorporation was inevitable. On 6 November 1944, a combined meeting of the Medical and School Committees was held, at which Purdon Martin reported on discussions with representatives of the BPMS, where it had provisionally been agreed that the medical school should be incorporated so as to have a separate legal existence and then affiliated within the BPMF. However, not until 21 March 1946 was a separate governing body of the medical school finally constituted.[14]

Although the severing of the medical school from the National Hospital and the foundation of the Institute of Neurology were at one level a consequence of the recommendation of the Goodenough report, they can more broadly be seen as symptomatic of the massive reorganisations of British society in the period, new levels of intrusion of the state in matters of health, the tendency to absorb small institutions into larger configurations, the postwar financial pressures on the health services and the bureaucratisation of state ownership.

At the time, to many of the National Hospital physicians, the loss of the medical school was in effect the main casualty of the war. But there was a silver lining, for, as a consequence of its incorporation into the BPMF, as both Greenfield and Ewart Mitchell had correctly predicted, the Institute was formally recognised as a teaching institution by the university and, when the NHS came into being in 1948, this recognition allowed the National Hospital to be categorised as a 'teaching hospital' within the new service, thereby bringing many attendant privileges. The fears of the senior physicians that loss of the school would diminish the National Hospital were thus proved groundless. Indeed, incorporation of the school into the BPMF salvaged the hospital's position as a 'national asset'.

The Institute of Neurology 1950–1997

The foundation of the Institute of Neurology and its incorporation into the BPMF turned out to be of immediate benefit to the National Hospital as it conferred teaching hospital status and removed the financial burden of education from its shoulders.[15] The forming of the Institute within the BPMF and University of London allowed access to modern research facilities and an enlarged portfolio.

The Early Years of the Institute 1950–1962

Once the University had assumed responsibility for management of the Institute, new investments were made, modern research facilities provided, classrooms opened for the study of pathology and neuroanatomy, and new laboratory space leased in 23 Queen Square for psychological, histological and biochemical research. The library was extensively reorganised and improved (now named the Rockefeller Library) and, by 1951, it

---

[14] Made up of six members of the medical staff and six others, to include members of the Board of Management, the director of the BPMS and a representative of the University of London. The Board of Management of the National Hospital was then asked to delegate the function of maintaining the medical school to this body.

[15] Here we give a brief summary of the evolution of the Institute of Neurology from its establishment in 1950 to its incorporation into University College London in 1997. Biographical details of individuals no longer living and academic and clinical contributions of members of the Institute are to be found in Chapters 9, 10, 11 and 13.

had 1,200 books and subscribed to 80 journals. A museum of neurology was founded in the academic year 1952–3. A Committee of Management was formed, replacing the Medical School Committee, together with an Academic Board that produced annual reports.[16] In summary, the Institute of Neurology was quickly developing into a fully fledged university facility.

In these early years, there remained a strong emphasis on teaching, with much the same format used in the former medical school. The programme was divided into short-term courses for doctors working for higher degrees (such as the MRCP or DPM) and longer-term tuition for others including those 'from the provinces, dominions or abroad considering a career in neurology or neurosurgery'. Teaching took the form of clinical clerkships and attendance at outpatient clinics, with biannual lecture series, ten-week full-time courses in neurology, set courses in neurosurgery and EEG, neuroradiology rounds, neuropathology and neuroradiology sessions, and clinical demonstrations. This mixture of lectures, demonstrations and clerkships, although now organised more formally, took an essentially similar pattern to that introduced by Beevor in 1895. The 'clerkships' were a rather distinctive Queen Square phenomenon and greatly valued by both the physicians and the students. Between 1946–7 and 1950–1, it was recorded that between 336 and 351 doctors from 55

countries had attended the school annually, the largest numbers coming from the Dominions, but with 58 students from the USA during that quinquennium and smaller numbers from other non-Empire countries.[17] The Wednesday and Saturday clinical demonstrations were more popular than ever, with 744 attendees in the academic year 1950–1.[18] Student numbers for courses, clerkships and demonstrations continued at much the same levels through the decade.

However, the main effect of replacing the medical school with an Institute of Neurology linked to the University of London was to start the slow process of remediation of research. Gradually, research superseded teaching as the primary activity of the Institute. The connection with the MRC was to prove important in this regard. Two free-standing MRC units had already been established: one in clinical neurology under the leadership of Carmichael – only the second MRC unit to be established in Britain; and the second in neuro-otology. Further MRC groupings were established over the next few decades, including the Applied Neurobiology Group (1964, led by John Cavanagh), and the Unit in Developmental Neurobiology (1975, led by Robert Balazs), and a number of influential MRC external scientific staff were sited at Queen Square. The most important of all the academic developments during this critical period, however, was the establishment of the university department of clinical neurology, which gradually addressed the issue of research in neurology, generally confined to small projects without significant findings or in many cases not leading to publication of results.[19]

---

[16] The Committee of Management, formed in 1951, was chaired by Sir Ernest Gowers, who also served as chairman of the Board of Governors of the hospital. This was a shrewd move, allowing the two to work seamlessly together. On the new Board, there were two other representatives of the National Hospital Board of Governors (the Countess of Rothes and W. H. Taylor), a representative of the university (J. Z. Young), two representatives of the BPMF (Aubrey Lewis and Russell Brain), five nominations of the Academic Board (Cawthorne, Cumings, Ironside, Logue and Meadows), Walshe (as an appointee) and three ex-officio members (Critchley as dean, Elkington as chair of the Academic Board, and Hamilton-Turner representing the chairman of the BPMF). The predominance of National Hospital staff showed how great was the fear that influence would be lost when federation with the BPMF was forced on the Institute. The Academic Board comprised initially the 37 consultant staff of Queen Square and Maida Vale, and was chaired by Elkington. By 1961, it had grown to 50 members but still only allowed medically qualified staff (with the exception of Professor Zangwill). Non-clinical academics such as Morton were not included at this time, and nor were the medically qualified scientists Dawson and Merton. The Academic Board continued to exist until it was summarily disestablished (without much thought about the implications) around 2010.

[17] Essentially, apprenticeships ('sitting at the feet of the giants of British neurology', as Walton put it) and the clerkships are a form of teaching that has stood the test of time, and are only now under threat from the weight of NHS management bureaucracies. The greatest numbers were (in order) from India, South Africa, Australia, Canada and New Zealand.

[18] These were the renowned Wednesday and Saturday demonstrations, open to the public, which had been started once-weekly by Collier in 1925 and taught by the physicians in rotation. The schedule became bi-weekly in 1946. Eventually these clinical demonstrations petered out, and were finally abandoned in the 1990s, to the regret of the more sentimental and historically minded physicians.

[19] There were, of course, exceptions to this, and notably the work in cerebrovascular disease (led by John Marshall and David Shaw) and on spinal cord function, pain and tremor by Peter Nathan and Marion Smith. These were initiated in the 1950s and flourished further when incorporated within the university department of clinical neurology.

This change, from a medical school promoting teaching into a research-intensive university institute, required a culture change, and it took several more decades for the research effort to realise its potential. Initially, even in the professorial departments of neuropathology, neurology and neurosurgery, clinical work and training were the first priority, and research was bolted on. Slowly, this changed.

It is notable that research in this early period was almost entirely human-based, apart from a small primate research laboratory maintained by Ettlinger. This situation changed gradually and, by the 1970s, animal experimentation had again become an important part of work carried out by academics at Queen Square, as in the nineteenth century. Much of the human research in this period was physiological in nature, with basic and applied clinical work by the non-clinicians Morton and Sears, and the academic clinicians Gilliatt, Thomas, Fullerton, Nathan, Smith, Halliday, Merton and Dawson. Physiological work was also carried out at Maida Vale, including early work on computerised analysis of the EEG. All this was very much in the British tradition of applied human neurophysiology.

Macdonald Critchley, appointed to the medical school in 1948, served as the first dean of the Institute until 1953. The precedence given to teaching is evident from his reports. In 1950/1, for instance, the leading article in the annual report was on the history of teaching at Queen Square (by Gordon Holmes). In his first dean's report, Critchley noted that 337 men and 57 women, from 39 different countries, attended the various courses or teaching events, in addition to 744 attending the Saturday and Wednesday clinical demonstrations. Research was not mentioned in his report and, in the departmental reviews, only 41 publications were listed as having been published in that year, of which less than half reported research findings, with most being descriptive clinical observations.

In October 1953, Michael Kremer replaced Critchley as dean of the Institute, and he served in this post until 1962. The Institute grew during his tenure, with the first three professorial departments formed, the two departments of neuropathology and, crucially, the university department of clinical neurology which he worked hard to create. In Kremer's years, teaching still remained the main focus of the Institute, but the research portfolio began to grow. Although not an academic himself, Kremer encouraged research whenever an opportunity was presented.

The Institute of Neurology from 1962 to 1992 and its Evolution into a Research-intensive University Department

The year 1962 was a turning point in the history of the academic renaissance at Queen Square. On 6 January of that year, Roger Gilliatt was appointed professor of neurology. This was the first established chair in neurology in the country, although it was then followed by others in Oxford and Glasgow.[20] In the same year, James Bull was appointed dean, remaining in post until 1968, and Lord Aldington became chairman of the Committee of Management of the Institute, replacing Sir John Woods and remaining in post until 1980, when he was replaced by Sir John Read. Gilliatt's appointment with the administrative support of Aldington and Bull resulted, over the next three decades, in a sustained growth of research activity, an evolution into a fully research-intensive university department, and restitution of the reputation of Queen Square as a world-leading neurological centre. The initial fears of the clinicians that, once severed from the hospital, the Institute would be swallowed up by the bureaucrats of the university were not realised, and the influence of the clinicians was recognised by their strong representation on the Committee of Management, which included ten consultants amongst its initial 21 members (and a further five who were ex-officio).[21] Nevertheless, it is easy to forget how small the Institute was in this period, with income in 1964/5 of only £75,177 and with an Academic Board, chaired by Denis Brinton, of only 44 persons. There were still only 17 physicians at Queen Square and Maida Vale, and only four appointees to the university department of neurology at the time of its formation (professor, Roger Gilliatt; reader, John Marshall; and two senior lecturers, Robin Willison and P. K. Thomas[22]).

Although teaching still dominated, research activities began to flourish and, in the two years of 1963–4,

---

[20] Others had previously held the title of professor, but through personal promotion or other forms of designation.

[21] The clinicians were M. L. Rosenheim, C. F. Harris, G. H. News, E. A. Carmichael, J. N. Cumings, H. Dimsdale, R. W. Gilliatt, V. Logue, J. Marshall, M. Critchley; and, ex-officio, M. Kremer, Russell Brain, D. Brinton, C. Hamilton-Turner and Sir J. Paterson Ross.

[22] Personal professorships in the Institute were conferred on John Marshall, Ian McDonald and P. K. Thomas in the 1970s.

for instance, the Institute produced 168 publications, of which around one-third were full research reports. In 1964, the MRC established its research group in applied neurobiology, led by John Cavanagh, and agreed to fund this until 1972, a vote of confidence in the academic future of the Institute of Neurology.

In 1968, Reginald ('Reg') Kelly took over from Bull as dean. There were now 24 consultant physicians (16 at Queen Square and eight at Maida Vale – five of whom, including Kelly, had appointments at both hospitals, but only three held substantive academic positions), and 64 members of the Academic Board. Kelly was determined to enhance research, and the profile of teaching began to lessen. In 1970/1, 177 students (164 men and only 13 women) were registered with the hospital, about half the number of 20 years earlier, although the Wednesday and Saturday clinical demonstrations were as well attended as ever. There were no taught degree courses (MSc or Diplomas) but, for the first time, university research degrees (MD and PhD degrees) began to be awarded for work at Queen Square. In that year, 185 publications were produced from the Institute, but this output included a significant number of reviews, chapters and case reports rather than original research.

The 1970s were to prove a tempestuous time for the nation and the Institute. The country's finances weakened and the NHS and universities had entered one of their periodic cycles of financial crisis. Central funding of the Institute had tightened, and research had become increasingly dependent on external grants and charitable donations. On 18 October 1971, the Brain Research Trust was created largely through the initiative of Denis Williams. Its object was to support research into neurological diseases, but funding was restricted to work carried out at Queen Square. This became a major source of financial support, raising over £220,000 for the Institute in its first 4–5 years.[23] The Wolfson Foundation provided £48,000 for rebuilding the banked lecture theatre in the Queen Mary wing, which was officially opened in October 1971 and still remains the place where

teaching at the Institute is delivered. In the academic year of 1973/4, there was a quinquennial visit of the University Grants Committee and they were impressed by the renewed research activity, concluding that a 'wind of change' had blown through the Institute of Neurology.[24] However, major problems were caused by delays in the phase 1 redevelopment plans (the rebuilding of Queen Square House), due largely to endless bureaucracy and postponement of funding from the Department of Health, the plague of NHS reorganisation and the waves of industrial action that spread throughout the country. Kelly's last annual report in 1973/4 had a distinctly melancholic flavour, as he mentioned how the building workers' disputes had damaged the Institute's forward plans, that investments had fallen in value, and that at least one major benefactor had withdrawn his promised donation because 'government action will make it impossible for him to find the money'. He continued:

> Within the Institute [there is] a labour force that continues to be loyal and which is prepared to continue to put up with poor working conditions and with a wages and salary structure that imposes upon them permanently a lower standard of living than they could achieve by joining in the militant scramble for more money and less work which seems to be the accepted standard outside, and which seems to be encouraged by the politicians who are prepared to make promises they cannot fulfil for vote catching reasons only and who are prepared to lay the blame for our present state on the oil sheiks and any other bogey man they can think of rather than accept the responsibility that is basically theirs and their failure to govern.[25]

Peter Gautier-Smith[26] took over as dean in 1975, and remained in post for seven years. In 1976, the

---

[23] At the time of writing, the Brain Research Trust has raised more than £30 million for research activities at the Institute of Neurology since its foundation. In parallel, in 1984, the hospital also established The National Hospital Development Foundation, which later adopted the working name National Brain Appeal, and this has raised over £40 million for equipment, buildings, clinical work and research at the National Hospital.

[24] Kelly disliked the metaphor, arguing that this 'wind' was an illusion and previous UGC inspections had not appreciated the transformation that the Institute was undergoing, with the current position representing the culmination of 15 years' strategic planning.

[25] For the development of the Institute, see Institute of Neurology annual report 1973–4, pp. 2–7. Kelly then goes on to castigate politicians for making 'a bogey man' of private practice.

[26] Peter Claudius Gautier-Smith had worked as senior house physician to John Marshall in 1960 and then as Macdonald Critchley's senior registrar before being appointed jointly to a consultant post at the National Hospital and St George's Hospital in 1962. He served as dean of the Institute of Neurology from 1975 to 1982 and retired from the hospital staff in 1989. His clinical practice

freehold of St Johns Mews was purchased for the Institute, and some academic activity delayed by the Queen Square House industrial action moved there. By the time that building work was finally completed and Queen Square House opened by the Queen Mother in 1978, seven years after she had laid the foundation stone, the economic difficulties of the country were taking their toll on the university system. The three-day week of 1974 and the winter of discontent in 1978 provided signs of deep-seated national economic problems. In addition to building problems and the country's poor financial performance, teaching and research were hampered by the continual stream of reports and changing policies in relation to the NHS and the London Postgraduate Institutes (see Chapter 14). Funds were never adequate for the ambitions of the Institute during this period, and cuts in the university block grant and the effects of inflation in the 1980s also led to more problems. In his bleakest annual report, in 1981, Gautier-Smith admitted:

> The academic year 1980/81 has proved a difficult one. Uncertainties about the future administration of the Postgraduate Institutes and Hospitals combined with a cut in the University block grant and the effects of inflation have led both to feelings of insecurity amongst our staff and grave difficulties for our administration in balancing our budget. In order to achieve the necessary saving, stringent economies have had to be made and maintenance grants to departments have been cut to the barest minimum, but despite this, many vacancies have had to be left unfilled to prevent redundancies. Inevitably, with lecturer posts being frozen, departments have become unbalanced and our future, which is so dependent on bright young people being attracted to the neurosciences, will be put in jeopardy if this trend continues.

was notable for the interest he took in all aspects of the lives of his patients amongst whom he had a devoted following. He was an excellent teacher, a stalwart of the hospital serving in many roles and on many committees. He was a gifted writer, incessantly curious and interested in the stranger corners of the human condition. His 31 novels, written in his spare time, are discussed later in this book, and his unpublished memoirs of his time at the hospital are full of rich anecdote. A devoted family man, the death of his beloved daughter Susan, a TV producer, of cardiomyopathy in 1996 was a grievous blow. A podcast of Gautier-Smith's thoughts on neurology is found at https://soundcloud.com/bmjpodcasts/neurology-and-detective-5 which was recorded a few years before he developed Alzheimer's disease.

Despite all this, a great deal was achieved. The award of Special Health Authority status confirmed on the National Hospital in 1977 was to an extent seen as recognition that Queen Square had regained national prominence in research and teaching. Advances in experimental medicine were creating many opportunities for neurology. In the early 1970s, the number of papers published annually ranged between 160 and 200, but in the academic year 1975, productivity again improved, with 242 publications to September 1975, increasing to 340 in 1977 and 450 in 1981 ('the highest ever'). This also was the first time that the growing external research grant income was published, in 1975 amounting to more than £1 million and reported to be 'half as much again' as the UGC block grant.

In 1982, Peter Gautier-Smith retired as dean and was replaced by John Marshall. Marshall wrote of Gautier-Smith's tenure, that

> It may seem platitudinous to say that no dean in the history of the Institute has had so difficult a time but in this instance it can be said without fear of contradiction. This is not because of circumstances peculiar to the Institute but because of events in the academic world as a whole. Frozen posts, so-called voluntary early retirement and the threat of redundancies have been the order of the day. The fact that the Institute is presently sound financially and that morale has been so well maintained is due to the efforts of our retiring Dean.[27]

Following publication of the Flowers report in 1980, five members of the BPMF were absorbed into one or other of the undergraduate medical schools and the Institute of Neurology considered itself fortunate to have survived this purge. With the bitter history of the 1930s now forgotten, links were formed with the Royal Postgraduate Medical School to strengthen Queen Square's position, and these included the appointment of Roger Gilliatt, who resigned as consultant neurologist at the Middlesex Hospital after 25 years in the post, to take up sessions at the Hammersmith Hospital. A joint lecturer post was also instituted at the Hammersmith and Queen Square to support Gilliatt, and Anita Harding was appointed. Links between the cerebral blood flow and neuro-oncology groups at Queen Square were made with the Positron Emission Tomography (PET) group based in the MRC Cyclotron Unit at the Hammersmith

[27] 'Dean's report', annual report of the Institute of Neurology, 1982/3.

Hospital. *The Times* had warned that, as central funding fell, universities would have to secure funds from elsewhere, suggesting a figure of 10 per cent income from non-UGC sources, but the Institute greatly exceeded that target with 75 per cent of its resources derived from non-UGC sources by 1983, including 55 per cent from grants.

Another initiative with which John Marshall was intimately involved was the creation of the National Hospitals College of Speech Sciences. In 1946, the hospital had considered establishing a school of speech therapy but discovered that one had recently been started by Ms Beryl Oldrey, a speech therapist at Queen Square, and Miss Marion Fleming. At first, they called this the National Hospital School for Speech Therapy but, as a commercial enterprise without any connection to Queen Square, the hospital objected and it was quickly renamed the Oldrey-Fleming School. In 1956, the Medical Committee rejected a proposal for merger, as it did with further invitations received in 1966 and 1969. When the closure of the West End Hospital in Dean Street was announced in 1972, the Board of Governors received requests to take over both the associated West End School of Speech Therapy and the Oldrey-Fleming School of Speech Therapy. This time they agreed, partly through the intercession of John Marshall who felt that the National Hospital should encourage speech sciences. This move was strongly supported by the DHSS which wrote that this 'would ensure the training of speech therapists took place in an appropriate clinical setting … and is in line with the recommendations of the Quirk Report[28], not only from the speech therapist's point of view, but also in improving the knowledge of doctors about speech and language problems'. The DHSS also noted that the isolation of speech therapy training from neurological departments had greatly hindered the evaluation of the therapy. Thus, with the Department's blessing, the two were merged as the National Hospitals College of Speech Sciences on 12 July 1973. Initially based in the old West End Hospital School at 59 Portland Place, with supplementary courses held at 84a Heath Street in Hampstead, the site of the Oldrey-Fleming School, the new College later moved to Wakefield Street, and John Marshall then arranged for the transfer of the MSc degree course in human communication, which had been based at Guy's Hospital Medical School since 1971, to the Institute of Neurology, where it became the first master's-level course taught at Queen Square. The College of Speech Sciences flourished and grew in size under the administration of the Institute of Neurology, and, then in August 1995, in parallel with the incorporation of the Institute into University College London, 'following a series of lengthy negotiations', it was transferred to UCL to become the department of human communication science in the faculty of Life Sciences.

Although research became the first priority for the Institute, encouraged no doubt in part by the potential to raise external funds which were then not available for teaching, the teaching portfolio was also enhanced under Marshall's deanship. For the first time since 1895, he switched the focus from internal stand-alone courses, which were the traditional Queen Square model, to university-taught courses offering master's-level degrees, and also laid a new emphasis on PhD and MD degrees. The first master's-level degree courses were the diploma of clinical neurology, introduced in 1983, which became a flagship for the Institute of Neurology, and the MSc in human communication offered by the Institute from 1984 to 1995.[29] By 1988, there were 33 students undertaking master's-level courses, many from Commonwealth countries. A steady increase in the number of graduate students (although still small by later standards) was now accommodated in the Institute, supported by central and research grants.[30]

---

[28] *Report of Committee of Enquiry into Speech Therapy Services* (London: DHSS, 1972). At the time, there were only 800 speech therapists in Britain, and the report recommended an expansion in their number.

[29] When the National Hospital's College of Speech Sciences was merged with facilities within UCL to form the new department of human communication science within the faculty of Life Sciences, the Institute of Neurology ceased to be responsible for this MSc degree.

[30] The Institute Registrar from 1973 to 1989 was Miss Pat Harris who was remembered fondly by numerous students in these years, and in whose memory an annual prize for the best MSc dissertation was instituted. She was replaced by Ann Newman, and then from May 1990 by Miss Janet Townsend as Assistant Secretary for Students. The post was the point of contact for all the students, many from foreign countries, and both Ms Harris and Townsend acted as friends, confidantes and advisers of whole generations of students from all over the world, and dealt with all the problems of settling into the strange environment they found at Queen Square. Elizabeth Bertram also joined the staff with responsibility for personnel issues in 1989, and remains in post at the time of writing. Pat Harris, Janet Townsend and Elizabeth Bertram all worked tirelessly for many years on behalf of the students and the Institute staff.

The funding of medical research began rapidly to rise in the 1980s and 1990s in Britain, with increasing government interest in the outcomes of academic research and recognition of the economic benefits of science and medicine to the country. There was much public debate about the state of science funding (a sustained campaign entitled 'Save British Science' was particularly influential) and research grants not only became more readily available but were also more focused on public benefit and evidence of effectiveness. Academics were exhorted to seek larger and more ambitious grants and were being, for the first time, judged on their ability to attract funds. Commercial collaboration was encouraged and was another sign of changing university priorities. In 1984, the University Grants Committee announced that it would undertake approximately five-yearly assessments of research in order to allocate central funds according to the quality of research. The Institute did well in this new environment, and when the Medical Sub-Committee of the University Grants Committee visited in 1985, the Institute was congratulated on its vigour, the enthusiasm of the staff, the ability to garner external funds, and the leadership. However, the UGC grant increase in the next year was only £14,000 on a total of £944,100, leaving a deficit of £140,000 that 'cannot be met by economies and efficiency savings, important though these are'. For the first time, substantial external support from the pharmaceutical industry was obtained. A small laboratory had been established in 1956 with assistance from May and Baker, looking into the role of 5-hydroxytryptamine (serotonin) in the central nervous system, but in 1986 a substantial grant was obtained from the Swedish pharmaceutical firm Astra and, with this and assistance from the Brain Research Trust, the Institute acquired a large property in Hunter Street, which was previously part of the Royal Free Hospital Medical School, and established a joint research unit with Astra within the department of neurochemistry. This joint venture (the Astra neurosciences research unit) occupied two floors of the refurbished Hunter Street building, and Dr Richard Green from the MRC Clinical Pharmacology Unit in Oxford was appointed as the first director. The work of Julian Axe, the Institute secretary, was instrumental in obtaining the grant from Astra and negotiating the purchase of the Hunter Street premises, and the new building was formally opened by Princess Anne,

the Chancellor of the University of London, on 4 December 1986. The neurochemical laboratories which were located in St John's Mews also moved into the new premises in 1987 and, in the next year, a Brain Bank funded by the Parkinson's Disease Society was established there. The potential benefits of linking with the neurological charities was also fully appreciated, and the Institute benefitted from these, especially in the fields of movement disorders, multiple sclerosis and epilepsy. The focus of research was necessarily changing and, from the mid-1980s, had shifted towards molecular biology, movement neurophysiology and structural and functional neuroimaging. The output of papers from the Institute was also increasing and in 1983, for example, 567 papers were published by the Institute staff, with a further increase to 657 in 1986.

The year 1987 was another one of change. John Marshall retired as dean in September, and became the temporary general manager at the National Hospital for a year. His was a very successful term of office during which the academic staff grew to the extent that, on his retirement, there were 14 professors and readers, and five university departments. He had negotiated severe economic conditions with great skill and sown the seeds of rapid growth. Under his stewardship, changes were initiated that set the Institute on an upward trajectory of personnel, funding and research productivity. This was a time of change since Julian Axe[31] also left the Institute in the summer of 1988, after five years assisting Marshall in the Institute administration, and Roger Gilliatt had retired a few months before. Under their leadership, leaving aside any personal distance, the Institute had grown considerably in strength and importance. Marshall's last report was upbeat, although it did note that the recurrent grant from the university was 'now so small a percentage of our income (less than a quarter) that it is insufficient to maintain the infrastructure necessary for a postgraduate Research Institute'. He thanked the Brain Research Trust for making up the deficit.

---

[31] Dr Julian Axe was a very popular figure at the Institute. He was the first Institute secretary with a university degree, and his research experience in biochemistry as well as his administrative training contributed to his understanding of the Institute affairs and its research. He went on to become registrar and secretary to St Bartholomew's Hospital Medical School. His post was filled by Sylvia Sterling until 1990 and then Robert Walker.

Nevertheless, by 1985, the country was in the early stages of a sustained economic boom with new grants becoming available and funding streams improving.

Marshall was replaced by David Landon as dean, who surprisingly did not include any word of thanks to Marshall in his first report. A few months earlier, in June 1987, David Marsden had taken over the chairmanship of the university department of clinical neurology. With his appointment came the Parkinson's disease brain bank and a new MRC Human Movement and Balance Unit, into which, in October 1988 on Hood's retirement, the remnant of the MRC Neuro-otology Unit was incorporated. Landon had to deal with the growing bureaucratic and administrative burden on university institutes, not least from external reviews, and, from the start, it was Marsden rather than Landon who drove the intellectual direction of the Institute. Marsden presided over great changes in the research emphasis of the department, which switched its predominant interest from peripheral neurology to movement disorders and neurodegeneration. These moves took the sting out of the often-quoted barb of the 1970s that the Institute should be called the Institute of Peripheral Neurology. Marsden also encouraged subspecialisation and work in other neurological areas, so that 11 sections were formed within the department over the next year, each focusing on one disease or area of research and with its own section lead and a mandate to grow that particular area of interest.[32] Marsden's style of letting each section lead work independently was a marked change from the Gilliatt years and, as a result, there was rapid acceleration in research activity and output. A Wellcome Trust grant of £1.37 million was made in 1988 to support the MRI unit in multiple sclerosis, and this marked the beginning of growth in neuroimaging research which was in future years to be a dominating feature at Queen Square.

---

[32] There were 11 sections in 1988–90: movement disorders; multiple sclerosis and NMR and cellular neurobiology; neurogenetics; neurocytology; muscle disease; epilepsy; experimental psychology; cerebral oedema; peripheral nerve and protein chemistry; functional imaging; neuropsychiatry. The department also contained the MRC Human Movement and Balance Unit, the brain bank and the drugs and therapeutics laboratory. There were also close links and joint appointments with the department of neurological sciences at the Royal Free Hospital, and the MRC Cyclotron Unit and Royal Postgraduate Medical School at the Hammersmith Hospital. In 1990/1, a section on neurorehabilitation was added, and links formed also with the National Hospital's DNA laboratories and autonomic unit.

In the last years of the1980s, an annual rolling five-year academic plan was produced, perhaps in response to the increasing number of external reviews of the postgraduate institutes. These plans, excessively bureaucratic, listed activity but lacked strategy or any synoptical vision, and seem to have petered out after 1994.

In 1989, the Research Selectivity Exercise by the Universities Funding Council (a body which had replaced the University Grants Committee in that year) gave the Institute its highest grade ('5') reflecting improvement from the UGC exercise in 1986 when the Institute was graded only as 'above average'. This was a significant achievement and the Institute was one of only four institutions in the field of clinical medicine in the country to receive this endorsement (and the BPMF as a whole was awarded a '4'). There had been more than 600 publications by Institute staff in 1988/9. The dean's report for that year for the first time listed the research grants gained by the Institute staff, indicating that total income had more than doubled over the previous decade from £2,769,000 in 1979/80 to £6,247,000 in 1988/9, of which research grants accounted for £3,124,000 (50 per cent). In the same period, the contributions from endowments (5–6 per cent) and tuition fees (4–6 per cent) were mainly unchanged but, as the Thatcher years progressed, the university block grant reduced from 39 per cent to 18 per cent of total income by 1995.

The international cachet of Queen Square had grown enormously under the leadership of Gilliatt and Marsden and, at a time when academic neurology was advancing worldwide, Queen Square had regained its place in the top division. Its academic activity had largely switched from the pre-1950 emphasis on teaching to research. Student numbers had increased (although still small by later standards) and, in 1988, there were 24 PhD, 16 MD and 19 MPhil students. The students in the five years between 1984 and 1988 were from 63 different countries, and the diploma course in particular had a good reputation in the countries of the Commonwealth.

In 1992, the Institute scored '4' in the Research Assessment Exercise, marking a reduction from 1989, an outcome that was received with much disappointment. The dean attributed this partly to technical factors: 'Viewed from within, there is every evidence that the Institute had maintained its momentum across the full range of its activities, as our increased grant income, major new developments and the production of over 700 research publications clearly attest.'[33]

His assessment was largely accurate and the Institute's research trajectory was clearly on a rapidly climbing course. In 1994, the Functional Imaging Laboratory began to be commissioned, with funding over five years of £20 million from Wellcome and £3.6 million from the Leopard Muller Trust. It opened in 1995. In the same year, a research MRI unit also opened at the Chalfont Centre for Epilepsy, integrated with the Institute of Neurology, with a £3 million award. In 1996, Astra vacated their laboratories and ended the collaboration that had started ten years earlier. A Centre for Cognitive Neurology opened at Queen Square, with Tim Shallice as its director. The Wellcome Trust awarded a large programme grant to attract Peter Goadsby and his team from Sydney to establish a headache unit. The advisory committee set up to review the R&D performance of the Special Health Authorities (SHAs) in 1995 was also complimentary about the Institute of Neurology, praising particularly the work in movement disorders, epilepsy, neurogenetics, imaging in multiple sclerosis and neuropsychology.

Tomlinson and the Absorption of the Institute into University College London 1992–1997

The series of reports that were set to perturb the Institute of Neurology, described in more detail in Chapter 14, began with the Tomlinson report in 1992.[34] This recommended that all institutes of the British Postgraduate Medical Federation of London University be directly linked to a multi-faculty university. This proposal was met with widespread dismay at the Institute, which valued its independence and had grown strongly in the preceding years. There was a general feeling that the report had ignored the Institute's submission and its recent achievements, and had taken a generic approach to activities that had many domestic flavours and might best be

considered individually for ideological reasons, and had ridden roughshod over their particular strengths. There followed a rear-guard action at Queen Square, but the days of the fully independent Institute of Neurology, metaphorically surrounded by a moat, were numbered. Over the next few years, many negotiations and discussions were held prior to absorption of the Institute of Neurology into University College London. David Landon's deanship ended in 1995 with this outcome, which was at the time widely regarded as disappointing.

David Marsden replaced David Landon as dean in 1995 and, with the unexpected death of Anita Harding who had been appointed as Marsden's successor, Ian McDonald took over chairmanship of the university department of clinical neurology. By then, the formal absorption of the Institute of Neurology within University College London had been finalised as part of the wholesale reorganisation of London medicine (and, at the same time, the National Hospital was absorbed into University College London Hospital). The BPMF was dissolved by Act of Parliament on 31 July 1996, and the Parliamentary bill to unite the Institute of Neurology with UCL received Royal Assent on 4 July 1996. The Institute of Neurology was formally incorporated into UCL on 1 August 1997. At the time, the mood of the hospital and the Institute was muted. There was much apprehension about how the hospital and the Institute would fare as part of a larger and more acquisitive organisation. There was a fear that this would signal the end of an existence that, despite many vicissitudes, had maintained autonomy and excellence in clinical neurology, teaching and research for over 100 years.

Nevertheless, the staff could look back with satisfaction at what had been achieved since the Institute of Neurology was founded as a limited company in 1948, and its first professorships of chemical pathology and neuropathology were appointed in 1958, at a time when there were only 20 staff. By 1997, the metrics were impressive. In that year, there were 25 professorial staff members and a total complement of just under 300. The income for that year was £14.6 million, which included research grants of over £9 million (63 per cent of total income) from 62 individual awards, including 10 from the MRC and 16 from the Wellcome Trust. There were 124 students registered for PhD, MPhil or MD/MS degrees. The publication output in the seven years 1990–6 from the university department of clinical neurology alone was 2,243 journal articles, 484 book

---

[33] 'Dean's report', annual report of the Institute of Neurology and National Hospital for Neurology and Neurosurgery, 1992/3.

[34] B. Tomlinson, *Report of the Inquiry into London's Health Service, Medical Education, and Research* (London: HMSO, 1992).

chapters and 59 books.[35] In the 1996 Research Assessment Exercise, the Institute was again given a '5A' rating, one step below the 5* grade which it was to achieve in the exercise four years later.

At a time when academic neurology was growing worldwide, the decision by the Institute to expand its academic base, secure external grant income and set research priorities had paid handsome dividends.

Queen Square had regained its international reputation by switching from the pre-1950 emphasis on teaching to research. As it was to turn out, following its absorption into UCL, the Institute continued to grow strongly and benefitted from the enhanced facilities of UCL, becoming within ten years unambiguously one of the jewels in the crown of the university. The academic record of the Institute of Neurology and the National Hospital in the clinical neurosciences now competes favourably with that of any other institution in the world.[36]

---

[35] The university department of clinical neurology was the largest in the Institute throughout this period, and its metrics over the ten-year period of 1990–9 were summarised in a separate report and included: 257 research grants totalling £17.5 million, over 200 PhDs and MD research degree students, and a total of 591 research workers. In 1999, there were 19 professors, 20 readers/senior lecturers, 8 lecturers and 151 junior faculty.

---

[36] In 2014, QS World Rankings of Universities rated neuroscience research at Queen Square and UCL second only to Harvard.

Chapter 13

The Rise of Academic Neurology at Queen Square 1962–1997

Although university professorships had been established in October 1958 at the Institute of Neurology in chemical pathology and neuropathology, the crucial step in the resurgence of academic work at Queen Square was the establishment first of a readership and then, in 1962, a professorship designated as head of the new university department of clinical neurology. These developments were achieved only after a prolonged struggle between individuals having different ideologies. In retrospect, it is clear that the future of the National Hospital and its Institute was threatened, and if academic development had not occurred, and the balance between research, teaching and clinical work remained unchanged, it is doubtful whether the National Hospital would have survived. Five names jostle for attention in the evolution of this saga: Francis Walshe argued often and loudly against the need for change; Arnold Carmichael might have led a resurgence but accepted that it would not happen for him; Derek Denny-Brown spurned the opportunity of returning to Queen Square and developing a university department; John Marshall, the victim of Machiavellian manoeuvres, saw the professorship slip away; and Roger Gilliatt was appointed and held the post from 1962 until retirement in 1986. The story of the professorial department at Queen Square is, ultimately, the story of Gilliatt. His personality and role as academic leader were complex. During Gilliatt's long tenure of the professorship, it could be argued that excellence in academic neurology at Queen Square rested not so much on his shoulders as on those of the few clinician scientists who worked around him, loyally but still somewhat in isolation from front-line clinical activities of the National Hospital, and with varying degrees of enthusiasm for the environment in which they functioned. As with Gilliatt, several began their independent research careers as consultant neurologists employed by the NHS and active in private practice. Together, this community, contributing at different times of their careers and in different ways,

ensured that the pulse of academic neurology continued to beat at Queen Square across a crucial transitional period.

Ian McDonald drafted notes on these events for a proposed (but unwritten) history of Queen Square, and wrote:

In decade and ½ following 2nd WW it was a commonplace to say that QS was not what it was. The problem was that it was what it was – immensely distinguished clinically, with physicians of highest calibre who were selected by great figures of the earlier 20th century but as replicas of themselves. What it lacked was imagination and flexibility. The major contributions were not in neurology but in pathology. Greenfield was at his zenith and radiology grew in stature under Hugh Davies and James Bull. The major reason for neurology being static at QS was the lack of a proper academic base. This was largely due to opposition of older staff to the notion of a professor. When Carmichael was offered a chair, as a junior physician and secretary of the medical committee, he was told that it was the wish of his colleagues that he should decline it. RWG [Gilliatt] said that Walshe campaigned actively against … and by 1961/2 an ultimatum was delivered by the University to Queen Square to the effect that if they did not appoint a professor of clinical neurology, they would withdraw their existing support … In any event the decision to have a chair was taken. Denny-Brown declined the invitation … His letter was influential because so great was Denny-Brown's prestige that the powerful forces of clinical reaction yielded when it was managed with consummate skill by Gilliatt and the deans early in his period … Marshall was the heir apparent but the affair of the book broke. As RWG once told me, poor Queen Square was just recovering from the blow of the Marshall affair when the story of [RWG's] divorce broke (Penelope went off with John Osborne) … But pressure from the University led them to advertise. Denny-Brown vouchsafed that RWG was the only hope for QS … RWG consulted MK [Michael Kremer] who ascertained that all but one – William Gooddy – would support him … Gooddy who had a mistress in town and a wife in the country objected to RWG on moral grounds!!![1]

Although development of the university department of clinical neurology dates from 1962, the story of academic neurology at Queen Square starts with the MRC unit run by Carmichael, and the machinations relating to establishment of the readership and then the professorship in clinical neurology.

Arnold Carmichael and the Medical Research Council

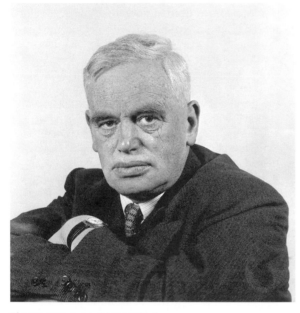

Figure 13.1 E. Arnold Carmichael.

Edward Arnold Carmichael (known as Arnold)[2] was a key figure in the renaissance of academic work at Queen Square, although mainly as an enabler. As Denis Williams wrote:

> His contribution was not so much in the weight or substance of his personal research, but in the influence he had upon the thought and attitudes of young postgraduates in all the neurological specialties who came to Queen Square from the then Empire, the Commonwealth, and the Western World ... His formal ward rounds and seminars became essential parts of each postgraduate student's week ... His emphasis on the physiological approach to medicine of Sir Thomas Lewis, and the physiologically orientated attitude of the Medical Research Society was, though, rather out of step with his colleagues' more direct bedside or purely clinical approach.[3]

Although others also conducted research from the position of an honorary consultant appointment, Carmichael was the first dedicated academic neurologist of the mid twentieth century working at Queen Square. He became somewhat isolated, never achieving presidency of the Association of British Neurologists or direct involvement with *Brain*, to each of which he aspired, and settled for editorship of the *Journal of Neurology, Neurosurgery, and Psychiatry*. For neurologists training in the late 1960s, he was already a forgotten figure beaten by a system that was opposed to the emergence of academic neurology, and not a personality to force that change. However, Carmichael was crucial to the hesitant and stuttering development of academic neurology at Queen Square. He played an

---

[1] McDonald opened his notebook with some anecdotes: the arrogant style of the 1950s; Mrs Greenfield saying in 1967 when she had lunch with McDonald and his mother that 'she had never been to Queen Square'; Kinnier Wilson telling his colleagues that it would not be necessary for them to write a textbook of neurology since he had the matter in hand; and anger over the precociousness of Russell Brain in writing a textbook of neurology when he was not a member of the staff at Queen Square. In retrospect, McDonald considered that the key postwar events relevant to academic neurology at Queen Square were the establishment of Carmichael's MRC unit with John Bates, Pat Merton, George Dawson and Martin Halliday; the closure of the animal house; and the contributions of Slater, Purdon-Martin, Hallpike, Davies and Bull. McDonald archive: manuscript, dated July 1987; an earlier version of this narrative in notes for a lecture on the history of Queen Square given in Dallas on 21 October 1986; and annotations written in his copy of Gordon Holmes, *The National Hospital Queen Square* (1954).

[2] Edward Arnold Carmichael was born, educated, graduated in medicine (with a gold medal) and worked as a junior doctor in Edinburgh. He served in the infantry in the First World War and was appointed resident medical officer at Queen Square in 1923. He was awarded a Rockefeller Travelling Fellowship to the USA and returned to be appointed as assistant physician to the outpatients in 1930, and to the new post of director of the neurological research unit of the Medical Research Council in 1932. During the Second World War, his research was focused on military issues and he was appointed CBE for these contributions. After retirement, Carmichael spent much time in America, as 'an able ambassador of British neurology', teaching in what, according to Williams, he felt was a less repressive and reactionary environment: see Anon., 'Edward Arnold Carmichael', *Lancet* **398** (1978): 18, and Anon., 'E. A. Carmichael', *British Medical Journal* **1** (1978): 51.

[3] D. Williams, 'Edward Arnold Carmichael', *Munk's Roll*, Vol. **VII** (London: Royal College of Physicians, 1984), pp. 91–2.

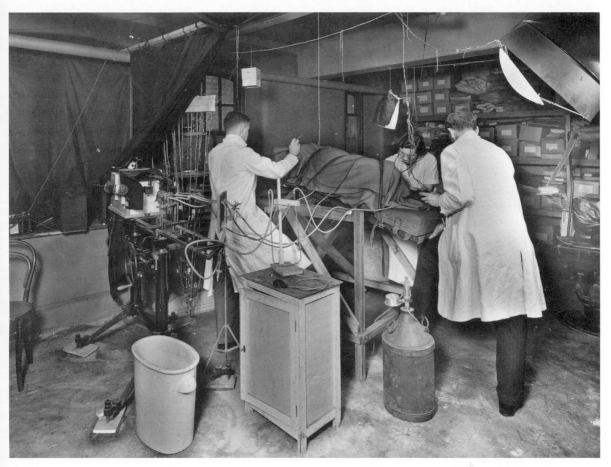

Figure 13.2 MRC neurological research unit, experiments on intracranial pressure, 1936.

important role in securing the grant from the Rockefeller Foundation in the late 1930s that reaffirmed the importance of research for the future of the National Hospital. Carmichael had worked with Julia Bell, geneticist at University College London, but his own research included studies of respiration, cerebrospinal fluid pressure, vascular responses, eye movements, otology and pain, some carried out with Greenfield.[4]

The origins of his MRC support lay in a controversial affair involving Kathleen Chevassut and the neurologist Purves-Stewart. Chevassut was trained in basic science at Bedford College for Women and hoped to study medicine but was discouraged by Purves-Stewart. He wanted Chevassut to follow up on work by William Bulloch, who claimed to have identified an agent associated with multiple sclerosis that he transmitted from humans to rabbits using spinal fluid. Chevassut followed up this observation and reported that *spherula insularis* could be cultured from the cerebrospinal fluid of more than 90 per cent of patients, but not controls. She then made a vaccine that Purves-Stewart used in human clinical trials. But their relationship deteriorated and each published

---

[4] This collaboration included publication of *The Cerebrospinal Fluid in Clinical Diagnosis* (1925). Perhaps the strangest experiment was his work on referred pain in the testicle (H. H. Woollard and E. A. Carmichael, 'The Testis and Referred Pain', *Brain* **56** (1933): 293–303). He and Woollard noted that the testicles were the most 'accessible of the internal organs to investigation' and experimented on themselves by compressing their testicles with a graded selection of weights, assessing the pain this produced and the effects of blocking the various pudendal nerves. Thus, for instance, they found that 300g produced slight discomfort in the right groin, 650g caused severe pain on the right side of the body, and >800g caused a sickening pain

spreading across the back. Anaesthetising the nerves of the testicle did not abolish the pain. This self-experimentation showed a dedication to science in the tradition of Head (who severed his radial nerve) and Merton (who subjected himself to repeated transcranial magnetic stimulation).

separate accounts of the work.[5] The Medical Research Council had supported her work and asked Carmichael to investigate the findings. He and Walshe came to the conclusion that they could not be reproduced. The implication was that Purves-Stewart had benefitted financially from the work by charging patients, and that Chevassut had colluded in providing unreliable data. The report was damning and Chevassut was declined further funding from the Medical Research Council. She was, however, offered support by the son of Sir Halley Stewart, who administered his father's philanthropic foundation and offered to set Chevassut up with research facilities at 30 Chesterford Gardens, North London. The staff at the National Hospital were also keen to secure these funds from the Halley Stewart Trust. Therefore, Walshe tried to undermine Chevassut in a letter to Dr Halley Stewart, urging him to suspend their support for a year: 'I wager that by then we shall be marvellously in agreement in believing that feminine charm and inconsequence and a light-hearted disregard of accuracy are fatal endowments for one engaged in scientific research.'

The secretary of the Medical Research Council, Walter Morley Fletcher, contacted Halley Stewart, who then dissociated himself from Chevassut's research when confronted with the fact that she had been receiving financial support from the MRC and his own Trust for the same work. *Spherula insularis* disappeared abruptly from interest after an episode at the Royal Society of Medicine in 1931 when, as Denis Brinton recalled, Carmichael reported his inability to confirm the findings. Chevassut left the meeting in tears and was not subsequently encountered in neurological circles.

However, the episode was important for the future of research at Queen Square, and it provided further evidence for the ambiguity of Walshe's manoeuvrings – fundamentally against research, but also keen to promote the interests of the National Hospital by any means. The suggestion was therefore made that the research facilities intended for Chevassut might be used by Carmichael, rather than see no return from

investment by the Halley Stewart Trust. There followed an elaborate proposal drafted by Walshe and Carmichael for starting a Medical Research Council unit comprising ten beds, nursing staff, a biochemist, and a medically qualified scientist as director. The inclusion of a clinical facility was not accidental since Walshe knew that this would make 30 Chesterford Gardens unsuitable for investment by the Halley Stewart Trust. He also sensed that Fletcher was supportive of Carmichael, as were representatives of the Rockefeller Foundation in Europe, which was also now in discussions on supporting research at Queen Square. As matters seemed to stall, the National Hospital offered to share the costs of the unit and support the clinical facilities, with Carmichael as director. Walshe continued to make flattering noises about the lavish equipment at 30 Chesterford Gardens and, as a result, the Halley Stewart Trust offered support for Carmichael processed through the Medical Research Council. Eventually, this included an annual endowment and a research fellowship. The MRC clinical neurological research unit duly opened in 1932. Carmichael encouraged many younger people to visit from elsewhere and assisted in the training of those who worked in the unit. These included John Walton from Newcastle, David Shaw and Ian Simpson from Edinburgh, and Norman Geschwind from Boston. Christopher Pallis was appointed to an honorary lectureship in the unit in 1954, and replaced by P. K. Thomas in 1959.

Carmichael invited Martin Halliday,[6] who had devised a method for measuring tremor as a surrogate for fatigue in pilots at risk of sudden sleep during the Berlin airlift at the end of the Second World War, to join the neurological research unit at Queen Square. Initially, Halliday studied tremor and myoclonus (contributing an important paper on its categorisation),

---

[5] See K. Chevassut, 'The Aetiology of Disseminated Sclerosis', *Lancet* **215** (1930): 552–60; J. Purves-Stewart, 'A Specific Vaccine Treatment in Disseminated Sclerosis', *Lancet* **216** (1931): 560–4. In writing this account, we have benefitted from, and periodically reproduced – not always with further attribution – material contained in S. T. Casper, *The Neurologists: A History of a Medical Specialty in Modern Britain c. 1789–2000* (Manchester University Press, 2014).

[6] Anthony Martin Halliday was born in Liverpool, educated at Dauntsey's School and qualified in medicine from Glasgow. In the RAMC, he was posted to the physiological section of the British Army's operational research unit where his work was noticed by Carmichael who recruited him to the MRC neurological research unit on demobilisation in 1953. In addition to his work at Queen Square, Halliday served as president of the EEG Society (now the British Society for Clinical Neurophysiology) and was awarded the society's Grey Walter Medal in 1989. He died in 2008 from pulmonary fibrosis. Other members of the department of applied physiology who served as president of the EEG Society/BSCN were Carmichael, Dawson, Cobb and Murray, demonstrating the esteem in which its members were held.

and in 1961 he was appointed consultant in clinical neurophysiology. He then became interested in the development and application of evoked potentials, and this is the work for which he is best remembered. Using the newly developed computers, Halliday transferred the analogue principles worked out by Dawson and devised a method for electronic digital averaging.[7] He worked with Jack Pitman, Dawson's technician, and the more sensitive and faster digital technologies allowed him to explore various modalities of evoked potential. From the clinical point of view, the most important work was the evaluation, with Ian McDonald, of pattern-reversal visual evoked potentials in providing laboratory support for the diagnosis of multiple sclerosis through the demonstration of subclinical involvement of the optic nerve in patients who had not experienced visual symptoms. By 1965, Halliday had perfected the technique for recording evoked potentials using digital signal averaging, and clinical applications began a few years later, starting with the demonstration of their delay due to demyelination in optic neuritis.[8] Halliday's many contributions, establishing Queen Square as an important international centre in the use of evoked potentials, were summarised in a monograph published in 1982.[9]

Peter Nathan influenced the ideas and practice of neurologists for more than 50 years. Nathan served in the RAMC in various units and was then drafted to St Hugh's in Oxford where he met Carmichael, and he joined the MRC unit in 1946. His grandfather, Joseph Edward Nathan, had founded a pharmaceutical company (Glaxo) in Bunnythorpe, New Zealand, in the 1850s, and the firm was further enriched by the sales of dried milk as a safe baby food and 80 per cent of the penicillin used towards the end of the Second World War. As a beneficiary of his grandfather's estate, work for Nathan was a hobby rather than a necessity, but he lived simply and without any affectation, giving considerable parts of his wealth to charity.[10] Nathan worked with Pat Wall on neurological aspects of pain and carried out a trial of transcutaneous electrical nerve stimulation for herpetic neuralgia. He tested the efficacy of acupuncture for pain relief and introduced its use into the NHS. With Marion (Mai) Smith, Nathan published a series of 20 classical papers defining pathways in the spinal cord involved in movement, pain, sensation and bladder function. Their contribution was definitive, although this precipitated one of Walshe's characteristic polemics.[11] Nathan and Smith's major contribution was based on studying patients undergoing spinal tractotomy for intractable pain, often followed through to neuropathological examination. This, in effect, led to the establishment of the first pain clinic in the UK. This was very much the work of a physician who sat in the shadow of the influential clinical neurologists who dominated Queen Square at that time. Nathan was a refreshing maverick, with no aspirations whatsoever to lead or be an administrator, but he was humorous and highly intelligent. He saw patients but, in typical Queen

---

[7] Arguably, Dawson was responsible for the most enduring work of the neurological research unit in the early 1950s. The Institute of Neurology annual report for 1951–2 concludes that 'Dr Dawson has been investigating mechanism of epileptic seizures, particularly he has studied the electrical activity of the brain evoked by voltage of somatopic sensory impulses. These evoked responses are small in relation to the spontaneous activity of the brain and a special method has been developed to record these.'

[8] See A. M. Halliday *et al.*, 'Delayed Visual Evoked Response in Optic Neuritis', *Lancet* **311** (1972): 982–5; and Halliday *et al.*, 'Visual Evoked Response in Diagnosis of Multiple Sclerosis', *British Medical Journal* **4** (1973): 661–4.

[9] A. M. Halliday, *Evoked Potentials in Clinical Testing* (Edinburgh: Churchill Livingstone, 1982).

[10] Peter Nathan was born in London, educated at Marlborough and the Middlesex Hospital Medical School. He was appointed a member of the MRC external scientific staff in 1947, and became honorary physician at the National Hospital in 1948. Geoff Schott (Obituary: Peter Nathan MD, FRCP, *Pain* 2003 102:217–220) describes Nathan as 'perhaps the last of the British neurological giants who had acquired an over-arching knowledge of the nervous system and psychiatry, yet at the same time he achieved pre-eminence in his chosen fields of interest and research, particularly pain.' He details Nathan's training, his formative time with Cairns at St Hugh's, and assesses his wide-ranging work and lasting contributions particularly in the field of pain. Nathan's work on pain was scientifically imaginative, profound and wide-ranging. His last paper was published in Brain at the age of 87, and with it he declared that his life's work was complete. He was a remarkably generous person, interested in the arts as well as sciences and, for instance, paying for production of the *Canterbury Tales* when the production at Oxford moved to London. Nathan's enduring legacy is his corpus of important papers, especially in the field of pain, and his three books: *The Nervous System* (London: Penguin books 1969), *Retreat from Reason* (London: 1955) and, after a chance conversation during the 1930s with the rising Adolf Hitler in a Bierstube which gave him a lifelong loathing of fascism, *The Psychology of Fascism* (London: Faber and Faber, 1943).

[11] F. M. R. Walshe, 'The Babinski Plantar Response, Its Forms and Its Physiological and Pathological Significance', *Brain* **79** (1956): 529–56.

Square style, these were under Gilliatt's care. Ian McDonald remembered that:

> When he saw a new publication he liked he would often send the author a short note on a scrappy piece of paper (headed notepaper was not to be wasted) using an ancient typewriter, which he referred to as his 'tripewriter'. The text was sprinkled irregularly with upper and lower case letters and numerous spelling mistakes. He would comment that since people knew what he meant, there was no point in wasting time with corrections ... Peter Nathan must have been one of the last private scholars of medicine. He used his personal wealth to further his work and to support a remarkable range of causes and individuals in medicine and the arts. His scientific contribution, made at Queen Square, is part of the fabric of neurology.

Marion Smith trained in neuropathology with Greenfield.[12] Her husband, Stephen Sherwood, was a neurosurgeon, and Smith's own research informed surgery for the relief of pain and stereotactic procedures for movement disorders. She was an outstanding experimental neuropathologist who helped to found, and was later president of, the British Neuropathological Society (1977–9). In retirement, she continued her research on the anatomy of the human brain, cerebellum and spinal cord, and pathology of the nervous system, at the Radcliffe Infirmary in Oxford, in close association with Peter Nathan.

John Bates worked on visual tracking and design of controls in tanks during the Second World War using his skills in mathematics, information theory, computer science and engineering.[13] Thereafter, his main interest was recording from the human brain and understanding the cerebral control of movement, working initially with Wilder Penfield and Herbert Jasper at the Montreal Neurological Institute. He joined Carmichael's unit in 1946, and held an honorary appointment as consultant neurologist at the National Hospital. Together with Wylie McKissock, he made recordings of electrical activity in the brain and stimulated the motor cortex, internal capsule and thalamus in patients with epilepsy and infantile hemiplegia. As with Marion Smith, Bates adapted the techniques of Irving Cooper from New York in developing surgical lesions for the treatment of Parkinson's disease – work that was continued on his return from the USA with Ian McCaul, Harvey Jackson and Purdon Martin. Bates was a member and, later, president of the Electroencephalography Society (1976–8). A man of culture and humanity, Bates 'correctly diagnosed his own cerebral lesions as they occurred and observed his own decline with curiosity and equanimity'.

Surrounded by these clever scientists and clinicians who practised very little neurology, and with a series of visitors who subsequently brought distinction to institutions elsewhere, by 1960 Carmichael found himself attending a meeting of the Medical Research Council discussing the parlous state and dismal future of academic neurology in the UK. The subject was perceived to be in decline through lack of commitment to research. There was considered to be an urgent need for clinicians trained in experimental methods, experts recruited into neurological centres from other disciplines, and university investment in research units and departments of neurology. The MRC estimated that it had committed £317,000 to neurology in the previous quinquennium and the secretary, Sir Harold Himsworth, was surprised that so little had apparently been accomplished from so much expenditure. It seemed that work was being done by scientists in the name of neurology without involvement of the clinical neurologist. But Carmichael's legacy was appreciated at Queen Square and he was flattered when, in 1977, as part of the rearrangements of estate involved with the rebuilding of Queen Square House, the new laboratories on the first floor of the Queen Mary wing were named the Carmichael Laboratories, in recognition of his contribution to the construction of the wing. Unfortunately, the laboratories were moved in the early 1990s and both the name and commemorative plaque were lost.

The Readership and Professorship of Clinical Neurology

In 1951, the dean of the Institute of Neurology, Macdonald Critchley, told the Academic Board of his

---

[12] Marion Cecelia Smith was educated at Notre Dame High School in Glasgow and graduated from Glasgow University in zoology and then medicine, qualifying in 1944. Peter Nathan, her colleague and collaborator at Queen Square, provided an informative and moving obituary following her death from a pulmonary embolus after surgery for low-pressure hydrocephalus carried out at the National Hospital: see *Munk's Roll*, Vol. VIII (1989), pp. 476–8.

[13] John Alexander Vincent Bates, the son of a general practitioner in Colchester, was educated at Rugby and qualified in medicine from Cambridge and University College Hospital. P. W. Nathan, *Munk's Roll*, Vol. IX (1994), pp. 32–4.

discussion with the British Postgraduate Medical Federation (BPMF) asking the University of London to create professorships of neurology, neurosurgery, neuropathology and one in either experimental neurology, neurophysiology or biochemistry, to be held at the Institute.[14] Exactly 50 per cent of those present (17 of 34) favoured establishing the professorship of neurology. The rest did not, or abstained. As a result, the subcommittee charged with taking forward the overall proposal reported that there was no place for both a professorial unit of neurology and the existing MRC unit. They recommended that the former should replace the latter on the retirement of the director, expected in 1961, although the present incumbent, Carmichael, might meanwhile be offered a personal professorship for his remaining tenure. On 7 August 1953, a meeting of the Academic Board attended by 26 members resolved to establish professorships in one or more of neuropathology, neurochemistry, neuroradiology or neurophysiology, but to support neurology only with a readership.

It was noted that the costs of establishing a professorship in any one of the designated areas of research would be considerable, personal professorships could be appointed in these departments as an alternative to establishing new posts, and there was always the danger that the MRC might decide to extend the duration of the director's appointment beyond the retiring age. The subcommittee reported to the Academic Board on 26 October 1953 that the university be asked to specify in more detail its requirements for establishing a professorial unit. With these holding measures in place, battle commenced with three conflicting positions: that there should be no academic appointments; that, if this undesirable step was to be taken, in the case of clinical neurology the post should be at readership not professorial level; and, conversely, that the Institute should support the appointment of a professor of neurology leading a university department.

The dean, now Michael Kremer, subsequently reported that his discussions had raised difficulties over accommodation, and he favoured settling for a readership, funded by the BPMF, rather than a university professorship in clinical neurology. The subcommittee met on 2 March and 17 May 1954

but, given the diversity of views, some members were opposed to the recommendation not to press for a professorship.[15] On 5 July 1954, the subcommittee listed options for facilities needed to support academic neurology: 10–20 inpatient beds at Queen Square and nine at Maida Vale; two outpatient sessions per week; three junior staff, subject to an increase in establishment by the Minister of Health; and three laboratories at 23 Queen Square. They advised that the matter be discussed by the Medical Committees of the National Hospital and the Maida Vale Hospital. Presentations were made for and against the proposals at a meeting confined to the Management Committee of the National Hospital on 26 July 1954.[16] Those in favour of the professorship argued that the Institute was poorly represented on the Academic Councils of the BPMF, and neurology thereby disadvantaged as a medical specialty. The University Grants Committee and the University of London expected centres to have full-time teachers on their staff. Part-time clinicians could no longer be expected to maintain the hospital's reputation for research. The subcommittee expressed the view that, in settling for the readership, a junior person would probably be appointed to a post mainly carrying teaching responsibilities and, although the reader might subsequently be promoted, research would be unlikely to flourish. Those against any form of academic development argued that the reputation of Queen Square had been established and maintained through the work of part-time clinicians over the entire period of its history and 'at no time has the reputation ... depended upon its academic (that is non-clinical) accomplishments'. A reader or professor differed only 'as a sprat differs from a herring', and neither would advantage the atmosphere of the National Hospital: 'Professors are very prone to have an inhibitory effect upon their colleagues, particularly the junior members of their own departments. The reader would become remote from general medicine surrounded by a team of juniors and [likely to become] twisted and narrow ... whole-time academic

---

[14] The minutes of the Medical Committee and the Board of Governors of the National Hospital for this period contain various documents which outline the arguments for and against the establishment of the readership and the professorship of neurology, and the following account is based on these.

[15] Significantly, the membership included Carmichael and Slater, each of whom had a vested interest in the establishments of professorships at Queen Square. The other members were Kremer, Henson and Hamilton-Paterson.
[16] The following extracts are taken from the arguments put forward at the Management Committee meeting (attached to the minutes of the Board of Governors of the National Hospital).

officers in hospitals seldom pull their weight on the clinical side.'

It was stated that a suitable candidate would probably not be found for 'so preposterous a unit', the university requirements were impractical, and locating the professor or reader on two hospital sites (National Hospital and Maida Vale) made no sense. The venture could not be afforded even with additional grants and, if academic neurology was to be introduced, this should wait until establishment of a fully funded and resourced professorship was realistic. Arguments relating to age were also offered.

A man or woman appointed to the readership would almost certainly be in the age group of thirty to fifty. Before that he would be too untried, after it too old. When appointed he would retain his appointment till sixty-five. He would of necessity be either a clinical neurologist or an experimentalist interested in physiology or pathology. If he were a neurologist it is difficult to see in what way he would differ from existing members of staff. If he were over forty, unless the post were taken by an existing member of our staffs, he would presumably have already been an unsuccessful applicant for a staff appointment. If he were under forty, he could still make whatever contribution was in him to make as an ordinary physician.

A view expressed by speakers on both side of the debate was well summarised by one unnamed member who spoke in favour of the proposal:

I would agree with those who say that there is something wrong with the present status of neurology. I am sure that there is a danger that neurology is becoming looked on as a sterile non-productive, rather rarefied subject. If this is so, it can only be the fault of the present practitioners in neurology, they must have given this impression to their colleagues in other branches of medicine, and if this is the case then a change must take place if the subject is not to deteriorate in importance. I am sure that closer association with the University would be one of the ways of preserving the high regard in which neurology should be held, and with the help of the University this could be expressed in a practical fashion by the promotion of more neurology and more neurologists in the country.

At the conclusion of the meeting, the vote was in favour of providing clinical facilities for a readership in clinical neurology (eight in favour and five against). The Medical Committee of Maida Vale Hospital endorsed this decision at its meetings on 1 and 22 November 1954. The Board of Governors considered the matter on 1 December 1954 and agreed to create the readership (eight in favour, four against and five abstentions).

Throughout these discussions, we hear the strident voice of Francis Walshe, whose memorandum had been tabled at several of these meetings and who despised the concept of the clinical professor.[17] Walshe prefaced his remarks with the challenge that what proved valuable in the past was no longer relevant to the present need, which was to understand the aetiology, pathogenesis and treatment of neurological disease. He maintained that this was the province of the clinical neurologist. Walshe was driven by a personal agenda. His major criticism was the conspicuous failure of neurophysiology to have made any useful contribution to research in clinical neurology. Walshe's suggestion, perhaps intended as a filibuster – but visionary, as it turned out – was that the future of the subject lay in promoting neurochemistry and metabolic studies of the nervous system.

Academic studies in the anatomy and physiology of the nervous system can never be the primary activity of a neurological hospital ... yet these subsidiary activities ... have in the past monopolised the time and energy of some of our best men ... despite the meagre returns they have made to practical medicine ... it is because we have become isolated from the active world of general medicine that we remain tied in thought and action to largely obsolete ... research ... that over the years ... has proved of relatively little value.

Walshe continued to argue that the clinical neurologist could not contribute to the discipline of neurochemistry, whether that person be an 'academic', courtesy of an arbitrary administrative act, or part-time clinician engaged in private practice. He pontificated that the dividend from establishment of clinical professors in Britain after the Second World War had been merely to expand administration, and little had been achieved by giving young neurologists nothing more than experience in classical neurophysiology or applied electronics. His solution was to train young clinicians in biochemistry before their return to clinical neurology, using the model recently introduced by the MRC. Walshe concluded that:

---

[17] The memorandum is attached to the minutes of the 1 December 1954 meeting of the Board of Governors of the National Hospital.

The present creation of a clinical readership or professorship would be a gesture of no significance to the future of neurological medicine. If neurology, and the National Hospitals as its centres, is to maintain its prestige, it will be by original work turned out by those working in them, and not by the lists of professors and readers that may adorn the front page of the Medical School's Annual Report.

Walshe's opinion on academic physicians was nothing new, and well known before this particular debate. He had published his excoriating attack on 'professors of medicine' in his annual address at the opening of University College London Medical School in 1947. As in other matters, he represented the traditional view that was, in many ways, having its last gasp. The subsequent course of academic neurology at Queen Square shows that, in one main respect, he took the wrong side in this, as in many other important debates, and the debacle over the professorship reflects how out of touch he was with the new mood of neurology after the Second World War.[18]

John Marshall

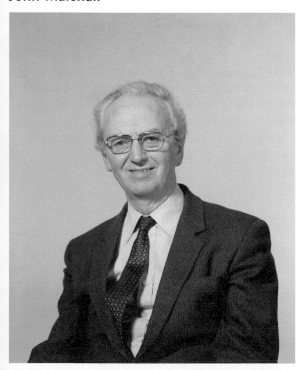

Figure 13.3 John Marshall.

John Marshall was appointed to the newly established readership in 1956.[19] Marshall grew up in Lancashire and was educated at a school in Bolton which had no tradition of tertiary education. He graduated in medicine from Manchester University in 1946 and worked in that city, the Maudsley Hospital, briefly as a research fellow at the National Hospital, and in Oxford and Edinburgh before returning to Queen Square. Eventually, he held a personal professorship between 1971 and 1987 in the Institute of Neurology. As a clinician, Marshall assessed a prodigious number of patients in record time through his visits to the West Middlesex Hospital in Isleworth, London. He led research at Queen Square in stroke (with Ralph Ross Russell, Lindsay Symon and George du Boulay). Marshall's work was wide-ranging: the introduction of rehabilitation; work on epidemiology and familial incidence of cerebrovascular disease; resolving mechanisms of tissue injury in transient ischaemic attack, preferring the concept of platelet embolisation to that of hypotension and arterial spasm; the development of intra-arterial and intravenous methods for quantifying blood flow; determining systems for distinguishing vascular dementia from Alzheimer's disease; conducting treatment trials of anticoagulation in ischaemic stroke, and aspirin in amaurosis fugax; early applications of the EMI scan and scintigram imaging in stroke; and the first nuclear magnetic resonance (NMR) scan in subdural haematoma. Throughout much of his academic career, Marshall was supported by a technician, Elias Zilkha, and secretary, Beryl Laatz, whom he regarded as 'priceless' and far more valuable than any research registrars.

Apart from his areas of research, mainly stroke, Marshall directed the intensive care unit at Queen Square, where he introduced negative pressure ventilation (the 'iron lung') for the treatment of poliomyelitis, using a design from the Cowley factory in Oxford,[20] and, subsequently, positive pressure ventilation. He supported speech therapy as a clinical and academic discipline based on techniques learned from the Australian therapist Lionel Logue, who had treated the stuttering King George VI, and it was Marshall who affiliated the College of Speech Sciences with Queen Square. Marshall served as dean of the

---

[18] Although this was the first chair in clinical neurology in the country, this was very late – and, for instance, a chair in radiology had been established at London University in 1920.

[19] John Walton was the unsuccessful applicant for the post.
[20] An inmate at one of Her Majesty's prisons revealed to Marshall's son-in-law that Queen Square was where he habitually 'nicked oxygen cylinders' destined for the Batten Intensive Care Unit.

Institute of Neurology from 1982 to 1987. In that capacity, he was instrumental in bringing David Marsden to Queen Square as Roger Gilliatt's successor. He prioritised appointments to the Institute of Neurology and National Hospital of clinician scientists, rather than applicants who were unlikely to make any academic contribution to the subject. In making this change, Marshall won some battles and lost others, but, throughout, his style and blunt manner made him something of an outsider, and the memories of events in 1962 surrounding the university professorship never entirely faded. In retirement, Marshall was chairman of the Board of Governors at the National Hospital for Epilepsy at Chalfont St Peter, and led the successful appeal for the magnetic resonance scanner dedicated to research in epilepsy.

The Catholic faith was the bedrock of Marshall's life. He was medical adviser to the family planning branch of the Catholic Church from 1951 to 1992, writing on contraception using temperature as a guide to abstinence[21] and periodically expounding his views on the Radio 4 *Today* programme. In 1963, he advised Pope John XXIII on the Vatican Commission on birth control, and Pope Paul VI on the more liberal approach to contraception issued in 1966, whilst still remaining true to the doctrine of natural birth control. In 1979, at the invitation of Roy Mason, then Secretary for State, Marshall served on a three-man committee investigating police behaviour in Northern Ireland. He served on the Warnock Committee which considered human fertilisation and embryology between 1982 and 1984. In 1985, Marshall was made Knight Commander of the Pontifical Equestrian Order of St Gregory the Great Knight. He was appointed CBE in 1990. Marshall had married Eileen, a US citizen, in the year he qualified in medicine. At home, Marshall was a dedicated father to five children (two were adopted), and an adventurous cook who might serve ostrich, kangaroo or crocodile meat (when in season). His children spoke movingly at an event to celebrate Marshall's life held at Queen Square on 24 June 2014, at which the Stroke Association announced their intention to name a lectureship in his honour.

Even though the investment by the BPMF in academic neurology had started to gather momentum by establishing the readership in the late 1950s, it was becoming clear that the doctrinaire style of clinical

neurology must change further as the National Hospital approached its centenary, if the subject and the institution were to avoid being left behind by advances in experimental medicine. Still Queen Square baulked at developing academically and, in the early 1960s, the University of London offered an ultimatum to the National Hospital on establishing a professorship of neurology. Now the consultant staff relented, ending a long and complex campaign of resistance.

One obvious option was to promote Marshall from the readership he had held since 1956. But those who opposed any investment in academic neurology still had not finished. In 1957, Longmans Green & Co. published *Physiology of the Nervous System* by Geoffrey Walsh and John Marshall. In 1959 appeared *Clinical Neurophysiology* by John Marshall. The preface explained that the book was intended for the clinician, enabling him (*sic*) to consider clinical practice from the standpoint of advances in neurophysiology: 'the pages have not been burdened with numerous references'. There was no mention of the earlier book and only a single reference to Dr Walsh's research papers. Many staff at the Institute of Neurology were acknowledged for having read and criticised various sections or loaned illustrations. But herein lay trouble ahead because, when the book was published, word spread that some of the material was too close for comfort to the contents of the book written two years earlier with Geoffrey Walsh. We have examined both texts and find little to justify this accusation, but whispers and hints of plagiarism were used by those opposed to the development of academic neurology in order to weaken the case that could be made to establish a professorship, given that Marshall was the likely appointee. Because of the perceived misdemeanour, Marshall agreed not to apply but changed his mind at the last minute, to the embarrassment of all, and was interviewed together with Laurie Liversedge (from Manchester) and Roger Gilliatt. Marshall remained silent on this episode and his support for Gilliatt was never in doubt. But their styles and social backgrounds were very different and the relationship appeared no more than cordial, at best, from the early 1960s until Marshall's retirement in 1987.

Derek Denny-Brown

It is an unfortunate gap in the archival records of Queen Square that no documents have come to light

[21] J. Marshall, *Catholics, Marriage and Contraception* (Dublin: Helicon, 1965).

that account for the transition from readership to professorship. But once it became clear that appointing a professor of neurology could not be avoided, the first thought was to invite Derek Denny-Brown.[22] He was a New Zealander who came to England in the 1920s to work with Sir Charles Sherrington and, trained in clinical neurology, he had been on the consultant staff of St Bartholomew's Hospital and the National Hospital in the 1930s. He had been in the United States, as professor of neurology at Harvard, since 1940 and, now the dominant figure in world neurology, was held in great affection by his former colleagues at Queen Square. Walshe wrote immediately to Denny-Brown reflecting, in passing, on the centenary celebrations, and dealing in derogatory terms with many colleagues at Queen Square:

> I had from another source a complaint that Russell B. was a 'stuffed shirt' and a 'Colonel Blimp'. He can talk of nothing but cervical spondylosis for the past few years – like Cairns who lectured on crash helmets for twenty years and Penfield on his C.E.S. for over twenty. In the end, Spillane has done much better work on this threadbare subject than R.B. The NH centenary went off amazingly well, but of course you should have been there and your absence was widely felt. The party was arranged by Critchley, rather round himself, and at the official dinner, Percival Bailey spoke for the American visitors and Monrad Krohn for the European visitors. Wechsler got no opportunity to speak, and I don't think any of us knew that he was the official delegate from the ANA. The main speech at the official dinner by the hospital chairman (Sir John Woods) was a major disaster, and the only two members of the hospital staff (alive or dead) that he mentioned were the two Rogers (Roger Bannister the four minute miler and Roger Gilliatt, Mr Armstrong Jones's best man). He then virtually invited the overseas visitors to contribute to a fund for rebuilding the hospital … Charles Symonds gave the Gowers lecture (75 minutes of heavy and mostly inaudible matter, good for reading, but hopeless to listen to). Norman Dott gave a Horsley lecture which I am told was awful and Critchley gave a good centennial lecture. I played for safety and turned up to the subscription dinner for all-comers – a very pleasant evening – and to the official dinner. The Duke of Edinburgh spent two hours in the hospital, going round the gadgets

(Carmichael's team being producers) and I am told he appeared to enjoy it all. My only effort was to present the Gowers medal to Symonds and I felt I had to cheer up the rather dispirited audience by some bright remarks. I seem to have succeeded. There is now being voiced a plan to rebuild the hospital in Fulham. An old Poor Law Hospital there is being pulled down and there is talk of a vast central postgraduate or rather specialist hospital being built on the site. I should hate to see us leaving Queen Square but the young men have no strong feeling for the place – and perhaps they are right – and if the Government can be interested the new century may be a new story for Queen Square. Having been attached to the place officially for 48 years of its first century, I am sure I don't belong to its second century. Still it was good while it lasted – though not so good of late years.[23]

And, of the same occasion, Denis Brinton also wrote to Denny-Brown:

> The lectures were good enough marred somewhat by the bedevilled acoustics of the BMA Great Hall which CPS in my view was unfortunately particularly unable to discipline; and the demonstrations laid on by the various departments at the National for the whole of the week were really very good. I do wish you could have been with us. I believe you might have been more convinced that we are not so old as we evidently lead some general physicians here to believe, although the other side of that coin is certainly that our public relations are rotten, and must be improved … I have had a ding-dong battle with Keith Murray who evidently approves the notion of us inviting you; a long evening thrashing things out with George Pickering who is similarly minded; and lastly, after consultation with John Woods, Russell Brain and Kremer, setting the stage for an inspired leak of what I should like. This has taken the form of a dinner with Roger Gilliatt, undoubtedly the potential leader of the youngest group at the N[ational] H[ospital], so that I could put fairly and squarely before him our problem as we see it. He is even now attempting to digest this strong man's meat with his infant's gastric juices. I have told him not to hesitate to talk to others since it is clear that we must <u>unanimously</u> invite you, if we are going to, and its no good beating about the bush any longer. I expect therefore that we shall debate the matter in committee(s) in the

---

22 Some details in this text are taken from D. A. S. Compston, 'Derek Denny-Brown', *Oxford Dictionary of National Biography* (2015), at https://dx.doi.org/10.1093/ref:odnb/107177.

23 McDonald archive: letter dated 2 August 1960. The menu and table plan of the more than 215 guests are in the Queen Square archive. Walshe is at the top table, but well separated from Brain and Penfield.

next month or two. I shall keep you informed. Roger Gilliatt, by the way, is a potential Prof[essor] [of] Clin[ical] Neurol[ogy] himself; but being a particular friend of John Marshall has at all events said that he does not want it yet. Whether he means what he says I am not so sure. He and others (EAC in particular) think of Ritchie [Russell] who I will strive against till the end as I have told Roger partly because I am sure that WRR's achievements have not even been better than second class and partly because for fifteen years at any rate he has been the chief of the slanderers of the N[ational] H[ospital] his alma mater. The results of this will be intriguing whichever way they go. I shall guard your interests, but, Good Lord, I hope that my colleagues see the light and that we get you on your terms. I was delighted to learn that you had accepted the Sherrington lecture. That committee was the pleasantest to chair that I have met. You chose yourself or rather Liddell started the ball rolling and I didn't have to do a thing. John Eccles and some quaint foreigner whose name I have forgotten but whose English is not so hot and who anyhow suffers from logorrhoea were puny runners.[24]

Denny-Brown was educated at New Plymouth High School in the Taranaki region of the North Island in New Zealand, and attended the University of Otago Dunedin School of Medicine, graduating in 1924. After qualification, he was briefly assistant to (William Percy) Gowland, professor of anatomy at Otago, working on comparative anatomy of the nervous system. Arriving in England in 1925, Denny-Brown was a student at the National Hospital before securing a Beit memorial fellowship working with Sherrington in Oxford, between 1925 and 1928. His DPhil thesis was 'On the Essential Mechanisms of Mammalian Posture' (1928), in which he illuminated the respective roles of fast pale and slow red muscles in movement and posture, respectively, correcting an error in Sherrington's previous research. Loosely inserted in a stray book from the library of E. G. T. Liddell, Sherrington's successor as Waynflete professor of physiology in Oxford, is a note in manuscript:

It amuses me to reflect that round about 1925, CSS [Sherrington] ... refused ... to consider that red and white muscles might have different duties but a current class book showed that their myograms were different in character. But then an eager young [man] who had worked his way from NZ as a ship's doctor came to England/Oxford/CSS cap in hand ... to study their differences. After the young man had come in to be interviewed and explained himself ... S's mood changed in a flash. So DB came to Oxford. But this is a naughty story.

After further training in neurology at the National Hospital, Guy's and St Bartholomew's, Denny-Brown was appointed assistant physician to the National Hospital, neurologist at St Bartholomew's Hospitals (1935–41) and physician to the Central London Eye Hospital (1936–41).[25] Denny-Brown saw patients, had a private practice and conducted research at the weekends. He shared consulting rooms with Symonds but was always late, the patients having to wait in the dining room, so that Symonds often had to delay their dinner. But, unlike his mentor Holmes, the clinician-researcher Denny-Brown had a different approach to research that leaned on his training with Sherrington: 'In drawing on inspiration for active laboratory work from contact with patients [Denny-Brown] was a new breed slowly being recognised in academic medicine ... the administrative arrangements of earlier periods had failed to keep pace with the needs of this new type of scientific clinician.'[26]

In 1936, Denny-Brown had visited John Fulton at Yale, supported by a Rockefeller Fellowship, and thus began his involvement with American neurology. After Tracy Putnam moved to New York, the chairman of the search committee for his replacement in Boston, Stanley Cobb, sent a telegram to Symonds, in January 1939, asking if he could ascertain whether Denny-Brown wished to be a candidate for the professorship of neurology at Harvard. Elected on 23 June 1939, he was returning by boat to England on the day that the Second World War was declared. Denny-Brown delayed his move to Harvard, working at the Head Injuries Hospital in Oxford from January 1940 and studying the physiology of concussion with Ritchie Russell. He had joined the Territorial Army section of the Royal Army Medical Corps on 9 December 1933 as

[24] McDonald archive: letter dated 7 August 1960.

[25] Sir Cyril Clarke recalled seeing Denny-Brown sprinting along the corridors at Guy's Hospital when Symonds' car was approaching, so as to be in place at the door for his arrival. Denny-Brown's referees for the consultant posts included Sherrington, Greenfield, Symonds and Holmes, each of whom made clear that Denny-Brown was a clinician scientist of extraordinary promise.

[26] *Harvard Gazette*, 27 January 1984, p. 4.

lieutenant, promoted to captain in 1934, and transferred to the list of reserve officers on 5 March 1938. Denny-Brown achieved the rank of lieutenant-colonel (1945–6), and had been awarded the OBE (Military) in 1941. In that year, expressing gratitude for the American war effort to James Conant, president of Harvard and an emissary of Franklin D. Roosevelt, Winston Churchill asked whether anything could be done in return. He was told that releasing a certain British medical officer so that he could take up his post in Boston would be appreciated. Evidently, Churchill turned to his Paymaster General (Maurice, Baron Hankey): 'Hankey, see to it.' Denny-Brown duly arrived in Boston in 1941 as 'agent of a foreign power', serving on the committee on aviation medicine, National Academy of Sciences, Washington (1941–5). But he was again summoned back to organise neurological services in India and Burma, finally settling in Boston from 1946 as professor of neurology, Harvard University.[27] In retirement, Denny-Brown worked as chief of neurophysiology and associate director at the New England Regional Primate Centre (1967–72) and as Fogarty Scholar at the National Institutes of Health (1973). He continued with experimental work and lectures until 1980. Denny-Brown died from multiple myeloma at home in Boston on 20 April 1981.

Denny-Brown's philosophy was that questions formulated in the clinic should be answered by experiments in the laboratory, especially through the application of neuropathology and neurochemistry. In formulating ideas, such was the force of his opinion on the probable underlying neuropathology that any discrepancy at the weekly brain-cutting session was blamed on 'the brain having got it wrong'. Denny-Brown was irascible but admired and influential. It was estimated that, by 1961, he had trained 19 of 41 chairmen of US departments of neurology. At a time when the distinction was unresolved, he promoted neurology as a specialty separate from internal medicine and psychiatry. Many of Denny-Brown's doctrines (and the scientific achievements of his clinical career) are rehearsed in his Shattuck lecture (1952):

Neurology, like any other branch of medicine, must continue to base its methods and philosophy on clinicopathological correlation ... neurology sprang from internal medicine ... in time it was no longer possible to keep abreast of all branches of medicine and the genus neurologist was born ... from the beginning of the budding process the neurologist has occupied a position that is thought to be somewhat academic – the impractical collector of static curiosities and geographer of abstruse anatomic networks, with more than the usual specialist's ritual of cabalistic signs ... the rise of neurosurgery soon encroached on what had been considered the neurologist's field and by the 1930s there were many who predicted the extinction of the genus neurologist. Some professed neurology as an appendage to neurosurgery or psychiatry ... the stock in trade became restricted to 'degenerative' diseases, multiple sclerosis and epilepsy ... such an attitude springs from a wrong conception of neurology and an erroneous conception of the structure of medicine. Neurology ... must mean neurological medicine and as such comprise all diseases that in any way affect the nervous system ... the neurologist must first be an internist ... a specialist is only a specialist by virtue of special ability to contribute ... the right to special facilities has to be earned by progressive contribution to the effectiveness of medical practice ... where neurology has been set up with special facilities in splendid isolation it has tended to wither. For progress it requires its own hospital beds and budget; for inspiration it must work with internal medicine.[28]

He went on to explain the work with which he had been involved: treating Wilson's disease with British anti-Lewisite (BAL); his work on mechanisms of transient cerebrovascular disease and disorders of the dynamics of cerebrospinal fluid and 'otitic hydrocephalus'; and research on primary muscle disease.[29] Sylvia Denny-Brown also recalls that her

---

[27] See S. Shulman and J. Vilensky, 'How Denny-Brown Came to Harvard', *Harvard Medical Alumni Bulletin* **71** (1997): 46–50; J. A. Vilensky *et al.*, 'Derek Denny-Brown (1901–1981): His Life and Influence on American Neurology', *Journal of Medical Biography* **6** (1998): 73–8.

[28] D. Denny-Brown, 'The Shattuck Lecture: The Changing Pattern of Neurologic Medicine', *New England Journal of Medicine* **246** (1952): 838–46.

[29] Denny-Brown also edited *The Selected Writings of Sir Charles Sherrington* (1939, reprinted 1979), published by the Guarantors of *Brain*. He published *Reflex Activity of the Spinal Cord* (1932: with Creed, Eccles, Liddell and Sherrington); *Diseases of the Basal Ganglia and Subthalamic Nuclei* (1946); *Handbook of Neurological Examination and Case Recording* (1946); *Diseases of Muscle: A Study in Pathology* (1953: with Raymond Adams); *The Basal Ganglia and Their Relationship to Disorders of Movement* (1962); and *The Cerebral Control*

husband made a suggestion to Mary Walker, who was distressed that she was not able to improve the condition of her patients with myasthenia gravis: 'Perhaps it will help you to know that the disease is like curare poisoning. The next time they met she had looked up curare poisoning in some medical encyclopaedia and followed the instructions suggested and now gleefully showed him patients who were vastly improved.'[30]

This led to the use of anticholinesterases (physostigmine) as symptomatic treatment for the condition. Denny-Brown described the pathophysiology of conduction block in peripheral nerves, and electromyography of fasciculation in muscle; he made contributions to hereditary and paraneoplastic sensory neuropathies, illuminated mechanisms of head injury, characterised nutritional deficiencies of the nervous system, and studied cerebral function and motor control in humans and non-human primates. He was not averse to experimenting on himself, studying reflex control of bladder and bowel function in man with E. Graeme Robertson, each using the other as a subject. He had Dupuytren's contracture and, after deciding to have one of his fingers amputated, had the digital nerve crushed several days before surgery to allow subsequent histological examination. Later, there was discussion in the literature between Graham Weddell and Denny-Brown as to how long after crush the nerve was examined, to which Denny-Brown retorted: 'Well, it was my bloody finger!'

On receipt of the invitation from Sir John Woods, Denny-Brown wrote, on 2 January 1961, to Michael Kremer, in his capacity as dean of the Institute, declining the offer but, in so doing, offering an analysis that brought a sense of realism to the strategists at Queen Square, and served thereafter as a manifesto on what constitutes a professor of clinical neurology.

My Dear Michael

I received your letter of December 5th safely, together with a letter from Sir John Woods, regarding the proposed Professorship of Neurology at Queen Square. It is a tremendous compliment that the staff should wish to interest me in applying for this post, and should express such cordial goodwill. It is very heartening to be so regarded, and I for my part can truly say that Queen Square is for me a sort of spiritual home, and I would be eager to do anything in my power for the institution that gave me my early training and stimulus.

For me to move to London at this stage in my career would be a very considerable dislocation of my family and of my scientific work. Before I can decide to do so I would like to be more sure that there would be a reasonable chance of accomplishing what would be expected of me, and what appears to me to need to be done.

The whole present situation of British Neurology that has led to the need for such a full-time chair is a complex one that involves a number of general considerations as well as the more practical details of organisation of the professor's department.

I think the staff of the hospital should agree on some statement of policy that could serve as a basis for all this change. Otherwise I can foresee difficulties of all kinds in the future. If for example the hospital wishes to concentrate on training consultants for the NHS, to serve in this or that regional area, then one or two years of training in clinical resident status, with a year or two at registrar level, would suffice. Queen Square does a superb job in this kind of training as it is, and does not need me for it. But there are many places, especially the undergraduate hospital units that could do this.

It is possible to make very few advances now without some sort of type of laboratory technique. The coming young men must have experience of such techniques. Queen Square has very good laboratories of neuropathology, neurochemistry, EEG, yet the present system does not attract the young clinician into the laboratory. A clinical professor may try to excite their interest, but unless he is himself working in the laboratory he could not accomplish much.

---

of Movement (VIIIth Sherrington lecture, 1966). An archive was created at the Indiana University School of Medicine, Fort Wayne, Michigan, preserving 2,200 100-foot rolls of film recording experiments on 450 monkeys performed between 1948 and 1972, and a further 500 films recording patients under Denny-Brown's care at the Boston City Hospital from 1942 to 1967. J. Vilensky et al., 'The Denny-Brown Collection: A Research and Teaching Resource', Annals of Neurology 36 (1994): 247–51.

[30] In 1931, Denny-Brown, considered by his host to be a rising star in British neurology, attended a party for trainee neurologists from Queen Square at the home of James Collier. There, Denny-Brown met Collier's niece, Sylvia Marie Summerhayes, daughter of John Orlando Summerhayes, DSO, physician and missionary doctor. It was the pursuit of his career, rather than Sylvia's judgement that Denny-Brown 'was a hopeless dancer', that delayed their marriage until 17 March 1937.

The plan outlined in your letter seems to me to envisage a clinical unit more or less segregated from the rest of the hospital. This is, I know, the principle on which the Professional Units of Bart's and St Thomas' were founded. Yet, it is I think, most undesirable, for it creates a rift between the 'part-timers' and the 'full-timers'. It automatically excludes the professional unit from all the rest of the clinical material, and it sets up research on entirely the wrong footing as an activity peculiar to one 'firm'.

How would the staff regard a mandatory year of neuropathology residency, following two years of clinical residency, for every resident accepted for the hospital? Is there any way of paying residents for a third year of this kind? How would the neuropathologist regard a clinical professor who wanted to assist him in 'slide sessions' as well as the usual 'brain-cutting' sessions, once a week? Neuropathology is the essential science of neurology, and unless the neuropathology laboratory is a place where everybody works in some degree no scientific progress can be made, and no progressive training of the few who are to be the future leaders of neurology can be undertaken. To a less degree neurochemistry and EEG should in part be common ground, though the material here is less unique.

Your professor of neurology in other words cannot be a pure clinician. He should have laboratories of his own where he can study his problems in his own way. Experimental neuropathology almost certainly would be an interest, and hence a need for histological, histochemical, autoradiographic, and electrical recording equipment. He should be free to follow his problems wherever they lead him, and his associates. But in addition he has to take an active part in teaching conferences in all these other subjects, and may have particular interests that are for example purely neuropathological.

I have written this out at some length because the present intention regarding the function of the professor is not clear. The great tradition of English neurology is clinico-pathological correlation. How is this to be carried on in the proposed set-up? Which seems to me to have all the limitations that hampered the work of Arnold Carmichael's Unit for so many years.

Of course the professor cannot take over direct responsibility for neuropathology, neurochemistry, or other existing laboratory departments, the heads of which have a well defined responsibility for routine reporting, as well as their own space and opportunities for research and teaching. What is needed is more clinically orientated advanced teaching and research, and these necessarily impinge on all the other activities. This is the principle that must be recognized and supported, if one is to avoid such

ridiculous possibilities as the head of a laboratory department refusing the right of a clinical professorship (or other clinicians) to the use of routine reports or material, regarding cases of common interest. The clinician must of course also recognise the right of the laboratory head to make special studies in his own way and to use these as he wishes. Goodwill should solve most problems, but if the principles are recognized the problems need not arise. The clinical professor should also not be just one who is to come and do all the clinical research of the hospital, but one who transforms, little by little, the magnificent opportunities of Queen Square into a milieu where everyone is playing some part in advancing neurological medicine each in his own way. The professor also has to be the main sparking force in the training of a group of strongly motivated young men, who are chosen from those who have shown some special aptitudes and ability in their third (neuropathology) year, and who then begin special fellowships in research for one to three more years.

I am not sure that I myself could at my age and in the relating short period of five years achieve the full potential of all this. But without some general realisation by the staff of the nature of the problem it would not be worthwhile even beginning. To attempt to transfer my present activities to Queen Square, setting up in a relatively segregated unit then would be impossible. It would take two years to get going again and without the elaborate interlocking arrangements I have here with neuropathology, and an enormous amount of expensive equipment, one could not get far. On the other hand, the challenge of Queen Square, and ones interest in furthering British neurology is very real.

And now some specific details. Taking them up in the order they come in your letter I would like some more information as to the number of beds. You say that 30 have been allotted the Academic Unit. Are these the same that are now allotted to Dr. Marshall, or are they 30 beds in addition to his? Later you say that the Unit consists of a Reader (presumably Dr. Marshall), and then a 'Reader and Lecturer paid by the University' – is this one person or two, and who are they? Then there are two other Lecturers – so the Professor and Reader, and 3 Lecturers between them supervise 30 (?60) beds. 30 beds for all of them would seem to me to be adequate, for the professor presumably will do only one 'grand round' once a week, and the others in turn conduct the daily rounds. If the professor is expected to do ward round each day in addition to two ½-day out-patient sessions a week, a hospital clinical conference, at least one neuropathology combined conference, as well as faculty meetings etc. he had better give up all idea of research, and particularly of training young men in research. This last activity takes at least 2 days a week for the first month, and ½ to 1 day a week for the rest of the year, for each young man beginning a research project.

Your first paragraph on page 2 mentions the University contribution. Where are the running expenses of the Academic Unit to come from? Even if we were to teach Latin we would need office expenses, initial cost of typewriters, the recurrent cost of repairs, publishing expenses, the purchase of technical manuals etc. Does the professor have to provide Bunsen burners, glass ware, basic chemicals, animals for pilot experiments, their food, photographic supplies? Does he have to provide his own microscope, camera, ovens? Does the University not realise that any laboratory has to have basic equipment and a basic budget for running expenses (at least £1500 a year)? No grant or Foundation that I know of will provide running expenses.

The space mentioned in your letter is difficult to assess. Six rooms on the first floor of the old east corridor are occupied by the present Unit. I can remember three of them, all very cramped. 'The rooms on the next two floors' – how many of them are there? Would it be possible to convert 2 or 3 of them to laboratories, do they have running water, electric power, is there a dark room, and would the professor have an office? What has happened to the space occupied by Carmichael's Unit, and its equipment? Has Carmichael's group entirely vanished, or are some left, and where do they stand? I cannot comment without this information. I understand the necessity of keeping some beds at Maida Vale, and provided that not more than one half day a week is spent at that hospital I think it would be a reasonable arrangement.

It is not that the facilities are poor or inadequate, Michael, for we are used to two or three men working at different projects in the one small room. I would like to be assured that both the staff and University fully understand what Academic Neurology really means in the modern world. I have trained 8 full professors, and 36 of various other academic ranks, here at Boston City Hospital, not counting those that have gone into private practice as neurologists, and I think I know. If some doubt my insistence on full-time training in neuropathology ask them to look up the records of Wilson, Collier, Holmes, Symonds and Adie.

It is in fact a very expensive business for a University, but then so is any modern technical training. Britain cannot expect to keep up with the Americans, or the Russians, or West Germans, with the set-up of the 1930s. The running budget of the Neurological Unit in Boston City Hospital from the University last year was $57,000 [£20,355] (includes salaries), with grants totalling approximately $113,000 from various sources. Yet this has 26 beds (85 chronic cases in a hospital for chronic disease), and about 2,600 outpatients, and 2,300 consultations in other parts of the hospital. I feel sure that the expensive equipment could ultimately be purchased from grants to Queen Square, but the basic framework must be soundly designed and well supported.

I shall look forward to having your comments and your answers to my questions. I wish this was all ten years ago, and I would have come like a shot. Now there are many complications, but rest assured that I would like to come, but would like to see some better chance of real success.

With my best regards,
Sincerely, Denny

P.S. You may show this letter to whomever you wish, or circulate it to the staff. Denny.[31]

In fact, there may have been a more practical reason for declining the offer. Sylvia Denny-Brown told McDonald that a trustee of the National Hospital visited him in Boston and was asked by Denny-Brown whether the date for retirement could be extended, because otherwise he could not accept the post. The answer was 'no': 'Denny never regretted the decision to stay at the BCH [Boston City Hospital] even though Ray Adams behaved in a peculiar fashion about the whole thing, which was a personal disappointment to him.'[32]

McDonald concluded that knowledge of the existence of this letter and its contents played an important part in securing the change in attitude that led to the transformation of Queen Square in the 1960s and 1970s. Later, Walshe wrote again to Denny-Brown:

I am sorry I shall not hear your Presidential address, and I sympathise with you if you have to sit next to our B [Russell Brain] at dinner. He is famed for being absolutely incapable of conversation. Nor need you be afraid of him, he cherishes beneath his florid countenance an inferiority complex in respect of Queen Square trained men – as he has every right to do. I

---

[31] The original is retained in the minute book of the Academic Board for 2 January 1961.
[32] McDonald archive: letter dated 15 March 1992.

have never taken him seriously and he knows it. It would be a mistake to do so. I have always held – and sometimes said – that the Queen square trained neurologists (that is, men who have been through the house) are the regulars and the Maida Vale products merely territorials – Saturday afternoon neurologists. RB is now primarily a committee man – urged on to public activities by a devoted and ambitious wife. He really is her creation, and but for her pushing him into medicine, would now be an obscure history don at Oxford. As you see, I still dislike the milk of human kindness, but I do know an image with clay feet when I meet one. I got an amusing letter from St Louis about our 'best man', offering me a copy of the American novel 'What made Sammy run' to pass on to RG [Roger Gilliatt]. Here is another man with a very ambitious wife, a journalist (and an assistant editor of Vogue) who moves in the Chelsea set. How RG likes all this publicity I don't know. Nobody should write on two sides of thin notepaper, so I will stop my scurrilities. PS I am getting back into fighting form again.[33]

Sir John Eccles considered that, in his work on the neurophysiology of inhibition in the control of movement and posture, Denny-Brown was the most brilliant experimentalist in the Oxford department. McDonald recalls a conversation between himself and Eccles:

It can't be emphasised enough the importance of [Denny-Brown's] influence in moulding modern neurology on both sides of the Atlantic. The major chairs in neurology in the United States in the post-war period were occupied more by pupils of Denny-Brown than pupils of any other teacher. His influence was no less important in this country. Amongst the generation of senior neurologists now, there are men who have described to me how important it was their coming into contact with Denny-Brown at St Hugh's during the war and the influence that he had in training them in the examination of the nervous system has remained to this day. Later, a number of neurologists in this country went to America to spend a period of time with him and I regard this as one of the most important facets in my own development. But he has a further role too and that was that he stated explicitly what he believed was the role of academic neurology and what the necessary prerequisites were. What I say now cannot be published but I have no doubt at all that the renewed vigour of Queen Square since the 1960s was directly

related to the esteem in which Denny was held because his views, which he stated explicitly, were what in fact have been put into effect over these last few years.[34]

All that Queen Square could salvage from this attempt at recruitment was the naming, in 1984, of new research laboratories after Denny-Brown. Sylvia wrote to John Marshall: 'Thanks for the photos which speak for themselves. Roger with his inimitable gesture, having conjured the name plate out of space, Chris Earl's humorous complacency and Ian obviously dubious about the whole occasion. Such spice is noticeably absent on this side of the Atlantic, but an appropriate and promising beginning for the lab.'[35]

Roger William Gilliatt

After refusing the professorship at the Institute of Neurology, once the appointment was made, Denny-

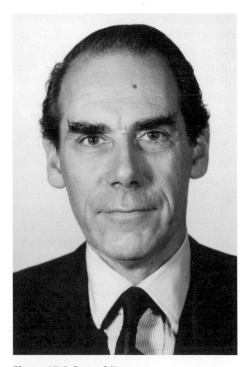

Figure 13.4 Roger Gilliatt.

---

[33] McDonald archive: letter dated 12 May 1962.

[34] McDonald archive: transcript of taped conversation, undated.

[35] McDonald archive: correspondence dated 27 January 1985.

Brown told McDonald that Gilliatt 'having the right priorities, being of the establishment, and likely to succeed in moulding the place to his purpose was the only hope for Queen Square'. As McDonald wrote later of Gilliatt:

> Thus at a time when other branches of medicine expanded, progress in neurology slowed and Queen Square polished its halo. Neurologists were still advised to go to Queen Square but it was not what it was. The transformation from 1 reader, 1 senior lecturer, 1 secretary and 2 technicians to 5 professors, 9 senior lecturers, 8 lecturers and grants of £1.5 M pa depended on three factors: Gilliatt's vision of neurology; his ability to harness goodwill and manage opposition; and the Denny-Brown factor and legacy of the letter to Michael Kremer. Gilliatt's method was rarely to be absent from Queen Square; to prepare for difficulties; to select and prepare allies; to use logical arguments; and occasionally to surprise. This came from his military background and his love of history and literature.[36]

Gilliatt[37] was born on 30 July 1922, the son of Sir William Gilliatt, surgeon to King's College Hospital, who attended the births of HRH Prince of Wales and HRH Princess Anne. After leaving Rugby School, he interrupted his undergraduate education in Oxford by enlisting with the King's Royal Rifle Corps in 1942. His war record was distinguished. Near Kloppenburg, he went forward on foot alone and rescued the crew of a burning tank, despite being subjected to heavy small-arms fire. The citation for his Military Cross spoke of 'Lieutenant Gilliatt's very great leadership … outstanding personal courage, [and his] great coolness under heavy shelling proving the greatest inspiration to his men'. Returning to Oxford on demobilisation, Gilliatt graduated with first-class honours in physiology (1946) and was then research assistant at the Spinal Injuries Unit, Stoke Mandeville Hospital, and the University Laboratory of Physiology, Oxford. After qualification in medicine from the Middlesex Hospital in 1949, Gilliatt trained in neurology there and at the National Hospital. He was appointed to the consultant staff of both hospitals

in 1955 and also began to develop a successful Harley Street private practice.

Hospital rounds were conducted with military precision. The sister placed the patients at attention in their beds, a chair at the foot for Gilliatt's bag. A luckless houseman at the Middlesex mentioning that a patient with tabes dorsalis had acquired syphilis in the First World War was taken aside and reprimanded for the indiscretion: 'when speaking of antecedent causes, leprosy "yes"; syphilis "no"'. Oliver Sacks described his time as houseman to Kremer and Gilliatt at the Middlesex Hospital in 1958:

> Gilliatt was much more forbidding: sharp, impatient, edgy, irritable, with (it sometimes seemed to me) a sort of suppressed fury that might explode at any moment. An undone button, we housemen felt, might provoke him to a rage. He had huge, ferocious, jet-black eyebrows – instruments of terror for us juniors … I was terrified of Gilliatt and became almost paralyzed with fear when he asked me a question. Many of his housemen … had similar reactions … Kremer and Gilliatt had very different approaches to examining patients. Gilliatt would have us go through everything methodologically: cranial nerves (none to be omitted), motor system, sensory system etc., in a fixed order, never to be deviated from. He would never leap ahead prematurely, home in on an enlarged pupil, a fasciculation, an absent abdominal reflex or whatever. The diagnostic process, for him, was the systematic following of an algorithm … Gilliatt was pre-eminently a scientist, a neurophysiologist by training and temperament. He seemed to regret having to deal with patients (or housemen), though he was, I was later to learn, a completely different person – genial and supportive – when he was with his research students.[38]

The same style was maintained at Queen Square. His weekly round began precisely at 10.30 a.m. with a cup of coffee and one dry biscuit. The registrar stated the facts, the senior registrar offered an interpretation, and the senior house officer was advised to remain silent. Gilliatt spoke awkwardly to the patient and very few decisions or changes in management were made. Behind the austerity lay the combination of intellectual superiority and an apparent reluctance to display his clinical skills alongside those of the full-time neurologists at Queen Square.[39] But sometimes, and

---

[36] Annual report, Institute of Neurology, University of London, 1992.

[37] Some details in this text are taken from D. A. S. Compston, 'Professor Roger Gilliatt', *Oxford Dictionary of National Biography* (2011), at http://dx.doi.org/10.1093/ref:odnb/49652.

[38] O. Sacks, *On the Move: A Life* (London: Picador, 2015).

[39] But he did win their affection, perhaps in recognition of his courage. In this respect, two letters from Sir Charles Symonds may be revealing. On 10 September 1966, Symonds writes from Field House, Ham, Marlborough:

especially if the case came from one of the neurologists practising neurology in a large swathe of the countryside – Cornwall (Anthony Herring) and Essex (Fred Lees) being particular sources of referral – Gilliatt indicated that he would visit the patient later in the week and 'make a note'.[40] These showed clinical skills and a sympathetic attitude to patients that Gilliatt did not reveal at other times.

Professional life changed for Gilliatt in 1962 when he was appointed to the foundation professorship of clinical neurology in the University of London. That Gilliatt was eventually able to effect the transformation of academic neurology depended on his vision of the field and ability to manipulate goodwill towards his own preferred position. He gave up his private practice and as the elite of between-the-wars neurology retired, Gilliatt began to dominate policy and strategy at the National Hospital and the Institute of Neurology. His method was to deploy his military training and skills to achieve what Gilliatt considered to be in the best interests of Queen Square. At times he considered that views in opposition to his own were a challenge to battle that had confronted his considerable powers of persuasion. Gilliatt was at ease with, and greatly admired by, those who worked in his immediate vicinity. He was hospitable and socially attentive of overseas students. But his waspish tongue became legendary and he appeared less relaxed with British trainees, among whom he had a fearsome reputation for aloofness and acerbity.[41] By

nature of his role in an institution that still retained a monopoly on the training of neurologists, Gilliatt nurtured most academic neurologists in the UK in the decades that followed appointment as professor of neurology, although these remained very few in number until the 1990s.

Understandably, given his training in Oxford, Gilliatt's vision for research was physiology as the basis for understanding disease mechanisms; physiology on the pedestal that had served clinical science so well from the time of Sherrington; and physiology as the holy grail of scientific discovery that was more elusive and desirable than clinical practice. This was a formulation that, in all respects, Walshe had already dismissed as not suitable for contemporary neurology. Perhaps Walshe was correct because, in seeking to emulate the Oxford school of physiology, Gilliatt's own work never delivered the moment of excitement to which he aspired. He did, however, bring rigour and discipline to experimental studies on mechanical and toxic injury of the rabbit peripheral nerve, to which a series of trainees in neurology were assigned, and he espoused the ethic of clinical science whereby a problem identified in the clinic is taken to the laboratory, investigated systematically, and the insights gained used to improve the management of patients. But his stance was mainly attuned to the romance rather than the reality of scientific discovery.[42]

The photograph of his last teaching session at Queen Square on 29 June 1987 appears to show a sombre mood, with Gilliatt flanked by Ian McDonald, Anita Harding and P. K. Thomas. Close by are Pamela Le Quesne (née Fullerton), Martin Halliday and Raymond Hierons. Significantly, at the back of the room are some of the scientists with whom Gilliatt worked: David Landon, Ed Thompson, Alan

---

'Dear Gilliatt ... '; but 2 February 1973, a letter congratulating Gilliatt on the brilliance of his experimental work conducted with Jose Ochoa on compression of myelinated axons is addressed 'Dear Roger ... '; and Gilliatt kept many presentation copies of Symonds' papers inscribed 'with best wishes Charlie'.

[40] This usually occurred on a Saturday when he would travel to Queen Square in a more leisurely way, stopping off at bookshops on the way home to search for copies of works by Anthony Trollope. He had hoped to write a book on the characters in Trollope in retirement but that did not materialise.

[41] On a draft paper in which the results could not be substantiated, Gilliatt wrote: 'There should be a black book listing the names of those whose papers we need never read again.' Reflecting on a clever and articulate applicant for a post at Queen Square: 'when discussing a case with him I feel rather like Bertie Wooster being reproved by Jeeves for wearing unsuitable socks'. An example of his style in a letter: 'Without wishing to put a damper on your recent discoveries, could I suggest that before you and George Bonney invent any more Greek names, you have a further look at the literature.' In wry appreciation of this letter, McDonald

reminded Gilliatt how he had discussed results obtained during an all-night session of recording when McDonald could not concentrate on the arguments, even though these led to a description of the refractory period of transmission.

[42] So much so that, in counselling a young trainee disappointed at not securing a prestigious post at Queen Square, and who was clearly threatening to respond in an eccentric manner by withdrawing from London neurology, Gilliatt suggested rationalising this behaviour for others on the basis that the young man's plans for a career as a consultant neurologist in London had stopped because 'something had broken in the lab' – the bemused and plainly sulking trainee wondering why dropping a glass pipette should be considered to exercise such influence on a young man's career prospects.

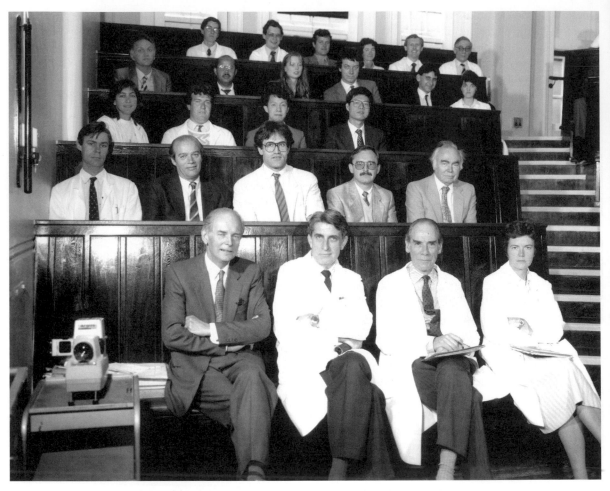

Figure 13.5 A-room lecture theatre, 1987 (left to right: front row – Thomas, McDonald, Gilliatt, Harding).

Davison and Tom Sears. Speaking after dinner on the occasion of Gilliatt's retirement, McDonald emphasised the transformation of Queen Square under his guidance. This might have seemed inevitable, but McDonald concluded that Gilliatt saw clearly how the style established in the 1930s had to change as neurology evolved.[43] Reflecting on his career at Queen Square, following the occasion of the unveiling of his portrait, Gilliatt confided:

> I tend to talk as if I were impervious to such things but in fact the whole portrait sequence has been a great prop and stay – I think that without your efforts I might have had a slight feeling that I was being kicked out and pensioned off by a not very grateful Institute. As it is I can look back on all those years in

the department with the feeling that we did really achieve something, all of us together.[44]

In retirement, Gilliatt moved to the USA and was appointed consultant in clinical neurophysiology, National Institute for Neurological Disease and Stroke, National Institutes of Health, Bethesda. He wrote to McDonald less than a month before his death on the topic of his publications. The attached list was incomplete and lacked two papers with Robin Kennett on cold injury, a letter to *Muscle and Nerve* on conduction block, and abstracts that he intended to have presented at a forthcoming meeting of the American Neurological Association and the American Association of Electrodiagnostic

---

[43] McDonald archive: manuscript notes, undated.

[44] McDonald archive: letter from Roger Gilliatt, dated 14 October 1988.

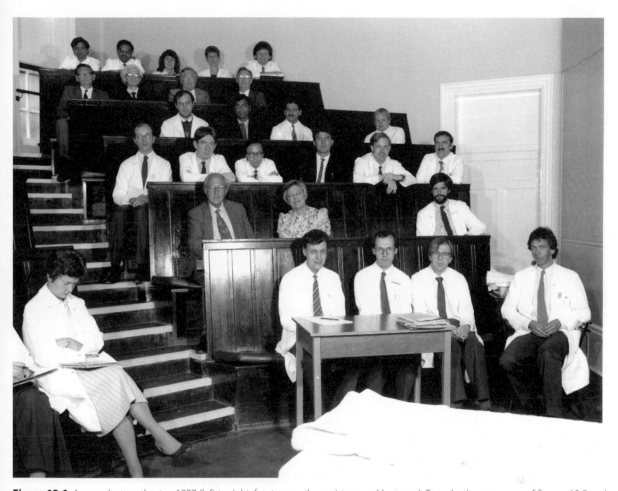

Figure 13.6 A-room lecture theatre, 1987 (left to right: front row – the registrars and lecturers). To make the panorama of figures 13.5 and 13.6, the photographer needed to take two shots, and in the interval, Anita Harding seems to have fallen asleep.

Medicine. Also missing was a very last-minute piece on double crush with Asa Wilbowra. This list and the reprints thereof were to be bound in four volumes and deposited with Gilliatt's DM thesis in the library at Queen Square, together with a slim volume edited with Art Asbury and translated into Russian.[45] Gilliatt died from pancreatic cancer on 19 August 1991 in Washington DC.

As with Marshall – but with an important difference – Gilliatt had also been caught up in the type of perceived scandal that, with much hypocrisy, Queen Square loved to disparage. Outside the world of science and medicine, Gilliatt was known for having

been best man at the marriage of Mr Antony Armstrong-Jones and Princess Margaret in Westminster Abbey in 1960.[46] Gilliatt was himself married to Penelope (née Conner), journalist and writer, in 1954, and there was sympathy at the subsequent break-up of the marriage of this quietly spoken and distinguished doctor, and public disapproval 'because Penelope Gilliatt had walked out on someone who had been best man at a Royal

---

[45] A. K. Asbury and R. W. Gilliatt, eds., *Peripheral Nerve Disorders*, Vol **I**, Butterworths International Medical Reviews: Neurology (London: Butterworth-Heinemann Ltd, 1984).

[46] The *Daily Express* ran a feature on him in the week before the wedding. The columnist (Anne Sharpley) wrote of Dr Gilliatt's presence, the ease with which those who met this quiet man soon found themselves involved in long discussions and arguments, and the 'nerve-wracking task of having the eyes of the world on him for a tricky courtly role usually carried out by members of the hereditary peerage'. He was, in fact, the second choice as best man, as Jeremy Fry had had to withdraw due to a scandal.

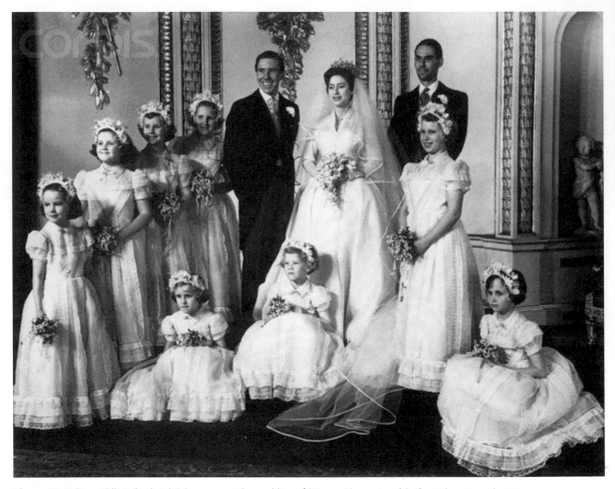

Figure 13.7 Roger Gilliatt (back right), best man at the wedding of Princess Margaret and Anthony Armstrong-Jones.

wedding'.[47] The gossip columnists made much of this, delighted to get back at her for a searing article written for *Queen* magazine attacking them for the inaccuracy and scurrilous nature of their columns.

The Earl of Snowdon (Mr Anthony Armstrong-Jones) read from 1 Corinthians 13 at the memorial service for Gilliatt on 18 October 1991. Princess Margaret was unable to attend due to a commitment to perform public engagements in Scotland. In his

address, McDonald emphasised the markers of Gilliatt's success: the highest ratings in the University Grants Committee and Research Assessment Exercises, and the foresight that allowed Queen Square and the Institute of Neurology to justify their existence and survive the Health Service reforms of the 1990s:

> How are we to understand a man whose biting tongue was legendary, yet who enjoyed the irony of being caught out himself ... a man who could say with relish that there was nothing like the prospect of a weekend in the country with a valet to unpack his clothes before dinner ... a man who drank orange juice in committees but brought 3 bottles of champagne when visiting ... a manifestly brave man of whom a wartime

---

[47] Gilliatt returned from a visit to the USA to learn that his wife had left and was living with the playwright John Osborne. After separating from his second wife, Mary, the mother of his two children, Gilliatt's later years were spent with Patricia Stolar in Washington DC, with whom he found much happiness.

comrade [said] 'No-one's tears flowed faster when a soldier died'?[48]

He had a complex character. Despite his military work, Gilliatt marched with the Campaign for Nuclear Disarmament, and despite his establishment credentials supported the Labour party. Pat Wall wrote privately that the obituaries of Gilliatt had not described the man he knew. Wall and Gilliatt had been together in Oxford and at the Middlesex. Wall outlines the difficulty of having an authoritarian parent, condemned to following the same profession and being sent to a public school:

> I saw him as the equivalent of Robert Graves in *Goodbye to All That*. He had the misfortune to have David Whitteridge as his tutor in Oxford. Whitteridge is one of those poisonous characters who lacking all originality uses his talent to sneer at originality … this passes in England for critical ability. There was one original man in the group, George Dawson but he was a softy and put in his place. In about 1970, Roger and I went to Russia on a government mission. We were making our way across Red Square with difficulty because of ice underfoot and vodka inside, and we were howling with laughter. He stopped laughing long enough to shout orders at the puzzled guard on Lenin's tomb. We resumed our laughter at them, at ourselves and at the world. It was gentle and innocent and so was he on occasions.[49]

For all his own foibles and complexities, Gilliatt supported and nurtured the academic activities of a small number of neurologists who worked at Queen Square from the 1960s and, through his patronage, academic neurology survived the crisis and probable demise that the attitudes of the 1950s had risked.

---

[48] As spoken and written in draft, the eulogy had a final paragraph that McDonald removed from the published version. This reads: 'I think one important answer is that above all he was a man who cared and cared deeply – about the lives of the soldiers in the burning tank, about the standing of his Hospital and Institute, about the standards in his profession, about his subject, and how his students contributed to it, about the happiness and welfare of his friends and above all his loved ones. We are all, as Donne said, diminished by Roger's passing. But he had a zest for life, and it is proper that we should rejoice in his. Roger had a powerful sense of historical continuity. His place in the history of Queen Square and of neurology in this country is secure as it is in the hearts of all those whose lives he touched.'

[49] McDonald archive: typescript dated 3 January 1992.

The University Department of Clinical Neurology 1961–1997

In addition to John Marshall and Roger Gilliatt, a number of other outstanding academics contributed to the reputation of the university department of clinical neurology in this period. Some of these researchers were the residue of Carmichael's medical research unit; some were loyal to Gilliatt and worked close to him; some were independent but compliant with Gilliatt's direction and leadership; some were outwardly supportive but needed distance from Gilliatt; and some were trainees in no position to bid for independence whilst apprenticed to Gilliatt and Queen Square, but who subsequently developed their own reputations.

Peter Kynaston Thomas

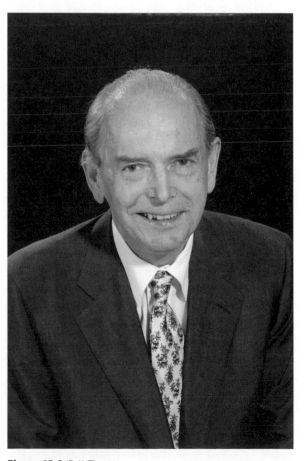

Figure 13.8 P. K. Thomas.

The work on peripheral nerves that dominated research in the decade after Gilliatt's appointment was driven largely by Peter Kynaston Thomas, with the assistance of Paddy Fullerton. Thomas,[50] universally known as 'P. K.', was born and educated in Swansea and graduated in medicine from University College London in 1950. From 1947 to 1950, he worked as part-time demonstrator in anatomy at University College and lecturer in physical anthropology at Birkbeck College, London. During National Service with the Royal Army Medical Corps as a clinical physiologist, Thomas was secretary to the Military Personnel Research Committee (1952 to 1954). After training in neurology at the National Hospital (1957–61), he moved to Canada as assistant professor of neurology at McGill University, Montréal (1961–2), before returning to London as consultant neurologist to the Royal Free Hospital Group (1962–91), the National Hospital (1963–91) and the Royal National Orthopaedic Hospital (1965–74). With the establishment of a professorial unit at Queen Square, Gilliatt maintained the appointment of Thomas as senior lecturer, previously held in Carmichael's unit, and P. K. held a professorship in the University of London based there and at the Royal Free Hospital School of Medicine from 1974 to 1991.

Starting in the 1950s, P. K. showed that nerve fibre diameter, myelination and internodal length determine the speed of electrical conduction. With Gilliatt, he described neurophysiological features that distinguish degeneration of peripheral nerve fibres from those disorders primarily causing loss of the surrounding myelin sheath. Thomas' lifelong interest in structure and function of the peripheral nervous system began through contact as an undergraduate with J. Z. (John Zachary) Young, who encouraged him to study the lateral line nerve of the trout. Although grounded in the classical discipline of neurophysiology, Thomas was quick to apply new techniques to the study of human peripheral nerve disease as experimental neurology

flowered from the 1960s. His use of nerve biopsy, electron microscopy, tissue culture, experimental models of common disorders such as the neuropathy that often complicates maturity-onset diabetes, and eventually transgenic mouse models of human peripheral neuropathy meant that his work over five decades remained innovative, creative and influential. He was early in his grasp of the importance of the new genetics in the study of peripheral nerve disease and a pioneer also in this field. In these important respects, his research epitomised the need to move on and adopt the modern technologies for which Walshe had argued. But P. K. was also a versatile, experienced and intuitive clinical neurologist who drew effortlessly on a vast range of knowledge in shaping his clinical opinions and writings, and his advice on the rarest or most complex cases was widely sought. His clinical descriptions involved careful clinical and laboratory examination, sometimes performed in remote places: loss of vision and sensory neuropathy attributed to nutritional deficiency in Cuba (where evidently Fidel Castro took something of a liking to P.K.); hitherto unrecognised disorders of the Roma gypsies in Bulgaria; and, in the last clinical study with which he was directly involved, climbing to 15,000 feet in remote regions of the Peruvian Andes to perform nerve biopsies and conduction studies for research on altitudinal neuropathy.[51]

P. K. attended the teaching round, held each Wednesday afternoon in the small seminar room attached to Gowers ward at Queen Square, where Gilliatt, who was well briefed on the case in advance, usually deferred to Thomas for an initial opinion and formulation of the problem. This gladiatorial event had many rules and regulations that were part of the folklore of the time, foremost among which was that seating in the room was hierarchical with the front row reserved for a select team made up of members of the professorial unit, a paediatric neurologist from Great Ormond Street Hospital (Edward Brett), selected consultant neurologists from outside Queen Square (notably Raymond Hierons and Michael Espir), occasional visitors from outside the UK, Ian McDonald, John

---

[50] Some details in this text are taken from: D. A. S. Compston, 'Professor Peter Thomas', *Oxford Dictionary of National Biography* (2011), at https://doi.org/10.1093/ref:o dnb/100176; 'Professor Peter Thomas', *Munk's Roll*, 2015:-http://munksroll.rcplondon.ac.uk/Biography/Details/6075; and A. K. Asbury *et al.*, 'Professor PK Thomas: Clinician, Investigator, Editor and Leader – a Retrospective Appreciation', *Brain* **134** (2011): 618–66.

[51] P. K. Thomas *et al.*, 'Hereditary Motor and Sensory Neuropathy-Russe: New Autosomal Recessive Neuropathy in Balkan Gypsies', *Annals of Neurology* **50** (2001): 452–7; O. Appenzeller *et al.*, 'Acral Paresthesias in the Andes and Neurology at Sea Level', *Neurology* **59** (2002): 1532–5.

Marshall and P. K., and sometimes another consultant neurologist from the National Hospital if his (there were no women) case was being discussed. P. K. was often entrusted to elicit the physical signs. Thomas was a beacon of common sense and clinical wisdom whose contributions were invariably illuminating. That he brought glad tidings of contemporary clinical science being championed in another institution leavened the atmosphere of the Gowers' round and proved subtly influential in the crucial transitional phase of academic neurology at Queen Square. Although loyal to the National Hospital, the school of clinical neuroscience that he nurtured at the Royal Free started the process of devolving modern academic neurology away from the exclusivity of the National Hospital. Thomas was foundation president of the European Neurological Society, which he helped to form in 1988, served as president of the Association of British Neurologists in 1990–1, and was awarded the ABN Medal in 1997.[52] He married Anita Harding after the death of his first wife, Mary, but after several happy years in which her youth and vitality rejuvenated P. K., he became a widower for the second time. Later, he had a large, non-dominant, ischaemic stroke resulting in dense left hemiplegia and loss of spatial awareness. Although house-bound and cared for by his third wife, P. K. continued to spend time thinking and editing because, in reality, apart from music, skiing and travelling in order to work and be in the company of his many professional friends around the world, he knew no other way of life. P. K. has claims to

have been, in the opinion of many, the outstanding clinical neurologist of his generation.

John Morgan-Hughes

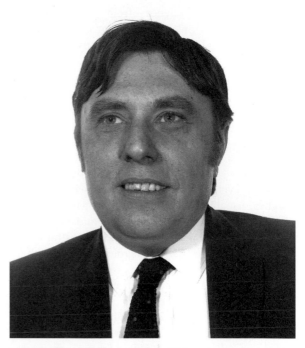

Figure 13.9 John Morgan-Hughes, 1971.

The tradition of the consultant neurologist who illuminated the science of neurology, which made Queen Square famous in its first period and which continued to flicker thereafter, did not change altogether once the work of the university department of clinical neurology gathered momentum in the 1960s. Marshall, as someone who held the first academic post in neurology, and, later, as dean, was keen to ensure that all consultants at the National Hospital saw research as one of their main responsibilities. In making that stipulation, he could not have had a more prominent example than John Morgan-Hughes who, in several respects, represented the type of neurologist for whom Walshe had argued in his polemical memorandum – challenging the need for academic investment, while at the same time extolling the virtues of abandoning physiology in favour of new disciplines if Queen Square was to remain a force in national neurology. Morgan-Hughes used metabolic studies of the nervous system as the basis for pioneering work in the

---

[52] Thomas was a prodigiously energetic and diligent editor of neurological journals. He served with Marco Mumenthaler as co-chief editor of the *Journal of Neurology* (1979–81: formerly *Zeitschrift für Neurologie*); and subsequently as editor of *Brain* (1982–91) and the *Journal of Anatomy* (1990–2001). Colleagues remember him weighed down by his shoulder bag in which papers currently under consideration were carried; anywhere and everywhere – airport lounge, conference auditorium, restaurant, in lectures, before and after an outpatient clinic, and at any time when no other essential activity was taking place – he would be altering, polishing and invariably improving the style and narrative of these manuscripts. Filling in for delinquent authors and committing to rigorous copy-editing of manuscripts were skills honed in the 1970s, when Thomas co-edited, with Peter Dyck and Edward Lambert, the monumental and landmark monograph on *Peripheral Neuropathy* (1975; 4th edn 2005), and the definitive work, edited with Peter Dyck, on *Diabetic Neuropathy* (1987; 2nd edn 1999).

entirely new discipline of muscle respiration and mitochondrial disease. Arguably, he was the most brilliant and original of the investigators who remained close to Gilliatt, and Morgan-Hughes retained the respect of those who were appointed to academic positions at Queen Square.

Morgan-Hughes obtained a first-class honours degree in natural sciences from Trinity College, Cambridge (1954), worked as senior house officer at Queen Square (1961), spent a formative year as an MRC-funded international post-doctoral fellow with Dr King Engel at the National Institutes of Health (Bethesda, USA, 1966) and was consultant neurologist at the National Hospital from 1968 to 1997. Morgan-Hughes was an enigmatic figure who caricatured himself as an amateur clinician scientist. He was overweight, had a distinctive hair-style and unusual mannerisms, and was almost never without a cigarette. But even a brief conversation with Morgan-Hughes, usually awkward and laced with cynicism, made clear that here was a man of formidable intellect and individuality who was not to be constrained by convention or the traditional role of the consultant neurologist at Queen Square. He remained a part-time consultant with a private practice, and provided services at the district general hospital in Bedford where he held enormous clinics dealing with all aspects of neurology. These sessions lasted well into the evening, and the on-call registrars at Queen Square were used to his telephone calls describing another interesting patient who needed urgent attention that he was transferring. His patients adored him, and did not complain about the long waits in his over-booked clinics. He took a keen interest in their lives and registered many personal details in his extraordinary memory. He also was very supportive of his junior staff; indeed, uniquely in academic neurology, a person about whom no one spoke ill behind his back.

By the early 1970s, patients had been described with muscle weakness present from birth or with later onset, having various morphological abnormalities of mitochondria. From this began to emerge a syndrome characterised by progressive ptosis with external ophthalmoplegia. In a first contribution to the subject published in *Brain*, Morgan-Hughes and W. G. P. (William George Parker) Mair added four examples of this disorder, with histochemical and ultrastructural changes confined to muscle mitochondria. In his career, John Morgan-Hughes looked at more than 12,000 muscle biopsies, of which samples taken from the triceps muscles of these four cases were among the earliest: 'The most striking abnormality was the presence of scattered muscle fibres containing excessive accumulations of sarcoplasmic material … dark red in colour with the modified Gomori trichrome stain … confined to the subsarcolemmal regions … or form[ing] a coarse reticular or punctate pattern which extended over the whole cross-sectional area of the fibre.'[53]

By 1982, the concept of mitochondrial disorders affecting muscle and the nervous system had broadened to include various encephalopathies with onset in childhood manifesting as learning disability, movement disorder and other motor deficits, visual failure, epilepsy and the features of oculoskeletal myopathy, sometimes with neuropathy. Associated with these protean manifestations of mitochondrial disease were raised lactate and pyruvate, and deficiencies involving the pyruvate dehydrogenase complex, cytochrome *b*, cytochrome *c* oxidase and impaired reduced nicotinamide adenine dinucleotide (NADH) oxidation. On this basis, Morgan-Hughes and his colleagues proposed a classification listing 19 disorders, in the categories of defects of mitochondrial substrate transport or utilisation, and those of the respiratory chain or energy conservation and transduction. Each had a likely but not fully predictable phenotype. In 1987, with Ian Holt and Anita Harding, Morgan-Hughes showed that mitochondrial DNA deletions, detectable only in DNA extracted from skeletal muscle, can cause human neurological disease and, with this demonstration of heteroplasmy, established an entirely new concept in medicine.[54]

John Morgan-Hughes was ahead of the game in realising that the concept of mitochondrial disease might become one of the great discoveries of late twentieth-century neurology – not only important in understanding muscle disease but also with implications for optic neuropathy, encephalopathy and neurodegeneration.

---

[53] J. A. Morgan-Hughes and W. G. Mair, 'Atypical Muscle Mitochondria in Oculoskeletal Myopathy', *Brain* **96** (1973): 215–24.

[54] I. J. Holt *et al.*, 'Deletions of Muscle Mitochondrial DNA in Patients with Mitochondrial Myopathies', *Nature* **331** (1988): 717–19.

John Michael Newsom-Davis

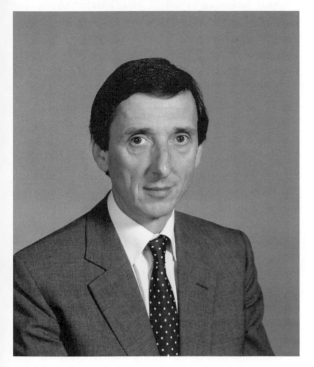

Figure 13.10 John Newsom-Davis.

Another consultant neurologist who contributed to the reputation of Queen Square for research in the 1970s was John Newsom-Davis.[55] With Morgan-Hughes, he took on the challenge of using new disciplines to inform the scientific basis of neurology. Because he invested in immunology and molecular medicine, he was considered to be the most important person in Britain who forced the emancipation of academic neurology as an authoritative discipline benefitting from modern scientific developments. Most of his rivals for that accolade were tainted by the old accusation of being applied physiologists. And yet that is precisely where his own academic career had started.

Newsom-Davis came late to medicine, having flown Meteors during National Service (1951–3), and at one point considered a career in the Royal Air Force. After Cambridge, he qualified in medicine

from the Middlesex Hospital Medical School in 1960. Moran Campbell fostered Newsom-Davis' interest in investigative medicine, and Michael Kremer attracted him to neurology. However, seeking an audience with Gilliatt in order to discuss his career, unexpectedly and disappointingly Newsom-Davis was advised to specialise in industrial medicine.[56] This rankled and – perhaps as a result – unlike Morgan-Hughes, he never felt close to Gilliatt and eventually based his laboratory work with P. K. Thomas at the Royal Free Hospital. His partial, and eventually complete, removal from Queen Square led to the perception that he was disloyal to his *alma mater* and 'bit the hand that had fed'. This was unjustified, although, as a young man, Newsom-Davis was not comfortable with the uncritical hagiography that characterised the hospital, being branded a 'communist' when, as resident medical officer in 1968, it fell to him to inform the Medical Committee that payments to junior staff looking after private patients would now be required.

Newsom-Davis first studied the neural control of breathing in patients with lesions of the spinal cord with Tom Sears at Queen Square, as lecturer from 1967 to 1969 in the university department of clinical neurology. He then spent a year as a research fellow at Cornell Medical Center, New York, working with Fred Plum. Newsom-Davis joined the consultant staff at Queen Square and the Royal Free Hospital in 1970. His expertise in the neurology of breathing led to him directing the Batten Unit at the National Hospital, where patients sometimes spent months dependent on assisted ventilation. At that time, he interacted with the leading neurophysiologist Ricardo Miledi, who wanted access to human intercostal muscle. Among others, Newsom-Davis provided a

---

[55] Some details in this text are taken from D. A. S. Compston, 'Professor John Newsom-Davis', *Munk's Roll* (-2015): http://munksroll.rcplondon.ac.uk/Biography/Details/5840.

[56] This conversation has a footnote in history. In 1970, Newsom-Davis published *The Respiratory Muscles* with Moran Campbell and Emilio Agostini. A copy of the book, inscribed 'To Roger Gilliatt/with compliments/John Newsom Davis', was found in a cardboard box outside the shop of Peter Eaton in Notting Hill, London, on 5 April 1984, purchased for £1 (reduced from £2) and brought to Newsom-Davis' attention. The 'find' was described in detail by Newsom-Davis during his contribution to Gilliatt's Festschrift in 1986. In the postscript to a letter addressed to the present owner, dated 2 October 1987, Gilliatt wrote 'PS. I sold some journals but no books when I left England so if you find any mementoes in second hand book stores, this is someone else's private enterprise!'

sample from himself, which led to an acute pneumothorax described to his wife during the night on which it developed as 'like a wet fish flapping around in my chest'.

Newsom-Davis' work changed direction in 1976 when conversation with a senior house officer who had recently worked at the Hammersmith Hospital led him to introduce plasma exchange as a novel therapy for myasthenia gravis.[57] This was the event that took Newsom-Davis back to school, studying for an MSc in immunology with Ivan Roitt and Deborah Doniach at the Middlesex Hospital Medical School. The availability of antibody removed from patients with myasthenia gravis undergoing plasma exchange provided experimental opportunities that benefitted from Newsom-Davis' background in experimental neurophysiology. With Angela Vincent, who joined him at the Royal Free Hospital School of Medicine in 1977, the group systematically unravelled disease mechanisms in many different categories of myasthenia gravis. The work was recognised by appointment, in 1980, to the first MRC clinical research professorship, held at the Royal Free Hospital and the Institute of Neurology. In 1981 came the second major discovery when another, hitherto unknown, autoantibody responsible for a closely related disorder, the Lambert–Eaton myasthenic syndrome, was identified, also helping to explain many mysterious disorders that constitute the remote effects of cancer. In 1987, Newsom-Davis was elected Action Research professor of clinical neurology in the University of Oxford. There followed a highly productive decade for the loyal group that moved with him from London. A third immunological discovery was added in the form of a novel autoantibody implicated in a rare disorder, acquired neuromyotonia (Isaac's syndrome). More was to follow with the realisation that the autoimmune ion-channel disorders have effects in the brain as well as on nerve and muscle.

Newsom-Davis represented the acceptable face of academic neurology for a broader community in the age of molecular medicine. His scientific achievements were recognised by election to FRS (1991), Foundation Fellowship of the Academy of Medical Sciences (1998)[58] and Foreign Associate Membership of the National Academy of Medicine of the USA (2001). He was appointed CBE in 1996. Few could rival Newsom-Davis as a communicator. Lectures were carefully crafted: the preparation was meticulous, the delivery lively, the arguments presented with impeccable logic, the language precise but never indulgent, and the recognition of good performance sincerely given and gladly received. He understood and could guide younger colleagues through the many and complex vicissitudes of academic life – the ups and downs of giving presentations, crafting papers and securing funding, and the uncertainties of career advancement.

In retirement, from 1998, Newsom-Davis needed new challenges. As a former secretary (1981–4) and medallist (1999), it was natural that he should be elected president of the Association of British Neurologists (1999–2000). He felt that the Association had drifted away from its origins in 1932 as a forum for discussing the best of British scientific neurology, and took several steps in the direction of merging the interests of an expanding membership focused on providing a high-quality clinical service with pride in presenting the best clinical neuroscience being carried out in the UK. From 1997 to 2004, he edited *Brain*. He introduced electronic processing and online publication well ahead of other journals in the field. His interest in clinical science did not wane. For over 40 years, removal of the thymus gland had been performed as a treatment for myasthenia gravis but without formal evidence either for efficacy or safety. In association with experts in the USA, Newsom-Davis obtained funding from the National Institutes of Health to conduct a multicentre trial involving over 80 centres. His death occurred in a road accident at Adjud, Romania, on 24 August 2007, after visiting a participating hospital in Bucharest.[59]

---

[57] Anthony Pinching, who later worked as a clinical immunologist at the Royal Cornwall Hospital, Truro. Pinching had worked with Keith Peters and Martin Lockwood at the Hammersmith Hospital, where plasma exchange was introduced for the treatment of immune nephropathy.

[58] The Council rooms of the Academy of Medical Sciences, Portland Place, London W1, are named after Newsom-Davis in recognition of a donation from the Welton Foundation, which he served as trustee for many years.

[59] The study was completed in 2017 and demonstrated the therapeutic effect of thymectomy. G. I. Wolfe *et al.*, 'Randomised Trial of Thymectomy in Myasthenia Gravis', *New England Journal of Medicine* 75 (2016): 511–22.

William Ian McDonald

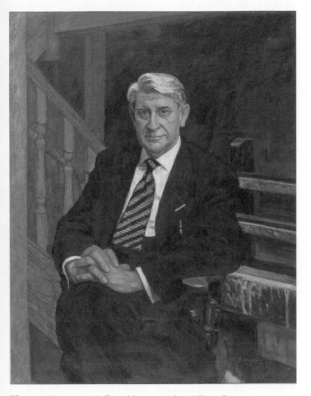

Figure 13.11 Ian McDonald, portrait by William Bowyer.

Ian McDonald[60] also came from the tradition of physiology as the basis for the study of neurological disease that Gilliatt espoused, but McDonald took that discipline into a modern era of mechanistic studies in the context of demyelinating disease. It was a source of personal anguish for McDonald that Marsden had been preferred as Gilliatt's successor in 1986, and he did not intend to contest the post again, even when the much younger Harding was appointed in 1995.[61]

---

[60] Some details in this text are taken from D. A. S. Compston, 'Professor Ian McDonald', *Dictionary of National Biography* (2009), at http://dx.doi.org/10.1093/ref:odnb/97538; and D. A. S. Compston, 'William Ian McDonald: 1933–2006', *Brain* **134** (2011): 2158–76.

[61] Ian McDonald, the disappointed applicant, was incensed to find Marshall (who had orchestrated Marsden's appointment) lounging in an armchair at his club, the Garrick, and was wont thereafter to quote an unflattering passage from Kenneth Grahame's book *The Wind in the Willows* (1908), where a passing badger leaves a trail that the other animals find unpleasant. It led to a rather obvious nickname that McDonald used for Marshall when wanting to discharge

But when she died, and with only a few years remaining before his own retirement, McDonald accepted the post that he had coveted secretly for so many years.

McDonald was born in Wellington, New Zealand, and graduated in medicine from the University of Otago in 1957. He worked first as research officer of the New Zealand Medical Research Council with Archie Macintyre, obtaining his PhD on 'The Effects of Experimental Demyelination on Conduction in Peripheral Nerve: A Histological and Electrophysiological Study' (1962), having already written a dissertation on 'Ascending Long Spinal Reflexes' (1955). Appointed lecturer in medicine at Otago, McDonald found that academic life in New Zealand had its limitations and, in 1963, he moved to London where his aesthetic interests were cultivated and his personality more easily expressed. McDonald's talents were quickly recognised at Queen Square, where, from the outset, he understood better than others the strategy being developed by Gilliatt for advancing academic neurology in the UK. McDonald was ever loyal to Gilliatt and acknowledged his role as handmaiden and custodian of this essential and awkward change.

After proleptic appointment as consultant neurologist to the National Hospital in 1966, McDonald worked for three years on muscle spindles in Boston with Denny-Brown, to whom most of the brightest neurologists training at Queen Square were usually sent at that time to broaden their experience of experimental neurology. This contact consolidated McDonald's interest in studying the pathophysiology and pathogenesis of demyelination affecting the central nervous system. But McIntyre wanted him back in New Zealand.

> I'm very glad you got the fellowship even if it means you must return to Queen Square for a while. However, there may be ways out of this – such arrangements aren't usually binding. Anyway, should there be a possibility of your coming here, please let me know … things often have to be jacked up well in advance, especially research posts.[62]

McDonald had no wish to return and the remainder of his career was spent in London: as consultant neurologist at Queen Square and Maida Vale

---

tension over the way that he felt he had been treated at Queen Square after Gilliatt's retirement.
[62] McDonald archive: letter, 12 February 1965.

Hospital, consultant physician at Moorfields Eye Hospital from 1969, and professor of neurology in the University of London from 1974. McDonald was one of very few neurologists active in experimental work in the 1960s. Working at that time with Tom Sears, McDonald characterised the physiology and morphology of demyelination and remyelination in the central nervous system. In the 1970s, with Halliday, he pioneered the use of evoked potentials, bringing objectivity to the diagnosis of demyelinating disease. In the 1980s, McDonald realised that magnetic resonance imaging and spectroscopy could be used to illuminate the nature of inflammatory brain disease, and his work provided laboratory measures for charting the efficacy of the first wave of disease-modifying treatments for multiple sclerosis introduced in the mid-1990s. Each of these achievements was substantial: together, the work represents a major and lasting contribution to clinical neuroscience.[63] McDonald was sought after as a clinical opinion and renowned for his expertise and knowledge of multiple sclerosis and neuro-ophthalmology. He trained by example, lifting less gifted colleagues and reflecting with generosity and uncomplicated pride on their achievements. Apparently easy performance, in his lectures and writing, concealed meticulous preparation and attention to detail. McDonald was adept at synthesising a complex story, and retained perspective and modesty about his own achievements set in the historical context of the illustrious predecessors whom he so much admired.

Inevitably, there were professional disappointments. The Institute of Psychiatry invited McDonald to replace Marsden after his move to Queen Square, but McDonald declined when it became clear that no one in a position of influence would support his continued involvement with the NMR Research Unit at the Institute of Neurology, which, by that time, had become the major focus of his research.[64] McDonald had already declined offers of several chairmanships in the USA, where he retained many friends from his time in Boston. A point often made in replying to enquiring deans was frustration over the extent to which clinical responsibilities in London restricted his research. When McDonald applied formally for one of two professorships supported by the National Fund for Research into Crippling Diseases, setting out his credentials and manifesto, his post to be held at the Institute of Neurology, the dean (Reginald Kelly) rejected, as out of the question, McDonald's request that he should have access to 21 hospital beds in which to manage his patients.[65] That application set out his plan to develop work in physiological, morphological, behavioural and clinical aspects of the visual system and spinal cord, because of their relevance to the clinical problems of visual failure and paraplegia. There was no mention, at the time, of multiple sclerosis.

In 1973, Professor E. J. (Ephraim) Field was removed from his post as director of the MRC Demyelinating Diseases Unit in Newcastle by the secretary of the MRC, Sir John Gray. On the advice of a subcommittee, with John Walton and Gilliatt as members, Gray offered McDonald the position: 'Council have long hoped that clinical work would develop but unfortunately this has not happened in recent years. They would certainly encourage the plans you outlined to me to combine clinical research with laboratory studies in the general field of demyelinating disease. Council do not confine this term to multiple sclerosis.'[66]

McDonald declined, again, not because of difficulties that had arisen with respect to his role as a neurologist in Newcastle, but for a different and surprising reason:

> I am a career academic neurologist with an interest in the pathophysiology of demyelinating disease. This has led me recently to an increasing interest in multiple sclerosis, but this has been a secondary interest arising from my primary research activities. Having read around multiple sclerosis a good deal in the past three months, and in particular having had the good fortune of attending the MS symposium in Barcelona which was so splendidly summed up by Sabin, it is clear to me that the answer to the problem is most

---

[63] From 1962 to 1985, McDonald published 31 papers on the physiology and neurobiology of demyelination and remyelination. Five papers that introduced the technique of evoked potentials appeared from 1972, and these techniques were used in much subsequent research. McDonald published 11 papers on the genetics of multiple sclerosis from 1976. But in the early 1980s he made a strategic change in direction, and thereafter carried out almost no further experimental work in animals. The opportunity to make that transition was provided by the introduction of magnetic resonance imaging, and most of his further work used that technology, with 102 original papers published from 1984 until after his retirement in 1998.

[64] McDonald archive: letter, 11 February 1987.

[65] McDonald archive: letter, 17 May 1973.

[66] McDonald archive: letter, 20 July 1973.

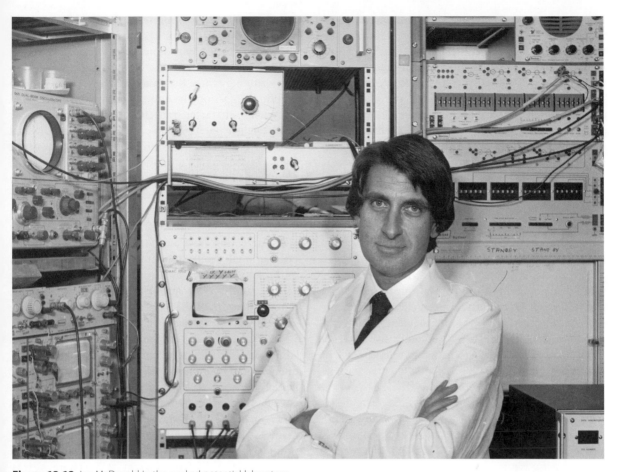

Figure 13.12 Ian McDonald in the evoked potential laboratory.

likely to come from virology, most probably with an immunological contribution as well ... I have no personal experience in these two fields.[67]

But other moves were actively considered. McDonald always maintained that his unsuccessful application for the Action Research professorship of neurology in Oxford in 1970, when Bryan Matthews was elected, foundered on the casting vote of a clergyman who felt that his nervous system would be in more sympathetic hands with Matthews than with McDonald. Although he never received formal notification of that decision, McDonald was informed by the university that his subsequent application for the same post, when Newsom-Davis was elected to replace Matthews, had not been successful.[68] Eventually, with the death of

Harding in 1995, McDonald was appointed as head of the university department at the Institute of Neurology, remaining in post until reaching the retirement age in 1998.

McDonald co-founded the European Neurological Society and served as its president (1994–5), and as president of the Association of British Neurologists (1994–5). Among many international prizes was the Charcot Award of the International Federation of Multiple Sclerosis Societies (1991), and McDonald was particularly pleased to be elected Foreign Member of the Venetian Institute of Science, Arts and Letters. McDonald edited *Brain* from 1991 to 1997, having earlier brokered the financially successful move of that journal from Macmillan to Oxford University Press, achieving financial security in the process, and thereby allowing the Guarantors subsequently to distribute significant resources in support of

---

[67] McDonald archive: letter, 8 October 1973.
[68] McDonald archive: letter, 15 April 1986.

young people training in the neurosciences. In retirement, he served as Harveian Librarian at the Royal College of Physicians of London, editing *Munk's Roll*; seeing through to publication the final volume of the *History of the Royal College of Physicians of London*;[69] and, with others, editing an illustrated history of *The Royal College of Physicians and its Collections* (2001). Over several decades, McDonald mixed with people active in music, dance, the visual arts, literature and history. These friendships outside medicine provided a counterpoint to his professional work and a rich source of information and anecdote that McDonald used in conversation, and in his writings and lectures. His passion was music, and it was therefore poignant that a small stroke in 2004 removed, for a while, his ability to understand music, read a score and play the piano. Later, he published, in *Brain*, a characteristically erudite account of this intensely personal episode.[70] Ian McDonald died suddenly from a coronary thrombosis at home in London on 13 December 2006.

Charles David Marsden

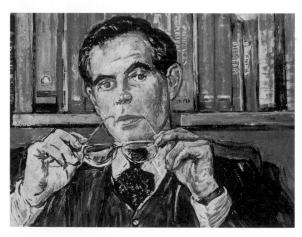

Figure 13.13 David Marsden, portrait by David Graham, 2000.

David Marsden was appointed professor of neurology at the Institute of Neurology when Gilliatt retired in 1986. His achievements in neurology were precocious and widely recognised. The definitive account of his life, written by three loyal pupils who remained close to him professionally and socially, concludes that Marsden's character reflected his background as: 'Part English public-school, part Greek, part British colonial Antipodean ... archetypal British with a Gypsy streak ... handsome, in a slightly Mediterranean way, with luxuriant dark eyebrows ... short in stature but such was his presence and charisma that few noticed this.'[71]

Marsden's combination of intellect and drive, communication skills and forceful personality, led to international leadership in the establishment of movement disorders as a subspecialty of neurology, encapsulated in his prolific publications and the monograph, published posthumously, *Marsden's Book of Movement Disorders* (2011).[72]

Marsden was the son of an Australian surgeon who married an English nurse in India and moved the family to many places around the British Empire. Largely brought up by grandparents in England and educated at Cheltenham College, Marsden trained at St Thomas' Hospital Medical School where he won many academic prizes and maintained a high sporting profile, having already captained England schoolboys at Rugby football. His progress at St Thomas' was meteoric and, after qualification in 1963, he advanced rapidly, but without a formal academic training other than an MSc on pigmentation in the substantia nigra completed as an undergraduate (1960). Marsden worked at Queen Square as a trainee between 1968 and 1969. When the Institute of Psychiatry decided to invest in academic neurology, Marsden was appointed (on the recommendation, among others, of Gilliatt) as senior lecturer in 1970, and as professor in 1972, aged 34 years.

Marsden's years at the Institute of Psychiatry in London and at King's College Hospital, as a neurologist and scientist, were happy and successful. The

---

[69] A. Briggs, *A History of the Royal College of Physicians of London*, Vol. **IV** (Oxford University Press, 2005).
[70] I. McDonald, 'Musical Alexia with Recovery: A Personal Account', *Brain* **129** (2006): 2554–61.

[71] Niall Quinn *et al.,* 'Charles David Marsden, 15 April 1938 – 29 September 1998', *Biographical Memoirs of Fellows of the Royal Society* **58** (2012): 203–28.
[72] Marsden published 1,368 papers, including more than 800 original articles, or one per week across most of his academic career (1975–98), and double that rate throughout 1986. He listed his recreation in *Who's Who* as 'the human brain'.

clinical contributions from that period of his academic career, and later, were the study of motor fluctuations in association with the use of L-3,4-dihydroxyphenylalanine (levodopa) derivatives; trials of novel agents that address the neurochemistry of Parkinson's disease and the possibility of cell-based therapies; non-motor manifestations of that disorder, especially cognitive impairment; structural and functional imaging in movement disorders; and the nosology and genetics of these conditions.

His experimental work in physiology, originally with David Owen (later Lord Owen and Minister of Health in the Government of Harold Wilson) and John Meadows at St Thomas' Hospital, focused on the measurement of tremor and an explanation of its dynamics through perturbations of long latency (spinal and cortical) stretch reflexes involving the transcortical loop, rather than defects of a central oscillator; the pathophysiology of myoclonus; systematic accounts of organic physiological defects in the context of disorders that were then considered to be psychological rather than manifestations of neurological disease; and the introduction of transcortical magnetic stimulation and motor-evoked potentials in clinical practice.

In neurochemistry and neuropharmacology, the achievements were recognition that transmitters other than dopamine are involved and can be targeted in the treatment of Parkinson's disease; identification of the scientific basis for focal stereotactic and electrical stimulation of nuclei within the basal ganglia in redressing the balance of inhibition and facilitation in the pathophysiology and treatment of movement disorders; and definition of the role of reactive oxygen species and heavy metals in the pathogenesis of neurodegeneration.

Marsden's understanding and philosophy of movement disorders were encapsulated in his use of Wilson's dictum for the basal ganglia, 'the dark basements of the brain', and the conclusion in his Robert Wartenberg lecture (1982) that the basal ganglia are responsible for the 'automatic execution of learned motor plans'.[73]

What would Walshe have thought of this now-legendary figure in British neurology? On the negative side, his training was in physiology, largely self-taught but with assistance from Pat Merton and Bert Morton.

But Marsden's experience and commitment to clinical neurology were never in doubt and commenting on cases remained the anchor of his professional life. Furthermore, the interplay between psychiatric disease and treatment with neuroleptic drugs, and the movement disorders that these patients manifest or develop in response to therapy, provided fertile ground for the development of neuropharmacology and neuropsychology based on tissue pathology, made available through the brain bank that Marsden developed at the Institute of Psychiatry. In that sense, he transcended the perceived limitations of the old-style physiologist and made his escape from the description of physiological performance in peripheral nerves to which Gilliatt's university department of clinical neurology remained largely committed.

For many of those who worked with him at that time, Marsden had an enormous presence, but he was remote. Undoubtedly, he inspired loyalty and devotion amongst people close to him and with whom he felt comfortable. He saw many patients and expressed authoritative and dogmatic views on their illnesses. It would now be agreed that he swung the pendulum too far in favour of an organic basis for some movement disorders. He taught in the grand style of nineteenth-century neurology: book rounds in which his own and other consultants' patients were discussed by large groups of doctors, with selected patients paraded before them. Marsden had a manner that usually engaged the person with neurological illness, but a ward round at the Maudsley Hospital (Mapother House) might be interrupted by the patient, sensing humiliation, losing control and hurling plates and flower vases at Marsden. As with many brilliant and much admired doctors, he did not always bother to suppress his irritation and, apart from the band of laboratory workers and research staff based in Windsor Walk – supported by plenty of smoke and beer in nearby public houses[74] – those around him were wary of intimacy. He sustained a hectic schedule encouraged by the coterie that shared Marsden's stamina for late nights and 'fast' living. Chancing on some of his staff while walking in Soho, London, Marsden might insist on a visit to Ronnie Scott's club where he ordered three bottles of Dom Perignon champagne and then left (having paid the bill). But, in general, those who worked with Marsden

---

[73] C. D. Marsden, 'The Mysterious Motor Function of the Basal Ganglia: The Robert Wartenberg Lecture', *Neurology* **32** (1982): 514–39.

[74] Favourites were the George Canning and the Phoenix and Firkin, close to Denmark Hill railway station.

remained somewhat detached from him, much as they never became close to Gilliatt.

There is no doubt that his major scientific achievements and the fabric of his life were formed at the Institute of Psychiatry, where he worked for 17 years. By contrast, the move back to Queen Square as Gilliatt's successor was evidently not entirely fulfilling. On arrival, Marsden wrote to McDonald, who had been much disappointed by the failure of his own application, making it clear that, although some independence was in order, McDonald should not develop an entirely separate academic unit, as was his preferred arrangement.[75] Marsden explained that exposing trainees and visitors solely to his own world of 'funny jerks and jumps' would not provide a sufficient experience of neurology. Later, as their relationship deteriorated, and reflecting more generally on his experience leading academic neurology at Queen Square, Marsden expressed concern that too few clinicians were committed full-time to the hospital and so able and willing to contribute to administration of the hospital and Institute, warning McDonald that he had a responsibility to serve in one administrative capacity or another.[76] In fact, McDonald had already been asked to become dean of the Institute of Neurology in 1986, soon after Marsden's election to the professorship, but had declined and, in so doing, had exposed the still sore wound:

> I have always found administration a chore but … accepted the necessity … in order to develop my clinical and research interests and to provide for my research students … I decided in 1983 … that I wished in principle to be considered for the Chair. I believed that the personal sacrifice of my research activity … would have been outweighed by the influence of neurology as a whole … in the event that sacrifice has not been necessary.[77]

With much energy and sense of purpose, Marsden rapidly modernised the university department, and his appointment ushered in a period of great change. As with Gilliatt, although not the dean, Marsden's was the decisive voice and, under his leadership, academic neurology at Queen Square retained its dominant position in the Institute of Neurology, and with a high national and international reputation. On taking over as head of department in 1987, there were five professors, one reader, nine senior lecturers and 32 attached workers, but under his leadership there was extraordinary expansion. On Marsden's retirement from the position in 1995, the department comprised ten professors, five readers and 164 research workers,[78] and it had been reorganised into 19 sections and units.[79] Each section had its own leadership and a mandate to grow their areas of interest, with far more freedom of action than had featured during Gilliatt's reign. Marsden's arrival meant a change from the focus on peripheral neuropathy to movement disorders. He brought from the Institute of Psychiatry an MRC Human Movement and Balance Unit, with its attendant scientific and clinical staff, which flourished at Queen Square. He trained neurologists in movement disorders and ensured the prominence of that subspecialty in UK neurology. He wrote a great deal (becoming one of the top cited neurologists in the world) and co-edited an influential textbook of neurology.[80] A brain bank, modelled on that at the Institute of Psychiatry, was started at Wakefeld Street, which focused on studies of neurodegeneration.

Marsden was considered a brilliant clinician scientist and he was elected to FRS, aged 45 years, in 1983. But for all the academic growth and success at Queen Square, he seemed increasingly unsettled and was badly affected by the early death of Anita Harding, for whom he had great affection and admiration, and in whose company he liked to relax. Marsden had

---

[75] Perhaps as compensation for what he knew to be a disappointment over his own appointment, Marsden offered the readership to a neurologist working outside London, whose field of interest matched that of McDonald, and indicated that the pair would be well placed to apply for an MRC unit in demyelinating disease to take up where E. J. Field had left off in Newcastle. In the event, Anita Harding was appointed to the vacant readership at the Institute of Neurology.

[76] McDonald archive: letter, 27 January 1989.

[77] McDonald archive: letter, 19 May 1986.

[78] These figures exclude visitors, students, technical and administrative staff.

[79] The sections and units were: autonomic disease, dementia, demyelinating disease and NMR, epilepsy, experimental psychology, headache, movement disorders, muscle, neuroepidemiology, neurophysiology, neuropsychiatry, Raymond Way Unit, rehabilitation, outcome measurement, Parkinson Disease Society Brain Research Centre, peripheral nerve, pharmacology and therapeutics, uro-neurology, MRC Clinical Sciences Centre.

[80] W. G. Bradley et al., eds., Neurology in Clinical Practice, 2 vols. (Boston, MA: Butterworth-Heinemann, 1990).

resigned from the professorship at Queen Square in 1995 to become dean, in part so that Harding could be appointed as his successor. However, she soon faced an uncertain future after developing carcinoma of the colon and died before taking up the post in October 1995, as intended, leaving Marsden marooned without his preferred ally and in a role for which he no longer had much appetite. During his three-year tenure as dean, Marsden became unwell with depression and 'difficulties with home life', taking time away from the Institute of Neurology and the National Hospital. Eventually, he decided to spend a year as Fogarty Fellow at the National Institutes of Health with Mark Hallett, a former fellow at the Institute of Psychiatry. Shortly before he left for the USA, Marsden confided that he had lost faith in research and wished to spend his remaining years writing on clinical neurology. This was apparent from his activities at the time: three clinics, a ward round, 'book round' and Gowers' teaching round each week. Others considered that his early and prodigious successes in the field of physiology, which had dominated research at Queen Square and in neurology more generally, had led him to expect more in terms of accolades than he did achieve. Realising that some of the esteem to which he aspired might not materialise led him to re-evaluate the currency of success in academic medicine. Marsden died suddenly, aged 60 years, in his apartment in Washington, soon after arriving in the USA for this sabbatical leave.

McDonald gave an address at the funeral held on 9 October 1998 at Medway Crematorium, UK. He spoke of Marsden having been appointed to 'the house' at Queen Square without having worked previously at the National Hospital, bringing a fine reputation from St Thomas' both for research and for his remarkable clinical abilities. After 17 years away from Queen Square, Marsden led the National Hospital and the Institute of Neurology in both activities. His patients knew that their concerns came first, and his colleagues that they could rely on his judgement, however complex the problem; and his research was by now of international renown. McDonald referred to Marsden's role as head of the university department of clinical neurology, ever sympathetic to the aspirations of its members, and nurturing the burgeoning subspecialties with an invaluable capacity to identify future leaders. As an administrator, and man of vision, he shepherded the difficult union of the National Hospital with the wider University College Hospital London Trust, and the

Institute with University College London. In all of this, he perceived and protected the unexpressed interests of others, timed his interventions in committee, and led a disparate group towards sensible decisions. McDonald ended with a comment on Marsden as being a lover of good living and having a gregarious nature while retaining privacy that left a distance, despite the admiration and affection in which he was held by a large number of neurologists around the world.[81]

Anita Elizabeth Harding

Anita Harding[82] was appointed successor to Marsden as professor and head of the university department of clinical neurology at the Institute of Neurology, and was due to take up the appointment in October 1995 but she died from disseminated carcinoma of the colon shortly before her 43rd birthday, having been ill for only five months. With an indefatigable zest for life, an earthy sense of humour, feet placed firmly on the ground despite a soaring reputation, possessing a rare talent for friendship among the many and varied people with whom she interacted, and having a natural flair for sensing and patrolling the complex and mysterious ingredients of elite professional success, her early death denied Harding the many accolades and appointments that her combination of personality and ability would inevitably have yielded. And, in turn, neurology never benefitted to the full from the many further contributions and outstanding leadership that she would surely have provided. Harding's clinical wisdom, enthusiasm, talent for research and extraordinary personality epitomise all that is valued most in a clinical scientist. She was an ambassador for British neurology, who patrolled the far corners of a still significant empire, which had its roots at Queen Square, where she worked and was happy. A pioneer

---

[81] McDonald archive: manuscript dated 9 October 1998. In a typescript that differs from the text in manuscript, McDonald highlights the mentorship of Anita Harding, and the 'shadow that her premature death' cast over Marsden's later years, which, for a time, seemed to diminish the energy that he had customarily expended in university, hospital and broader scientific activities – the shadow beginning to lift with the opportunity to return to original work on the award of the Fogarty Fellowship at the National Institutes of Health: a year that promised also to be satisfying at the personal level.

[82] Some details in this text are taken from D. A. S. Compston, 'Anita Harding (1952–1995)', *Advances in Clinical Neurology and Rehabilitation* **9** (2009): 28–30; and (supp.) (2009): 30–31.

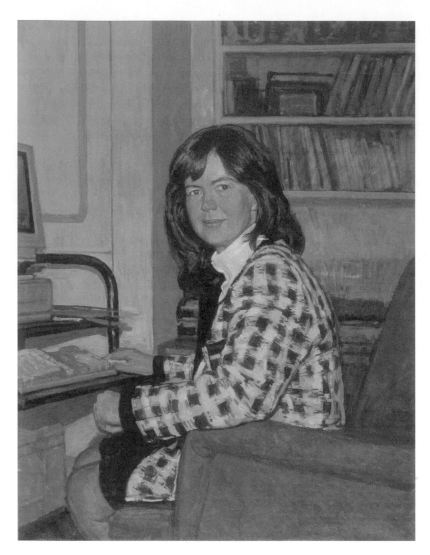

Figure 13.14 Anita Harding.

of neurogenetics, she is remembered for the insightful way in which she anticipated the entry of molecular genetics into neurology. Not everyone would have predicted that the field was heading for such prominence in medicine from the 1990s. Despite her vision, Harding was unable to participate in the discoveries that modern molecular medicine made possible, and a generation of neurologists trained since the mid-1990s lost the opportunity of mentorship and supervision by an outstanding clinical neurologist. There is no sense in which these losses might be considered speculative or judged ambiguous. Anita Harding was on a trajectory to greatness that was unstoppable. Her achievements in a career that was active from 1977 until a few days before her death were already outstanding and, as the leading clinician scientist of her

generation working in the UK, Harding already ranked as a major figure in late twentieth-century world neurology.

Born in Ireland, and adopted by parents who lived in the Midlands, Anita Harding grew up in Birmingham and was educated at the King Edward VI High School for Girls before training in medicine at the Royal Free Hospital School of Medicine, where she graduated in 1995, winning a number of undergraduate prizes. As a student, she visited the neurological department of the Montréal General Hospital. After hospital appointments at the Royal Free with Professor Dame Sheila Sherlock and P. K. Thomas,[83]

---

[83] Harding married P. K. Thomas, as his second wife, in 1977. They were well suited: at Harding's memorial service,

and in Oxford, she worked first at the National Hospital in 1977 and subsequently joined Cedric Carter as a research fellow in the MRC Clinical Genetics Unit at the Institute of Child Health. Thus began the work that was to shape her short career. First, she classified monogenic diseases of the nervous system, with an emphasis on the hereditary ataxias and peripheral neuropathies. These studies formed the basis for her doctoral thesis on 'The Hereditary Ataxias and Paraplegias: A Clinical and Genetic Study'. Later, she reworked the text into a monograph on *The Hereditary Ataxias and Related Disorders* (1984). Her single most important discovery, published in *Nature* with Ian Holt and John Morgan-Hughes in 1986, was the first identification of a mitochondrial DNA mutation in human disease and the concept of tissue heteroplasmy of mutant mitochondrial DNA. But Harding also published on the spectrum of trinucleotide repeat disorders in neurodegenerative disease, and on the population genetics of diseases showing ethnic or geographical restriction.

In the year before taking up her post as senior lecturer and honorary consultant at the Institute of Neurology in 1986, Harding visited laboratories in Cardiff (UK) and the California Institute of Technology, Massachusetts General Hospital, Seattle, Duke and Denver (USA). These visits proved pivotal in matching her clinical expertise with a knowledge of the emerging discipline of molecular genetics. The subsequent rise in her career was rapid. She was appointed reader in the University of London and honorary consultant neurologist to the National Hospital in 1987, elected to a personal professorship in 1990, and to the post she never occupied as head of the university department in 1995.[84] With her death, the succession passed to McDonald who,

buffeted by the earlier disappointment and the turbulence that the premature resignation of Marsden and the death of Harding had caused, swallowed his pride and took the post he had assumed would be his on Gilliatt's retirement in 1983.

Harding's position in such elite and exclusively male company deserves comment. With the establishment of the university department in 1962, Gilliatt had transferred the discipline and methods of clinical neurology into investigative work and, largely through others, schools developed and strategic programmes emerged. Harding was in the vanguard of the second wave in this process and she came to epitomise its style and activities better than any of her contemporaries. Through her marriage to P. K. Thomas, Harding witnessed at first hand the diffusion of academic neurology away from the Institute of Neurology and, as a close confidant of Gilliatt, she saw at the same time the long-term significance of Queen Square as a national hospital. Her special trick was to balance the need to nurture communities at Queen Square and elsewhere, and to export and maintain excellence and influence through a network of clinical, scientific and personal collaborations. As she provided what every patient wants – knowledge, experience, interest, time and hope – her clinical opinion was extensively sought. Harding blossomed in the warmth of good doctoring and she was immensely popular – indeed, loved by all.

Harding was a devoted worker for British neurology. The trappings of academic life were heaped upon her because, as a person with inexhaustible energy, she met deadlines and delivered. These were remarkable achievements for a woman in a traditionally chauvinist specialty.[85] That so much was achieved by the age of 43, in a career that was fully active for only ten years, is sobering; that it was done in a style from which respect and friendships grew exponentially is a mark of her personality; and that it was not done at the expense of domestic pleasures was to the advantage of her husband, family and friends.

P. K. gave one of the three addresses and explained that she was in some ways like a daughter to him, and, when asked whether it was cruel of nature for her to die so young, replied that nature 'was not cruel, just indifferent'.

[84] Paradoxically, and despite her ambition, this appointment seemed to come too easily for Harding, and she sought advice from friends on whether to accept the nomination without even having to submit an application or to enjoy the frisson of interview and decision in her favour over other candidates. This was not gladiatorial, but somehow the whole process felt flat. Sadly, in the event, there was no time for these formalities; nor, in the opinion of those to whom she spoke, much point in toying with competition when everyone wanted and expected only one outcome.

---

[85] As a trainee neurologist at Queen Square, Harding challenged the conventional sartorial uniformity of her male colleagues. Later, she dressed with style: Armani suits for the clinic and designer jeans for assigning genes. More than once she was found absent from a scientific meeting through having disappeared with another female professor (Professor Dame Kay Davies), to which accusation she retorted 'when the going gets tough, the tough go shopping'.

Outwardly self-assured but never over-confident, Harding was privately self-effacing and there always remained that endearing hint of the *gamine*. xThese were essential qualifications for her type of success, and they were traits that endeared her to neurologists throughout the world. She excelled in conversation and revealed a breadth of interests – football and cricket in season, contemporary literature and popular culture. She was a tease without malice or waspishness, but loved gossip. She maintained her network of informants by telephone. Sunday was her night for collecting information, and correspondents could rely on leaks reaching their intended destinations early on Monday morning. Her style did not change with success. By chance, a conversation was overheard on the London Underground shortly after her death, in which reference was made to Harding's obituary in a national newspaper: she was described as having spent time with each of her staff and professional dependants planning their lives during the last few days of her own, and wryly commenting that it would not now be necessary for her to master Windows 95. 'She must have been a wonderful person', remarked the unknown conversationalist. She was.

Chapter 1

Never, Never, Ever – Change and Integration 1962–1997

The Winds of Change

'What is most needed at the present time is the prospect of a period of stability.' So stated the Minister of Health, R. H. Turton, commenting upon the Guillebaud Committee report, in the House of Commons on 25 January 1956.[1] However, the hope for stability was not to be realised and, in the years between 1961 and 1997, there turned out to be almost constant change to the organisation and administration of both clinical and academic medicine in Britain, from which neither the National Hospital nor the Institute of Neurology escaped unscathed.

In 1961, London medicine had adjusted to introduction of the National Health Service and the often-praised tripartite arrangement seemed reasonably sound,[2] and there was much to celebrate in terms of improved access to and improvements in health care. The National Hospital was a stand-alone entity within the National Health Service, and the Institute of Neurology was an affiliated member of the British Postgraduate Medical Foundaation (BPMF). Each was managed independently by their own Boards of Management. In 1962, the then Health Minister Enoch Powell announced his ten-year plan for dealing

---

[1] *The Report of the Committee of Enquiry into the Cost of the National Health Service (Chairman C. W. Guillebaud)* (London: HMSO, 1956). The Guillebaud Committee had been set up by the Treasury in 1953 to assess expenditure in the NHS, and found that there had been a fall in spending from 3.75 per cent of the gross national product (GNP) in 1948, to 3.25 per cent in 1954.

[2] The tripartite system comprised: (i) Hospital Services, with non-teaching hospitals administered by 14 Regional Hospital Boards, and teaching hospitals by Boards of Governors; (ii) Primary Care Services, comprising GPs, dentists, opticians and pharmacists who were independent contractors administered by Executive Councils; and (iii) Community Services, such as maternity and child welfare clinics, health visitors, midwives, immunisation, health education and ambulance services, administered by local authorities.

with the deteriorating fabric which the National Health Service had inherited, pledging £570 million for a national network of new hospitals. As he stated in the House of Commons on 4 June 1962, we have 'an opportunity to plan the hospital system on a scale which is not possible anywhere else, certainly not this side of the Iron Curtain'.

However, in the years that followed, all sense of optimism vanished as medical services became more and more centralised and constrained by government policy, buffeted by repeated financial crises, and confronted by a convoluted series of directives and administrative reorganisations. Self-determination and freedom of decision-making were lost as the National Health Service trundled towards introduction of the internal market and a business-oriented style of management. Health became a political football, with each election manifesto promising investment and improvement that could only be managed centrally.

The impact of the administrative reorganisations and funding deficits were particularly acute in London, where the overall trend was for forced amalgamation of smaller institutions into larger conglomerates. The many hospitals and medical schools, each with a distinguished history and powerful friends, lobbied hard and steadfastly resisted change. Several disappeared and the existence of the National Hospital was repeatedly threatened. The view that the National Hospital and its Institute of Neurology were too small to be economically efficient was not new. Similar concerns dated from at least the 1920s when the King's Fund and other official bodies and committees had argued for their absorption into larger federal institutions. Although not unused to fending off such threats, eventually the forces proved unstoppable.

At the beginning of this period, the privileged status of Queen Square, with a Board of Governors directly accountable to the Secretary of State, and no intermediate authority, seemed to promise significant protection from the administrative perturbations beginning to affect many other hospitals. Nevertheless, as the National Health Service embarked upon its innumerable policy shifts and managerial contortions, the National Hospital was caught up in the maelstrom, and forced to adapt and respond by near-constant fire-fighting.

Financial crises often loomed and it was this fiscal pressure that eventually proved to be the main driver for change. Despite the stability hoped for by Turton, and steady increases in funding, expenditure continuously outstripped investment.[3] Many forces contributed to the financial pressures – some due to scientific and medical developments, some the result of societal change and central government policy, and some that were internal. The science of neurology made huge advances in this period, in diagnostic capacity (notably due to the advent of CT and MRI scanning) and in treatment, with the introduction of novel drugs and technical developments. The public expected to benefit from such innovations, and, as a result, health care costs rose much faster than the general rate of inflation. Furthermore, the rise in consumerism altered the relationship between doctor and patient. Rigidities of the British class structure were gradually eroded from the 1960s and less deference shown to authority, including the hospital consultant, a change which was manifested by the *Patient's Charter* produced by Secretary of State William Waldegrave in 1991, outlining the rights of patients to expected qualities of service, especially in terms of waiting times. The rise of scientific medicine also encouraged subspecialisation within neurology, adding to cost pressures. This trend had not been condoned by the earlier generation of neurologists, who opposed specialisation and favoured retaining the link to internal medicine. But change became inevitable in the later decades of the century.

Another factor causing difficulties in this period was the poor quality of under-maintained estate, which added to the cost burden, and the inexorable need for new buildings and more space. The temptation for any hospital that did manage to accumulate a surplus to engage in a programme of new building, sometimes without heed to the extra ongoing costs of maintenance, seemed impossible to resist.

The propensity for central government to respond to financial pressures by proposing 'reorganisation' was a profound change from the pre-1948 situation, and repeatedly challenged the position of the hospital and Institute. Top-down management was deemed necessary by central government, to achieve fiscal stability. The paternalistic nature of the Boards of Management went out, and a professional managerial culture came in. Hospitals were swamped by an avalanche of bureaucracy requiring legions of regulators, auditors, professional managers and accountants. These organisational and management changes came with their own costs that in turn contributed significantly to the parlous state of funding in the National Health Service. The clinical input and influence of physicians diminished, not least because restraint and budgeting were not skills that came naturally to medical practitioners. Resource allocation seemed to be in conflict with the primary responsibilities of clinical staff to do their best for individual patients and to advance neurological science. The ethos of service as the foundation of medicine was starting to unravel.

These issues were felt throughout the country but the planning of services in London posed particular problems, including socio-demographic issues, the high levels of deprivation, the poor quality of existing building stock compounded by the high cost of land and renovation, the inheritance of poorly coordinated services prior to the National Health Service, and the complex requirements for teaching and research. Each of these added to its difficulties and worked against the role that Queen Square saw for itself.

Between 1960 and 1997, there was a dizzying sequence of reports and reviews concerning hospital services and postgraduate teaching. Amongst those that impacted directly on Queen Square, and to which it had to respond, were (and this list is not exhaustive):

1960:   *Report of the Royal Commission on Doctors' and Dentists' Remuneration*

1961:   *Report of the Joint Working Party on the Medical Staffing Structure in the Hospital Service* (the Platt report)

---

[3] As a proportion of gross domestic product (GDP), government spending on health had risen from 0.5 per cent in 1900, to 1.14 per cent in 1921, 3.07 per cent in 1948 and 3.5 per cent in the early 1960s. The spending brake was then released a little and the figure was 4.98 per cent by 1970. A period of flat-line spending followed with a figure of 4.88 per cent in 1988 and 4.9 per cent in 1998. There was then a rapid rise to 8.01 per cent in 2009 and 6.2 per cent in 2016 (www.ukpublicspending.co.uk/pastspending).

1962: Enoch Powell's Hospital Plan; *Porritt Report on Medical Services*

1966: *Report of the Committee on Senior Nurse Staffing Structure* (Salmon report)

1967: Cogwheel report on the organisation of doctors in hospitals

1968: Kenneth Robinson's Green Paper on *Administrative Structure of the Medical and Related Services in England and Wales*; Royal Commission on Medical Education (Todd report); Seebohm Report

1970: Second Green Paper on NHS by Richard Crossman

1971: Revision of Crossman proposals by Sir Keith Joseph

1973: NHS Reorganisation Act

1974: Reorganisation setting up 14 Regional and 90 Area Health Authorities, which eventually led to the redesignation of Queen Square as an AHA(T) in 1977

1974: Halsbury Committee report on pay and conditions of nurses

1975: Merrison report on the regulation of the medical profession; London Co-ordinating Committee report

1976: Report of the Health Resource Allocation Working Party

1977: NHS Act 1977 designating postgraduate hospitals, including the National Hospital, as Area Health Authorities (Teaching) (AHA(T))

1978: Report of the Howie Committee into safety in clinical laboratories and post-mortem examination rooms

1979: Report of the Royal Commission on the NHS (Merrison Committee); publication of the consultative document on the recommendations of the Royal Commission, *Patients First*. These led to the 1982 NHS Reorganisation Act and redesignation in 1982 of the National Hospital as a Special Health Authority (SHA)

1980: Black Report on health inequalities; Flowers report on London medical education; London Health Planning Consortium Report, *Towards a Balance*, and their accompanying reports on postgraduate hospitals and on neurology and neurosurgery in London

1981: Short Report (Social Services Committee); London Advisory Group report; Parliamentary statement that six postgraduate hospitals (including the National Hospital) would be designated as Special Health Authorities

1982: NHS reorganisation abolishes Area Health Authorities; first of the six reports of the Körner Committee on Health Services Information

1983: Griffiths report on management structures in the NHS

1985: Enthoven report on the management of the National Health Service

1986: Hospital medical staffing report *Achieving a Balance*

1987: White Paper, *Promoting Better Health*; GMC Education Committee on Training of Specialists

1989: White Paper, *Working for Patients* – the proposal for the creation of an NHS 'internal market'

1990: NHS and Community Care Act – which enacted into law the reorganisation which created the internal market

1991: White Paper, *Health of the Nation*; *The Patient's Charter*; King's Fund Commission report; Peckham strategic review of Research in the NHS

1992: Tomlinson report into London's Health Services; PFI (Private Finance Initiatives) introduced into the NHS; *London Health Care 2010*, King's Fund report

1993: London Implementation Group report, *Making London Better*; London specialty review of neuroscience; Expert Advisory Group report, *Hospital Doctors: Training for the Future*

1994: NHS reorganisation, with NHS regions replaced by eight regional outposts, with two for London; Queen Square Locality review; *Supporting Research and Development in the NHS* (the Culyer report)

1997: White Paper of the new Labour government, *The New NHS: Modern, Dependable*; King's Fund report, *Transforming Health in London*; Turnberg report, *Health Services in London – a Strategic Review*.

The National Hospital had safely negotiated the first waves of reorganisations introduced in the 1970s and 1980s, but the storm clouds continued to gather. Whilst clinging to its special status as a 'London teaching hospital', Queen Square was exposed to the instabilities of management and governance arising from both the meanderings of National Health Service policy and postgraduate education in London University. By the 1990s, all sense of security had faded. The policy changes of the Thatcher government, which introduced the internal market, meant that funding now depended on income derived from the number of referrals contracted from primary care. Located in central London, Queen Square did not have a natural catchment and its geographically better-placed competitors jealously guarded their own referral bases. Critically, NHS and university policy remained hostile to small and specialised units. Central funds for academic work were reduced, and research became increasingly dependent on external sources. It is little wonder that, with this plethora of reviews, reports, policy changes and reorganisations, life at the National Hospital, and elsewhere, was considered to be in a state of 'permanent revolution'. It was thus to some extent with a sense of inevitability that the National Hospital and its Institute of Neurology were eventually absorbed into larger institutions (University College Hospital NHS Trust in 1996, and University College London in 1997, respectively), both losing their independent Boards and autonomous control over domestic affairs. In retrospect, it is perhaps surprising that Queen Square survived the endless round of changes in direction and policy for as long as it did.

Hospital Life in a Period of Change

In the early 1960s, these perturbations lay ahead and, as that liberal decade unfolded, there was an initial sense of enthusiasm and hopefulness about the future of hospital care. The 1959 election manifestos of all three parties had promised relaxation of postwar austerity and a period of economic expansion. For those who knew Queen Square across this period and nurtured its tradition, the impending changes initially seemed remote, and life at the hospital and its newly built Institute of Neurology proceeded much as before.

At the first meeting of the Board of Governors in 1962, chaired by Sir John Woods, with Geoffrey Robinson as secretary, the appointment of Roger Gilliatt to the professorship of neurology was ratified with a start date of 1 April, although he did not return from two months visiting neurological centres in the USA and Canada until June. The professorial department was allocated 30 beds, of which 24 were at Queen Square and six at Maida Vale. A special meeting of the Academic Board was scheduled in response to the request by the chairman of the Institute of Neurology, Lord Aldington, to prioritise suggestions for other new departments to the University Grants Committee (UGC), and all agreed that the immediate priority was neurosurgery, but that psychiatry, psychology and pathology should be developed. It was an optimistic time.

In 1960, the routine of work at Queen Square might have seemed little different from that experienced 50 years earlier. The neurological service was delivered by five firms, each with one senior and two or three junior consultants. The senior registrar organised outpatients and saw cases each day of the week but had no responsibility for inpatients. He (or rarely a she) allocated the best cases for teaching, in which the patient was interviewed and examined in a tiered lecture theatre (A-room) with up to 30 students observing. Teaching was undertaken by the second consultant on the firm, the senior physician being excused all NHS outpatient work (this changed after Gilliatt, as always leading from the front, was appointed to the chair of neurology). The resident medical officer looked after the wards, and was continuously present in the hospital, apart from one two-day weekend and one other allocation of leave from Saturday lunchtime every five weeks. Two assistant house physicians (equivalent to senior house officers) were assigned to each firm. Everything revolved around the ward rounds[4] in which all clinical decisions were taken. These occurred once, or in some cases twice, each week, with an entourage of attached doctors and students (the size of which depended on the consultant's reputation and sense of showmanship), and with the ward sister and senior nurses in attendance to make sure tea and sandwiches were available.

In 1966, hospital activity was reported to the Board of Governors, showing around 280 beds open (and 30 closed) with 4,500 admissions each year, bed occupancy at around 85 per cent, and average length

---

[4] One consequence of the subspecialisation and increase in numbers of consultants after the 1980s was the virtual disappearance of this ritualised consultant ward round.

of stay 19–20 days. The outpatient department was seeing over 8,000 new cases and around 40,000 follow-ups per year.[5] Over the next three decades, the neurological bed numbers fell, but the number of inpatients remained roughly the same, an equation made possible by progressive shortening of the length of stay. Outpatient numbers tended to fall over the period, despite an increase in medical staffing and in the number of clinics held, reflecting the longer consultation times in later years. Thus, at Queen Square in 1985, there were 201 beds – 129 allocated to neurology, 45 to surgery, 11 to psychiatry, 5 in the Batten Unit, and 11 private beds – and 4,169 discharges with an average length of stay of up to 13.2 days. There were also an additional 84 beds at Maida Vale.[6] There were 1,415 surgical operations carried out in that year, 152 different clinics and 6,352 new outpatients. One quarter of the inpatients were from outside London, justifying the claim that the National Hospital was an important 'tertiary' centre and the 'last court of appeal' (although 94 per cent of the outpatients were from the Thames regions). By 1995/6, after the absorption of the work of Maida Vale Hospital onto the Queen Square site, the number of inpatient discharges at Queen Square had risen by 20 per cent to 5,181, despite a reduction in total NHS bed numbers to 228.[7] Of these, 61 per cent were from the North Thames region, 21 per cent from South Thames and 19 per cent from outside London. Roughly the same distribution was noted amongst the 37,820 outpatient attendances. This was the level of activity level that justified the application for NHS Trust status.

---

[5] Other activity figures were: 10,000 physiotherapy treatments, 8,000 X-ray examinations, around 2,500 neurophysiological tests (EMG or EEG) and 16,000 pathological investigations.

[6] Figures taken from the hospital 'strategy document 1996–1991' (itself a new phenomenon). The figures for Maida Vale were 52 neurology, 28 neurosurgical and 4 private beds, 1,789 discharges (average length of stay 14 days) and 659 surgical operations. There were also 27 rehabilitation beds at Finchley and 45 NHS beds in the new Special Centre for Epilepsy at the Chalfont Centre.

[7] These figures are taken from the National Hospital for Neurology and Neurosurgery (NHNN) joint trust application in April 1995 (and include the transfer of activity previously at Maida Vale to the Queen Square site); the bed count was: 98 neurology, 17 ITU, 46 neurosurgery, 18 neuro-rehabilitation, 10 neuropsychiatry, 6 epilepsy telemetry beds and 33 epilepsy assessment beds (at Chalfont). In addition, there were 11 private beds on Nuffield ward.

Throughout the 1960s and 1970s, expenditure at the National Hospital was increasing rapidly and this began to impinge on the hospital's ambitions.[8] The Department for Health noted this inflation and pointed to the fact that length of stay for inpatients at Queen Square was considerably longer than elsewhere, operating theatre costs appeared excessive, and expenditure on medical typing was high due to the unusually long and elaborate case notes, a matter of professional pride for neurologists. This was the opening gambit in what over subsequent decades led to continuous financial pressures.

As time passed, the National Hospital became increasingly concerned to justify its existence by adopting a more community-based focus, an issue that became of critical importance in the 1990s. The need to provide a district service had been first raised by Kenneth Robinson's 1968 Green Paper, and one method of achieving this, suggested in the Todd report of 1968, was to form linked appointments with other hospitals in and around London. Discussions were held directly with potential partners and via the North West Metropolitan Board for linked consultant posts. One of the earliest proposals would have been a very busy post combining Queen Square, Watford and Bedford, but this was never put in place. In fact, a joint appointment with Edgware General Hospital was the first to be implemented, with Roman Kocen appointed in 1969, having access to seven beds at Maida Vale but admission rights at Queen Square only by courtesy of the senior physician. Other links were later formed with a variety of district and teaching hospitals, and additional joint medical appointments made, giving the National Hospital the semblance of a community focus.

The need to improve medical education and training, both undergraduate and postgraduate, had been a powerful driver of change in the postwar years, and the idea that the modern doctor could be trained merely by apprenticeship – without any curriculum,

---

[8] Expenditure was: £833,589 in 1957, £1,536,761 (of which nearly two-thirds was used for salaries) in 1967, £1,973,574 in 1970, and £2,365,165 by 1972. At the end of our period, in 1996, expenditure was £41,579,000, representing £1.2 million less than income. The Royal Commission on the National Health Service set up by the Wilson Labour government in 1975 made the point that 'It would be unrealistic to suppose that the fortunes of the NHS can be insulated from those of the nation', an admission which was to become all too painfully evident in subsequent years.

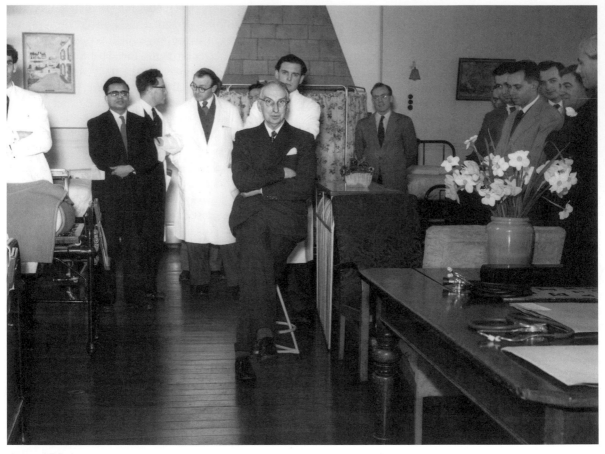

Figure 14.1 Purdon Martin's last ward round, 1958 (and the end of the era of Queen Square's 'Edwardian' style).

however informal – was becoming untenable. Senior registrar rotations were established with Great Ormond Street Hospital in January 1966, then with St Mary's, and later several other London teaching hospitals. But, by 1970, new arrangements were needed for the junior staff to improve their training. After 100 years, it was decided to abolish the posts of registrar to outpatients and the resident medical officer at the National Hospital, and to attach one senior registrar to each firm to supervise the care of inpatients and outpatient work on that firm's allocated day. The suggested staffing for each the five firms at Queen Square and the two at Maida Vale was now one senior registrar, one registrar and two assistant house physicians. One senior registrar was designated lecturer on the university firm.

The number of junior staff in the 1960s was still a matter for the hospital to decide, as it had done since the foundation 100 years earlier, but this freedom to appoint however many and whoever it liked ended

when, in 1973, a letter from the Department of Health described redistribution of registrar and senior registrar posts to allow more equitable national coverage. The Medical Committee protested strongly and a meeting was held on 28 January 1974 at Queen Square with Dr Tate from the Department of Health. The dean, Reginald Kelly, had prepared a document in which he made reference to the 1969 international directory of neurology, stating that 113 of the 130 practising neurologists in the UK had received all or a significant part of their training at Queen Square, as had the six existing professors of neurology and two more whose appointments were imminent. He pointed out that the National Hospitals had nearly 300 beds, 18 neurologists, 2 paediatric neurologists, 4 neurosurgeons, 4 neuroradiologists, 10 neurophysiologists, 4 neuropathologists, 4 neuro-otologists, 3 neuro-ophthalmologists and the only professorial department of neurochemistry in the UK, and that, in addition to the teaching and clinical work, there was considerable research activity: 'there is nowhere in the world where such exposure to so much expertise is possible both with regard to quantity and quality'.[9] Dr Tate explained that the current ratio of consultant to registrar/senior registrar in the UK was 10:7 but almost parity in London. Kelly countered by arguing that training posts at Queen Square were of very high quality since they required less service commitment: 'if the number of junior staff was reduced, the effect on the training facilities would be catastrophic and would be a set-back of 20 years'. The committee pointed out that many of the best US trainees were sent to the National Hospital for training, and not at the expense of the National Health Service. Queen Square improved the training of registrars from other units, mentioning as examples the centres in Liverpool, Stoke, Aberdeen, Cambridge and Southampton. In the face of this onslaught, Dr Tate retreated and left with the agreement to change one surgical registrar to senior house officer grade. The Royal Colleges of Physicians and of General Practitioners then published a joint report on general professional training and, on the recommendation of the Medical Committee, agreed to recognise nine neurology senior house officer posts at the National Hospital for general professional training.

A priority for Queen Square, throughout this period, was to remedy the poor condition of its estate. The prospects seemed favourable with the announcement in 1962 by Enoch Powell of the government's new Hospital Plan. Even though the primary focus of the ten-year schedule was on the development of district general hospitals, this encouraged the National Hospital's ambition for its own rebuilding. A huge amount of management and clinician time went into the plans, but progress was chaotic and for most of the period there were almost continuous revisions, new target-setting, disappointments and considerable wasted effort, so that, by the end of the 1970s, the endemic financial crises in the NHS prevented the hospital's ambitious redevelopment plan (see Chapter 2). Lack of investment in buildings was a national problem, and although temporary respite appeared possible in 1992 when Private Finance Initiatives (PFI) were introduced by the Conservative government of John Major as a means of funding hospital building

projects, the terms of these loans were punitive and the scheme became highly controversial. Fortunately, as it turned out, Queen Square was not involved in PFI and such building as did occur was part-funded by philanthropy, but its neighbour (and subsequent owner, University College London Hospital (UCLH)) did sign up to the largest PFI for hospital building in England, with payments indexed for 35 years. Peter Dixon, the then chairman of UCLH, later had to admit that this would have a distorting effect on health service provision in London for several decades.[10]

In the 1960s and 1970s, the Board of Governors had 30 subcommittees covering various aspects of hospital life. Of particular note was the computer committee, ahead of its time when constituted in 1966, which, in 1972 and again in 1974, proposed an ambitious facility to be shared between the National Hospital and Great Ormond Street Hospital, based around an ICL 2903 computer with data entered from punch cards, paper tape and teletape. This was a time when IT was being recognised as important in the health service, most of the proposed usage being concerned with hospital administration – salaries, costing and activity analysis, along the lines later proposed by the Körner report in October 1982.[11] The committee identified a range of potential other uses, including a diagnostic index, analysis of research data, and simulation studies in specialised management of patients. A computer room was set up in Guilford Street, the British-made computer programmed in Fortran, with eight remote data entry points. The capital cost was estimated to be £100,000 and the annual running costs £20,000. Despite this initiative, paper rather than electronic reports continued to dominate hospital administration for many years.

Other technological innovations were made. Geoffrey Robinson, as hospital secretary, made a tour of hospitals in the USA in 1967 and was impressed by the microfilming of records at Johns Hopkins Hospital and at the National Institutes for Health. This system was introduced in the department of neurophysiology at Queen Square. In passing, Robinson also 'gained a strong impression that the NIH enjoys immunity from financial restriction

---

[9] His figures could be thought somewhat overstated since they included the Maida Vale appointees (and beds) and also part-time appointments with other hospitals.

[10] Peter Dixon. https://www.theguardian.com/commentis free/2009/nov/13/pfi-hospitals.

[11] *Körner Steering Group on Health Service Information* (London: HMSO, 1982). The committee was chaired by the redoubtable Edith Körner. Its recommendations have stood the test of time and remain at the centre of much subsequent NHS data collection.

in respect of their research work'. Technology was not often discussed by the Board, although mention was made in 1970 of providing a link between the telephone exchange and junior staff bleep system allowing two-way communication. Previously, the hospital had used a multi-tone bleep arrangement installed in 1957, replacing an antiquated system dating from 1937 whereby junior doctors were alerted to call the switchboard by numbers on clock faces displayed in each ward which lit up according to a code allocated to each individual. This had the twin disadvantages that the doctor had to be looking at a clock to notice the call, and, unlike the bleep system, it did not reach the Queen's Larder, the pub on the corner of Queen Square which functioned as a surrogate junior doctors' mess.

A number of other issues had to be resolved in these years. In 1978, the National Hospital considered the report of the Howie Committee on safety in laboratories and post-mortem examination rooms.[12] The Department of Health had been put under pressure to act following clinical laboratory outbreaks of hepatitis in Edinburgh and smallpox in London, and the observation that rates of infection were higher in laboratory workers than the general population. Extending to three volumes, the 'Howie Code' was criticised for being unduly over-bureaucratic and demanding practices that were disproportionate and costly. Particularly relevant to the National Hospital was the request from the Department of Health to handle rabies. The Medical Committee was firmly opposed and, following correspondence between Roman Kocen and Mary Sibella, senior medical officer at the Department, it was resolved that specimens would be held at Colindale, and patients managed in a separate cubicle within the Batten Unit at Queen Square.

Another issue confronting the consultant workforce of the National Health Service at this time was the uneasy coexistence of public and private medical provision. In the early 1960s, the number of private beds had been tightly controlled, with a 15 per cent upper limit[13] for National Health Service hospitals. The charges for private beds, set by the Department of Health, rose sharply but, in 1966, the limitation on fees chargeable by

medical practitioners for private patients was abolished.[14] This infuriated the Labour party, which included in its manifesto for the 1974 election a pledge to ban private practice altogether in National Health Service hospitals, encouraging consultants to work full-time. Once elected, the new Labour government wrote to all hospitals on 12 May 1975 explaining its intention to phase out private beds, the stock to be allocated back to the NHS, and to negotiate a new contract for consultants. As might have been anticipated, the senior staff at Queen Square were not amused and considered sanctions, but, by a vote of 34 to 17, with one abstention, the decision was that no industrial action would be taken. Nevertheless, in December 1974, consultants did 'work to rule'. Despite its formidable Minister of Health, Barbara Castle, the Labour government then retreated, clarifying that it did not wish to abolish private practice but merely to separate it from the National Health Service. Another recurring issue was whether junior staff should be responsible for private patients. By 1986, those at Queen Square were accommodated at the Italian Hospital, and it was agreed that junior staff should not be required to attend cases during routine working hours. The junior staff at Queen Square also met to consider industrial action in relation to the imposition of a reduced 40-hour week, but this proposal was defeated by 32 to 18, with three abstentions. There was little support from the consultants, who considered the new junior staff contract, scheduled to be introduced from 30 September 1975, insufficient for the clinical needs of the hospital and training. In fact, analysis of the hours worked by the junior staff revealed that medical and surgical registrars at Maida Vale were working up to 100 hours per week, and not one of the junior staff worked less than 45. This period of unrest, for both senior doctors and trainees, marked the beginning of a more or less permanent state of distrust between medicine and government that has never gone away.[15] The mid-1970s was a

---

[12] DHSS, *Code of Practice for Prevention of Infection in Clinical Laboratories and Postmortem Rooms* ('Howie Code') (London: HMSO, 1978).

[13] For UK residents.

[14] Ministry of Health circular HM(66)91, and the Statutory Instrument 1966 no. 1553.

[15] It could be argued that, with a less than subservient workforce which still retained the trust and confidence of the electorate, and constant increase in medical interventions and people's expectations, government saw that it must wrest control away from doctors by increased scrutiny

time when the country faced many economic and industrial problems and groups of ancillary National Health Service staff began to take industrial action, including radiographers and National Association of Local Government Officers (NALGO) staff in 1974, despite the 'social contract' agreed between the Labour party and the Trades Union Congress.

The traditional fabric of life at Queen Square was maintained to some extent more by the nursing than the medical staff during these perturbations in the 1960s and 1970s. The old-fashioned rituals of nursing were safe under the beady-eyed tutelage of Matron Ling and stalwarts such as the legendary Sister Maggie Magnusson, who brought the mystery of Icelandic sagas to her love of Queen Square and her 'adoption' of the young men and their families whom she befriended,[16] and the wonderfully kind and courteous Sister Matai – a tiny woman from Ceylon who ran the male Bentinck ward. Miss Ling came to the National Hospital in 1943 as nurse–tutor and was appointed matron in 1946. She was a formidable but humorous and remarkable person, whose priority was the care of patients. She remembered their names and visited most on each ward once or twice daily. She employed young, often handicapped, women with epilepsy 'from good homes' as domestic staff in order to provide them with shelter, employment and a sense of dignity and belonging. Many of these women worked at the hospital for 30 or 40 years, despite having regular epileptic fits.[17] She did a round every day and knew everyone, including porters and kitchen staff and their stories, held tea parties each afternoon for selected doctors and senior staff members, and was known to take patients out in her vintage open-topped Sunbeam tourer for a ride around London. Every Christmas, she held a party for the children of staff and patients, which sadly also came to an end on

her death. She also played a prominent role in the organisation of the centenary celebrations[18] and was one of the hospital's most dedicated servants. Her influence extended beyond Queen Square and, in 1948, she had led a tour of nursing staff to the MRC Nutritional Field Station at Fajar in the Gambia. In 1950, Miss Ling visited the Claremont Hospital for Nervous Diseases in Belfast to investigate the possibility of providing assistance with training. A scheme was devised whereby a few trained nurses would be sent to Belfast, and Queen Square would receive many untrained nurses in exchange, at a time when the perennial shortage of nursing staff in London was particularly acute. This was a mutually advantageous arrangement and, in 1963, Miss Ling was made honorary life governor of the Claremont Street Hospital. Always preferring the title 'matron' and refusing to call herself 'chief nursing officer', she declined any official farewell or presentation on retirement in 1981. Margery Ling had made the hospital her life and she maintained the traditional values of nursing which had descended directly from Florence Nightingale. Because of her influence, nursing standards at the hospital were very high. By the end of the century, this nursing ethos, considered increasingly out-of-date, was disappearing nationally, and was one reason for the recruitment problems which were particularly acute in London. These caused major concerns at Queen Square and for Barbara Johnston who was appointed matron in 1981 in the place of Miss Ling. Nursing education was boosted in these years, in an attempt to aid recruitment and also in recognition of the increasing professionalism of nursing. An informal nursing school was established in Queen Square, but the nationwide emphasis on professionalism had the effect of reducing the sense of vocation, and in these years nursing changed considerably. The hospital made efforts to provide cheap on-site accommodation, but rued the failure in the earlier years to build a large nursing home. Overseas recruitment drives were another new strategy launched in these years. Despite all these efforts, staffing remained a continuous problem, not helped by low NHS pay rates and the costs of living in London.

The hospital also was fortunate in having a number of long-serving non-clinical and administrative staff whose dedication to Queen Square enriched the

---

and governance, each step towards central control being managed by periodically adopting Aneurin Bevan's tactic of 'stuffing their mouths with gold'. Largely, it has worked.

[16] Maggie Magnusson died in 2017, aged 101, suddenly, whilst sitting reading a book, having returned to a remote part of Iceland soon after her retirement from the National Hospital in the late 1970s. She kept in touch with some of her young men and their families by letter, always sending a present at Christmas, until a few months before her death.

[17] It was not to the credit of the National Hospital that they were all made redundant in the 1990s under a harsher management regime.

---

[18] The text of her lecture is preserved in the National Hospital archives.

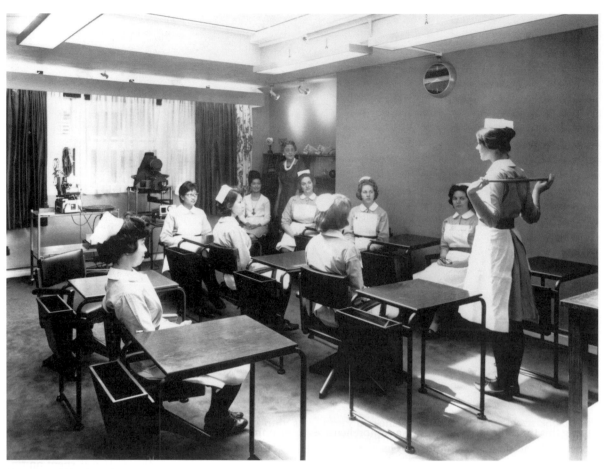

Figure 14.4 Teaching the nurses.

raising to provide for development of clinical services and investigative work became increasingly obvious as the constraints of NHS funding bit deeper and resources were directed elsewhere. The foundation, in 1971, of the Brain Research Trust was an important first step, and then, in 1984, the National Hospital Development Foundation was established. The Brain Research Trust was primarily focused on research funding and the Development Foundation on clinical services, although, of course, the distinction was often blurred. The Foundation financed building projects and the procurement of medical equipment including CT and MR scanners for service use, and these were profoundly important in the battle to maintain the position of Queen Square in leading research. Over the years, the Foundation raised over £45 million and, without it, the redevelopment of the Chandler wing in 1990 and the provision of a large variety of hospital services would not have been possible. The setting up of the Development Foundation as a charity was intended to separate fund-raising from NHS management control. The Foundation was assisted particularly by royal patronage, notable from Diana Princess of Wales, who was patron of the hospital between 1986 and 1996, and who, during this time, made nine high-profile visits to Queen Square. Her father, Earl Spencer, had had a stroke and was a patient at the hospital, and she was invited to become patron by John Young, then chair of the Board. She visited the hospital first in October 1986 to open the new Harris Intensive Care Unit,[21] and became renowned for her empathy and rapport with patients and staff. In June 1987, she hosted a Development Foundation reception at the Guildhall which attracted 600 guests. Other visits were made in this period by Princess Anne and

---

[21] The Harris Intensive Care Unit was state of the art at the time, and was funded by a gift from Philip Harris (subsequently Lord Harris of Peckham) who was a member of the hospital Board.

Prince Charles, keeping up the tradition of royal patronage of the hospital which dated from its foundation.

In 1988, the question of whether the name 'National Hospital for Nervous Diseases' was a disadvantage for the hospital was raised by the Foundation. It argued that nervous diseases were not well understood by the public and the Foundation considered that the confusion with psychiatric disease might hamper fund-raising. This issue had surfaced periodically over the decades, although the Medical Committee view in the past had been that any perceived confusion should best be resolved by education of the public rather than changing the hospital name. In 1988, extended discussions were held, and members of the Medical Committee were split on the matter. Some favoured the status quo and others considered such variants as the 'National Hospital, Queen Square', the 'National Hospital Queen Square', the 'National Hospital for Neurology' and the 'National Hospital for Neuroscience'. Roman Kocen, ahead of his time, teasingly suggested 'Neurocare'. The Board of Governors also supported the 'National Hospital for Neuroscience', at their meeting on 17 November 1988, although admitting that this might be equally unappealing to the public at large. The 'National Hospital for Neurology' was strongly opposed by Lindsay Symon, in his capacity as neurosurgeon. The problem was that no term covered all the neuro-specialties, and the hegemony of neurology, so long part of the hospital fabric, was now an anachronism. The chairman of the Board undertook to discuss with the fund-raising trustees whether 'neurosurgery' was needed in a revised name, and in the end the 'National Hospital for Neurology and Neurosurgery' was chosen, despite its lack of aural attractiveness and the fact that it did not acknowledge the other neuroscience specialties. It was an expedient, not a professional, choice, underlying the new realities of medical finances in the late twentieth century. Patients and the medical profession continued referring to the hospital as 'Queen Square' or 'the National', and still do. Eventually, the designation 'National Hospital for Neurology and Neurosurgery' was laid before Parliament early in 1990, and formally agreed in May of that year.

The distinguished record of the Development Foundation was potentially blighted in 1991 when a widely publicised scandal was exposed. It became apparent that the deputy director was forging the director's signature on cheques. Rosemary Aberdour was a flamboyant figure who masqueraded as offspring of the fictitious Earl of Morton, but was actually the 29-year-old daughter of an Essex radiologist. The newspapers had a field day and she was the subject of *Scam!*, a 30-minute documentary on the BBC – notoriety Queen Square could do without. It was claimed that 'Lady Rosemary' kept a personal staff of five, a green turbo-charged Bentley complete with chauffeur, spent £50,000 on creating a Chinese temple at the Savoy hotel, £200,000 on jewellery, and over £1 million on parties with dancing girls (for whom it was said she had a particular predilection) flown in from St Lucia and drag queens hired from a West End cabaret. She had forged cheques with John Young's signature and, when challenged on one occasion by the bank, attributed the shaky script to the chairman's Parkinson's disease (another fiction). On 12 June 1991, she was dismissed from her post and fled to Brazil. On her return, Ms Aberdour pleaded guilty to 17 charges of deception, theft and forgery, and, in 1992, was convicted of embezzling £2.7 million and jailed for four years. Her barrister, Graham Boal, told the court that 'the cars and jewels have gone back to their rightful owners and the pretty balloons have long since burst and the party is over'. Fortunately, the majority of the embezzled funds was recovered and the Foundation managed to overcome embarrassment by assigning blame elsewhere (largely to the bank). The Foundation remains an important part of the hospital fabric.[22]

Ethics

Until the 1960s, clinical research had largely been at the discretion of the individual physician, with very little governance or ethical supervision. In 1968, the Board of Governors received the Ministry of Health circular HM(68)33 on 'supervision of the ethics of clinical investigations'. The immediate response was that there was already advice provided by the medical members of the Joint Research Advisory Committee. Adverse publicity in 1972 drew attention to the potential conflict of interest in decisions taken largely by the funder and researcher and to the fact that change was needed. Public disquiet focused on accusations of experimentation at London teaching hospitals, especially the Hammersmith and Royal Free Hospitals. A BBC programme had aired allegations made by Dr Maurice Pappworth and, in 1973, it was stated in a House of Commons debate that 'the nation was

---

[22] Although changing its name in 2011 to 'the National Brain Appeal'.

disturbed' by the idea that National Health Service patients were being used as human guinea pigs.[23] The agreed response from Queen Square was that the hospital had an ethics committee comprising the medical members of the Joint Research Advisory Committee. It was proposed that a lay member should be involved, but this suggestion was dropped as some felt that it would be difficult for that individual to understand the science. When the matter was reconsidered, the question of formal written consent for participation in research was put on hold on the basis that the form would need to be so vague that oral explanation by the research investigator was preferable. Only in 1973 was it finally agreed that an ethics committee should be formed as a joint subcommittee directly responsible to the Board of Governors. Thus, despite reluctance, by 1976, an Ethics Committee that might be regarded as shifting the interests of the research towards those of the participants, and with lay membership, had evolved. The emerging importance of ethics reflected the much greater commitment to research than teaching as the function of the Institute of Neurology – a change in emphasis that was fully in place by the end of the 1980s.

The dignity of patients extended beyond research ethics. Patients were much better informed and came to the National Hospital with preformed ideas on diagnosis and treatment, rather than accepting avuncular directives. The old-style public demonstrations held on Saturday mornings disappeared in the 1980s and teaching became less impersonal and more sensitive, with patients' rights to privacy better protected. Although the celebrated Gowers' round continued with clinical presentation to a large audience, this now required explicit and informed consent in writing, with the patient often remaining present for the discussion. Patients were involved as members of ethics committees adjudicating on research projects.

The Changing Practice of Neurology 1962–1997

From the 1960s onwards, changes occurred in the practice of neurology which to a large extent reflected the transformation taking place in British society as much as the exigencies of the NHS. These were decades marked by rising egalitarianism and consumerism, increased informality, lessening of respect for convention and the questioning of authority. The reputation that neurologists had earned in pre-war years for elitism and arrogance slowly disappeared, and their style of practice became less paternalistic and rigid. In parallel, the opposition amongst physicians to the NHS (amounting to the threatened BMA boycott at its introduction) largely dissolved, and most became supportive and content to work within the system. The ability to be employed part-time and retain some private practice was important, especially to the surgeons who were able to earn large sums in addition to their NHS salaries. For most neurologists, private-practice income was far more modest, although boosted by the considerable number of patients from overseas, notably the Middle East, who visited private clinics and hospitals in London. Outside London, the pickings of private practice were less rich, and Henry Miller, in polemical style, when referring to the special hospital (i.e. Queen Square) was dismissive about what he saw:

> The lack of more than a handful of full-time appointments in neurology is disastrous for the development of the subject. A professional life largely spent in a motor-car travelling between multiple hospitals is incompatible with intensive application to the development of the subject ... we present a somewhat faded daguerreotype, with our black-and-white striped ambience and our flag nailed by historical circumstance to the creaking mast of the part-time appointment. Important though it is to extend the benefits of modern British Neurology to the denizens of the Persian Gulf, it is not enough.[24]

This was an unfair parody of the situation at Queen Square, where relatively few of the staff had large private practices and only one or two gamed the system. What Miller did not comment upon, or seemingly notice, however, was the most important development – that of the rise in influence of the medical academics. They did clinical work on a part-time basis, but this was in order to carry out research and teaching and not primarily the pursuit of private practice. This was to become an influential pattern of practice at Queen Square. It heralded a much more

[23] See J. Seldon, *The Whistle Blower: The Life of Maurice Pappworth: The Story of One Man's Battle Against the Medical Establishment* (University of Buckingham Press, 2017).

[24] H. Miller, 'The Organisation of Neurological Services and Neurological Training', *Proceedings of the Royal Society of Medicine* **61** (1968): 1004–10.

significant and portentious change as the reins of leadership at Queen Square were wrestled away from the hospital clinicians and vested almost totally in the academic appointees, whose employment contracts were held by the Institute not the hospital.[25]

Although clinical arrangements in the hospital were still largely dictated by deliberations of the Medical Committee, and the hospital still exercised relative independence in most medical matters throughout the 1950s and early 1960s, there was one area in which the government intervened immediately, and this was in relation to the numbers of doctors. Not least this was because consultant numbers had increased markedly at the inception of the NHS and this inflation in staff numbers was perceived to be unaffordable. Thus, approval was required for any new consultant post, and strict medical manpower rules were put in place, representing a significant departure from pre-war days. This caused a crisis in the ranks of the junior staff, and many senior registrars who were unable to find consultant posts left the country. Although the Platt report of 1961 recommended staffing increases, with four new consultant posts in neurology around the country each year,[26] this did not materialise. In the later decades of the century, though, there was a more rapid rise in consultant numbers at Queen Square in part due to the appointment of medical academics, with their salaries largely funded by the university, and, from the early 1980s onwards, the number of neurologists began to increase.

In the years between 1860 and 1948, a new neurological appointment was made only every two years or so. Between 1948 and 1977, 20 neurologists (about one post a year) were appointed, and in 1978–97 a further 32 (roughly three posts every two years). Thus, in the first 30 years of the hospital's existence, there had been 10 or fewer neurologists on the staff at any one time, and in the years between 1887 and 1947 fewer than 13. By 1967, the number had risen to 18, and by 1997 to 29, of whom 11 held whole-time academic appointments (and then, after this, the trickle turned into a flood). There was a similar increase in consultant numbers in other neuro-specialties and, by 1996, there were 105 consultants on the hospital staff (including a number of honorary appointees), of whom 20 held professorial positions. Another consequence of this rise in numbers was loss of the rigidly hierarchical structure of the clinical firms, and of the sense of omnipotence among the senior physicians, which had been maintained up until the 1960s but had almost completely disappeared by the mid-1990s.

This rise in consultant numbers was partly stimulated, and made possible, by the creation of positions with clinical costs of the appointees shared between the university and the NHS. The first of these academic physicians were Gilliatt (appointed in 1955), Marshall (in 1956), P. K. Thomas (in 1962) and Ian McDonald (in 1966), and then in the early 1980s the number began to increase.[27] The distinction between hospital and university work became increasingly blurred and indeed this fusion, and flexibility, lay at the heart of the success of the Queen Square during these years. When David Marsden assumed the leadership of the university department, he strongly encouraged the development of subspecialisation in clinical work and in research. This changed the pattern of practice of the academic physicians, who progressively reduced their general neurology commitments in favour of specialised clinics – for instance, in epilepsy (Shorvon, Duncan, Fish), multiple sclerosis (McDonald), movement disorders (Marsden, Lees, Schapira), autonomic medicine (Mathias), pain (Nathan), urology (Fowler) and peripheral nerve and muscle and ataxia (Thomas, Harding, Morgan-Hughes). In many ways, this was salvation for the hospital which, through such practice, was thus able to differentiate itself from departments of neurology being formed throughout the

---

[25] The full-time academics held Institute contracts of employment, with payment for the proportion of their time (typically, in the 1980s and 1990s, 3–5 weekly half-day sessions) spent on hospital clinical work vired from the National Hospital to the Institute of Neurology.

[26] *Report of the Joint Working Party on the Medical Staffing Structure in the Hospital Service* (London: HMSO, 1961).

[27] The full-time academic physicians appointed after 1980 were Shorvon (1983), Harding (1986), Marsden, and Schapira (1987), Duncan (1989), Frackowiak, Miller and Quinn (1990), Goadsby and Wood (1995), Hanna and Collinge (1996) and Kullmann (1997). After David Marsden's arrival, other NHS physicians also started taking up academic sessions and some later transferred their contracts of employment entirely to the Institute of Neurology, and others had payments for sessions vired from the hospital to the institute, sometimes within block grants. Clarifying the source of funding of some contracts became extremely confused. The key was flexibility in the allocation of duties as well as funding. The system worked very well and was much to the benefit of Queen Square.

country, in which subspecialisation was less easy because of manpower constraints until expansion of the workforce occurred from the mid-1990s. At Queen Square, the academic physicians initially ran both specialised and general neurology clinics, but later new appointees tended to reduce the commitment to general neurology, and some gave this up altogether. The academic neurologists tended to have little (or no) private practice, to conduct 2–4 clinics a week, and focus for the rest of their time on teaching or research. For the surgeons, the rewards of private practice were generally too great to ignore, with only Valentine Logue forgoing this financial luxury.

The rise of the academic physician had a further, perhaps surprising, consequence at Queen Square, that teaching lost its pride of place. In earlier periods, this had been a cornerstone of the practice of the hospital neurologists at Queen Square, but it assumed a much lower priority after the 1980s. With funding of the Institute increasingly dependent on external income and research achievement, the acquisition of grants became a priority for many academics. Grant writing became increasingly an end in itself, a tendency fuelled in part by the Research Assessment Exercises, which relied on easily quantifiable metrics. This led to short-termism and unhealthy gaming, over-exaggeration of research findings and the denigration of teaching. As had happened in nursing, the ethos of research changed irrevocably in these years, with business and volume replacing the previously more donnish and contemplative style.

General neurology remained at the core of work for consultant neurologists appointed by the National Health Service,[28] and, although some did develop subspecialist interests and became celebrated in the field,[29] most retained their entire practice in general neurology, in some cases helping to maintain high levels of referral in their private practices. The

hospital (NHS-employed) neurologists also almost invariably had posts linked to other hospitals. Of course, in the pre-NHS days, this was true of all the physicians, whose links were with the old-established London teaching hospitals, but in the post-NHS days new links were formed with the district and regional hospitals, such as Bedford (Morgan-Hughes), Watford (Schott), Whittington (Scadding), Northwick Park (Rudge and Blau), Edgware (Kocen) and Whipps Cross (Clarke), as well as the teaching hospitals. These links became of great importance when the NHS internal market introduced competition for patient services, and were encouraged by the hospital as a survival strategy in the face of criticisms of elitism and lack of relevance. Some academics, too, had links with other hospitals – for instance, the Middlesex and later the Hammersmith (Gilliatt), West Middlesex (Marshall), Royal Free (Thomas) and Moorfields (McDonald). For many of the neurologists, therefore, their working lives were a patchwork, reflecting to some extent the fragmented nature of London medicine. The same applied in the surgical field. Valentine Logue's attachment to St Thomas' Hospital was another linked appointment, albeit on the basis that all neurosurgery would take place at Queen Square, and, in the 1970s, neurosurgery links were made with Great Ormond Street, and ENT surgical links with the Royal National Throat, Nose and Ear Hospital.

If Henry Miller was writing today, one suspects the target of his criticism would be the highly specialised nature of most academic practice, and the fact that limited time is spent on clinical work, carrying the real risk of deskilling the specialist. It was certainly true that the number of neurologists whose time was exclusively, or even predominantly, devoted to clinical practice declined significantly, and only a few of the rapidly increasing numbers of neurologists at the National Hospital could aspire to the levels of clinical acumen that were a defining characteristic of its work in the past. Perhaps the neurologist most widely admired for his clinical opinions in this period was Christopher Earl, the leading non-academic generalist, widely believed to be the only one who matched his mentor Symonds.

---

[28] The hospital neurologists appointed after 1962 were: Gautier-Smith and Blau (1962), Bannister and Ross-Russell (1963), Zilkha (1965), Morgan-Hughes (1967), Kocen and Newsom-Davies (1970), Rudge (1974), Schott (1978), Thomas (1980), Scadding and Wiles (1982), Lees (1983), Mathias (1985), Rossor (1986), Fowler (1987), Thompson, Harrison and Ormerod (1990), Plant (1991), Howard and Llewelyn (1992), Ball (1993), Kapoor (1994), Greenwood and Brown (1995), Clarke and Farmer (1996) and Manji (1997). (NB: for reasons discussed above, some of these appointees held paid Institute as well as hospital contracts).

---

[29] For instance, Morgan-Hughes, Lees, Rossor, Fowler Thompson. Some of those who did develop more specialist work tended also, later, to transfer their contracts and take up full-time university positions.

It was also in this period that, for the first time in the history of the hospital, the neurologists were outnumbered by other specialists – due to the rise of radiology, surgery, physiology, pathology, ophthalmology, otology, urology and psychiatry. The academic physicians, though, tended to lead the Medical Committee, which remained the conduit through which important decisions were processed and refined in these early years. Its work in the 1960s and 1970s became dominated by Roger Gilliatt, as chairman of the university department of clinical neurology and, to a lesser extent, by the professors of neurosurgery – Logue, and then Symon. The committee met monthly and attendance was considered mandatory. Discussions were predicated on the interests of the academic departments and this moulded the hospital's style and practice. It was only with the rise of the post-Griffith management structures in the mid-1980s that power shifted finally away from doctors altogether and settled with the professional administrators. The influence of the Medical Committee was diminished and then largely extinguished after the take-over of the hospital by UCLH.

Another striking feature of this period was the absence – because Queen Square did not have a casualty or emergency service – of 'acute neurology': the emergency treatment of such conditions as meningitis, encephalitis, coma, trauma or stroke. Although efforts were made to provide a 24-hour service for urgent referrals from general practice or other hospitals in and around London, the lack of emergency neurology was often pointed out by those antagonistic to the stranglehold Queen Square exerted on training. Henry Miller, for instance, in his lecture delivered at Queen Square on 'Neurology in the General Hospital' strongly criticised the training provided by 'the special hospital' in contrast to that of the 'general hospital'. He argued that the special hospital affords unparalleled facilities for the collection and analysis of groups of rare cases, and work – superficially unpromising – that may throw unexpected light on commoner and more intrinsically important clinical problems. He contrasted the highly selective nature of patients in a special hospital with the more representative population of a general hospital, and made the point that this tended to distort the subspecialist's view of prognosis and natural history. He continued:

A second, immediately noticeable, difference is that in the general as opposed to the special hospital the

neurologist's patients are often acutely and sometimes catastrophically ill. Indeed perhaps the commonest of all the problems that the neurologist is asked to help his hospital colleagues to elucidate is that of the patient admitted unconscious ... it is clear that topographical neurology affords little help ... which emphasizes at once that the neurologist in the general hospital must be a physician even before he is a neurologist.[30]

There was force in his argument that, because the National Hospital lacked acute neurology and its cases were too highly selected, it could not provide comprehensive training. It was in response to this criticism that all senior registrar posts started to rotate between Queen Square and other London hospitals in the 1970s.

The relative prominence of the various subspecialty areas changed over time, often dependent on new technologies, discoveries or treatments. Thus, for instance, the work in epilepsy rapidly developed in parallel with advances in imaging and EEG telemetry and the introduction of a plethora of new licensed anti-epileptic treatments. Similarly, the work in multiple sclerosis was stimulated by imaging, movement disorders by advanced physiology and new drug and surgical therapies, and peripheral nerve and muscle disease by the rise in neurogenetics and biopsy-led neuropathology.

The second half of the twentieth century saw profound advances in the science and practice of medicine, from which neurology greatly benefitted. These often presented financial pressures, but it was essential for the National Hospital not to be left out of these developments in order to justify its national role and intention to continue leading British neurology. The tensions are well exemplified by levodopa, introduced in the 1960s but in short supply, and with delays in availability introduced with approval from the Dunlop Committee. A letter from the chief medical officer, Dr Godber, emphasised that levodopa was available only within the context of a clinical trial – a tactic frequently used subsequently to manage the introduction of new drugs. Notwithstanding this instruction, in 1970, 30,000 gm of levodopa were being provided nationally by the Department of Health each month. Similar attempts at rationing, sometimes by setting clinical criteria for use, affected the availability of disease-modifying therapies for

---

[30] H. Miller, 'Neurology in the General Hospital', *British Medical Journal* 1 (1958): 477–80.

multiple sclerosis from 1995, cholinesterase inhibitors for Alzheimer's disease, and the eight new anti-epileptic drugs and devices for brain stimulation, licensed for use in epilepsy between 1989 and 1997. Queen Square was also involved in the introduction of drug therapies for psychiatry in the 1960s. These accelerated closure of the large asylums, marginalised social psychiatry and brought mental illness centre-stage in public debate. But perhaps the most profound technological change was the introduction of non-invasive imaging, initially CT and then MR, which completely transformed protocols for accurate diagnosis, eroding the erstwhile unchallenged authority of the physical examination and its practitioner. The advent of medical imaging also shifted the focus from inpatient to outpatient management of neurological disease. Later, digital subtraction angiography reduced the need for contrast radiology, and interventional procedures altered neurosurgical practice. The need not to be left out of developments in Positron Emission Tomography (PET) and functional MRI (fMRI) diverted space and resources away from clinical practice towards research activities. Later, the rapid growth of clinical and molecular genetics allowed many obscure disorders to be diagnosed and classified, thereby shaking up the classical nosology of neurological disease. Entirely new mechanisms were shown to be responsible for conditions that had previously been considered under the old headings, *inter alia*, of toxic, infective and degenerative disorders. Mitochondrial neurology, and ion-channel and synaptic disorders came of age. Neuroplasticity was seen as a process to be manipulated in the management of otherwise chronic disabling conditions and rehabilitation. Improvements in neuro-anaesthesia brought dividends to intensive care and complex neurosurgery. New surgical procedures were introduced for movement disorders. There was much development of surgical equipment, starting with the operating microscope and continuing with various computerised navigation systems and stereotactic technologies. The use of electric stimulators would have brought a smile to the faces of those who worked the nineteenth-century electric room at Queen Square.

Paralysis and Epilepsy

In that spirit of past and future history, it seems appropriate to conclude an analysis of the practice of neurology at Queen Square after 1962 by considering the two conditions on which the hospital had been founded 100 years earlier. Each serves as an illustration of trends in neurology as the hospital embarked on its second century.

Stroke remained the main cause of paralysis in 1960 as it was in 1860. However, by 1960, stroke was hardly treated at the National Hospital. The small number of neurologists rendered this impractical and the care of patients with stroke had been ceded to general physicians and geriatricians. The general view at the time was that little could be done for patients with stroke, and it was often commented that stroke was a vascular not a neurological condition.[31] In 1860, general paralysis of the insane was also a notable cause, but this was no longer seen by 1960, and multiple sclerosis, which had only just been differentiated from other causes of paralysis in the nineteenth century, was by then the commonest cause of paralysis encountered in the hospital.

An important initiative in relation to paralysis, starting in the late 1980s, was the setting up of a rehabilitation unit. This was staffed by a consultant and two junior staff, a non-clinical research fellow and therapists, and was partly funded by the Brain Research Trust and the Development Foundation. It was based initially at Finchley, and then moved to the Albany wing of the National Hospital in the reconfiguration that followed the completion of the Powis wing redevelopment. The unit grew rapidly in size, occupying space made available through the reduction in the number of hospital beds at Queen Square and the closure of the facility at Finchley in 1999. In addition to providing a clinical service and training, from its inauguration, the work of the unit was linked to the Institute of Neurology. Its research aimed to develop and audit clinical and physiological outcome measures and make neuro-rehabilitation more focused and cost-effective. Close ties to the multiple sclerosis unit of the university department of clinical neurology were established since much of the research involved MRI and assessment, longitudinally, of

---

[31] This changed only at the beginning of the twenty-first century, by which time the neurological establishment had grown very significantly and, furthermore, treatments for acute stroke were being implemented. Suddenly, stroke became a desirable subject, and a turf war broke out, with neurologists trying to retake the ground. At Queen Square, a stroke unit, and a stroke section within the university department, were formed in 1999. This topic has since grown rapidly and stroke is now one of the crucial services in the hospital portfolio.

disability and this stimulated innovation in clinical practice in paralysis and rehabilitation.

Paralysis and epilepsy are essentially symptoms rather than specific diseases, and by the end of the nineteenth century, 'paralysis' had lost its identity as a single condition. Epilepsy, on the other hand, managed to preserve its designation as a specific pathological disorder and had a different trajectory in the twentieth century. Epilepsy remained central to the activity and intellectual life of the National Hospital from the time of its foundation until the First World War. Interest then waned, and no real development occurred until the introduction of EEG in the 1940s. This awakened a dormant field. Further technical developments began to occur in EEG recording, particulary in the USA and France, and Roger Gilliatt then placed a focus on epilepsy in the university department of clinical neurology in the early 1970s by initiating a programme of EEG telemetry and clinical research. In 1972, the Special Centre for Epilepsy, with 28 beds, opened at the Chalfont Centre, a move facilitated by publication of the Reid report and subsequent Parliamentary debates. Another important technical development was that of therapeutic drug monitoring (TDM). The first laboratory was set up in 1966 by Peter Lascelles in the department of chemical pathology and then in 1973, Alan Richens moved from his Wellcome research fellowship post at St Bartholomew's Hospital Medical School to the Institute of Neurology to take up a post as honorary lecturer in the department of clinical neurology and was promoted to a joint readership in neuropharmacology in January 1978. He carried out studies on phenytoin, largely at the Chalfont Centre for Epilepsy, which attracted international prizes.[32] Richens' relationship with Gilliatt was strained. In 1981, he was awarded a personal chair within the university department of neurology but a few months later left Queen Square to take up a professorship in Cardiff. Had he stayed, a department of neuropharmacology, focusing on epilepsy, might have evolved and this was another lost opportunity for Queen Square. When Lascelles retired in 1988, Philip Patsalos, whose PhD was conducted in Lascelles' laboratory was appointed, with grant support from the Sasakawa Foundation as head of the Drugs and Therapeutics Laboratory, and he too was awarded a personal chair in 2003. In 1978, Sir Jules Thorne had visited Gilliatt's department and awarded a grant of £300,000, the first of several from the Sir Jules Thorne Charitable Trust supporting work in epilepsy at Queen Square. This proved crucial in sowing the seeds of subsequent growth. In 1988/9, the epilepsy unit at the National Hospital and Institute were reorganised to provide a coordinated clinical and research programme on both the Queen Square and Chalfont sites, and agreement was reached to form a cooperative tripartite partnership between the National Hospital, the Institute of Neurology and the National Society for Epilepsy (the national charity which administered the Chalfont Centre), with each partner sharing resources. The National Society committed funds for medical salaries as well as clinical resources, and launched a successful £3 million centenary appeal[33] for an MRI unit (based around an IGE Horizon 1.5 Tesla scanner) for epilepsy research, which opened in April 1995. In January 1995, epilepsy telemetry expanded and a new Sir Jules Thorn Telemetry unit was opened at the National Hospital, part-funded by the Sir Jules Thorn Charitable Trust, and with an annual throughput which grew to about 500 patients. Other facilities included the establishment of a clinical trials unit and a pharmacology laboratory at the Institute of Neurology. The tripartite arrangement worked well and epilepsy clinical and research work expanded rapidly. By 1990, members of the group were seeing about 6,000 outpatients across both sites per year; there were 45 beds in the medical assessment unit at Chalfont; and an epilepsy surgery programme had been put in place at Queen Square, which grew to treat 100 cases per annum. In 1994, the group was granted WHO Collaborative Neuroscience Research and Training Status, and was offering medium-term rehabilitation, long-term residential care, counselling and psychological services, as well as inpatient and outpatient neurological facilities. By 1997, there were three neurologists, two neurophysiologists, two neuroradiologists, a neurospychiatrist and three neurosurgeons involved in the epilepsy group, in addition to a pharmacologist, three physicists and two psychologists. Between 1990 and 1997, 72 postgraduate fellows (51 of whom had medical qualifications) worked in the group, during which

---

[32] One of Richens' doctoral students was Emilio Perucca who was elected president of the International League Against Epilepsy in 2013.

[33] The 'Snapshot' appeal was launched in 1992, chaired by Sir Colin Chandler, the chief executive of Vickers, with Lord Ralf Dahrendorf as the honorary president.

time 376 peer-reviewed journal papers, 138 chapters and 33 books were published.[34]

Literary References to the National Hospital

The authorities may have wished that Ms Aberdour's exploits belonged in a fictional non-factual narrative of the history of Queen Square but, by virtue of its position and reputation, the physicians and surgeons of the National Hospital attracted many famous patients and, at a time of growing popular interest in the brain, the occasional celebrity wrote, directly or as fiction, of their experiences. For some, Queen Square was a frightening place full of austere and arrogant men limited in their ability to relieve suffering, and treating people as specimens. Others were more positive, as the doctor–patient relationship changed from condescension to partnership, and as neurology became more therapeutic. A few illustrative selections from this canon will suffice.

In 1959, whilst working as a lecturer in the Colonial Service in Brunei, Anthony Burgess had a 'brain storm'. He assumed that he had a malignant brain tumour with less than a year to live and was admitted to the National Hospital. The registrar, Roger Bannister, was instructed to address his patient as 'Dr Burgess'. During neuropsychological testing, the writer was asked to explain the difference between the words 'gay and melancholy' to which he answered that 'gay' had a French origin whereas 'melancholy' was Greek. He claimed that his investigations included trepanning (possibly a ventriculogram) and that he was pursued down the street when he tried to escape through the front door of the hospital. Burgess' experience of Queen Square appears in *The Doctor is Sick*.[35] Bannister is cast as Dr Railton: 'he used to be on the telly when he was learning to be a doctor, but as a trumpeter rather than an athlete'. Burgess satirises

the hospital's inhumanity and professional hierarchies. The consultant conducts his ward round like a 'pontifical high mass'. The health professionals form 'A subterranean world of female technicians … white-coated young women … jauntily self-assured … despite their lack of clinical knowledge … their mere narrow mastery of certain machines … they deferred to no one.'

Burgess is Edwin Spindrift, a linguistics lecturer with a PhD, who protests: 'You've got your work to do and you assume you're doing it with something inert, something passive. You forget that I'm a human being.' Finally, one evening, while his wife is distracted by disreputable acquaintances in a local pub, Spindrift absconds and experiences picaresque adventures in London's petty-criminal underworld. It is unclear whether this is a delusion induced by his neurological disorder or a dream sequence. Spindrift's tumour, like Burgess' in real life, was misdiagnosed and disappears.

In 1956, the author of the Gormenghast trilogy, Mervyn Peake, developed severe psychomotor retardation, insomnia and irritability.[36] After a consultation at the National Hospital, he was referred for electroconvulsive therapy at the Holloway Sanatorium in Virginia Water. He slowed down mentally and continued to be treated for involutional melancholia. He developed tremor and, after an embarrassing encounter with a theatre critic who accused him of being drunk, was referred back to the National Hospital. Peake's wife, Maeve, whose father was a medical practitioner, later described in her biography the distress created by the lack of sympathy given by the medical staff:

> One learns the big things in life sometimes in small ways. I had asked to see a doctor at the hospital, to know as far as anyone could know what lay ahead. I was told that the doctor attending him was busy, but if I would wait in the hall I could see him on the way out – almost as though I was about to ask him to tea not as though I wished to know something which would affect all our lives. A dreadful feeling of insignificance overcame me as I waited. Was it complete lack of imagination on the doctor's part that he told me the

---

[34] Details from S. Shorvon, 'Epilepsy: A Seven Year Report of the Clinical and Research Work of the Epilepsy Group of the National Society for Epilepsy, the National Hospital for Neurology and Neurosurgery and the Institute of Neurology' (Institute of Neurology, 1998).

[35] A. Burgess, *The Doctor is Sick* (London: Heinemann, 1960). Anthony Burgess was born in Manchester with the full name of John Anthony Burgess Wilson. He was a literary critic, poet and songwriter, as well as a novelist. Some of his other best-known works include *The Wanting Seed* (1962), *Inside Mr Enderby* (1963) and *Earthly Powers* (1980).

[36] Mervyn Peake was born in China, the younger son of Congregationalist missionary parents. He is best known for the Gormenghast trilogy (or quartet): *Titus Groan* (1946), *Gormenghast* (1950), *Titus Alone* (1959), and a novella, *Boy in Darkness* (1956), the canonical status of which is unclear. Peake was also a talented artist, poet and illustrator.

most devastating news I could hear of my husband standing in a hall, with the never-ending stream of people who pass and re-pass one almost somnambulistically in all hospitals? He said, 'Your husband has premature senility.' He was then forty-six years old.[37]

Peake continued to deteriorate, with spread of the tremor to his legs. He complained of a 'continuous block in his head'. With no guarantees of success, he and his family agreed to a left stereotactic thalamic ablation, which was carried out in 1960 as a private patient at Queen Square by Wylie McKissock. Postoperatively, the right-sided tremor and stiffness of gait had lessened but his speech was indistinct and he found it harder to express himself. He was confused, full of uncertainty and unable to write. Lord Brain was of the opinion that Peake should never have been operated upon.

Ian McEwan provides a more sympathetic, fictionalised, view of clinicians at Queen Square in his portrayal of Henry Perowne, based on shadowing a neurosurgeon, Neil Kitchen, when researching *Saturday*:

> He clipped the neck of a middle cerebral artery aneurysm – he's something of a master in the art – and performed a biopsy for a tumour in the thalamus, a region where it's not possible to operate. The patient was a 28-year-old professional tennis player, already suffering acute memory loss. As Perowne drew the needle clear from the depths of the brain he could see at a glance that the tissue was abnormal. He held out little hope for radio- or chemotherapy. Confirmation came in a verbal report from the lab, and the afternoon he broke the news to the young man's elderly parents. The next case that day was a craniotomy for a meningioma in a 53-year-old woman, a primary school headmistress. The tumour sat above the motor strip and was sharply defined, rolling away neatly before the probing of his Rhoton dissector – an entirely curative process. Sally closed that one up while Perowne went next door to carry out a multi-level lumbar laminectomy in an obese 44-year-old man, a gardener who worked in Hyde Park. He cut through four inches of subcutaneous fat before the vertebrae were exposed, and the man wobbled unhelpfully on the table whenever Perowne exerted downwards pressure to clip away at the bone.[38]

As for the novel, Perowne is busy and, rushing to keep to his schedule, crashes into the car of Baxter, a truculent and angry man whom he immediately diagnoses as suffering from Huntington's disease. Later that night, the troubled and murderous Baxter and an accomplice force their way into Perowne's home where his daughter, Daisy, is made to strip naked, revealing that she is pregnant. Learning that she is a poet, Baxter asks her to recite verse. She chooses Matthew Arnold's 'Dover Beach', which calms Baxter down sufficiently for him to listen to Perowne's encouraging account of new therapies for Huntington's disease. But, trying to leave, Baxter tumbles down the stairs and Perowne is summoned later to remove a subdural haematoma. Perowne muses that, despite the satisfaction in carrying out life-saving operations, he struggles to find meaning in his comfortable life. When interviewed by the *New Yorker*, Kitchen stated that he didn't see much of himself in the character of Perowne: 'I live in a small house in Islington, I ride a collapsible bike to work. I don't have a big Mercedes.'

On the night of 28 July 1995, Robert McCrum, editor-in-chief at Faber and Faber, woke with severe headache and was unable to move his left side. After a night in the intensive care unit at University College Hospital, he was transferred to the National Hospital, where it was established that he had an intra-cerebral haematoma. His memoir, *My Year Off: Rediscovering Life After a Stroke*, was partly an attempt to close the door on the 'insult to his brain' that had thrown him into a land of slowness, dominated for several years by dismal outpatient clinics and punishing physiotherapy:

> The irony of my condition as a neurological patient was that I'd often watched the results of brain surgery from my office. The Queen Square headquarters of Faber and Faber overlook this world-famous hospital. I'd stared out of my window at shaved and hideously scarred shuffling figures in pyjamas, like concentration camp survivors, and wondered about their fate. For so long I had faced this imposing red brick façade across the square. It was strangely intriguing finally to be wheeled into its shabby cavernous Victorian interior, as cool as a vintage wine cellar, though the unmistakeable mixture of hospital smells – hoovered carpet,

---

[37] M. Gilmore, *A World Away: A Memoir of Mervyn Peake* (1970).

[38] I. McEwan, *Saturday* (London: Vintage, 2006). McEwan was born on 21 June 1948 and lives in London. Two of his better-known books are *Atonement*, which was made into

an Oscar-winning film, and *On Chesil Beach*, for which he was awarded the Jerusalem Prize. He is known for meticulous research and interest in scientific themes: 'a chronicler of the physics of everyday life'.

disinfectant, wood polish and urine – is evocative only of disease, sickness and physical catastrophe.[39]

The left side of his face drooped badly for the first week and felt as if it had received an irreversible dental anaesthetic. He was unable to stand and his speech was slurred. Every few hours, he would be turned over in bed 'as if I was a slow-cooking roast'. He had profound fatigue and a marked sense of detachment from his hospital surroundings. As a way of coping, he began to construct a narrative in a large black notebook documenting what he and his wife gleaned of the medical profession's understanding of stroke. His descriptions illustrate how, largely as a consequence of social change, each new generation of doctors he saw at Queen Square become more sympathetic and communicative with the patients under their care:

> My doctor … an elegant soft-spoken neurologist of great warmth and wisdom, advised me to think of the bleed in my head as a kind of bruise; over time the scavenging macrophage cells would literally eat up the damage to the cerebral tissue, leaving that part of my brain permanently disabled … [He] reassured me that those parts of my brain which control memory, thought and personality were unaffected but Sarah was naturally concerned that I might have suffered a change of personality. The rehabilitationist, a tousled, academic style neurologist, widely acknowledged to be the top of his profession, sheepishly confessed to me that doctors are actually quite ignorant about the brain. It was oddly comforting. At least we were somehow all in this together.

Eventually McCrum came to terms with his deficits, realising that he had become a lightning conductor for a thunderstorm of physical calamity. His experience had made him realise that we are all in some senses in the doctor's waiting room and that, although hidden from the world at large, distress and pain, illness and loss are part of the human condition.[40]

One example of reference to the hospital estate is in *The Quick* (2007), written by Laura Spinney, the wife of a former consultant and dean of the Institute. The buildings are accurately described, and some characters bear striking resemblance to individuals on the medical staff. The story is centred around a single-minded neurobiologist, Sarah Newell, who conducts neurological research on a beautiful young woman, designated 'DL'. Newell feels barely suppressed adoration for her charismatic boss, Professor Mezzanotte. Several other leading characters see reflections of themselves in the mirage of DL, who has remained in the hospital for more than a decade in a chronic vegetative state. The novel describes a cold, dark clinical world where horrific liberties are taken with the almost-dead by their families and a negligent health system.

> But the hospital was older, more earthbound. It wasn't designed to draw attention to itself, but to shelter, or to hide, the most fragile of our brethren. It squatted at the heart of this giddy, gaudy, construction site, like a trapdoor you might stumble through by chance. Everybody knew about that grand old hospital, with its historic reputation: backdrop to some of the greatest discoveries in medicine. But ask them to point to it on a map, and they would shrug their shoulders and grin. It was all but invisible to the untrained eye, and this invisibility was only partly an accident of town planning. The front of the hospital, the tip of the iceberg, occupied one side of a pretty Georgian square which was reached by several cobbled alleyways. These narrow openings – just wide enough to admit an ambulance – were easy to miss. If you peered into them from the busy street outside, they looked dark and uninviting. So people carried on walking into the brightly lit theatre district, or in the other direction, to the museums and restaurants. They rarely came to the square without an appointment, unless they arrived by ambulance, or fell in drunk. And so it was cut off from the city that encircled and pressed in on it, like an eddy in a fast-flowing river … On passing through one of the narrow alleyways, and emerging into this peaceful backwater, the newcomer would be presented with a red-brick, rather austere building with a gabled roof and regimented rows of small windows. In fact that façade was deceptive, because grey, military style blocks stretched back for some distance behind it, fanning out in all directions. There was a wide entrance with a flight of shallow steps leading up to it, a long ramp for wheelchair users and ambulance bay on the street. Nowhere on the front of the building would you find the word 'hospital', something the reader might find hard to believe, until I explain it had no emergency department, and the administration wished to discourage the scourge of every casualty room – the hospital tourist – from dropping in.

Finally, to a more domestic theme – the novelist who wrote crime fiction whilst working as a

---

[39] R. McCrum, *My Year Off: Rediscovering Life After a Stroke* (London: Picador, 1998).

[40] R. McCrum, 'Memoirs of a Survivor', *Observer*, 19 June 2005.

consultant neurologist at the National Hospital. Peter Gautier-Smith made a bet with a friend that writing a cheap thriller would be far easier than the medical monograph on meningiomas that he was struggling to finish.[41] Under his *nom de plume*, 'Peter Conway' went on to publish 31 crime-fiction books, the last of which, *Web of Deceit* (2010), is about a neurosurgeon called Kershaw who is found murdered at his home. Although Gautier-Smith always denied that any of his literary characters were based around his colleagues at the hospital, several are easily recognisable, various neurological disorders feature in the stories, and there is the established preference of the medically qualified detective author for poison over firearms.

In *Fallen Angel* (1985), a pharmacist is pushed to his death from the second floor of the hospital where he works. The description of the crime scene is a very accurate depiction of the entrance hall at the National Hospital when Gautier-Smith was appointed to the staff in the 1960s:

> The facts are that both the night sister, who was standing in her office on the first floor and the head porter, who was at that counter over there, heard a cry and the latter saw the body first hit the banisters and then the table. The cause of death seems to have been lower medullary compression due to a fracture dislocation of the upper part of the cervical spine, with an associated head injury. I will, of course, have to do a full post-mortem, but I have observed one or two points of interest already. The body was not moved at all before my arrival – most unusual these days, when everyone likes to have a go at resuscitation.

The detective notices something on the carpet, puts it in a container and then decides to take a look up the stairs with his assistant. He notes that the main staircase of the hospital winds upwards in a clockwise direction from the front hall. The banisters are stoutly made of iron, topped by a polished wooden hand-rail, and on each side of the three floors there is a stone balustrade, which protects the stair-well. On the first two floors, there are wide passages connecting a pair of wards on either side with doors leading off that house to the nursing administration. On these two levels, the balustrade is painted light blue and in a good state of repair, but at the top it is a very different matter. There, the stone-work extends on two sides of the landing and everywhere the paintwork is cracked and peeling; as

well as that, the floor-covering is stained and curling at the edges and the adjacent rooms are obviously only used for storage, being full of beds, mattresses and old chairs. The building is a good deal narrower at the top, the ceiling lower. As the detective pushes the fire door at the end fully open, he sees an iron walk-way leading to an adjacent part of the hospital: 'Looking down from the vertiginous view the detective assistant could see the dead body in the main hall and a glimpse of the porter. After this inspection Newton concluded that it would have been simple and require little strength to tip the unfortunate pharmacist over the balustrade to his death.'

The pharmacy mentioned in the book is also modelled on that at Queen Square, adjacent to the outpatient department of the main hospital at the back of the building. In another of his books, called *Unwillingly to School* (2007), one of Gautier-Smith's characters visits an institution called the National Neurological Centre to track down the records of an autopsy performed in 1944, saying 'they're very proud of their records at the Neurological Centre, especially in the Department of Pathology'.

> I went through the main entrance of the Neurological Centre's research block and was directed to the pathologist's office on the fifth floor. Alastair Henderson was a large, rumpled-looking man; his white coat, the pockets of which were weighed down by an assortment of notebooks and small bottles, had a large coffee stain on one sleeve and I noted with quiet amusement that one of his socks was inside out. The autopsy confirmed tuberous sclerosis, which had been diagnosed in life by Sir Henry Rawlence, a neurologist at the Centre, in 1938. But just to make things more complicated, head trauma and arsenic poisoning were both possible causes of death.

So much for the atmosphere and gentle evolution of hospital life at Queen Square, and the writings of those who experienced the hospital, before and during the period in which external events systematically forced radical change.

The Turbulent 1960s and 1970s – the Todd Report, and Remaining Independent in the Face of Procrustean Methods

The fundamental problem for the National Hospital after 1948 was that it did not fit neatly into the structures of the NHS, either at the start or in any of the

---

[41] P. C. Gautier-Smith, *Parasaggital and Falx Meningiomas* (London, Butterworths, 1970).

service's frequent reorganisations. It was a small but expensive square peg in an increasingly cash-strapped round hole. This problem was the elephant in the room, affecting every major decision and reappearing each time that NHS reorganisation was proposed. In the end, it was the issues of lack of fit into NHS structures, and economic and fiscal restraint that were to bring about the hospital's loss of independence.

Early skirmishes were brushed aside by the Board of Governors. In 1966, a letter from the Minister (Mr Robinson) concerning informal discussion about the possibility of the hospital being administered by a regional health board was received, but the idea judged 'not advisable' by the Board on the basis that the work of the hospital was distributed with 55 per cent derived from outside London. The Cogwheel Report of 1967 proposed the formation of medical divisions to facilitate change in hospitals,[42] but, unwise as a defence, Queen Square considered itself too small to benefit from this innovation. It was, however, the report of the Royal Commission on Medical Education published in 1968 (the 'Todd report') that most obviously threatened Queen Square.[43]

Ever since the 1920s, postgraduate medical training in London had been viewed as failing to realise its potential through lack of coordination and efficiency. In neurology, the National Hospital and its Institute retained a near-monopoly on education, and jealously guarded their independent status even though this frequently came under threat. Once the Todd Committee inquiry was underway, the National Hospitals, the British Postgraduate Medical Federation, the Institute of Neurology and the Association of British Neurologists were among the 500 or more organisations and individuals that gave evidence. The hospital and Institute submitted a 35-page document that sought to establish the special and unique nature of neurology. Although perhaps potentially risky, given the importance to Todd of undergraduate education, the document eschewed the teaching of pre-qualification medical students, which it was considered should be carried out by

neurologists working in large, fully staffed teaching hospital departments. It endorsed the 1965 Royal College of Physicians report on neurological services recommending a doubling of consultant posts, and all its recommendations on postgraduate education. It did not support the institution of a diploma, quipping that 'neurology is a specialty which views the epidemic of diplomatosis – unique to medicine in these islands – with embarrassed dismay'. It recommended experience of research as an essential part of neurological training, with more emphasis on the basic sciences. It argued for creating a centre, similar to the National Hospital and Institute of Neurology, outside London, and for expansion in professorial departments throughout the country.[44] In relation to Queen Square, the document urged expansion in partnership with the Institute of Neurology, supported the idea of a single university hospital with one governing body, and recommended that the University of London assume full financial responsibility for the educational and research programmes of the Institute of Neurology.

In the event, the hospital's recommendations were largely ignored, and formal publication of the Todd report in 1968 caused utter dismay in the Queen Square bunker. The report noted that the Goodenough report of 1944 had recommended that each of the special hospitals should be affiliated with a larger undergraduate medical school, but the University Grants Committee had pulled back from this, in 1962, recognising the 'considerable fear' of the staff that their identity would be lost. The Todd Committee reformulated this suggestion and proposed that the 12 undergraduate medical schools in London should be 'paired' into six multi-faculty clusters and that the postgraduate institutes in London should each be attached to one of these paired undergraduate medical schools. Furthermore, the report suggested that the institutes should ultimately become part of the undergraduate medical schools, the Royal Postgraduate Medical School (RPMS) should develop an undergraduate course, and the special hospitals

---

[42] *The First Report of the Joint Working Party on the Organisation of Medical Work in Hospitals* (London: HMSO, 1967).

[43] *Royal Commission on Medical Education* ('Todd report') (London: HMSO, 1968) (see paragraphs 440–58, and Chapter 9 generally, for the discussions most relevant to the National Hospital and the Institute of Neurology).

[44] The document noted that there were only two university departments of neurology, London and Glasgow, and that the post in Newcastle was a personal professorship. The continued dominance of neurological training at Queen Square was reflected in the agreement, at the time, from the Association of British Neurologists that the National Hospital be used as its permanent address.

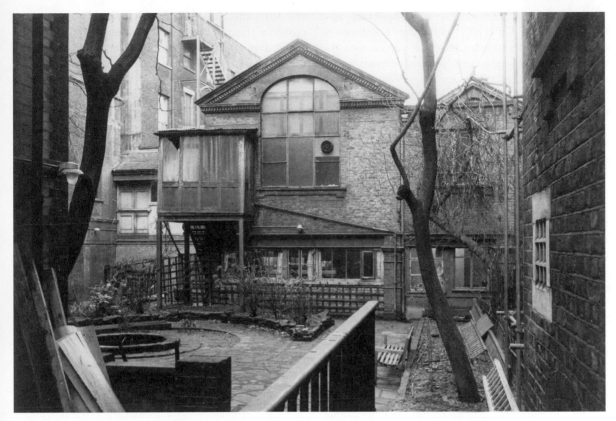

Figure 14.5 Hospital garden and telephone exchange, before demolition, 1969.

should be associated with or absorbed into the larger general teaching hospitals.

In a step too far, the report also proposed that the National Hospital and Institute of Neurology should be moved to south London and paired with the Maudsley and King's College Hospital. Todd noted that, although 'the plans are well advanced for rebuilding [the facilities at Queen Square] on the present site, this seems to us to have no particular virtue except that it happens to be available'. This suggestion utterly horrified the hospital staff and galvanised opposition.

The report also recommended reconsideration of the decision, dating from the inception of the National Health Service in 1948, that teaching hospitals should retain their Boards of Governors: 'London teaching hospitals have not provided facilities for medical education either efficiently or economically … the Boards of Governors of the teaching hospitals generally have not represented University opinion adequately … have not been responsive to the needs of their medical schools … have been insulated from the pressure of district service'.

Although the Medical Committee and Board of Governors had already commented on a draft, when the final Todd report was published on 4 April 1968, its recommendations came as something of a thunderbolt. A joint subcommittee was formed with the Institute of Neurology, and an extraordinary meeting of the Academic Board convened. After years working on the plan for redevelopment on the island site at Queen Square, their response was unambiguously dismissive: 'The proposals for reorganization of London teaching hospitals generally appear to be based on unsupported foundations.' The subcommittee agreed that association with an undergraduate teaching hospital was desirable on condition that the identity of the National Hospital and Institute of Neurology was preserved, and that any link should be with University College and the Royal Free Hospitals, and not Guy's or King's College. The National Hospital and Institute of Neurology belonged at Queen Square. Links with Great Ormond Street Hospital and the Institute of Child Health should be strengthened. The phase 1 development should not be held up, nor teaching or research compromised.

An outraged and hostile response was also recorded by the University of London pointing out that although it trained almost 30 per cent of the nation's medical students, it had not been invited to give oral evidence. When its voice was eventually heard, the report was already drafted and the object of the hearing was to 'try out on the dog' some of the conclusions about the reorganisation of the medical schools in London.[45] The Teaching Hospitals Association was equally dismissive of the conclusions relating to London teaching hospitals.

The paralysing effect on activity was made clear when the secretary of the hospital, Geoffrey Robinson, received a telephone call from the Ministry instructing him not to place an order for the internal automatic telephone exchange without prior approval, in view of the recommendation of the Todd report.

In its submission to the Todd Committee, the hospital had noted its desire to strengthen links with Great Ormond Street and the Institute of Child Health. It is not clear what background discussions may have taken place but, in response to the letter of 1 July from the Board of Governors, K. G. Moyse of the Department of Health replied on 7 August 1968:

> You will have been aware of passages in paragraph 453 of the report to the Royal Commission on Medical Education, which suggests that the joint development of the National Hospital for Nervous Diseases and the Hospital for Sick Children should not take place. I am now able to inform you that the Department has given careful consideration of this matter and has come to the conclusion that the development of both hospitals should be carried out as a joint project on the combined site. I am writing in similar terms to Mr Piller at the Hospital of Sick Children, and copying this letter to Mrs Williams at the University Grants Committee.

This was a reprieve for Queen Square but the indignation did not subside immediately, and the minutes of a further joint subcommittee meeting on 2 October 1968 recorded the comments of the Academic Board: 'We have been here for over a century, as all the world of medicine knows, "Queen Square" is a household term the world over, and no cogent reasons have been given to justify a wasteful and unprofitable move.'

With this, the Todd report, at least in so far as it directly affected Queen Square, was effectively put on hold, but at the price of much anguish and wasted time. Nonetheless, the seeds had been sown and the ideas in relation to London medicine as whole, and for the postgraduate hospitals in particular, were in many ways re-invented later in the reports of the Flowers Committee, the London Health Planning Consortium, and the Tomlinson Committee.

In November 1967, whilst the deliberations of the Todd Committee were still being finalised, the then Minister of Health, Kenneth Robinson, announced a review of National Health Service administration, publishing a Green Paper on the *Administrative Structure of the Medical and Related Services in England and Wales* (1968) that proposed the abolition of National Health Service regions and the nearly 700 separate authorities (executive councils, regional hospital boards, boards of governors and hospital management committees), replacing them with 40–50 Area Health Boards. Not unreasonably, the London teaching hospitals saw the transfer of their control to a Health Board as a further threat to their special status, and a loss of influence. The Teaching Hospitals Association convened a meeting at which a series of 'non-negotiable' principles was agreed: the need for a direct relationship between the Ministry and the London medical schools; the right to appoint their own staff; the need for adequate financial support to reflect teaching and research activity; and retained control over endowment funds. Joint subcommittees of the National Hospital and Institute considered the Green Paper, and unanimously opposed its proposals. One objection was that, since 39 per cent of patients came from outside the immediate geographical catchment area, Queen Square was entirely different from a district general hospital. The Secretary of State met with the Teaching Hospitals Association on 24 February 1969, and Lord Cottesloe specifically raised the problems faced by the postgraduate institutions in the new structure.

Robinson's Green Paper was eventually withdrawn, but substituted in 1970 by a second Green Paper prepared under the auspices of the new Minister for Health, Richard Crossman. He proposed that Area Health Authorities report directly to the Secretary of State (and not to local government) and that inner London should be organised as five central areas with an outer ring of 10–12 zones. The Teaching Hospitals Association and London Postgraduate

---

[45] Letter from the principal of the University of London, 25 May 1968.

Committee met again and emphasised the need to safeguard the postgraduate hospitals, retain authority over the appointment of their own staff and for the level of consultant manpower to reflect additional district clinical responsibilities. Their arguments were won at the time, and the governance of the teaching and postgraduate hospitals was left unchanged.

In 1972, the Teaching Hospitals Association contracted SCICON Management Consultants to undertake a study of proposals for areas and regions in London. This was the start of the tactic for engaging outside management consultants, often at great cost, in developing policy to front-up battles with the government. SCICON then undertook a study of the postgraduate London hospitals at a cost of £18,000, of which £320 was provided by the National Hospital. Their report considered five possible options for management of the postgraduate hospitals: (1) to retain Boards of Governors; (2) to create a single separate authority for the postgraduate hospitals; (3) to go along with full integration into a Teaching Area Health Authority; (4) to accept administration under a Regional Health Authority; and (5) to consider direct administration by the DHSS. Not surprisingly, the preference was to retain the Board of Governors and, failing that, to join a separate authority for the postgraduate hospitals.

The 1973 NHS Reorganisation Act replaced the old tripartite structure (which had existed since 1948) with a system of 90 Area Health Authorities reporting to 14 Regional Health Authorities. However, it was also agreed that the Boards of Governors of the London Postgraduate Teaching Hospitals would be retained for a further three to five years and be directly answerable to the Minister, but this would then be reviewed. Thus, in 1977, six of the postgraduate institutions, including the National Hospital, were each designated as Teaching Area Health Authorities (AHA(T)s) to reflect their combined academic and clinical roles. Once again, the London postgraduate hospitals had escaped radical change.[46] This

reorganisation was obfuscated by management jargon, and the medical profession remained cynical. Straining with mixed metaphors, the *Lancet* opined:

> We are at last coming in sight of the Great Day when, according to the prophets, a second coming of the NHS is going to cause the rooting out of all that is bad in the present system and lead us into some therapeutic Heaven, where all will be perfection, peace and light. But the whole business is being viewed with much less than fervent optimism by many of us who actually come into contact with patients – the 'grass roots' of the service. And let's face it, grass roots puts us in our place, as low down as you can get. From our lowly viewpoint the NHS looks like a particularly nervous colony of ants which has just had a particularly large garden fork shoved in and stirred around. Individuals race hither and thither, carrying little schemes with them and giving them to others, who carry them a little further and pass them on in their turn. Of course the trouble is we don't understand. We are unable to share the enthusiasm of our administrative colleagues as, with the schoolboy eagerness of modern Druids waiting for the midsummer sun to rise at Stonehenge, they prepare for the New Day.[47]

Leslie Williams had been appointed chairman of the Board of Governors in 1974 and, in the protracted negotiations with the Department of Health, he defended Queen Square's corner with great skill.[48] At a meeting of the postgraduate hospitals hosted by the Brompton Hospital, Williams asked the DHSS to provide clarity on why abolition of the Board of

---

[46] The 1974 NHS reorganisation of the NHS was based on the principles enunciated in the Green Paper: of integrating the three strands of health services, involving clinicians in management and encouraging consensus decision-making; 14 Regional Health Authorities and 90 Area Health Authorities were set up. This change had been planned by the Conservative government of 1970–4, but the economic crisis in the country, exacerbated by a sudden rise in oil prices in 1973, resulted in significant industrial unrest and

the 'winter of discontent'. The government fell just before the reorganisation was due to be implemented. The incoming Labour government was faced with a disastrous economic situation but considered that to abandon the planned reorganisation at this late stage would cause chaos. Important from Queen Square's point of view was the fact that the new junior Health Minister, David Owen, was a qualified doctor who had trained in neurology with David Marsden, and Owen was sympathetic to the National Hospital.

[47] 'In England Now', *Lancet* **303** (1974): 61.

[48] Sir Leslie Williams CBE was a civil servant and trade unionist who served the National Hospital for many years. He was also chairman of the London Postgraduate Committee, which was a powerful lobby at the time, largely due to Williams' skill, despite an unassuming and gentle manner, in bringing conflicting opinions to a consensus at difficult meetings. His obituary in the *Independent* of 23 October 1993 described him as having 'an intellectual and forensic skill that would have earned him a fortune as a barrister'.

Governors was necessary, stating that 'there was no virtue in "equality of misery"'.

Over the next few years, the government commissioned a spate of further reviews regarding the postgraduate hospitals. The basic problem was put, some years later, succinctly by Sir Reginald Wilson, chairman of the Board of Governors at the National Heart and Chest Hospital, in a letter to Sir Patrick Nairne, permanent secretary at the DHSS:

> So far as change has occurred during the last five years, it has been in the direction of making it even more difficult, except by Procrustean methods, to fit the postgraduate hospitals into the standard structure of the regionalised services.[49]

This did not, however, stop the government pursuing these increasingly 'procrustean methods'.

In March 1976, David Owen had suggested setting up a single authority to integrate the planning and management, and rationalisation, of services at the Great Ormond Street Hospital for Sick Children, the National Hospital for Nervous Diseases and the Royal London Homeopathic Hospital. A steering committee accepted the potential of this arrangement and it was cautiously supported by the National and Great Ormond Street Hospitals. One issue discussed was the relocation of Maida Vale. The department had stated that it was considering accommodating the Elizabeth Garrett Anderson Hospital in the Royal London Homoeopathic, but this had been earmarked for the transfer of Maida Vale, and the Board replied that this decision would jeopardise the latter's proposed move.

In 1976, a Royal Commission on the NHS, chaired by Sir Alec Merrison, had been established, and this reported in 1979 (the Merrison report). The Royal Commission was established to consider best use and management of the financial and human resources in the NHS, taking a UK-wide focus. Hundreds of recommendations were made, carrying major implications for the NHS in general, but with the question of governance of the postgraduate hospitals left to a further inquiry.[50] The government then published a consultative paper *Patients First* (1979). This report noted that the first objective of the National Health Service 1974 reorganisation was to improve the integration of services for patients in hospital and the community, and, although partially achieved, there had been widespread criticism that the reorganisation resulted in too many tiers, too many administrators, failure to take quick decisions, and money wasted. *Patients First* then set out the government's proposals to abolish the Area Health Authorities that intervened between regions and health districts, and to strengthen unit management by greater operational delegation. In the place of the AHAs, District Health Authorities serving areas similar to the old health districts were proposed. With regard to London, the paper continued:

> Underlying the Royal Commission's recommendation (No. 93) that there should be an inquiry into the problems of the health service in London, was its concern about the excessive concentration of teaching and research facilities and the influence of this upon the provision of Health Services. Much of the work necessary is already in hand. Reports are soon to be published on a wide range of developments in the health services in London; and the University of London's working group chaired by Lord Flowers which is considering the future disposition of the University's medical and dental schools and postgraduate institutes, is expected to report in February ... the lead [for postgraduate hospitals] will be left with the Department ... [it] will need to take into account the recommendations of the Flowers working party and other reports ... It follows that if London is going to follow the rest of the country, an important range of decisions affecting the future organisation and pattern of services in London must be taken by December 1980. This is a tight timetable and there well could be an advantage in establishing an advisory group with an independent chairman.

On 28 September 1979, the London Postgraduate Committee had written to the DHSS after meeting to consider the Merrison report. Sir Reginald Wilson pointed out that the proposal for an independent inquiry into the so-called London problem should be firmly discouraged. The postgraduate teaching hospitals and their particular form of constitution and operation must be accepted as an integral, if not standardised, part of the National Health Service, and justice still remained to be done on the matter of pay and status for the staff of postgraduate hospitals: 'While the Boards of Governors are not blindly dedicated to maintaining the status quo, they felt it vital to strengthen the hand of local governance and management at hospital level.'

Nevertheless, two further bodies had already been established and these both reported in 1980 – the

---

[49] Board of Governors 13/78 Appendix K.
[50] It recommended a special inquiry on London and its postgraduate hospitals (paragraph 17.5 of the report), which was to take concrete form in the shape of the Flowers report.

London Health Planning Consortium and the Flowers Committee on medical education. Both these reports were to have an important impact on the position of the National Hospital.

Surviving the 1980s – the Flowers Report and London Health Planning Consortium, the London Advisory Group, the Special Health Authority and the Griffiths Report

The planning of health care and medical education over this period can be seen as a patchwork of extraordinary confusion, contradiction and prevarication. Of course, the most significant underlying cause was the deteriorating financial position of Britain, which impacted not only on the National Health Service but also the universities. Planning was chaotic, but signalled the principles of change that eventually did come about with the much wider restructuring that was to follow.

The Flowers report, commissioned by the University of London, was published in 1980 and was a dramatic essay in reconfiguration of postgraduate education in London.[51] Anyone hoping for time in which to allow existing structures to mature was in for disappointment. The report recommended momentous changes. An editorial in the *British Medical Journal* summed up feeling in London at the time:

> Doctors have grown weary of organisational reform: in the past decade they have had to struggle to continue their day-to-day work against the upheavals caused by the reorganisation of the NHS and the restructuring of nursing by Salmon, find their way through a maze of ever-proliferating committees and bureaucracy … and so an initial response to Lord Flowers's proposals for a new framework for medical education in London will be to ask 'why more change?'[52]

The journal continued by wryly noting that, in contrast to earlier proposals for the reorganisation of London medicine, the Flowers report recommendations seemed likely to be carried through in some form simply because the University of London

'holds the purse strings'. And so it was to prove, at least in large part.

The Flowers report restated many of Todd's (and Goodenough's) conclusions, but in a revamped form. It recommended that the 34 dispersed providers of undergraduate and postgraduate medical education in London be grouped into six schools of medicine and five postgraduate institutes, that the other institutions should lose their separate identity, the British Postgraduate Medical Federation should be dissolved, and the Royal Postgraduate Medical School at the Hammersmith Hospital joined with St Mary's Hospital Medical School. The Flowers Committee recommended that the National Hospital should be included in the University College Hospital group,[53] and designated a 'university hospital', and the Institute of Neurology should remain on the Queen Square site, taking over the relocated neuro-otology department from the Institute of Laryngology and Otology.

The Flowers report was received in February 1980 and John Marshall, deputising for the dean, responded to the effect that the Institute of Neurology was in favour of integration but not without earmarked finance or at the expense of reduced academic independence.

The Flowers report conducted its work at the same time as the London Health Planning Consortium. This had been formed by the DHSS at the end of 1977 as a successor to the London Co-ordinating Committee and with wide-ranging advisory powers. These two bodies were independent and looking at different aspects of London medicine, but the groups had individual members in common and their reports were undoubtedly the result of close liaison. The Consortium's terms of reference were: 'to identify planning issues relating to health services and clinical teaching in London as a whole, to decide how, by whom and with what priority they should be studied; to evaluate planning options and make recommendations to other bodies as appropriate; and to

---

[51] *London Medical Education: A New Framework* (University of London, 1980) (the Flowers report).
[52] Anon., 'London's Medicine', *British Medical Journal* **280** (8 March 1980): 665.

[53] The University College School of Medicine and Dentistry group was to comprise the following institutions: University College Faculties of Medical and Clinical Sciences, the London School of Hygiene and Tropical Medicine, and the Institutes of Child Health and Neurology. In addition, the following were to be absorbed into the University College Medical School and no longer to have a separate status: the Middlesex Hospital Medical School, the Royal Free Hospital Medical School, and the Institutes of Orthopaedics, and Laryngology and Otology.

recommend means of coordinating planning by health and academic authorities in London.'

The Consortium's headline report was published in 1980 in tandem with the Flowers report, and was entitled *Towards a Balance: A Framework for Acute Hospital Services in London Reconciling Services with Teaching Need*. It was concerned almost entirely with acute hospital services and undergraduate teaching in inner London, and had little directly to say in relation to postgraduate hospitals, other than that:

> It has been the policy to consider wherever possible, their relocation in much closer association with general teaching hospitals. It may be, therefore, that our proposals for the general teaching hospitals (particularly those concerning The Middlesex and University College Hospitals and St Thomas' and Westminister Hospitals) will offer opportunities for implementing that policy. We propose to review the position in the light of any recommendations by the Flowers Working Party about the future of the Institutes.

The report concluded that London had more acute beds than was needed for the provision of services. This was partly because of the falling population in central London. Although the teaching hospitals claimed in counter-argument that they received patients from all over the country, the Consortium did not agree that this justified so many extra facilities, and produced numbers to prove its point. Furthermore, the Resource Allocation Working Party (RAWP) formula was beginning to bite and money for the four Thames regions was being diverted to the Home Counties. The Consortium also felt that there were too many under-sized units in some specialties and rationalisation was needed. It recommended a number of mergers of hospitals and their medical schools and, with most teaching hospitals providing linked services to district general hospitals, that offered a sufficient catchment for service and teaching. It recommended that specialties such as neurology be concentrated on fewer sites, but made no specific recommendations about Queen Square.

The London Postgraduate Committee responded to *Towards a Balance*, writing to the Secretary of State and the vice-chancellor of the University of London reiterating the need to retain the identity of specialist hospitals and postgraduate institutions and restating the dangers of being absorbed into larger undergraduate medical schools. The committee concluded that the hospitals and their institutes were indivisible, played an important role in development nationally and

internationally, and acted as referral centres for difficult cases, providing specialist education and training for large numbers of doctors, centres for research, and leaders in their specialties. These were different responsibilities from those of the undergraduate teaching hospitals, which could not be met if absorbed into those organisations, because of competition for funds, loss of identity, less specialist clinical work, reduced ability to fund research and loss of morale for loyal staff. The Institute of Neurology defended independence for the National Hospitals, with administration through the Special Health Authority, as of 'vital importance to the future prospects and prosperity both of the Hospital and Institute, which are interdependent'. In passing, the preference was expressed for maintaining Boards of Governors and, if that was not possible, creating a London Post-Graduate Hospitals Authority.

After publishing *Towards a Balance*, the London Health Planning Consortium then proceeded to look at three high-cost specialties (cardiology; radiotherapy and oncology; and neurology and neurosurgery) and, in 1980, published the *Report of the Study Group on Neurology and Neurosurgery*. This noted that there was neurological activity in 50 hospitals (some also offering neurosurgery) and recommended that services be concentrated in combined neurology/neurosurgery centres, each providing the full range of facilities as part of a major general hospital, with each neurologist based at the neurology centre, even if some sessions were also delivered elsewhere. The report recommended that rationalisation should take place and that nine centres should be created in or close to London: the National Hospital, the Royal Free, Charing Cross, Atkinson Morley, Hurstwood Park, the Maudsley, Great Ormond Street, the Brook/Oldchurch and London/Bart's. The move of Maida Vale to Queen Square was strongly supported, as were links between neurology at University College and the Middlesex Hospitals. Neurosurgery was to move from the Middlesex to Queen Square but to remain active at the Royal Free,[54] and Queen Square was to continue providing services for St Thomas', leaving arrangements at the Hammersmith and St Mary's unchanged. The report made positive comments about the National Hospital and endorsed its position as a regional centre, a secondary referral centre, a neurosurgical centre, and a centre

---

[54] After 2010, neurosurgery did begin to move from the Royal Free to Queen Square, and the neurosurgical unit at the Royal Free was finally closed in 2013.

for postgraduate teaching and research. The Consortium advised that, in order to implement its recommendations regarding high-cost specialties, working parties led by clinicians from outside London should advise on the provision of each specialist service.

These two bodies, Flowers and the London Health Planning Consortium, were clearly coordinated and acted like a pincer movement, their interlocking proposals proving hard to ignore, especially with reduced income in London due to the application of the RAWP formula. Both recognised that the rationalisation proposed would be difficult to implement, but, as the Flowers report concluded, the alternative was 'to let economic and demographic forces take their inexorable and indiscriminate toll', and urgent action was needed.

In its response to the Flowers and London Health Planning Consortium reports, the government signalled its intention of setting up an implementation group. On 2 May 1980, the Minister of Health, Dr Vaughan, duly announced that a London Advisory Group had been formed, with Sir John Habbakuk, principal of Jesus College, Oxford, and vice-chancellor of Oxford University, as chairman. Leslie Williams was a member, which was of vital importance to the National Hospital. The body was tasked with devising a practical mechanism to move the existing proposals forward.

The group visited each of the postgraduate hospitals and considered their management. It produced an 'admirably' short report which recommended that some of the hospitals and institutes could be rehoused and merged into existing general hospitals and medical schools, but that others would retain their autonomy, and these hospitals would be best designated as Special Health Authorities (SHAs) and would retain their existing management boards.[55] On receiving the report in February 1981, the National Hospital learned with some relief that it was included in the second category. In the event, five other institutions which had been part of the BPMF were moved from their existing premises, fully integrated into undergraduate medical schools and thereby, in effect, abolished.[56] The National Hospital survived this purge,

and a letter from Habbakuk to the Secretary of State on 27 February 1981 explained:

> We were impressed by the ability of the Boards of Governors to act as focal points of loyalty for staff in the hospitals for which they are responsible. The arguments for their retention were put to us forcibly by the Boards themselves and also by Sir Leslie Williams, who rightly acted as their advocate throughout our discussion. And in the case of six of the Boards, we have recommended that they should stay.[57]

It was a relief to the Board at Queen Square that the hospital survived, and furthermore that the Todd report recommendation of a move to Camberwell was not reiterated. The London Postgraduate Committee met on 8 April 1981 and Williams was congratulated for his work, although there was understandable disappointment for those postgraduate hospitals that were to be closed down. Although the Secretary of State confirmed in a Parliamentary statement on 15 July 1981 that the six surviving postgraduate hospitals would become Special Health Authorities, retaining their Boards of Governors and having direct access to the Department of Health without the interference of a regional authority, there was still local concern at Queen Square over the relative lack of medical representation on its Special Health Authority, which was to have a chairman and 19 members – to include two Institute of Neurology nominees, not necessarily physicians, and two consultants nominated by the senior medical staff.

The next major change occurred in 1982 with the NHS Reorganisation Act which, enacting recommendations of the Merrison report, abolished the Area Health Authorities, and set up 192 District Health Authorities reporting to 14 Regional Health Authorities. Arrangements for the surviving

---

[55] *Acute Hospital Services in London*. Report of the London Advisory Group to the Secretary of State for Social Services. January 1981. The six Institutes to remain as separate entities were: Neurology, Psychiatry, Child health, Ophthalmology, Cardiothoracic, and Cancer research, as was the Hammersmith Hospital.

[56] The postgraduate Institutes losing their separate identities were: Dermatology, Laryngology and Otology, Orthopaedics, Urology, and Obstetrics and Gynaecology. A decision was delayed on the Dental Institute. The future of the Institute of Basic Medical Science was felt not to lie with the University.

[57] The six were: Great Ormond Street, the National Hospital, Moorfields, Bethlem Royal and the Maudsley, the National Heart and Chest, and the Royal Marsden. The Hammersmith Hospital had indicated that it wished to be managed by the North West Thames region and found to its surprise that it too was reconstituted as an independent Special Health Authority.

postgraduate hospitals (the Special Health Authorities) were left relatively unchanged, with their Boards of Governors preserved. Once again, the National Hospitals survived the cull largely inatct. At the Board of Governors' meeting of 19 November 1981, Williams indicated his wish to resign as chairman once the new arrangements had taken effect, and John Young[58] was then appointed by the Minister of Health from April 1982, with Tom Oakman as vice-chairman.

Documents arrived regularly from the Department on governance, standing orders and financial instructions for the postgraduate teaching hospitals, but the direct lines of communication with the Department did allow a new round of capital acquisitions. An offer of £1.375 million for the examination halls at 8–11 Queen Square was accepted, with funding from the Department of Health and Social Security conditional upon Maida Vale moving to Queen Square, with anticipated savings of £0.5 million p.a. The Al Maktoum family (rulers of Dubai) provided a £2 million donation to improve accommodation for private patients,[59] and the Harris family provided £623,000 towards the new intensive care unit, which opened on 1 October 1986.

There were exploratory discussions around potential new clinical links triggered by creation of the District Health Authorities. Thus, Haringey approached the National Hospital for joint appointments with St Anne's and the Prince of Wales Hospitals, and the Medical Committee considered a link with the North Middlesex Hospital. An approach by Redbridge Health Authority to link with St George's, Ilford, was considered, but a link with Oldchurch Hospital, Romford, was preferred. In the event, none of these materialised. Soon after, the North East Thames Regional Health Authority

published its strategic planning guidelines for 1983–93, providing yet another perceived threat to the specialty by suggesting that neurologists working exclusively away from centres for neurology and neurosurgery should be regarded as general physicians.

The next tremor to shake the National Hospital was publication in February 1983 of the Griffiths report on management of the NHS, proposing yet further management change. Sir Roy Griffiths, then director of J. Sainsbury plc, is best remembered for his statement that 'if Florence Nightingale was carrying her lamp through the corridors of the NHS today, she would almost certainly be searching for the people in charge'. His report recommended the establishment of a full-time NHS Management Board, the appointment of general managers, and a move away from consensus to a performance management model. The Board of Governors expressed considerable concern over the radical change in culture to John Patten, Parliamentary Under-Secretary of State for Health, who visited the hospital on 20 December 1983. The Board subsequently commented to the Department:

> The relationships between a firm and its customers are in principle so fundamentally different from those between the NHS and its patients, that parallels with industry are misleading ... The 1974 and 1982 reorganisations emphasized team management as the key to the management process, whereas the general management concept has now become the latest panacea.

Nevertheless, Griffiths' proposals were accepted, and Peter Zimmerman was recommended for the role of general manager at the National Hospital.[60]

At this stage, North West Thames and North East Thames Regional Health Authorities each began to develop strategic plans for creating neuroscience regional centres, and this had clear implications for the National Hospital. The Board of Governors supported the development of Charing Cross as a centre. However, since 40 per cent of activity in North West Thames was provided at the National Hospital and further increase was expected following the move of

---

[58] John Young was an extraordinary man. He was a fighter pilot in the war and owned Youngs Brewery in Wandsworth, which he ran with brilliant elan. He was a bubbly extrovert with a very attractive personality, enormously kind and thoughtful. On his retirement from the Board, he took on the Development Foundation, working tirelessly and unceasingly on behalf of the hospital. He raised and donated large sums of money, and was also a close friend and confidant of Princess Diana, and encouraged her close involvement with the hospital. On his death, a ward in the new block was named after him

[59] The mother of the Al Maktoum family, the rulers of Dubai, had died in Queen Square, and the gift was from her sons in her memory.

[60] Peter Zimmerman had replaced Geoffrey Robinson as secretary in 1980. The Board of Governors supported Geoffrey Robinson's request for his salary to be extended by six months so that he could write *The National Hospitals for Nervous Diseases 1948–1982* (London: The Board of Governors of the National Hospitals for Nervous Diseases, 1982).

Maida Vale, there was concern that this workload might be adversely affected. More directly of importance to Queen Square, and obviously welcomed, was the decision by North East Thames to close three of its six regional centres – Bart's, the Middlesex and the Whittington – with Bloomsbury Health Authority recommending that neurosurgery from these hospitals should transfer to the National Hospital by the end of 1987. Less welcome was the planned reduction of neurology beds in Bloomsbury by 50 per cent.

No doubt in response to the increasingly uncertain future, the hospital began in 1986 to produce annual five-year 'strategy documents'. Annual updates continued for a number of years, but ended up being a litany of pious aspiration, and the absence of any clear-cut strategy or priorities no doubt increased the hospital's only too obvious vulnerability. It was only after 1992 that strategy in its true sense was developed, by the Board and, in particular, by the formidable duo of Anthony Wheatley and Elizabeth Howlett.

1990–1992 – the NHS and Community Care Act and the Tomlinson Report

Towards the end of the 1980s, despite the deluge of reports and reviews that had to be endured, the Boards of the National Hospital and Institute of Neurology could both reflect with some satisfaction that, thus far, their relative independence had been retained. They had successfully parried the recommendations for merger, amalgamation or closure made by a whole series of government-commissioned reports, including the Goodenough, Todd and Flowers reports, and had survived the large-scale reorganisations in the structure of health care of 1948, 1973–4 and 1980–2. Any complacency that might have been felt, however, was to prove utterly misplaced. In the next few years, the NHS was to undergo a further massive reorganisation, and the London hospitals and institutes faced another momentous reconfiguration, this time in the wake of the 1990 NHS and Community Care Act and the 1992 Tomlinson report. The co-ordinated changes recommended by the Act and in the report effectively brought to an end the independent existence of the National Hospital and Institute of Neurology.

The passage into law of the 1990 NHS and Community Care Act resulted in the most radical change in the organisation of medical care since the introduction of the National Health Service in 1948. Its ideology was derived from the report, commissioned by the Nuffield Trust and published in 1985 by Professor Alain Enthoven, a professor of private and public management at Stanford, entitled *Reflections on the Management of the National Health Service: An American Looks at Incentives to Efficiency in Health Services Management in the UK*. Enthoven proposed an 'internal market' as a way of countering the resistance to change in the National Health Service, and its many perverse incentives. His market-driven idea was enthusiastically adopted by the Conservative government under Margaret Thatcher. In November 1989, *Working for Patients, NHS Reforms* was published as a White Paper proposing a purchaser–provider split, in which general practitioners became fund holders and bought or contracted health services on behalf of patients. With the 1990 Act, health authorities ceased running hospitals but functioned as purchasers of care from their own or other authorities' hospitals. The providers (the hospitals) were to become 'NHS Trusts',[61] and these formed a contract with the purchasers to provide services. The position and role of the London special hospitals in this new internal market was to begin with somewhat unclear. The White Paper was discussed by the Board of Governors, and the consequences of the Act and its progeny, the NHS internal market, dominated the Board's agenda over the subsequent years. The Act also changed the structure of the Board, which then consisted of six non-executive members and six executives drawn from the administrative and clinical staff of the hospital. A number of managerial reforms were also introduced,

---

[61] This was not a Trust in the usual legal sense, but a public-sector corporation which was established under the Act to provide medical care (egregious newspeak in our view). Most Trusts were hospitals, but some were ambulance or community care organisations. Each had a Board of Management and was chaired by a non-executive. In their original form, NHS Trusts were, at least in theory, relatively independent organisations whose assets had been transferred from the government to be held by the trustees, with a debt of equivalent value held by the Treasury. They were directly accountable to the Secretary of State for Health, and special NHS Management Executive 'outposts' were set up to monitor them. They were in theory able to set levels of remuneration and decide on staffing numbers, but were heavily restricted in terms of capital expenditure. They were required to make an at least 6 per cent return on their assets, break even, and stay within external financing limits. The first wave of 57 Trusts was established in 1991, and a further 105 Trusts approved in 1992. The third phase of 168 Trusts was formed in April 1993 and the fourth targeted for completion in 1994. The concept of Foundation Trusts, with more financial and operational freedom, was announced in 2002, and the first ten Foundation Trusts designated in 2004.

such as resource management, medical audit, quality assurance, and the establishment of a monitoring group for referral of patients. Initially, the Special Health Authorities were told to express an interest in becoming Trusts by May 1989, but later plans deferred their loss of central funding until after other hospitals had completed their transition. Later, the Secretary of State for Health, Virginia Bottomley, confirmed that central funding for the Special Health Authorities would continue to March 1994.

The *coup de grace*, as it turned out for Queen Square, proved to be publication in October 1992 of the *Report of the Inquiry into London's Health Service, Medical Education, and Research* (the Tomlinson report),[62] coming hot on the heels of the 1990 Act. The recognition of London's unique problems was not new, and indeed, in 1920, a *Lancet* editorial had noted 'The embarrassing position of London in matters of health administration has always been recognised by those who study local organisation and the problems of developing and, where necessary, remodelling that administration, where the health of so vast and heterogeneous a population is concerned is admittedly one of unending difficulty.'[63] This did not, however, stop more attempts to do just that.

The Tomlinson Committee was set up 'to advise on the organization of, and inter-relationships between, the National Health Service and medical education and research in London'. Its purpose was to advise the Minister how to fit the inner London health services into the new 'internal market'. The report, published in October 1992, was an earthquake which shook the foundations of the National Hospital. A criticism of the many previous analyses, including those of the Goodenough and Todd

Committees, was that they were too long, too detailed, and gave no clear guidance on implementation, and therefore not surprisingly many of their recommendations had not been enacted. No such criticism could be levelled at the Tomlinson report. The committee was given only one year to complete its deliberations and asked not to produce a lengthy report (it was less than 30,000 words) but, rather, to focus on the immediate management action needed without getting involved in 'speculative or longer-term planning'. To what extent its findings were predetermined in advance by the government is unclear, but it is difficult to believe that there was not extensive briefing before the work began and that the major decisions had not already been taken in principle. The report had not a single critical word to say about the concept of an internal market, but 'attached great importance to developing a programme for change from the "bottom up", building upon consensus, rather than merely devising our own blueprint for action'. This was a smokescreen of double-talk, for a blueprint for action was exactly what the report proved to be.

The starting point was that change was inevitable, owing to the forces of the internal market: 'if not managed firmly – and in certain cases, urgently – the result will be a serious and haphazard deterioration in health services in London'. Relevant to Queen Square was the conclusion that London had too many hospital beds, as proclaimed by the London Health Planning Consortium. Tomlinson averred that, within ten years, between 2,000 and 7,000 could usefully be lost: 'a managed run-down of the most vulnerable hospitals therefore becomes essential to remove surplus capacity in an orderly way'. This process targeted Maida Vale Hospital and the Middlesex Hospital, both of which had neurological and neurosurgical links to Queen Square, and neither survived.[64] The report further determined that the Special Health Authorities were a 'distorting factor' in the inner London internal market, centrally funded as they were and not subject to market forces and contracts with purchasers. In Tomlinson's view, 'the

---

[62] B. Tomlinson, *Report of the Inquiry into London's Health Service, Medical Education, and Research* (London: HMSO, 1992). Sir Bernard Tomlinson was previously professor of neuropathology in Newcastle, and had NHS management experience as chair of the Northern Regional Health Authority (from 1982), and the Joint Planning Appointments Committee of the DHSS (1986–90). He trained in medicine at UCL, and held junior training posts in Nottingham, Ashford and Newcastle, but must have been one of the few neuropathologists never to have worked at Queen Square. In 1991, he was invited to chair the review by William Waldegrave, Secretary of State for Health, and as part of his work visited Queen Square in the spring of 1992, meeting the chairman of the Board of Governors, Elizabeth Howlett.

[63] Anon., 'The L.C.C. and M.A.B.', *Lancet* **196** (1920): 359–60.

[64] In the case of the Middlesex, this brought to an end the tradition for neurology that had enthused undergraduates and young doctors for more than 100 years and trained a significant proportion of consultants occupying prestigious clinical and academic positions throughout the country. The staff, expertise and resources of Maida Vale Hospital were effective absorbed into Queen Square, but without any of its beds.

services of the SHAs should be subject to the same rationalisation as the other inner London hospitals', and it was as a direct result of this recommendation that, in 1996, the National Hospital was incorporated into the University College Hospital Trust.

The report also recommended a reduction in the intake of medical undergraduates, and merger of London medical schools under the aegis of four multi-faculty colleges of London University (UCL, Imperial College, King's College and St Mary's/Westfield College, with St George's left on its own), and that the nine postgraduate institutions should also then be integrated into these four colleges.

The committee paid lip service to the complexity of London's health needs, noting that population density was higher than in many other parts of Britain, with a large number of transient residents, high population turnover, and extremes of poverty and wealth; that the Jarman deprivation score[65] was significantly higher than average in all the inner London districts; that the population was culturally diverse, with English often not the first language, and with refugees and homeless people; that deaths from AIDS in the Thames regions were found to exceed those in the rest of the UK put together; and that there were high hospitalisation rates for emergency mental illness and high rates of deaths from accidents, poisoning or violence and substance abuse. However, the solution to these problems, in the committee's view, should not be to provide hospital beds but rather the 'gradual and systematic transfer of resources from the acute sector to Community Health Service and Family Health Service budgets in London'. In relation to neurology, the committee noted that there were 13 neuroscience centres, and they were strongly of the view that single-specialty hospitals could not provide the best cost-effective care. They viewed the single-specialty hospitals as a formula for duplication of services and 'plainly inefficient', and decided that each Special Health Authority should be part of a major hospital complex, and service development subject to formal approval by the relevant purchasers on a pan-London basis. The committee, with extraordinary over-simplification, noted that the

> Well-intentioned efforts of the special trustees of the teaching hospitals and SHAs who are able to marshal

sometimes huge wealth in support of priorities … may not always accord with the health needs of the population … We place great importance on the inclusion of the SHAs' capacity in the rationalisation of inner London's acute sector capacity. We therefore *recommend* that steps be taken immediately to ensure that the SHAs are brought into the internal market within an appropriate funding framework.

The committee advised that clinical research be concentrated on fewer sites, with close links to basic science, a process that would be made easier by the 'rationalisation' of specialty centres and hospitals.

> Increasingly it will make less sense, both for research and service, to maintain a number of separate single-specialty clinical research centres in London. There is strong concern among the postgraduate schools that they would require ring-fencing to survive in a multi-faculty environment, and that research priorities would be altered by integration into a faculty of medicine. We have considered these arguments carefully, but we have not found them ultimately persuasive. We believe that the research potential of all the postgraduate schools, including those which are already strong, can only be fully realised through integration in multi-faculty colleges. Research selectivity gives all universities a strong incentive to sustain the best research.

The mention of research selectivity was a reference not only to the quinquennial Research Assessment Exercises but also to the 1991 strategic review of the research programmes in the NHS, which included the Special Health Authorities, being undertaken by Professor Peckham, the new Director for Research and Development in the NHS. The Institute and National Hospital provided a joint strategy paper on their planned R&D to the review, which was commended, whilst noting the lack of research on common disorders such as trauma and stroke.

The Tomlinson Committee considered that the cost of health care in London lay partly in 'top-heavy' medical staffing in many London hospitals, in excess of that justified by present or future service requirements or academic commitments. If the inner London undergraduate teaching hospitals were to match the number of consultants per episode of care as the average teaching hospital elsewhere, 450 fewer consultants would be needed. This analysis proved too simplistic for, as the NHS subsequently evolved, emphasis has been placed on consultant-led care. However, at the time, it seemed one way of

---

[65] The Jarman index was developed, as a measure of general practice workload, by Brian Jarman (later professor of general practice at St Mary's Hospital Medical School) in 1984.

balancing inadequate funds available to the internal market, albeit by ignoring issues of quality. The message from Tomlinson was greeted with widespread dismay, and it is obvious in retrospect (and to many at the time) that most of the committee's recommendations were the result of the inadequate funds provided for the internal market and not any issues of quality improvement. To argue otherwise was a triumph of rhetoric over reason.

In order to bring about these profound changes, the report recommended that specialty reviews should be carried out and a 'high-level Implementation Group' established to drive through change as quickly as possible. In fact, the government had already announced that it was setting up a dedicated 'London Implementation Group' before the report was published.

The Tomlinson report was criticised for being short on detail and lacking any sophisticated cost or resource analysis. It can be argued that the loss of beds has resulted now in profound under-supply in London, with the recurring crises of inadequate acute care, and that the loss of medical school numbers has contributed to the severe under-provision of doctors in Britain over subsequent decades. The report also rode roughshod over the many examples of high-quality performance, which had sometimes taken years to put together, and many of which were damaged or destroyed by the massive rearrangements. There are many who consider the Tomlinson report to have been responsible for a series of future calamities in NHS provision, but at the core of the problem was the establishment of an under-resourced internal market. Tomlinson, in this sense, is best considered not the judge or lawmaker but merely the executioner. The report was admirably concise and very clearly written, and its clear strategic approach appealed to politicians and, as such, was easy to translate into action. From other perspectives, it could be argued that it set London medicine on its upward trajectory, and in the nick of time – history will judge.

1993–1997 – the Trust that Never Was and the Mergers with University College London and University College London Hospital, the Final Act

The pace then quickened. The government's Special Health Authority Management Unit (SHAMU) indicated that there would be pressure on the National Hospital to achieve Trust status by 1 April 1994. There followed a period of frenetic management activity, during which the threat of imminent closure of the National Hospital, or loss of its identity through absorption into a neighbouring Trust, loomed continuously. The Board had to focus on its application for Trust status at a time when other reviews were under way, and during 'the period of greatest uncertainty' as the general manager put it. Furthermore, the Board also had to provide responses to numerous other ministerial requests for information, annual business plans to be devised, strategic plans provided and continuously updated, and option appraisals, audits, and targets for hospital activity, personnel issues, quality assurance and risk assessment supplied. Financial reports were considered at monthly intervals and the convoluted process of redeveloping the estate still needed to be worked through. It is striking, though, how few clinical issues were discussed by the Board, a sign of the extent to which the new NHS had lost sight of quality, and indeed its mission, in the interests of finance and management. John Young retired in 1986 and Tom Oakman was appointed as chairman of the Board of Governors. Peter Gautier-Smith and then John Marshall had been acting general managers before the formal appointment of Rear Admiral Anthony Wheatley, who took up post on 23 August 1988. Dealing with these many issues was largely devolved to Wheatley and the new chairman of the Board of Governors, Elizabeth Howlett. A huge and impressive number of papers, reports, analyses and documents inundated the agenda of the Board. It is doubtful whether other members of the Board, including its medical representatives, were close to the details, and these two carried heavy responsibility for negotiating what was in essence a battle for survival.

The government published another paper in February 1993, entitled *Making London Better*. This outlined its policy in the wake of Tomlinson, stating that 'no change is not an option for London'. In relation to the Special Health Authorities, the document made clear that

> The Special Health Authorities need to be in the NHS internal health market and better integrated with other educative and research institutions. It is Government policy that SHAs should join the internal health market with other hospitals from April 1994 (as NHS Trusts, subject to consultation) and thereafter to participate in a national research

market. We have commissioned two studies to address the impact of new funding arrangements on research. The first, by CASPE Consulting Ltd, compared the excess costs of SHA patients' services with similar hospitals and analysed these excess costs. The second study, initiated by the NHS Management Executive Director of Research and Development, involved the establishment of a research review of each SHA to assess the quality of its research and its overall contribution to the NHS. Each SHA's scientific and R&D contribution is being examined using external and independent peer review. These reviews are due to report in the summer.

In *Making London Better*, the government also announced how it would act to implement the Tomlinson recommendations. The first step was formation of the London Implementation Group led by Tim Chessells, chairman of the North East Thames Regional Health Authority.[66] This was immediately integrated into the NHS Management Executive (NHSME), the high-level governmental body in overall charge of the National Health Service, and it had the ear of the Minister. The London Implementation Group then initiated the series of specialty reviews recommended by Tomlinson and *Making London Better*. Thus, simultaneously, four bodies were being asked by the Ministry to produce reports relevant to the National Hospital and to make recommendations about its fundamental structure: CASPE Consulting Ltd, the Expert Advisory Group, the London Implementation Group, and its Specialty Review panel for neuroscience.

The process began with the Expert Advisory Group. This was formed by Michael Peckham, as Director of Research and Development of the NHS Management Executive, to assess each of the London Special Health Authorities. The neurosciences group included several neurologists, a neurosurgeon and an expert in rehabilitation. The Institute of Neurology submitted evidence in advance of a meeting with the group on 15 April 1993.[67] David Marsden met one of the neurologists from that panel and expressed the view that neurology was best served by developing a

British identity for the subject, in which 'the skills of everybody within the United Kingdom are harnessed towards a common aim'.[68] Briefing papers for the meeting included a factual report and a manifesto from the National Hospital setting out a secure future for itself, within the context of the Tomlinson report and *Making London Better*. Taking the North Thames Region as its logical responsibility, Queen Square argued that the existing six regional centres should be reduced to three – the National Hospital for Neurology and Neurosurgery (with a satellite at the Hammersmith Hospital), the Royal Free Hospital and the Royal London Hospital, losing Charing Cross, the regional centre at Oldchurch, and St Bartholomew's Hospital. The difficulty that Queen Square could not offer services for major trauma was finessed by recommending closer links to the Middlesex (which had yet to close) and University College Hospitals. At its meeting in April 1993, the group focused on the need for the National Hospital to make more impact on research and development relevant to the National Health Service, such as into stroke and trauma, integrating that contribution with activities of the Institute of Neurology in neuroscience. In terms of regional responsibility for a local population, strategic location within that catchment area, sufficient critical mass to sustain junior staffing and training, provision of out-reach services, contact with other medical disciplines, links to a university, and the ability to secure contracts within the internal market, the situation for the National Hospital did not appear entirely secure.

A large number of referees were asked to comment, widespread consultation was undertaken, and the exercise became over-burdened by detail. The many referees of the document submitted by Queen Square had not been well briefed on the importance of judging the research by the criterion of its clinical relevance. There was, however, a clear view that some disciplines, including neuropathology, neuropsychiatry and neurosurgery, were in decline at the time, and others facing uncertainty with the imminent retirement of distinguished members of staff. Where the panel felt that Queen Square had left itself vulnerable was in the lack of investment in basic scientific infrastructure at the National Hospital and Institute of Neurology, by comparison with some of its competitors. The minutes of the Expert Advisory Group meeting drew attention to a rather poor submission by the National Hospital,

---

[66] Sir Tim Chessells had a controversial career in business but was much in favour in the higher echelons of the Conservative government. He was memorably described in conversation by Dr Peter Harvey as 'made of asbestos and painted blue'.

[67] *Submission to Director of Research and Development of the NHS Management Executive*, March 1993, 55 pages, with figure and six appendices.

[68] Letter from David Marsden to Alastair Compston, 17 March 1993.

which failed to deal with the stated purposes of the exercise. The issue raised by Denny-Brown decades earlier – that too many consultants were drawing on research funds and facilities, but not making any contribution – was identified, as was the need for a strategy that reduced the number of part-time consultants, and placed better emphasis on common conditions without necessarily compromising the status of the National Hospital as a tertiary referral centre. It was acknowledged that some deviation from the strict model of the internal market might be needed in order to achieve this balance.[69] But, above all, the Expert Advisory Group recommended reorganisation of existing research into groupings that better served the research and development agenda of the National Health Service.[70] The general manager wrote that the National Hospital had emerged from this review 'with credit and the potential of a promising future' and, as a result of the recommendations in *Making London Better*, negotiations were also begun with UCLH about the transfer of inpatient neurology from Gower Street to the Queen Square site.

In parallel with this exercise, the London Implementation Group established its six specialty reviews, including one on neuroscience. The group comprised seven members chaired by Mr Rab Hyde, a neurosurgeon from Glasgow. Each panel member had responsibility for an entire discipline. The terms of reference were to consider the current organisation and funding of the specialty; to take a position on what the individual patient should reasonably expect as a model of care in hospital and the community; to consider access to and timing of care; to reflect upon communication with patients and their families; to define the essential components of a tertiary centre and those to which it should have access; and to consider requirements for teaching and support of subjects allied to medicine. These were to form the basis for proposing a new system for the delivery of care in the neurosciences throughout London that optimised clinical performance. Change was considered inevitable;[71] and the group considered that

London, driven by its history rather than strategy in the modern age, had lagged behind reorganisations elsewhere in the country. The panel received submissions from each of 11 independent neuroscience centres in the London area and arranged site visits, touring the metropolis in a mini-bus on each working day during much of March and April. The group was given six months to complete its work, and the report was submitted on 31 May 1993.[72] Focus groups were hosted that tested the proposed models of care and their likely impact. These, and the preparedness of the group members to be contacted as individuals and receive correspondence following each visit, led to much special pleading on behalf of all 11 existing centres.[73]

The visit of the specialty review team to the hospital was not received well at Queen Square. It was noted at an emergency meeting of the Board of Governors on 8 July 1993 that 'The meeting had been disappointingly short and the team had seemed unreceptive to other than their own apparently pre-set views. It appeared that the group's agenda was in conflict with the recommendations of the DoH policy document *Making London Better* especially with regard to their perception of the future relationship of QS with the Royal Free Hospital.'

The Board characterised the specialty review model of the tertiary centre as very similar to that which already existed and felt that progress in rationalising services across the University College Hospital, the National Hospital and Great Ormond Street Hospital, with the agreement to transfer all neuroscience from University College Hospital to the Queen Square site, had not been appreciated.

In the event, the specialty review did not endorse the prior belief that London was over-provided with neuroscience facilities, but the group did favour a configuration in which there were fewer and stronger centres supporting a network of district general hospitals aligned to a university college strong in basic neuroscience, and with the capacity to adapt to future developments. The principle was a hub-and-spoke

---

[69] Minutes of the meeting of the Expert Advisory Group for the National Hospitals for Neurology and Neurosurgery (NHNN) SHA held on 15 April 1993.
[70] These were: clinical and molecular genetics; epilepsy and neuro-epidemiology; movement disorders; muscle and peripheral nerve; dementia, neuropsychiatry, clinical neuropsychology and cognitive neurology; multiple sclerosis, neuro-rehabilitation and neuro-urology; and neuro-oncology, stereotactic and skull base surgery.

[71] The neurologist and neurosurgeon on the panel were told by the Secretary of State, Virginia Bottomley, 'Don't worry about closing Queen Square.'
[72] *Report of the Neurosciences Review Group*, May 1993, 61 pages with 4 annexes.
[73] Summarised as *Report of the Neurosciences Review Group: Supporting Evidence Including Literature Review*, June 1993, 75 pages.

system of easy access to specialist facilities and seamless care across the community, district hospital and neuroscience centre. Based on this model, the specialty report set out in detail its vision of how neurosciences services might best be delivered by the year 2000. Like the Goodenough, Todd, Flowers and Tomlinson Committees, the report supported the principle of neuroscience centres as part of a major multi-specialty hospital, rather than stand-alone institutions. Whilst the existence of some nurse practitioners liaising with the community was praised, the report concluded that, despite its workload and its links with other hospitals, in most respects the National Hospital was remote from continuity of care with district hospitals and general practitioners. There was also concern that the level of funding available to the National Hospital under the Service Increment for Teaching (SIFT) formula would not prove sufficient after the award of Trust status, given the mismatch between income and high expenditure. The panel felt that Queen Square might not survive entering the internal market from April 1994 (as proposed at that time), unless scale was reduced and an economically viable regional catchment identified. It considered three options in relation to the National Hospital, including its closure and relocation to another site, but came down in favour of the establishment of a joint Royal Free and National Hospital NHS Trust, with its neuroscience services centralised on the Queen Square site. This recommendation was made in the knowledge that it 'breached the important principle that neuroscience centres should be based on general hospital sites' but considered that the benefits of a close union between the two hospitals, with retention of neurology on the Queen Square site, justified this departure from its stated preferred model. The report concluded:

> The National Hospital remains a national and international resource providing a service to the south east of England. Its clinical practice however is distorted by its major research interests and in some respects its patient care is less than optimal. Its major shortcoming is its isolation without established formal and practical links to a viable general hospital. The hospital currently has areas of expertise which are important to maintain.

The London Implementation Group accepted the specific recommendations of its specialty review panel that the 11 neuroscience centres should be reduced to six, and that central London be 'divided' into four quarters, each having a neuroscience centre located within, or linked closely to, a multi-specialty hospital and, as part of a university institution, providing expertise in basic science. Not surprisingly, it also accepted that the National Hospital should remain at Queen Square, that neurosurgery should move from the Royal Free to the National Hospital, and that these hospitals (the National Hospital and the Royal Free Hospital) should form a joint Trust.

On 13 May 1993, before the recommendations of the specialty review and the London Implementation Group were received, an emergency meeting of the Board of Governors was held, at which it was decided that the National Hospital should proceed with a fourth-wave Trust application on its own and not in tandem with any other hospital. The move was supported by the Special Health Authority Management Unit and the 'Eastern outpost' of the NHS Management Executive. The outline case had been submitted in March 1993 and the full submission was needed by July. SANA consultancy undertook reviews of the hospital for planning the Trust application. The excess cost of patient care in the NHS due to R&D and teaching had been estimated by CASPE Consulting to be 39 per cent, in their review carried out on behalf of the Department of Health. SANA surveyed the consultants at the National Hospital and estimated that 36 per cent of inpatient and 41 per cent of outpatient work could be classified as R&D. They also recommended the setting up of neurology and neurosurgery clinical directorates, with leadership selected in part by the Medical Committee, and a new clinical directorate of rehabilitation therapy services. These were put in place.

The situation became complicated by intervention of the North East Thames Health Authority, which recommended delay in the Trust applications for UCLH, Great Ormond Street and the National Hospital. It suggested that the National Hospital should combine with the Royal Free, and relocate to Hampstead, with UCLH and Great Ormond Street merging on the vacated Queen Square site. The chairman of the Board, Elizabeth Howlett, was furious and attended a meeting of the Regional Health Authority on 20 December, where, as she put it later to the Board, she 'defended our position robustly'. On the same day, she wrote to the Minister, Virginia Bottomley, saying that the Board and the executive of the National Hospital for Neurology and

Neurosurgery did not acquiesce in the recommendation to move to the Royal Free site, and that 'I would further wish to register with you our annoyance at the manner in which this recommendation was put forward.' The report containing this recommendation had been made without any financial appraisal of capital or revenue costs, and it had not arrived until the morning of the Board meeting. Mr Wheatley wrote to staff to say that the National Hospital was wholly opposed to the Regional Health Authority's proposal and the fourth-wave Trust application was going ahead. In his cool and understated way, he continued: 'The RHA's input is one of many that will be taken into account within the Department of Health before a decision is made at Ministerial level in January.'

Elizabeth Howlett then met Tim Chessells and Virginia Bottomley on 17 January 1994, and put her case, but the application to become a stand-alone Trust was rejected on 10 February 1994. Mrs Bottomley explained that this was because she considered it unlikely that the National Hospital would survive in the internal market as a single Trust, and did not have a realistic medium-term financial strategy. She indicated that she had asked the London Implementation Group to undertake a 'locality review' which would assess the possible co-location of all or some of the UCH services at Queen Square, compared to the costs of redeveloping the current UCH site. The hospital was precipitated into crisis. Mrs Howlett wrote back to Virginia Bottomley on 11 February 1994 expressing the Board's extreme disappointment that the Trust application had been rejected, and to Tim Chessells on 14 February saying that this decision was 'bitterly disappointing. The reasons for this decision are contentious and unclear, and certainly do not reflect any of the discussions we had with yourself or with the Secretary of State on 17 January 1994.'

Elizabeth Howlett wrote in her annual report of the Board that co-location of the National Hospital and Institute of Neurology was perceived locally as 'fundamental, but less well understood externally', and that, despite this, a full-scale Queen Square locality study had been undertaken, after a pilot earlier in the year, which would report to the Department of Health, together with the review of neuroscience in north central London. In December 1994, the locality study was published, suggesting that some women and children's activity could move to the Queen Mary wing at Queen Square. Needless to say, this was strongly opposed by the National Hospital.

An extraordinary meeting of the Board of Governors was called on 17 February 1994 to discuss strategy. Mrs Howlett met Sir Tim Chessells again on 22 February and reported to the Board on 1 March that this had been productive and cleared the air. Chessells had confirmed that the reason for Trust application rejection was the perceived inability of the National Hospital to remain solvent as protected funding in the internal market was reduced, and he also admitted the folly of physical separation of the Institute of Neurology and the National Hospital. He explained that it was up to the hospital to make proposals. He was happy for the National Hospital to lead in working out a 'neuroscience strategy for North London'. Mrs Howlett and the Board considered this indicator to be an important concession, and the Board agreed to commission a financial review of the medium- and long-term outlook, once Culyer research and development funds were withdrawn.[74]

Chessells wrote to Mrs Howlett on 3 March 1994, to the effect that the North East Thames Regional Health Authority had no jurisdiction over the National Hospital, and their recent pronouncement did not mean in any way that there were proposals to move the National Hospital away from the Queen Square site. This was important as, concurrently, the Development Foundation was trying to secure funding. Mrs Howlett was able to write to the Harris Trust, which had pledged £1 million for setting up a medical ITU in the new wing, that the the plans for rebuilding were secure and to acknowledge their generosity, which had met the shortfall in the £10 million required for the project.[75]

---

[74] The Culyer report had recommended that NHS funds for research facilities should be awarded on the basis of assessments of institutions made every three to five years. The recommendation was accepted and these funds were known as 'Culyer funds'. *Research and Development Task Force. Supporting Research and Development in the NHS* ('Culyer report') (London: HMSO, 1994).

[75] Letter, 15 March 1994, reported to Board of Governors on 17 March 1994. Redevelopment of the Powis wing was finally completed £3 million over budget and several years late, with delays largely caused by prevarications over the future of the National Hospital. Renamed the Chandler wing in November 1995, this was visited by HRH Princess Diana in March 1996, and formally opened on 22 March 1996 by John Horam on behalf of the Minister of State, Stephen Dorrell, who thought it prudent not to attend a week before the hospital officially ceased to exist.

The review of neuroscience in north central London was then considered by the Board in April 1994. This suggested the formation of a consortium with the Royal Free Hospital Trust, agreeing a common tariff in the new market for services at the two hospitals and including rotational training schemes with the Royal Free and UCLH. Work started on producing a 'blueprint' paper on this topic. A heads of agreement document was set out, and in June 1994, the outline concept and initial business proposals for the 'consortium' were agreed. This was viewed with approval by the medical staff, who saw the advantage of collaboration whilst retaining independence, although whether such an arrangement could have been successful (or even would have been allowed to succeed) in the increasingly competitive atmosphere of London medicine is unclear.

In April 1994, the postgraduate hospitals entered into 'the internal market' of the NHS, with the National Hospital retaining its Special Health Authority status. Completion of the Powis wing redevelopment meant that the National Hospital had a new ward block and operating theatres. This was timely, since expensive new facilities placed an important obstacle in the way of moving the hospital services away from Queen Square. When the new block opened, Maida Vale Hospital was decommissioned, the wards closing in December 1993 and the outpatients in February 1994, and the complex process of merging the staff at Maida Vale into Queen Square was undertaken by the Board. In line with the 'internal market' procedures, a clinical directorate was set up, as well as a support directorate to cover corporate development, estate planning, contracting, marketing and information. Contracts were formed with over 50 purchasing authorities and, although patient-flow characteristics did not assume 'steady state' in the first year, from April 1995 full market operation began. Income for the hospital was to be gained from contracts within the internal market for health services, and regionally arranged training and education funds. There was a transitional grant for excess costs, reducing to zero by 1997/8. How research was to be funded was not yet fully decided, but there were moves towards a market-orientated model here too.

Despite all the uncertainty, internal developments continued and, in 1993/4, a second MRI scanner was installed in the radiology department, the new EEG telemetry unit was built (opened in 1995 and funded largely through the Sir Jules Thorn Trust, as the original unit had been), a new pain relief service was opened, new therapy services facilities introduced, and a new dining room and coffee lounge provided. Quality assurance and clinical audit strategies were implemented and the hospital also finally acquired the freehold of number 33 Queen Square. At the Institute of Neurology, the creation of the Functional Imaging Laboratory was underway. This was an extraordinarily busy period for the administration, but under the guidance of Anthony Wheatley and the Board, headed up by Elizabeth Howlett, the work was completed with military precision.

Despite previous failures, the decision was then made, after much debate at Board level, to proceed with a fifth-wave Trust application, again as a standalone Trust. The decision was made partly because of the favourable conclusions of the independent assessment of the hospital's business position and prospects. The North Thames regional office undertook to carry out an informal assessment of the management and business plans to assist with preparation. In line with his previous advice, the chairman of the London Implementation Group, Chessells, again told Elizabeth Howlett that he would oppose single-trust status for the 'National Hospital for Neurology and Neurosurgery NHS Trust'. Nevertheless, the application was submitted. While awaiting the outcome, a substantial cost reduction was imposed on all the directorates in response to the precarious financial state of the hospital. This included the hitherto unthinkable change of the professorial Gowers ward from a seven- to five-day ward. Given the atmosphere and indicators, it probably came as no surprise that an extraordinary meeting of the Board on 14 March 1995 was told that the application for single-trust status had once again been turned down, and for the second time in less than a year. The Minister for Health, Gerald Malone, intimated once more to the chairman that they should seek a joint Trust application, to be operational by April 1996, and extended the hospitals' SHA status until then.

There followed a flurry of activity in the Academic Board, Medical Committee and the general management team considering potential partnerships, once the reality dawned that failure to acquire Trust status would mean the certain closure or take-over of the National Hospital. The option of linking with Great Ormond Street was favoured, but stalled since the Hospital for Sick Children intended to apply for its own single-trust status. It was then decided, by majority view, that a joint application with UCLH (and not the Royal Free Hospital) should be taken forward and negotiations managed by the chairman, general manager and medical director. A ministerial letter dated 10 March 1995 confirming rejection of the Trust application reiterated that the Minister was concerned about the wider market risks for the National Hospital and its high-cost capital-intensive base.

Many members of the medical staff continued to resist the idea of a joint Trust application, seeing this as the end of the 'National Hospital' and, as the tortuous managerial processes proceeded, efforts were made to resist change. The clinicians felt that tradition and independence were threatened by NHS reforms which required hospitals to compete for trade and resources. McDonald led a rear-guard action arguing that history and tradition should have placed the National Hospital above the vulgarities of the market. He asked several dignitaries to write to the Secretary of State for Health with the somewhat cryptic message 'We are what we were, not what we might be.'[76] She turned a deaf ear, even to Lord Walton of Detchant. From a briefing leaked to McDonald by a journalist from the *London Evening Standard* on 27 March 1995, it was learned that Junior Health Minister Baroness Cumberlege[77] had told the House of Lords that the National Hospital had been and would be refused Trust status unless it combined with another hospital of its own choosing that was equally committed to teaching and research, and that the most sensible marriage would be with University College Hospital.[78] However, she was

unable to confirm that neurosurgical beds in London, the perennial Queen Square 'lesion', would not be cut as part of the new contracting arrangements. Nevertheless, she stated in the House of Lords: 'This particular hospital and its institute have a very proud record. The hospital is, we believe, of world standing but we do not believe that its future is necessarily viable. That is why we are looking ahead. If it joins a Trust – as we are recommending it should – with another hospital, we would want to keep the excellence and the worldwide reputation and expertise embodied at Queens [*sic*] Square' and 'My Lords, it is our intention not only to protect and maintain the expertise within this hospital and within the Institute, but also to promote its excellence. We believe it is a remarkable institution and we want to see it strengthened.'[79]

Pressed by Lord Walton about whether he could be assured that the National Hospital would remain on the Queen Square site, she replied: 'My Lords, that is really for the Trust to decide once it is formed. I am aware that in the National Health Service it is a very dangerous thing to say, "Never, never, ever".'

A Board meeting on 31 March then determined to look into the possibility of a combined Trust application with UCLH (and the Eastman Dental Hospital). Discussions with UCLH began on 11 April 1995 and included the preconditions by the National Hospital that it should retain its identity and remain co-located with the Institute of Neurology on the Queen Square site. These were agreed by Charles Marshall, the chief executive of UCLH, on condition that there was a National Hospital division headed by a general manager accountable to UCLH. On 30 April 1995, a report was submitted to the North Thames regional chairman indicating that negotiations with UCLH would start as the National Hospital's preferred partner. A joint Trust application was then drafted on behalf of the National Hospital, Eastman Dental Hospital and University College Hospital. The benefits to the National Hospital were stated to be 'no immediate change in service provision, but it is anticipated that service quality will improve in some areas by redirecting savings from sharing overheads in patient care'. The National Hospital at that time was approximately one-third the size of UCLH, reporting an establishment of 1,094 staff,[80] compared with 3,133 at UCLH and 328 at the Eastman, and was clearly the junior

---

[76] McDonald archive: various correspondence dated 15 February to 22 March 1995. The correspondents were Sid Gilman, James Lance, Guglielmo Scarlato, Art Asbury, Guy McKhann, Hanjo Freund, Cesare Fieschi, James McLeod, Hans van Crevel, Bob Fishman, Gerard Said, Bud Rowland and John Walton.

[77] Baroness Julia Cumberlege was Junior Health Minister between 1992 and 1997. Her father was a doctor and, as she famously said in a debate on the NHS in 2000, 'My father joined it in 1948 and, since patients came to the house, in my home we literally had blood on the carpet ... We are all trapped in a marvellously pure ideology, the ideal socialist dream. We all have to have dreams, but this one does not work. It does not work because it is isolated in a brutally competitive world which generates the money for unreal dreams' (Hansard, 2 February 2000).

[78] McDonald archive: filed as 'Hospital survival: 'Dear Ian/ You will know all about this. I don't know exactly what your thinking on this is. It looks to me as if the Government is sneaking another dubious announcement out on the quiet. / P.'

[79] Hansard, 27 March 1995 (150327-02).

[80] A full-time equivalent complement of 34 consultants, 67 junior medical staff, 383 nurses, 222 admin. staff, 204

partner, but with the attraction of a large new block with 150 beds, intensive care unit and operating theatres, combined with a very highly rated academic record. UCLH was concerned to allay the anxiety at Queen Square that this was a take-over ending the identity of the National Hospital. This was reassuring and the UCLH Board deserved great credit for their tact and diplomacy.

In 1995, the hospital had managed to balance its books and even achieve a surplus,[81] but this was with the help of a £16.3 million block contract for R&D, which was planned to be withdrawn rapidly over subsequent years. Waiting times were reduced, but non-urgent patients still had an average delay of 3–4 months for an appointment. At the time, 90 per cent of income came from health authorities all over the country, and 5–19 per cent from GP fund-holders. Other developments that could be highlighted included a new personnel directorate, the opening on 3 January 1995 of the new EEG telemetry unit, the day care surgery unit, and the formal opening of the new Powis wing. At Chalfont, the new epilepsy research MRI unit opened in April 1995, and the Institute's Wellcome department of cognitive neurology was established at 12 Queen Square, incorporating the new Leopold Muller Functional Imaging Laboratory. Activity figures for the hospital in 1995/6 showed that in the year there were 5,181 inpatient episodes, the highest ever recorded in the hospital to that date, and 37,830 outpatient visits. It was on the basis of these figures that the hospital proceeded with yet another Trust application.

Matters moved quickly forward. Sir Ronald Mason, the chairman of UCLH, joined the Board of Governors of the National Hospital as an observer. Giltspur Communications Ltd was engaged to assist with the remarkably brief and sketchy combined UCL/NHNN/Eastman Dental Hospital application. An extraordinary meeting of the Board of Governors took place in August 1995 to review the final draft before submission to the North Thames Regional Health Authority and start of the consultation process. It was agreed that there would be three clinically based general management divisions of the joint Trust – medicine, surgery and the National Hospital for Neurology and

Neurosurgery – and a fourth non-clinical service support division. The two pathology directorates and physiotherapy at Queen Square remained accountable to the general manager at the National Hospital.

The formal application was submitted on 21 September 1995 and quickly approved by the government on 18 January 1996. Even so, Elizabeth Howlett expressed annoyance at the way in which she was notified that day through a phone call from the UCLH director of corporate development, and she informed the Board of Governors on 25 January that she had yet to hear directly from the Secretary of State. The Board expressed concern that, although the dean, David Marsden, had been appointed to the new Trust Board through the university, there was no one to represent the National Hospital. The National Hospital Special Health Authority dissolution order came with abolition of the Board of Governors at midnight on 31 March 1996, and on 1 April 1996 the National Hospital thenceforward formed part of the University College London Hospitals NHS Trust, along with the Eastman Dental Hospital, the United Elizabeth Garrett Anderson and Soho Hospital for Women, the Hospital for Tropical Diseases, the Middlesex Hospital and University College London. The old Board of Governors was dissolved and Elizabeth Howlett stood down as chairman on 1 April 1996. Various letters of thanks were sent to her, including one from Princess Diana. Gerald Stern, a non-executive member of the Board, wrote: 'Whilst it is the bittersweet end of an era I think you can be confident that you have secured the long-term future for the National Hospital. When I recall that at one stage the hospital's very survival seemed to be in jeopardy, I hope you will enjoy a feeling of profound and enduring achievement.'

In parallel with this re-alignment of the National Hospital with UCLH, the Institute of Neurology, originally formed in 1948 as a limited company, became affiliated in 1995 with University College London and the Institutes of Child Health and Ophthalmology, and relinquished ties to the BPMF which was then also formally dissolved. Then, on 1 August 1997, the Institute of Neurology was officially merged with UCL. Under the terms of the University College London Act 1996, the original companies incorporating the Institute of Neurology (Queen Square), the Institute of Child Health and the Royal Free Hospital School of Medicine were dissolved.[82] An enabling bill received

---

technical staff and paramedics, 150 auxiliaries and 32 senior managers.

[81] In 1994/5: the income was £39,248,000 and expenditure £34,361,000 (and a retained surplus of around £750,000). This compares to a deficit in 1990/1 of over £1.5 million.

[82] University College London Act 1996, c. iii, Section 4.

Royal Assent on 4 July 1996, and united the Royal Free Hospital and University College London Medical Schools, the Institute of Neurology and the Institute of Child Health. The Committee of Management also ceased meeting as of this date, although the individual identity of the Institute within the College was retained, as was the name 'Institute of Neurology'. The transition included the important agreement that clinical neuroscience activity in the Trust would be concentrated on the Queen Square campus.

Throughout this extremely chaotic period, the Institute of Neurology had nonetheless continued to expand. As Sir John Read noted, in the 17 years of his chairmanship (1980–97), annual income had risen from £3 million to £14 million, grant income from £1 million to £9 million, and staffing levels from 216 to 270, with a very large academic output. These achievements were matched by the financial solvency of the hospital. This was an outstanding outcome considering the stormy financial and administrative environment, and great credit was due to the leadership of the hospital and Institute. Furthermore, it was finally and unambiguously agreed to concentrate clinical neuroscience on the Queen Square campus – despite the numerous previous attempts to disrupt this arrangement – on the basis that close association and co-location of the Institute and the hospital were the best solution for the future of neurology at the National Hospital and its Institute of Neurology, for London and for the nation.

It has become clear to us, in preparing this history, that the co-location of the hospital and institute has indeed been fundamental to the success of Queen Square, as the Board in the 1990s recognised and fought hard to preserve. At the time of writing, this co-location is again threatened, and we venture the opinion that severing this link will result in loss of identity for the hospital in the medium term, and the ending of the unique brand of translational clinical research, based on the seamless intermingling of science and clinical practice, which has been the outstanding contribution of Queen Square over the years.

Policy documents continued to flow over the next few years and our period ends, in 1997, with the Turnberg report, the 23rd major twentieth-century inquiry into London's health services to be published. In contrast to Tomlinson, Turnberg's recommendations were more conciliatory. He called for 'a more coherent approach to London's health needs than the mere arbitrary cost-cutting of previous governments', and commented in his letter to the Minister, presenting his report in November 1997, with sentiments which also summed up the prevailing opinion amongst doctors at Queen Square: 'We found a health service under pressure. Services ... sorely stretched. Furthermore, there is evidence to suggest that the pressures are increasing. Despite all this, health care workers are doing the best they can and we found examples of good practice, even in circumstances of severe pressure.'

In 1997, the ten-year agenda of the new Labour government, in their report *The New NHS – Modern, Dependable*, was published, in which the Health Secretary, Frank Dobson, in whose Parliamentary constituency Queen Square lay, promised to bring the internal market to an end. Change and reorganisation continued but his promise did not materialise.

This tortuous peripeteia was, of course, a watershed in the history of Queen Square, and marked the formal end of independent management of both the National Hospital and its Institute of Neurology, the former 'medical school'. In reality, of course, ever since the 1950s, control of the destiny of Queen Square had increasingly been sliding towards central authority. As it turned out, and as those who contributed to the policy of change had anticipated, these seemingly final acts of 1996 and 1997 have had, from the present perspective, a clearly positive effect. Both the National Hospital and the Institute of Neurology retain their separate identities, in spirit if not absolutely in governance, and their combined activities have generally flourished, increasing in both range and quality. In the event, in 2018, Queen Square remains, despite its repeated trials and tribulations, the national treasure that the Chandler siblings set out to create in 1859.

Postscript

We began with the risky and ambitious decision taken by three obscure siblings to address concerns over the medical care of their grandmother by founding a hospital that took national responsibility for people with paralysis and epilepsy. The initiative attracted patronage from the business world and royalty, and the most distinguished doctors and surgeons of Victorian medicine, who took an interest in the brain and spinal cord, responded by working at Queen Square. Their legacy was maintained by an equally distinguished group of physicians born in the nineteenth century who carried forward the vision across the turbulent first half of the twentieth century. They inherited a tradition for expertise in clinical medicine and surgery, and some also advanced knowledge on the nervous system in health and disease. The spirit of independence that had always been fundamental to the ethic of the National Hospital and its medical school bred a degree of arrogance that excited criticism from outside and periodically left Queen Square isolated and out of touch with the times. The insistence on independence was not helped by recurring financial pressures and occasional erratic strategy. These various issues were brought sharply into focus with the advent of the National Health Service. But, for another 48 years, the original organisational structures survived on the basis of unambiguous excellence in what Queen Square did best – clinical neurology and neurosurgery. Just in time, reality dawned and self-satisfaction with parading things as they always had been was replaced by a new breed of visionaries who saw that the modern

centre of excellence had to perform at the highest level in clinical medicine, teaching and research. As regional centres began to develop and their integration of services with internal medicine matched the public appetite and political imperatives, Queen Square again had to think about itself and change or face closure. Taken to the water, the horse may have stooped reluctantly to drink, but drink it did. Queen Square flourished and now, as we write, is again a national centre of which London and the United Kingdom can be proud, and part of a university college that supports what is arguably the most successful neuroscience cluster in Europe, if not anywhere. The intimate association and co-location of the hospital and its institute have been the basis of their outstanding contribution to translational clinical neuroscience and their survival in the turbulent waters of British medicine. The story we have told is a saga of vision and triumph, sometimes against the odds, based on excellence in acquiring knowledge on diseases of the nervous system and applying that to the care of people with paralysis, epilepsy and much else besides. It celebrates the history of a fine institution and the people who worked tirelessly to ensure its success.

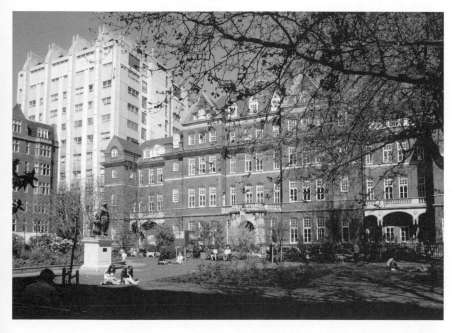

Figure 14.6 The National Hospital today

Appendix 1 Medical and Surgical Appointees to the National Hospitals and/or Institute of Neurology 1859–1997

Included in these lists are all the medical and surgical staff appointed to the National Hospital Queen Square and/or the Institute of Neurology since their foundation up until the absorption of the hospital into UCLH in 1996 and the Institute into UCL in 1997. We also include the staff based in the hospital at Maida Vale when it was absorbed administratively with the hospital at Queen Square in 1948, and those subsequently appointed to that hospital. The dates of appointment and retirement refer to the senior positions

of assistant physician/physician, assistant surgeon/surgeon or consultant.

After 1948, only salaried staff are included (i.e. not those with exclusively honorary positions). The dates of retirement are from their salaried position and do not include periods as emeritus or honorary staff.

The dates listed are taken from a variety of sources. In some cases, different dates are cited in separate sources, and the list is compiled from that which we consider most reliable.

KEY:
* Appointed to Maida Vale only
** Appointed to Maida Vale and Queen Square
*** Approximate date
n.a. At the time of publication, still in post
- Alive at the time of publication
n.k. Date not known

Physicians/Neurologists

	Year of birth	Year of death	Year of appointment	Year of retirement (or resignation/death in service)
C. Brown-Séquard	1817	1894	1859	1863
J. Ramskill	1817	1894	1859	1897
J. Hughlings Jackson	1835	1911	1862	1906
C. Radcliffe	1822	1889	1863	1889
Sir John Russell Reynolds	1828	1896	1863	1869
P. Bazire	1835	1867	1864	1867
Sir Edward Henry Sieveking	1816	1904	1864	1867
H. Bastian	1837	1915	1867	1907
T. Buzzard	1831	1919	1867	1906
C. Elam	1824	1889	1870	1877
D. Maclure	nk	1879	1870	1879
Sir William Gowers	1845	1915	1872	1910
Sir David Ferrier	1843	1928	1880	1907

(cont.)

	Year of birth	Year of death	Year of appointment	Year of retirement (or resignation/death in service)
P. Horrocks	1853	1908	1880	1883
J. Ormerod	1848	1925	1880	1913
C. Beevor	1854	1908	1883	1908
J. Anderson	1853	1893	1887	1893
Sir Felix Semon	1849	1921	1887	1909
H. Tooth	1856	1925	1887	1921
Sir John Rose Bradford	1863	1935	1893	1896
J. Taylor	1859	1946	1893	1924
W. Colman	1864	1934	1896	1898
J. Russell	1863	1939	1898	1928
F. Batten	1865	1918	1900	1918
W. Turner	1864	1943	1900	1925
J. Collier	1870	1935	1902	1935
Sir Edward Farquhar Buzzard	1871	1945	1905	1921
L. Paton	1872	1943	1907	1937
T. Stewart	1877	1957	1908	1942
Sir Gordon Holmes	1876	1965	1909	1941
C. Hinds Howell	1877	1960	1912	1942
S. Wilson	1874	1937	1912	1937
P Saunders	1877	1923	1916	1923
W. Adie	1886	1935	1921	1935
Sir Francis Walshe	1885	1973	1921	1955
J. Birley	1884	1934	1923	1926
Lord Brain*	1895	1966	1924	1960
D. McAlpine*	1890	1981	1924	1955
G. Riddoch	1889	1947	1924	1947
J. Martin	1893	1984	1925	1958
Sir Charles Symonds	1890	1978	1926	1955
M. Critchley	1900	1997	1928	1965
E. Carmichael	1896	1978	1930	1961
D. Brinton	1902	1986	1935	1965
D. Denny-Brown	1901	1981	1935	1941
R. Ironside*	1899	1968	1935	1965
S. Nevin*	1905	1979	1935	1970
J. Elkington	1904	1963	1937	1963
A. Feiling*	1885	1975	1941	1951
H. Dimsdale*	1907	1977	1945	1967
P. Sandifer*	1908	1964	1945	1964
M. McArdle	1909	1989	1946	1975

(cont.)

	Year of birth	Year of death	Year of appointment	Year of retirement (or resignation/death in service)
S. Meadows	1902	1993	1946	1967
D. Williams	1908	1990	1946	1974
M. Kremer**	1907	1988	1948	1973
E. Pritchard*	1899	1962	1948	1962
W. Gooddy**	1916	2004	1951	1981
J. Paterson	1915	1962	1951	1962
R. Henson**	1915	1994	1951	1981
R. Gilliatt	1922	1991	1955	1987
R. Kelly**	1917	1990	1955	1982
J. Marshall**	1922	2014	1956	1987
C. Earl	1925	2012	1958	1989***
N. Blau**	1928	2010	1962	1993
P. Gautier-Smith**	1929	2017	1962	1989
P. Thomas	1926	2008	1962	1991
R. Bannister	1929	2018	1963	1985
P. Nathan	1914	2002	1963	1979
R. Ross-Russell	1928	-	1963	1993
K. Zilkha	1929	-	1965	1994
W. McDonald**	1933	2006	1966	1998
J. Morgan-Hughes**	1932	2012	1967	1997
R. Kocen**	1932	2013	1970	1997
J. Newsom-Davis**	1932	2007	1970	1987
P. Rudge**	1939	-	1974	2005
J. Schott**	1944	-	1978	2010
D. Thomas	1943	-	1980	2006
J. Scadding	1948	-	1982	2003
M. Wiles	1948	-	1982	1990
A. Lees**	1947	-	1983	n.a.
S. Shorvon	1948	-	1983	n.a.
C. Mathias	1949	-	1985	2013
A. Harding	1952	1995	1986	1995
M. Rossor	1950	-	1986	n.a.
C. Fowler	1950	-	1987	2012
D. Marsden	1938	1998	1987	1998
A. Schapira	1954	-	1987	n.a.
J. Duncan	1955	-	1989	n.a.
R. Frackowiak	1950	-	1990	2009
M. Harrison	n.k.		1990	1999***
D. Miller	1954	-	1990	2014

(*cont.*)

	Year of birth	Year of death	Year of appointment	Year of retirement (or resignation/death in service)
I. Ormerod	1955	-	1990	1992
N. Quinn	1948	-	1990	2007
A. Thompson	1955	-	1990	n.a.
G. Plant	1952	-	1991	n.a.
R. Howard	1955	-	1992	n.a.
G. Llewelyn	1956	-	1992	1997
J. Ball	1953	-	1993	2005
R. Kapoor	1958	-	1994	n.a.
P. Brown	n.k.	-	1995	2010
P. Goadsby	1958	-	1995	2010
R. Greenwood	1946	-	1995	n.a.
N. Wood	1962	-	1995	n.a.
C. Clarke	1944	-	1996	2006
J. Collinge	1958	-	1996	n.a.
S. Farmer	1961		1996	n.a.
D. Kullmann	1957	-	1997	n.a.
M. Hanna	1963	-	1997	n.a.
H. Manji	1956	-	1997	n.a.

Neurosurgeons

	Year of birth	Year of death	Year of appointment	Year of retirement (or resignation/death in service)
Sir Victor Horsley	1857	1916	1886	1916
D. Armour	1869	1933	1906	1933
Sir Percy Sargent	1873	1933	1906	1933
J. Taylor	1889	1961	1931	1954
Sir Hugh Cairns	1896	1952	1933	1937
Sir Geoffrey Jefferson	1886	1961	1933	1939
H. Jackson	1900	1982	1935	1965
W. McKissock[**]	1906	1994	1946	1971
V. Logue[**]	1913	2000	1948	1977
L. Symon[**]	1929	-	1966	1995
L. Walsh	1916	1986	1966	1980
N. Grant	n.k.	-	1971	1990
D. Thomas[**]	1941	-	1977	2006
A. Crockard	1943	-	1978	2006
R. Hayward	1943	-	1981	1994
M. Powell	1950	-	1985	2012

(*cont.*)

W. Harkness	1955	-	1991	2005
N. Kitchen	1962	-	1995	n.a.
J. Palmer	1961	-	1996	1999

(Note: Three other surgeons were appointed between 1859 and 1880 – but did not carry out intra-cranial surgery. These were: Sir William Ferguson (1808–76; on the staff 1860–76); J. Z. Laurence (1828–70; on the staff 1860–1870) and William Adams 1820–1900; on the staff 1872–1890.)

Physicians in Psychological Medicine/Psychiatrists

B. Hart	1879	1966	1926	1946
E. Slater	1904	1983	1946	1964
H. Shorvon	1906	1961	1948	1961
P. Tooley	1912	1991	1948	1954
R. Grace	1896	1963	1952	1960
R. Pratt**	1917	1983	1954	1982
A. Elithorn**	1920	2013	1956	1986
R. Hunter	1923	1981	1960	1981
A. Lishman	1931	-	1964	1965
H. Merskey**	1929	-	1967	1976
M. Trimble**	1946	-	1976	2004
M. Ron	1943	-	1982	2009
R. Dolan	1954	-	1987	2018
M Robertson	1948	-	1987	2004

Assistant Pathologists

	Appointed
W. Colman	1889
J. Taylor	1890
W. Colman	1893
J. Russell	1896
F. Batten	1899
J. Collier	1900
F. Buzzard	1902
G. Holmes	1904
T. Stewart	1904
C. Hinds Howell	1908
S. Wilson	1912
E. O'Flynn	1924

(*cont.*)

	Appointed
R. Waller	1932
J. Cumings	1933
W. Blackwood	1946

(Note: From 1864 to 1914, the pathologists were junior staff appointments, and, between 1914 and 1948, assistant pathologists were appointed, but these were not full consultant posts.)

Consultant Pathologists

J. Greenfield	1884	1958	1914	1949
J. Cumings	1905	1974	1946	1971
W. Blackwood	1910	1990	1947	1976
W. McMenemey*	1905	1977	1948	1970
W. Mair	1913	2002	1958	1978
J. Cavanagh	1921	-	1962	1986
D. Mathews	n.k.	n.k.	1963	1965
R. Barnard*	1932	2005	1964	1991
M. Smith	1915	1988	1964	1973
D. Landon	1936	-	1964	2001
A. Dayan	1935	-	1965	1973
P. Lascelles	1930	-	1966	1988
P. Norman	n.k.	-	1970	1999
M. Erdohazi	1915	n.k.	1974	1983
E. Thompson	1940	-	1974	2005
L. Duchen	1928	1996	1977	1992
F. Scaravilli	1939	-	1978	2004
B. Harding	1948	-	1983	1994
T. Revesz	1948	-	1990	2013
M. Thom	1964	-	1996	n.a.

Clinical Neurophysiologists

W. Cobb	1913	1999	1946	1980
D. Hill	1913	1982	1946	-
G. Dawson	n.k.	n.k.	1948	1961
J. Bates	1918	1993	1961	1983
R. Willison	1925	2012	1962	1989
M. Halliday	1926	2008	1965	1991
K. Wynn Parry	1924	2015	1966	1989
B. McGillivray	1927	2010	1971	1989
D. Small	n.k.	-	1976	1980
N. Murray	1947	-	1980	2007
H. Townsend	1929	-	1980	1994
Sir David Fish	1956	-	1989	2010
S. Smith	1957	-	1989	2011
B. Youl	1957	-	1993	2003
G. Sheean	n.k.	-	1996	1997

(Note: At Maida Vale, clinical neurophysiology was performed by the neurologist Sam Nevin and, when he retired, the service at Maida Vale was subsumed into that at Queen Square.)

Consultant in charge of Uro-neurology Unit (founded in 1987)

C. Fowler	1950	-	1987	2012

Consultant in charge of Autonomic investigation Unit (founded in 1985)

Sir Roger Bannister	1929	2018	1963	1989
C. Mathias	1949	-	1989	2013

(Note: R Bannister retired from his hospital practice in 1985 but retained his position in the autonomic function unit until 1989.)

Neuro-otologists and ENT Surgeons

A. Cumberbatch	1846	1929	1886	1907
Sir Felix Semon	1849	1921	1887	1909
Sir Charles Ballance	1856	1936	1891	1908
S. Scott	1875	1966	1909	1939
T. Just	1886	1937	1921	1936
Sir Terence Cawthorne	1902	1970	1936	1967
C. Hallpike	1900	1979	1944	1965
W. McKenzie	1908	1981	1948	1975
M. Dix	1902	1991	1965	1976
M. Harrison	1913	2009	1967	1974
H. Ludman	1933	-	1968	1998
W. Gibson	1944	-	1977	1983
L. Luxon	1948	-	1980	2015
G. Brookes	1950	-	1984	n.a.
R. Davies	1955	-	1991	2015

Neuro-ophthalmologists and Ophthalmic Surgeons

R. Carter	1828	1918	1886	1899
M. Gunn	1850	1909	1886	1909
L. Paton	1872	1943	1907	1937
F. Williamson-Noble	1889	1969	1925	1954[***]
T. Lyle	1903	1986	1937	1968
H. Hobbs[*]	1910	1990	1946	1975
Sir Stephen Miller	1917	1996	1955	1977
M. Sanders	1939	-	1969	1999
D. Taylor	1942	-	1976	1989
J. Elston	1949	-	1987	1991
E. Graham	1949	-	1989	2014
J. Acheson	1955	-	1992	n.a.
J. Riordan Eva	1956	-	1995	1997

Radiologists

R. Reynolds	1880	1964	1919	1939
H. Davies	1905	1967	1939	1966
J. Bull	1911	1987	1948	1975
G. du Boulay	1922	2009	1954[**]	1984
D. Sutton	1917	2002	1950[**]	1984
B. Kendall	1929	2015	1967[**]	1994
I. Moseley	1940	-	1975	2000
G. Lloyd	n.k.	n.k.	1978	n.k.
J. Stevens[*]	1947	-	1983	2010
D. Kingsley	n.k.	-	1986	n.k.
W. Taylor	1956	-	1993	2002
H. Jager	1956	-	1996	n.a.

Anaesthetists

J. Silk, D. Buxton, R. Bakewell, Llewellyn Powell, Z. Mennell, J. Ryan, V. Hall, O. Jones, E. Taylor, R. Beaver, D. Aserman, A. Hewer[*], D. Wylie[**], M. Trapps[*], T. Roberts[*], H. Howell-Jones, D. Coleman, M. Bowen-Wright, J. McDonald, D. Jewkes[**], P. Painter[**], D. Ellis[**], L. Loh[**], G. Ingram, N. Hirsch, I. Calder, F. Kurer, M. Smith, P. Nandi, S. Wilson, J. Salt, A. Agastopoulou-Ladas (The anaesthetic department at Maida Vale was subsumed into that at Queen Square in 1976/7).

Other Clinical Staff

A number of other doctors were appointed on honorary contracts or in specialties not included in the tables above and/or had primary appointments elsewhere. Many were distinguished in their fields and had important attachments to Queen Square. These included: M. Baraitser, R. P. Beaney, R. Birch, M. Brada, R. Bradford, E. Brett, D. Brooks, A. Bronstein, T. Carlstedt, S. Daniel, L. Ginsburg, A. David, K. Friston, H. Harding, H. Hardwick, J. Hedley, D. Holdright, S. Hughes, H. Jackson Burrows, D. James, B. Jones, A. Kennedy, J. Laidlaw, J. Land, J. Lehovsky, C. Lockyer, W. McCullagh, P. Merton, M. Newton, B. Neville, M. O'Brien, J. O'Dowd, R. Orrell, J. Oxley, C. Pattison, G. Perkins, A. Randle, A. Ransford, A. Richens, J. Sander, P. Shaw, K. Shuttleworth, Sir George Smart, M. Sturridge, J. Surtees, W. Tate, S. Tucker, C. Williams, J. Wilson, R. Wise, J. Zakrzewska.

Appendix 2 Dates of Appointment of Senior Administrative Positions at the National Hospital/Institute of Neurology 1859–1997

Chairman of the Board of Management/Board of Govenors of the National Hospital

	Appointed	Retired (resigned or died in service)
D. Wire	1859	1860
W. Hale	1860	1872
T. Parker	1872	1873
J. Back	1873	1878
G. Porter	1878	1901
H. Wace	1901	1903
D. Power	1903	1905
Sir Frederick MacMillan	1905	1936
H. Styles	1936	1940
Lord Broadbridge	1940	1943
O. Blyth	1943	1946
Sir Ernest Gowers	1947	1957
Sir John Woods	1957	1962
K. Miller Jones	1963	1974
Sir Leslie Williams	1974	1982
J. Young	1982	1986
T. Oakman	1986	1992
E. Howlett	1992	1996

Secretary/General Manager of the National Hospital
i Hospital Secretary

	Appointed	Retired (resigned or died in service)
G. Reid	1859	1865
C. Edmonds	1865	1866
T. Boughton	1866	1866
B. Rawlings	1866	1901
T. Kirby	1902	1902
G. Hamilton	1902	1939
L. Thomas	1939	1945
E. Mitchell	1945	1958
G. Robinson	1959	1980
P. Zimmerman	1980	1985

ii Hospital General Manager

P. Zimmerman	1985	1987
J. Marshall	1987	1988
A. Wheatley	1987	1996

(The post of general manager was created in 1985 following the Griffith report.)

Chair of the Board of Management of the Institute of Neurology

Sir Ernest Gowers	1950	1957
Earl of Cromer	1957	1958
Sir John Woods (Dep. Chair)	1958	1962
Lord Aldington	1962	1980
Sir John Read	1980	1997

Secretary of the Board of Management of the Institute of Neurology

R. Gould	1950	1973
D. Sherwood	1973	1983
J. Axe	1983	1988
S. Sterling	1988	1990
R. Walker	1990	2015

Dean of Medical School (until 1950) and of Institute of Neurology (after 1950)

J. Ormerod	1880	1909
F. Batten	1909	1923
C. Hinds Howell	1912	1923
J Greenfield	1923	1943
J. Martin	1943	1948
M. Critchley	1948	1953
M. Kremer	1953	1962
J. Bull	1962	1968
R. Kelly	1968	1975
P. Gautier-Smith	1975	1982
J. Marshall	1982	1987
D. Landon	1987	1995
C. Marsden	1995	1999

Appendix 3 Physicians – National Hospital 1860–1997

The chart below illustrates the duration of service of physicians/neurologists on the staff of the National Hospital Queen Square between the years 1980–1997.

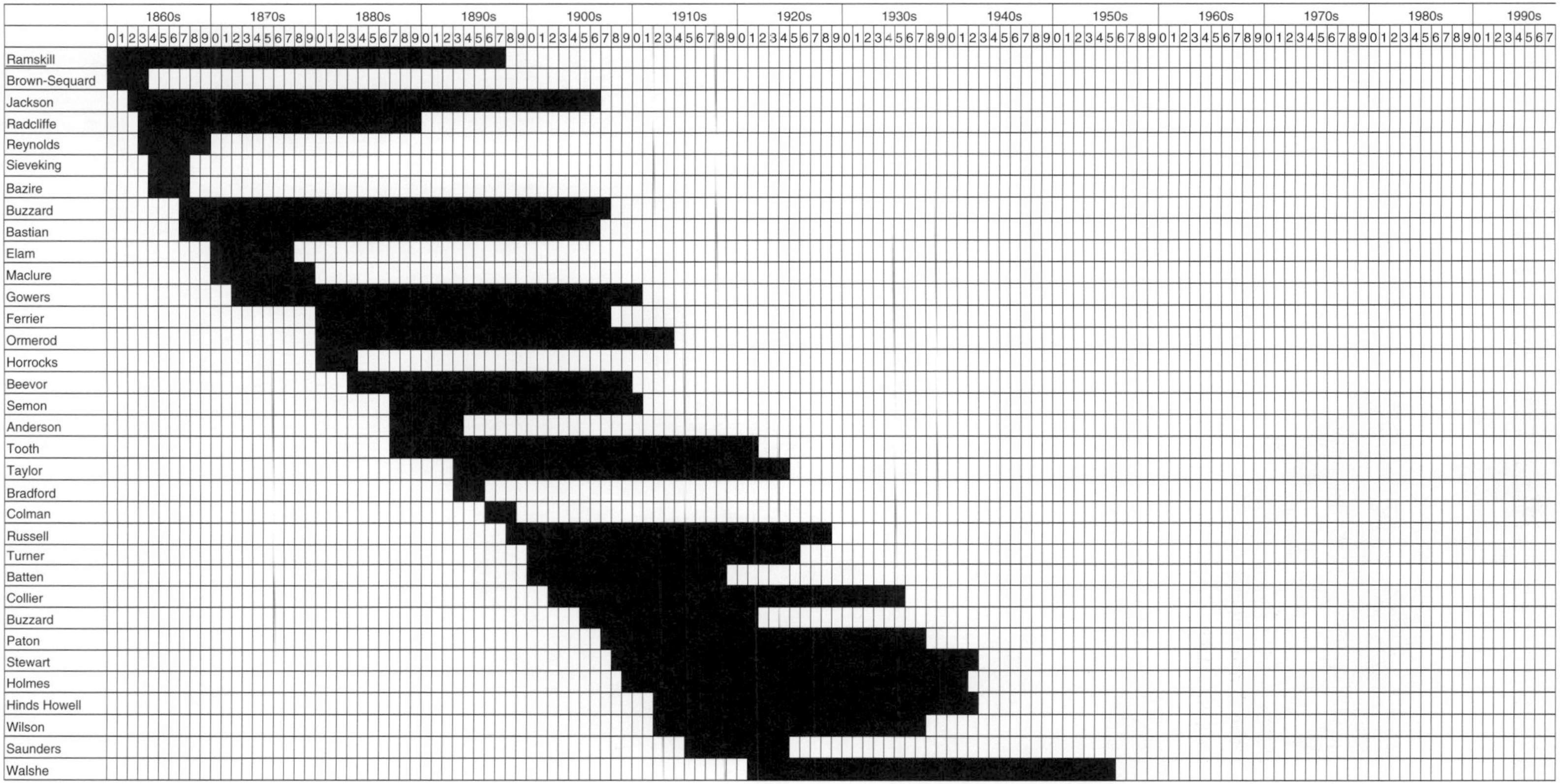
1860s
1870s
1880s
1890s
1900s
1910s
1920s
1930s
1940s
1950s
1960s
1970s
1980s
1990s
Ramskill
Brown-Sequard
Jackson
Radcliffe
Reynolds
Sieveking
Bazire
Buzzard
Bastian
Elam
Maclure
Gowers
Ferrier
Ormerod
Horrocks
Beevor
Semon
Anderson
Tooth
Taylor
Bradford
Colman
Russell
Turner
Batten
Collier
Buzzard
Paton
Stewart
Holmes
Hinds Howell
Wilson
Saunders
Walshe

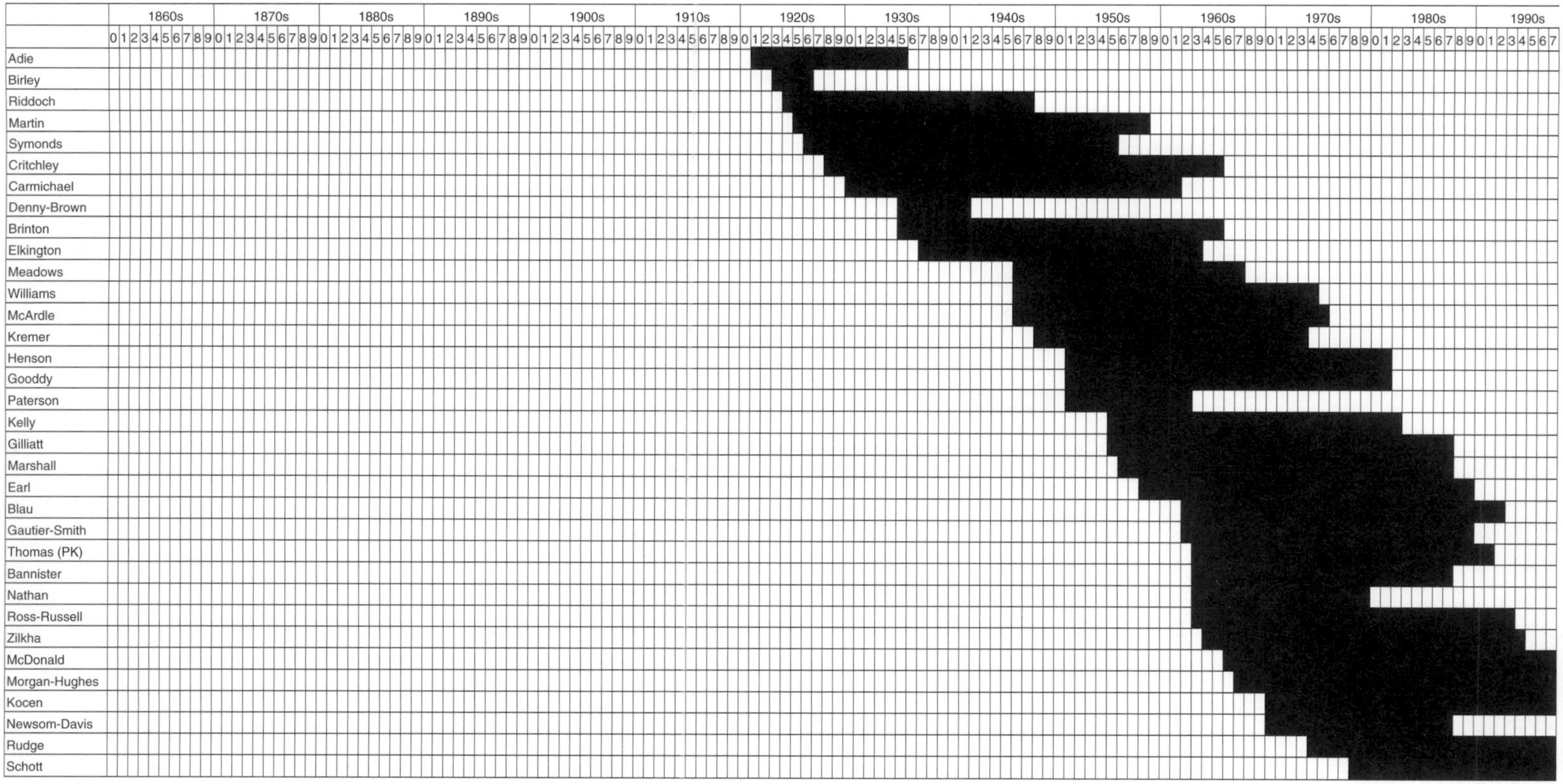
1860s
1870s
1880s
1890s
1900s
1910s
1920s
1930s
1940s
1950s
1960s
1970s
1980s
1990s
Adie
Birley
Riddoch
Martin
Symonds
Critchley
Carmichael
Denny-Brown
Brinton
Elkington
Meadows
Williams
McArdle
Kremer
Henson
Gooddy
Paterson
Kelly
Gilliatt
Marshall
Earl
Blau
Gautier-Smith
Thomas (PK)
Bannister
Nathan
Ross-Russell
Zilkha
McDonald
Morgan-Hughes
Kocen
Newsom-Davis
Rudge
Schott

1860s 1870s 1880s 1890s 1900s 1910s 1920s 1930s 1940s 1950s 1960s 1970s 1980s 1990s

0123456789 0123456789 0123456789 0123456789 0123456789 0123456789 0123456789 0123456789 0123456789 0123456789 0123456789 0123456789 0123456789 01234567

Thomas (D)
Scadding
Wiles
Lees
Shorvon
Matthias
Harding
Rossor
Marsden
Fowler
Schapira
Duncan
Frackowiak
Harrison
Miller
Quinn
Thompson
Omerod
Plant
Llewelyn
Howard
Ball
Kapoor
Goadsby
Greenwood
Brown
Wood
Clarke
Collinge
Farmer
Hanna
Manji
Kullmann

Index

NB: Names of individuals are listed with their years of birth and death (where relevant). Where no dates are indicated, the authors have not been able to verify the details.